CSF Rhinorrhea

Abdulaziz A. AlQahtani
Paolo Castelnuovo
Roy Casiano • Ricardo L. Carrau
Editors

CSF Rhinorrhea

Pathophysiology, Diagnosis and Skull Base Reconstruction

Springer

Editors
Abdulaziz A. AlQahtani
Department of Otorhinolaryngology
King Fahd Medical City
Riyadh, Saudi Arabia

Paolo Castelnuovo
Department of Otorhinolaryngology
University of Insubria, Varese
Varese, Italy

Roy Casiano
Department of Otolaryngology, Head and Neck Surgery
University of Miami, Miller School of Medicine
Miami, FL, USA

Ricardo L. Carrau
Department of Otolaryngology-Head and Neck Surgery
The Ohio State University Wexner Medical Center
Columbus, OH, USA

ISBN 978-3-030-94780-4   ISBN 978-3-030-94781-1 (eBook)
https://doi.org/10.1007/978-3-030-94781-1

This Springer imprint is published by the registered company Springer Nature Switzerland AG
The registered company address is: Gewerbestrasse 11, 6330 Cham, Switzerland

Foreword

As endoscopic skull base surgery has rapidly evolved over the last 25 years, the refinements in technique, technology, and anatomical understanding have been astounding. The partnership and collaboration between otorhinolaryngologists and neurosurgeons have dramatically synergized the field. Yet one of the major challenges continues to be the issue of skull base reconstruction and avoidance of cerebrospinal fluid (CSF) leaks and related complications such as meningitis, tension pneumocephalus, and prolonged hospitalization. As such it is appropriate and timely that we have an all-encompassing text that addresses these issues around CSF in a most modern and extensive fashion. The book is divided into 6 parts and 40 chapters that cover all topics related to CSF rhinorrhea led by four editors who are leaders in the field. Their all-star multidisciplinary panel of authors includes experts in rhinology, neurosurgery, radiology, and anesthesiology, some of whom are inventors of skull base surgical approaches and reconstruction techniques. The book is enriched by a wealth of high-quality figures and online videos that illustrate real-world clinical cases.

In totality, this textbook provides in-depth theoretical and practical knowledge related to the basic physiology of CSF, the various etiologies of CSF rhinorrhea, diagnostic techniques for detecting a CSF leak, the surgical and nonsurgical techniques for resolving CSF leaks, postoperative care and monitoring, and finally, an evidence-based assessment of managing CSF rhinorrhea, quality of life issues, competencies in CSF leak repair and related medicolegal issues. Appropriately, the editors focus the most attention on the surgical techniques and team approach for treating CSF leaks with chapters that cover all areas of the skull base, and the wide array of materials available for repair including autologous grafts, pedicled flaps, free flaps, and synthetic materials.

Looking at this textbook from the long perspective of where endoscopic pituitary and skull base surgery started in the mid-1990s, the progress in our collective understanding and management of skull base defects and CSF rhinorrhea is remarkable. When endoscopic endonasal surgery was in its infancy, postoperative CSF leaks after extended transsphenoidal approaches were ranging from 20% to 50% in multiple series at experienced centers. Through the pioneering and intrepid work by many involved in this textbook, those rates in 2022 are typically at 5–10% for extended approaches and 1–5% for sellar approaches, and they continue to decrease with increasing experience and innovation by surgical teams around the world. The importance of this most essential phase of an endonasal operation cannot be overemphasized. Having a clear and appropriate exit strategy in any skull base procedure of the anterior, middle, or posterior fossa is a must. While postoperative CSF leaks remain the "Achilles' heel" of an otherwise perfect operation, this impressive textbook is an outstanding summation of the current state of the art and an essential compendium for any practitioner in the field. The editors are to be congratulated for providing such an important work.

Daniel F. Kelly
Pacific Neuroscience Institute
Santa Monica, CA, USA

Contents

Part I

Skull Base Development and Anatomy

Dimitrios Terzakis, Vasileios Chatzinakis, and Christos Georgalas

1

1.1 Osteology of the Three Cranial Fossae

The base of the skull is one of the most fascinating and complex anatomical areas of the human body. It has been characterized as the region with the greatest histological diversity in the body according to the last WHO extensive classification [1]. It stands between the brain and other facial structures as it forms the floor of the cranial cavity. Five bones contribute to the skull base. The ethmoid, sphenoid, occipital, paired temporal and paired frontal bones. It is functionally and anatomically divided to three distinct regions: anterior, middle, and posterior cranial fossae (Fig. 1.1).

D. Terzakis · V. Chatzinakis
Endoscopic Skull Base Center, Hygeia Hospital, Athens, The Greece

C. Georgalas (✉)
Endoscopic Skull Base Center, Hygeia Hospital, Athens, Greece

UNIC, Medical School, University of Nicosia, Nicosia, Cyprus

1.2 Ventral Portion of Anterior, Middle and Posterior Cranial Fossa

1.2.1 Anterior Cranial Fossa

Three bones combined contribute to the anterior cranial fossa: The frontal, ethmoid, and sphenoid. Most of the lateral part of this fossa is formed by the frontal bones, specifically their orbital plates. In-between, stands the ethmoid bone (crista galli and cribriform plates supporting the olfactory bulbs). The posterior part of the anterior fossa is delimited by the sphenoid wings laterally and the sphenoid body medially. When accessed from the exocranial side, the lateral portion of the anterior skull base stands on top of the orbits and maxillary sinuses. Medially, it relates to the sphenoid sinus (posterior portion of the medial exocranial anterior surface) and ethmoid bone (medial and anterior thirds). The exocranial aspect of the anterior cranial fossa as well as the nasal cavity is divided along the midline by the bony part of the nasal septum, which is part of the ethmoid bone and attached to the sphenoid crest and rostrum [2]. Its boundaries to each orbit are defined by the lateral plates of the ethmoid bones. Important foramina and grooves can be identified in the endocranial and exocranial surfaces, transmitting vascular and neural structures (Table 1.1). Anterior and posterior

A. A. AlQahtani et al. (eds.), *CSF Rhinorrhea*, https://doi.org/10.1007/978-3-030-94781-1_1

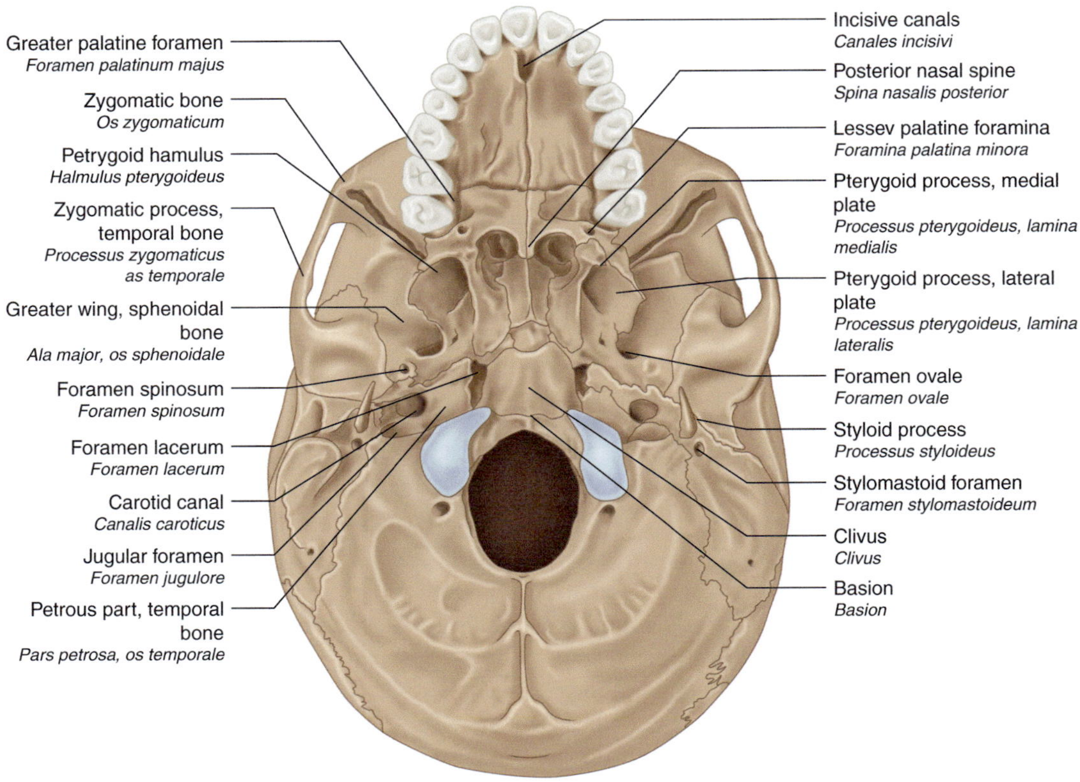

Fig. 1.1 Skull base, general aspect, inferior view. The most important anatomical landmarks are keyed

ethmoidal canals transmit the anterior and posterior ethmoidal nerves and arteries respectively and run between the frontal and ethmoid bones, along their suture line. Filaments of the olfactory nerve pierce through the cribriform plate. These perforations have dural invaginations which make this area very susceptible to iatrogenic and spontaneous CSF leaks (Fig. 1.2). Lateral to the cribriform plate is the lateral lamella that bridges the cribriform plate and the lateral ethmoid roof (fovea ethmoidalis). The lateral lamella is an extremely thin bone (0.05-0.2 mm) and the one most frequently perforated during sinus surgery. On the contrary, fovea ethmoidalis is significantly thicker. The cribriform plate and the lateral lamella are not always on the same level. If they are, the lateral lamella is short and horizontal. If, however, there is a considerable distance between the level of the cribriform plate and the lateral ethmoidal roof, the lateral lamella can be long and thin increasing the risk of an intraoperative injury—even more so, if it slopes horizontally, rather than vertically [3]. Consequently, the height of the lateral lamella defines the depth of the olfactory cleft which can be asymmetrical, inducing an extra risk for perforation. The first division of the trigeminal, trochlear, oculomotor, and abducens nerves as well as the superior ophthalmic vein are transmitted through the superior orbital fissure which lies between the sphenoidal wings. Finally, the optic nerve and the ophthalmic artery run along the optic canals, between the anterior and posterior roots of the anterior clinoid processes. Knowledge of all and identification of many of these anatomic structures is crucial during various endoscopic approaches to the anterior cranial fossa -and represent potential conduits for CSF.

Table 1.1 Foramina of the external surface of the cranial base and their content; Latin nomenclature. (Reproduced from Paulsen F, Waschke T, Sobotta atlas of human Anatomy, 16th ed., Munich: Elsevier GmbH, 2019)

Foramen	Content
Foramen incisivum	• N. nasopalatinus (N. maxilaris [V/2])
Foramen palatinum majus	• N. palatinus major (N. maxilaris [V/2]) • A. palatina major (A. palatina descendens)
Foramina palatina minora	• Nn. palatini minores (N. maxillaris [V/2]) • Aa palatinae minores (A. palatina descendens)
Fissura orbitalis inferior	• A. infraorbitalis (A. maxillaris) • V. ophthalmica inferior • N. infraorbitalis (N. maxilaris [V/2]) • N. zygomaticus (N. maxilaris [V/2])
Foramen rotundum	• N. maxilaris [V/2]
Foramen ovale	• N. mandibularis [V/3] • Plexus venosus foraminis ovalis
Foramen spinosum	• R. meningeus (N. mandibularis [V/3]) • A. meningea media (A. maxillaris)
Fissura sphenopetrosa, Foramen lacerum	• N. petrosus minor (N. glossopharyngeous [IX]) • N. petrosus major (N. facialis [VII]) • N. petrosus profundus (Plexus caroticus internus)
Apertura externa canalis carotici and Canalis caroticus	• A. carotis interna, Pars petrosa • Plexus venosus caroticus internus • Plexus caroticus internus (Truncus sympathicus, Ganglion cervicale superius)
Foramen stylomastoideum	• N. facialis [VII]
Foramen jugulare	Anterior area • Sinus petrosus inferior • N. glossopharyngeus [IX] Posterior area • A. meningea posterior (A. pharyngea ascendens) • Sinus sigmoideus (Bulbus superior venae jugularis) • N. vagus [X] • R. meningeus (N. vagus [X]) • N. accessorius [IX]
Canaliculus mastoideus	• R. auricularis nervi vagi (N. vagus [X])
Canaliculus tympanicus	• N. tympanicus • A. tympanica inferior

Table 1.1 (continued)

Foramen	Content
Canalis nervi hypoglossi	• N. hypoglossus [XII] • Plexus venosus canalis nervi hypoglossi
Canalis condylaris	• V. emissaria condylaris
Foramen magnum	• Meninges • Plexus venosus vertebralis internus (Sinus marginalis) • Aa. vertebrales (Aa. subclaviae) • A. spinalis anterior (Aa. vertebrales) • Medulla oblongata/Medulla spinalis • Radices spinales (N. accessorius [XII])

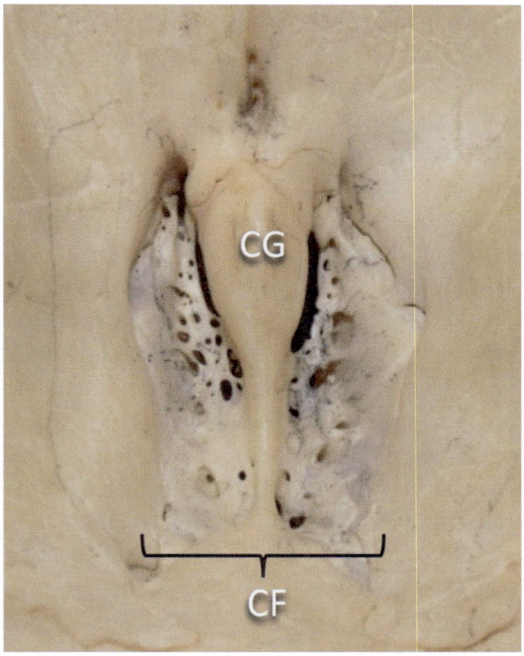

Fig. 1.2 Close-up view of cranial nerve foramina within anterior cranial fossa. *CG* crista galli, CF cribriform plate. (Reproduced from Edwards B, Wang JM, Iwanaga J, Loukas M, Tubbs RS. Cranial Nerve Foramina Part I: A Review of the Anatomy and Pathology of Cranial Nerve Foramina of the Anterior and Middle Fossa. Cureus. 2018;10(2):e2172)

1.2.2 Middle Cranial Fossa

The sphenoid and temporal bones contribute to the formation of the middle cranial fossa which stands in continuity to the anterior. The medial part is formed mainly by the body of the sphenoid, whereas the combination of sphenoid wings and squamous and petrous parts of the temporal bone contribute to the lateral parts. The sella is the medial portion of the middle cranial base, whilst the lateral portions are the temporal fossae. The small parasellar regions, one on each side, house the cavernous sinuses, thus being two of the most important -from a surgical point of view- skull base regions. Laterally, the sphenoid ridges are formed by the lesser sphenoid wings which, medially, also form the roof of the optic canal. In the middle of the sphenoid planum stands a remnant of the fusion of the ossification centers, called the sphenoid jugum. Posterior to the planum, the chiasmatic sulcus is found, which stands between the optic canals' openings. The last are superior to the optic strut, inferior to the orbital fissure. Between the chiasmatic sulcus and the sellar cavity stands the tuberculum sellae. The sella, especially its posterior limit is the actual boundary to the posterior cranial fossa, consisting of the dorsum and posterior clinoid processes. A number of important foramina are located at the area of the middle cranial fossa. Starting from anteromedial to posterolateral lie the superior orbital fissure, foramen rotundum, foramen ovale and foramen spinosum which transmit important nerves and vessels. Foramen lacerum lies posteromedial to the foramen ovale and carotid canal is formed from the articulation of petrous apex with the sphenoid and occipital bone. The innominate foramen and the foramen of Vessalius are two inconsistent foramina located medially to foramen spinosum and foramen ovale, respectively. Thorough understanding of the anatomy of this particular area is a critical step to understanding part of the course of the carotid artery (Fig. 1.3). Right after the artery leaves its canal on the petrous portion of the temporal bone it is encircled by the lingula, a protrusion of the sphenoid bone located at the junction of the body and the greater wing. The petrolingual carotid is divided from the vertical cavernous carotid segment by the petrolingual ligament, attached to the lingula [4]. Concerning the ventral middle cranial base, its medial part includes the sphenoid body and the upper basal part of the occipital bone. Its lateral part is formed by the greater sphenoid wing and the lateral pterygoid plate; the petrous, tympanic, squamous, and styloid parts of the temporal bone; and the zygomatic, palatine, and maxillary bones. Inferiorly to each cavernous sinus, an intermediate part corresponding to the area between the pterygoid plates extends from the pterygopalatine fossa anteriorly to the pterygoid fossa posteriorly. The pterygopalatine fossa is formed by the posterior wall of the maxillary sinus, the pterygoid process, the palatine bone and the sphenoid bone above. The fossa communicates with the infratemporal fossa and also with the nasal cavity through the sphenopalatine foramen. Its roof is divided into anterior and posterior parts by the passage of the chorda tympani, through the squamotympanic fissure. The lateral part of the middle skull base includes the infratemporal fossa, mandibular

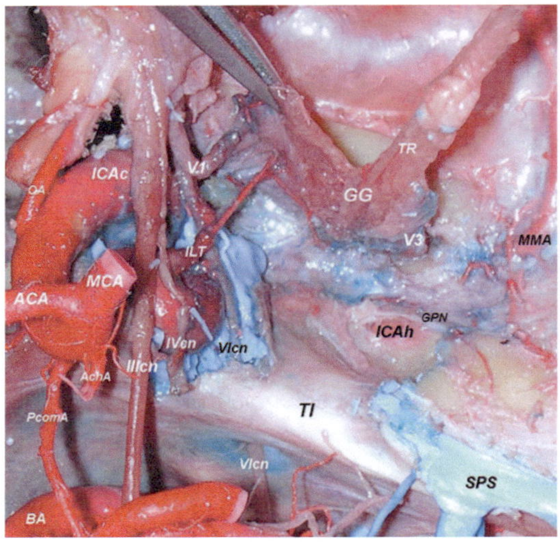

Fig. 1.3 Right middle cranial fossa from above. *ACA* anterior cerebral artery, *AchA* anterior choroidal artery, *BA* basilar artery, *GG* gasserian ganglion, *GPN* greater petrosal nerve, *ICAc* cavernous portion of the internal carotid artery, *ICAh* horizontal portion of the internal carotid artery, *ILT* inferolateral trunk, *MCA* middle cerebral artery, *MMA* middle meningeal artery, *OA* ophthalmic artery, *ON* optic nerve, *PcomA* posterior communicating artery, *SPS* superior petrosal sinus, *TI* trigeminal impression, *TR* trigeminal root, *V1* first branch of the trigeminal nerve, *V3* third branch of the trigeminal nerve, *IIIcn* oculomotor nerve, *IV* trochlear nerve, *VIcn* abducens nerve. (Reproduced from Castelnuovo P, Dallan I, Tschabitscher M. Surgical anatomy of the internal carotid artery. Springer-Verlag Berlin An; 2016)

fossa, and the parapharyngeal space which is not further discussed here. Important foramina in the area connecting the intracranial and extracranial spaces are the jugular foramen (containing the jugular bulb and transmitting branches of the ascending pharyngeal artery, the glossopharyngeal, the vagus, and the accessory nerves) and the carotid canal (transmitting the carotid branch of the ascending pharyngeal artery, the sympathetic nerves, and the carotid artery).

1.2.3 Posterior Cranial Fossa

The posterior cranial fossa is a complex anatomical area which is formed by sphenoid, temporal and mainly by occipital bone, with squamosal, condylar, and basal parts. The basal part along with the sphenoid, forms the clivus. The clivus is located in the midline of the anterior part of the posterior cranial skull base and is formed by the posterior portion of the sphenoid body (basisphenoid) and the basal part of the occipital bone (basiocciput) [5]. Its upper third extends from the posterior clinoids and dorsum sella up to the level of the floor of the sella. The middle third is located between the sella floor and the floor of the sphenoid sinus or the level of the nasal choana. It roughly corresponds to the part of the posterior sphenoidal wall, inferior to the sella and is bounded laterally by the vertical paraclival part of the internal carotid arteries (ICAs). The abducens nerve (CN VI) courses superolaterally through the Dorello canal at the midpoint of the paraclival ICA. The petrous apex is immediately deep to the paraclival ICA. Anterior to the petrous apex and posterior to the clivus sits the sulcus for the inferior petrosal sinus. The paraclival ICA extends from the anterior genu of the petrous ICA to the parasellar segment of the ICA. Anterior genu sits on foramen lacerum immediately adjacent to petroclival synchondrosis. This corresponds to the point where the horizontal petrous carotid runs anteromedially and turns superiorly to become the paraclival carotid. A key anatomical landmark for this is the vidian canal that extends posteriorly from the pterygopalatine fossa to the anterior genu of the ICA, running on the floor of the sphenoid sinus. The eustachian tube sits just below the foramen lacerum while its cartilage is attached to the lacerum cartilage. The cranial aspect of the clivus corresponds to the basilar artery and the prepontine cistern. The inferior third extends from the choana down to foramen magnum. It corresponds to the nasopharynx and consists mostly of the occipital bone. The posterior boundary of the fossae is formed by the squamosal part which is bridged to the basal part through the condylar part of the occipital bone. The endocranial and exocranial surfaces of the anterior limit of the posterior fossa, as part of the ventral skull base, can be approached endoscopically by working through the sphenoid sinus or the nasopharynx. The dorsal skull base, is better approached suboccipitally.

1.3 Skull Base Embryology and Development

The skull is divided into two parts. The cranium or neurocranium which surrounds and protects the brain and the facial skeleton or viscerocranium. The neurocranium is a composite skeletal structure made up from the cranial vault or Calvaria which encloses the brain and the skull base or chondrocranium. The bones of Calvaria and facial skeleton are formed by intramembranous ossification (nasals, maxillae, premaxillae, zygomatic, mandible-frontal, parietal, and squamous temporal) while the bones that form the base of the skull are formed mainly by endochondral ossification (ethmoid, basisphenoid, basioccipital, petrous temporal). Tissue origin of skull base is both from ectoderm and mesoderm. Development of skull base starts at fourth embryonic week. At first, the ectomeningeal capsule appears which is a mesenchymal anlage. This mesenchymal capsule starts to surround the brain and has distinct embryologic origin. It will form the skull base and calvaria. The anterior part which corresponds to the anterior skull base is derived from neural crest while the posterior part that will give form to the posterior skull base is from paraxial mesenchyme. The ectomeningeal capsule consists of 2 layers. The inner layer that will form the dura mater and the outer layer that will form the skull base and cranial vault. The chondrification of this capsule from many discreet chondrification centers that eventually undergo endochondral ossification and fuse together to form the skull base starts at 7th embryonic week. The cranial vault will undergo an intramembranous chondrification. Chondrification of the skull base proceeds from caudal to rostral from 3 main pairs of cartilaginous precursors that extend and fuse to each other: The parachondral cartilages are located posterior to the pituitary gland and are the precursors of the basioccipital, which corresponds to the part of the occipital bone around the foramen magnum and the clivus. The hypophyseal cartilages, lateral to pituitary gland, precursors of the posterior sphenoid body or basisphenoid. And the prechondral cartilages, anterior to the pituitary gland, which are the presphenoid, the orbitosphenoid and the alisphenoid cartilages. The presphenoid cartilages are the precursors of the anterior sphenoid body, and the orbitosphenoid and alisphenoid cartilages are the precursors of the lesser and greater wings, respectively. Prechondral cartilages give also rise to the nasal capsule (ethmoids-nasal septum-inferior turbinate) and the frontal bone. Of note, blood vessels, cranial nerves and eyes have already initiate to develop before the chondrification of the skull base from cartilage precursors. Thus, endochondral bone formation occurs around pre-formed skull base foramina [6]. Ossification of the cartilaginous skull base proceeds from posterior to anterior and from central to peripheral initiating from numerous ossification centers. However, some areas of the skull base remain cartilaginous in late fetal and postnatal life. Ossification of the skull continues postnatally until puberty or early adulthood where flexible fibrous joints separating the bones of the cranial vault, named sutures, are completely ossified. In the skull base there are similar joints which are cartilaginous and will be converted into bone before adult life. This type of cartilaginous suture is named synchondrosis. All these kinds of joints are important for the ongoing growth of the postnatal brain and skull but mainly allow the head to pass through the birth canal. There are three synchondroses encountered in the skull base which fuse in different ages. Mid-sphenoidal (perinatal fusion), spheno-ethmoidal (fusion at the age of 6-8 years) and spheno-occipital (late fusion during adolescence). The spheno-occipital synchondrosis is considered to be very important because of its late ossification and major contribution to postnatal growth of cranial base. Sometimes it may persist into adult life and may be mistaken for a skull base fracture or defect.

1.4 Sphenoid Bone and Sinus

1.4.1 Sphenoid Bone and Sinus Anatomy

The sphenoid bone, as part of the floor of all three parts of the skull base, the orbital apex and the lateral wall of the skull -as mentioned above- is one of the most complex structures of the cranium. It is butterfly shaped and its name is derived from the Greek "sphenoides", meaning wedge-shaped. It is composed of the body with the sphenoid sinuses developing in it- the lesser and greater wings and the pterygoid plates (Fig. 1.4). Of the sinus's eight sides, six sides face towards the endocranium and the other two sides toward the nasopharynx and nasal cavity [7]. The superior wall of the sinus is in direct contact to the olfactory nerves, optic chiasm and hypophysis, thus a major landmark during transsphenoidal hypophysectomy. The anterior wall can be displaced by highly-developed Onodi cells, but in general it is connected to the perpendicular plate of the ethmoid [7]. The floor of the sinus forms the dome of the choanae and of the nasopharynx. The lateral walls are immediately adjacent to the ICA, optic nerve and the cavernous sinus. In a well pneumatized sinus, the relations to the surrounding structures are closer than average and ridges corresponding to these structures can be identified, barely or highly noticeable. Pneumatization of the sphenoid sinus can extend to all directions. As a general rule, it spreads more often laterally than posteriorly and inferiorly. The three most accepted pneumatization patterns of sphenoid sinus are

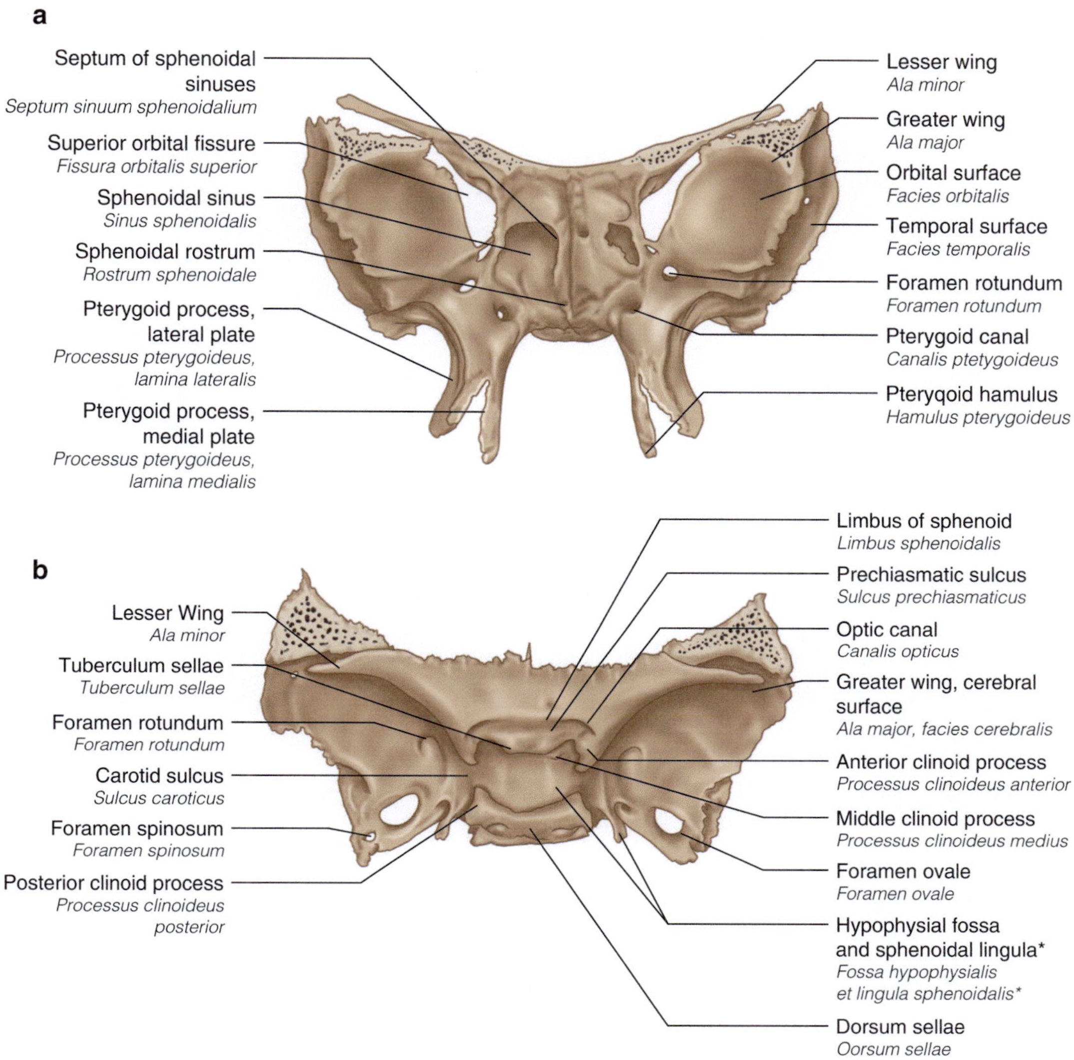

Fig. 1.4 (**a**) Sphenoidal bone—anterior view (**b**) Sphenoidal bone—superior view

sellar (80%), presellar (17%) and conchal (3%), while some authors add the postsellar type to the aforementioned configurations [8]. The conchal type or the fetal-type represents a small sinus anterior to the sella turcica, from which is separated by a thick layer of trabecular bone (Fig. 1.5). The presellar or juvenile type is pneumatized to the anterior level of the sella while the sellar type or adult type represents pneumatization of the sinus below the sella or further posteriorly (in postsellar type) [9]. The sphenoid sinus is present only in primates and develops postnatally. Pneumatization onset varies from 6 months to 4 years of life and is completed by 12 to 14 years of age with pneumatization of most sinuses reach the sella by the age of 7. The two sphenoid sinuses are usually separated by one or more bony septum(-a), often deviated laterally to one side or the other [10]. Extreme care should be taken intraoperatively before fracturing or removing these septa as the ICA or other important structures could be engaged. Thorough evaluation of the pre-operative CT-scans, minimize the risks of surgery.

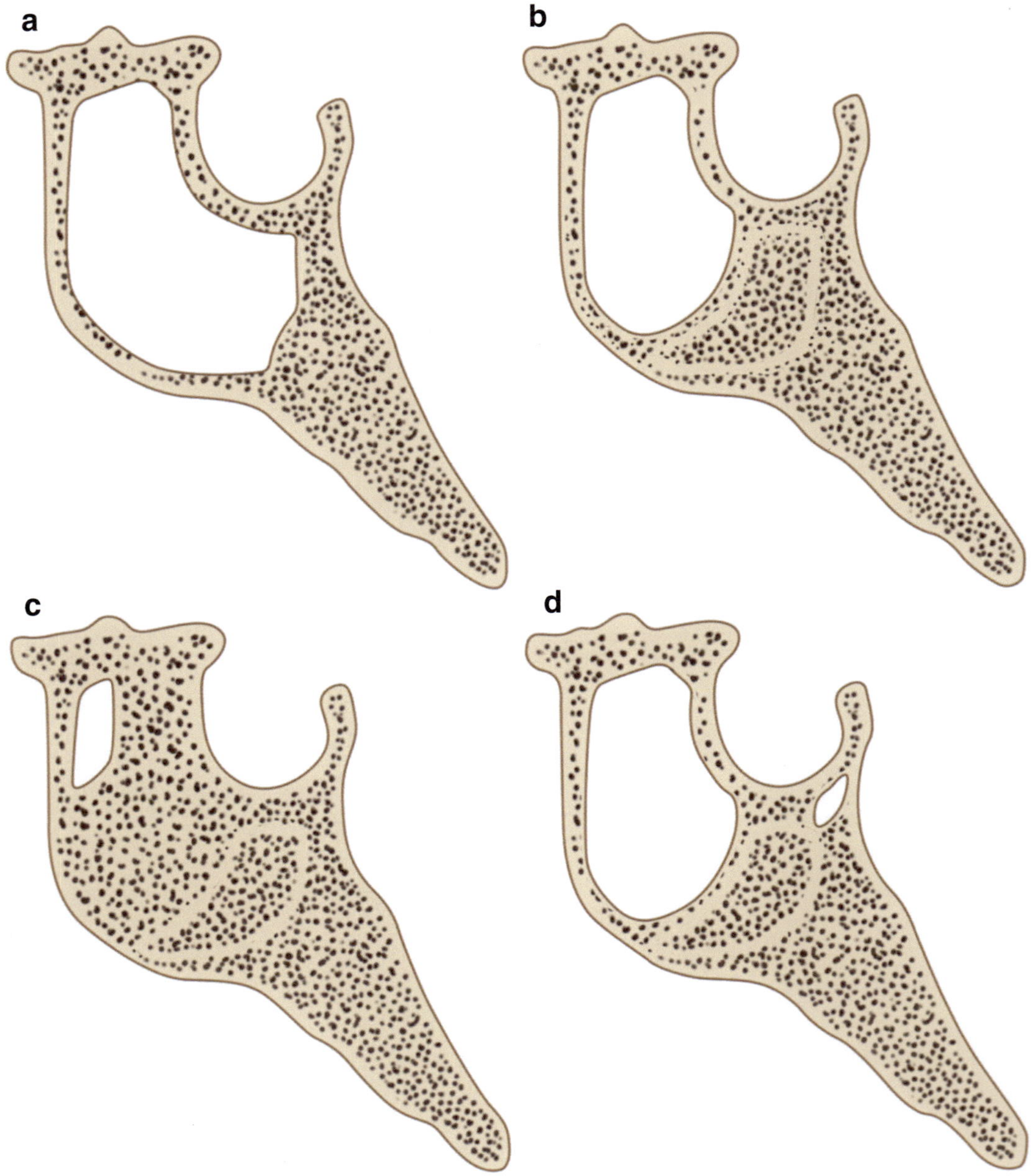

Fig. 1.5 Sphenoid pneumatization patterns. (**a**) sellar; (**b**) pre-sellar; (**c**) conchal; (**d**) post-sellar

1.4.2 Endoscopic Anatomy of the Sphenoid Sinus

In depth description of the complex anatomy of the sphenoid sinus is beyond the scope of this chapter. However, highlighting the major relations of the sphenoid sinus is of outmost importance for understanding the anatomy and performing endoscopic surgery. In the midline of the posterior wall of the sphenoid sinus one can see the sellar bulge. Inferiorly lies the middle third of the clivus which is separated from the sella by the sellar-clival junction while anterior and superior to the sella lies the planum sphenoidale. The tuberculum sella which is a bony protuberance, separates the sella from the planum sphenoidale and corresponds to the chiasmatic sulcus intracranially. Four main prominences and 3 recesses can be seen on the lateral sphenoidal wall depending on the extent of pneumatization. The 4 prominences starting from above are the optic nerve, the parasellar internal carotid artery, the V2 and the V3. The 3 recesses of the lateral sphenoid are the lateral OCR, the depression between the Cavernous sinus and the V2 and the depression between the V2 and V3. Onodi cells or posterior sphenoethmoid cells are a frequent variation encountered in the sphenoid sinus (7-25%). They are posterior ethmoidal cells that pneumatize posterior, laterall and superior to the sphenoid face placing the sphenoid sinus inferomedially. Recognizing their presence before and during endoscopic surgery is very important as there is risk of optic nerve injury and skull base penetration. There are embryological defects that pose potential risk for CSF leak such as the persistence of lateral craniofacial canal and ecchordosis physaliphora. The persistent lateral craniopharyngeal canal (Sternberg's canal) is a congenital osseous defect of the sphenoid bone, which has been consider by many authors as a potential cause of CSF leaks in the lateral recess of the sphenoid [11]. However, recent studies have shown that the majority of sphenoid CSF leaks are located in the lateral recess of a pneumatized sinus, laterally to V2 and not at the expected location of the upper opening of the canal which is located medially to the V2, right next to the sella [12]. It has been postulated that the arachnoid pits developed on the cranial aspect of lateral recess (or on the floor of the middle cranial fossa) due to increased intracranial pressure, when combined with attenuated lateral recess roof associated with lateral recess pneumatization are the main cause of CSF leaks in the lateral sphenoid [13]. Pneumatization has impact not only in anatomic variations but also in risk for CSF leak. Extensive pneumatization of the sphenoid sinus (pneumosinus dilatans) can play a role in the pathogenesis. Ecchordosis physaliphora is a rare benign congenital lesion originating from remnants of the notochord, normally located in the retroclival prepontine region. It is appeared usually as an osseous round defect of the posterior sphenoidal wall at the level of the midclivus. Although it appears that may be an asymptomatic condition it can present with associated CSF leak and meningitis [14] (Figs. 1.6, 1.7, and 1.8).

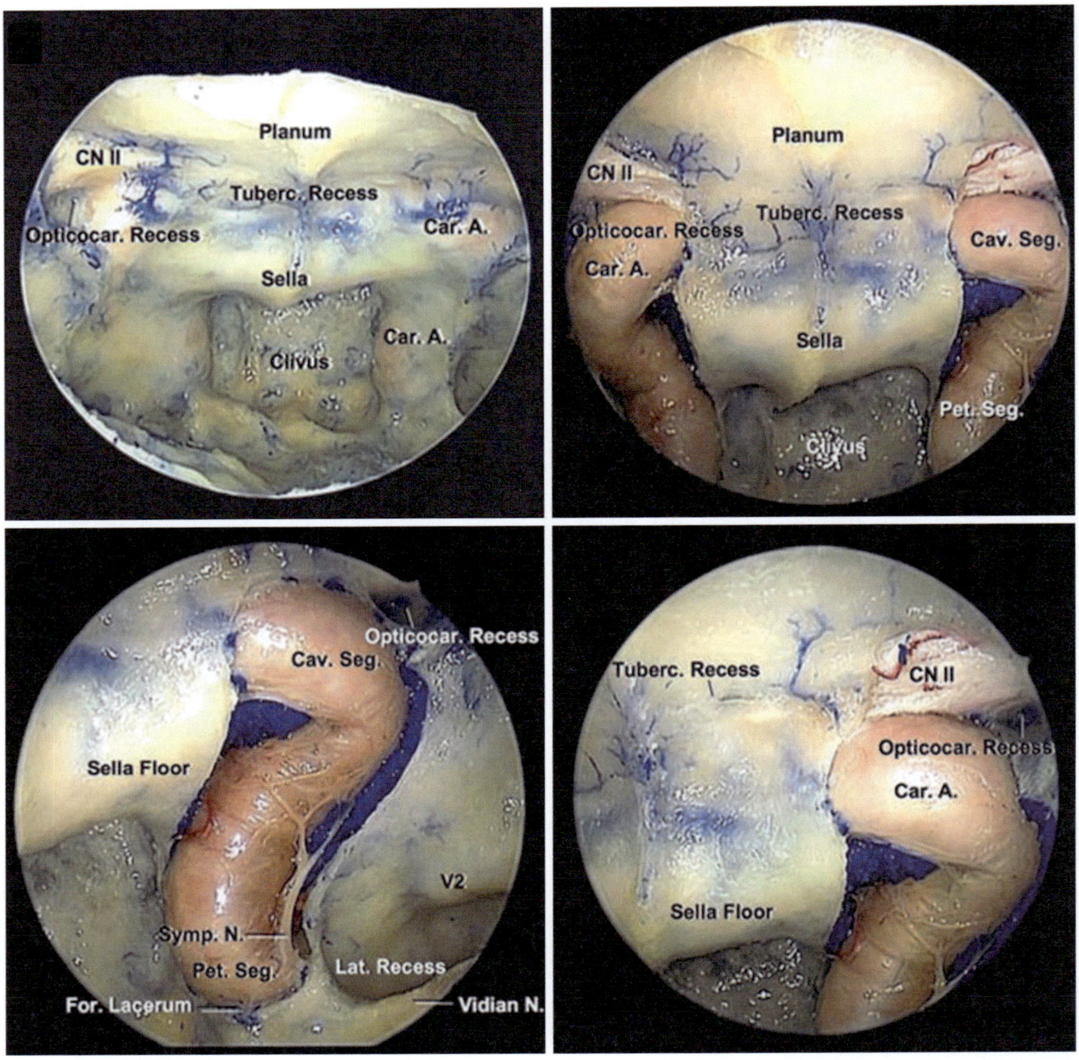

Fig. 1.6 Endoscopic views the relationships of the recesses in the sphenoid sinus to the surrounding neurovascular structures. (Reproduced from Wang J, Bidari S, Inoue K, Yang H, Rhoton A Jr, Extensions of the sphenoid sinus: a new classification. Neurosurgery. 2010;66(4):797–816)

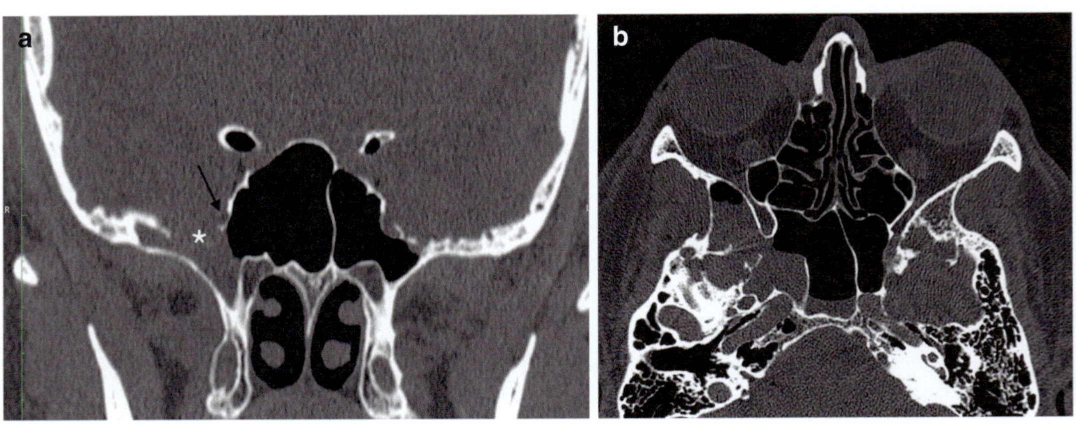

Fig. 1.7 (**a**) Spontaneous CSF rhinorrhea with associated meningoencephalocele in extremely pneumatized lateral recess of the sphenoid sinus. V2 nerve *(black arrow)*, skull base defect *(asterisk)*. (**b**) Same patient—axial view

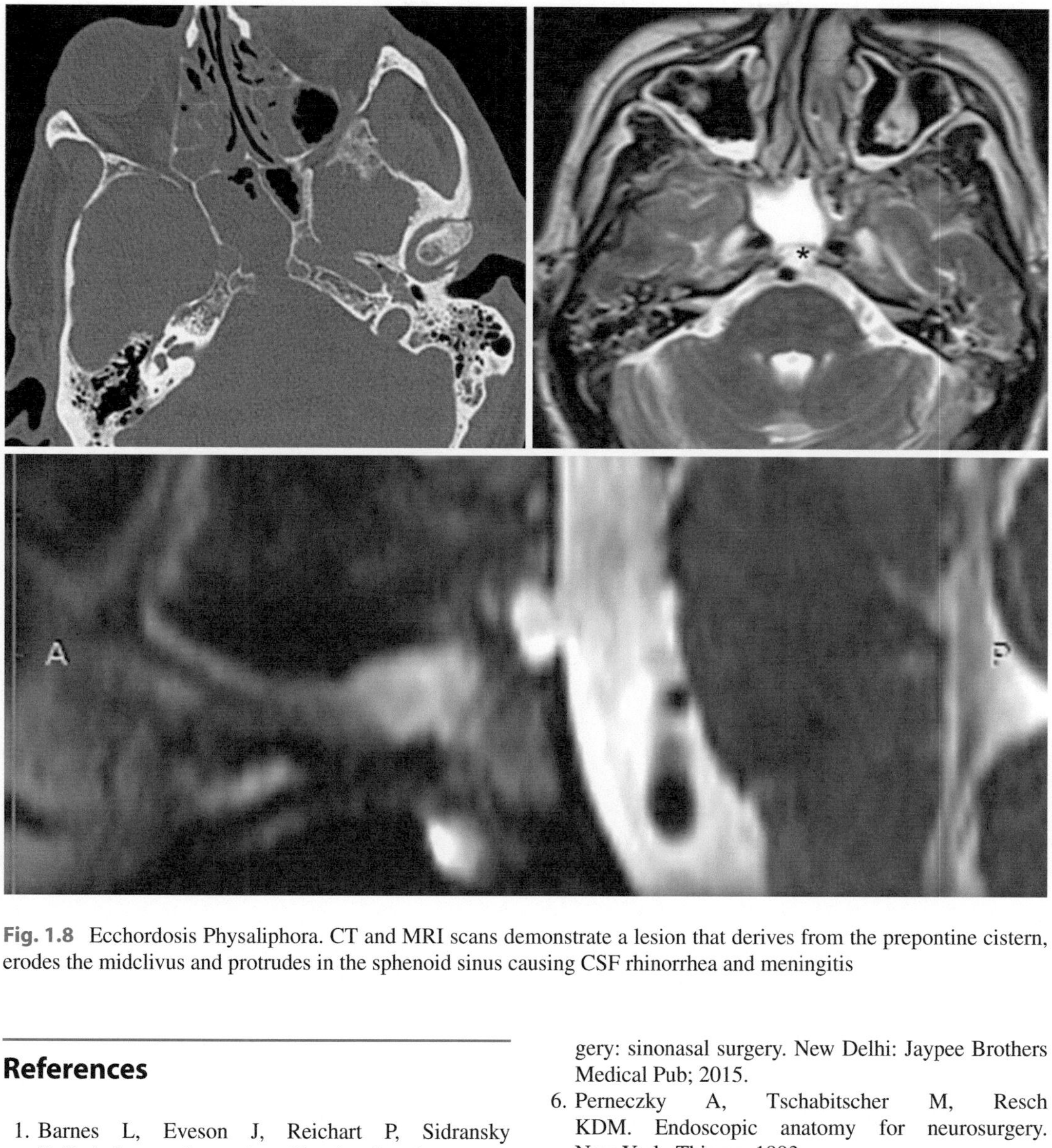

Fig. 1.8 Ecchordosis Physaliphora. CT and MRI scans demonstrate a lesion that derives from the prepontine cistern, erodes the midclivus and protrudes in the sphenoid sinus causing CSF rhinorrhea and meningitis

References

1. Barnes L, Eveson J, Reichart P, Sidransky D. Pathology and genetics of head and neck tumours. Lyon: IARC Press; 2005.
2. Stamm AC. Transnasal endoscopic skull base and brain surgery. New York: Thieme; 2019.
3. Gera R, Mozzanica F, Karligkiotis A, et al. Lateral lamella of the cribriform plate, a keystone landmark: proposal for a novel classification system. Rhinology. 2018;56(1):65–72.
4. Castelnuovo P, Dallan I, Tschabitscher M. Surgical anatomy of the internal carotid artery. Berlin: Springer-Verlag; 2016.
5. Payne S, Singh A, Sataloff R, Woodworth B. Surgical techniques in otolaryngology–Head and neck surgery: sinonasal surgery. New Delhi: Jaypee Brothers Medical Pub; 2015.
6. Perneczky A, Tschabitscher M, Resch KDM. Endoscopic anatomy for neurosurgery. New York: Thieme; 1993.
7. Budu V, Mogoantă CA, Fănuţă B, Bulescu I. The anatomical relations of the sphenoid sinus and their implications in sphenoid endoscopic surgery. Rom J Morphol Embryol. 2013;54(1):13–6.
8. Hamid O, El Fiky L, Hassan O, Kotb A, El Fiky S. Anatomic variations of the sphenoid sinus and their impact on trans-sphenoid pituitary surgery. Skull Base. 2008;18(1):9–15. https://doi.org/10.1055/s-2007-992764.
9. Levine HL, Clemente MP. Sinus surgery: endoscopic and microscopic approaches. New York: Thieme; 2005.

10. Wiebracht ND, Zimmer LA. Complex anatomy of the sphenoid sinus: a radiographic study and literature review. J Neurol Surg B Skull Base. 2014;75(6):378–82.
11. Tomazic PV, Stammberger H. Spontaneous CSF-leaks and meningoencephaloceles in sphenoid sinus by persisting Sternberg's canal. Rhinology. 2009;47(4):369–74.
12. Barañano CF, Curé J, Palmer JN, Woodworth BA. Sternberg's canal: fact or fiction? Am J Rhinol Allergy. 2009;23(2):167–71.
13. Illing E, Schlosser RJ, Palmer JN, Curé J, Fox N, Woodworth BA. Spontaneous sphenoid lateral recess cerebrospinal fluid leaks arise from intracranial hypertension, not Sternberg's canal. Int Forum Allergy Rhinol. 2014;4(3):246–50.
14. Georgalas C, Terzakis D, Tsikna M, et al. Ecchordosis physaliphora: a cautionary tale. J Laryngol Otol. 2020;134(1):46–51.

Physiology of CSF

2

Reda Kamel, Hussam Elbosraty, Mohamed Hafez, and Tarek Kandil

2.1 Historical Review

The existence of CSF has been known for centuries. Hippocrates was among the first to describe the fluid as water that surrounded the brain [1]. In 1914, Cushing published his article titled "Studies on the Cerebro-Spinal Fluid" and accredited the choroid plexus as a source for CSF [2]. Dandy, shortly after, conducted an experiment in which he ablated the choroid plexus of one lateral ventricle in a dog, then obstructed the foramen leading into the third ventricle; he discovered that the ventricle that was ablated and evacuated of CSF would collapse, while the ventricle that was not manipulated would expand [3].

Since then, this theory has been taken as fact (the classical theory), and many studies conducted on the choroid plexus and CSF secretion have revolved around this concept. The original theory of CSF production views 75% of all CSF being produced by the choroid plexus epithelium, while the remaining quarter being produced by other CNS structures such as the ependymal wall, cerebral parenchyma, and interstitial fluid (ISF) [4].

2.2 Nature of CSF

The cerebrospinal fluid (CSF) space consists of the intracerebral ventricles, subarachnoid spaces of the spine and brain (e.g., cisterns and sulci), and the central spinal cord canal [5]. Cerebrospinal fluid (CSF) is a clear, colorless ultrafiltrate of plasma located within the ventricles of the brain and the subarachnoid spaces of the cranium and spine (between the arachnoid matter and pia matter) [6, 7].

2.3 Volume and Pressure of CSF

In adults, the mean CSF volume is 150 mL, distributed among the ventricles (25 mL) and subarachnoid spaces (125 mL) [6, 7]. CSF pressure determines intracranial pressure with physiological values ranging between 3 and 4 mmHg before the age of 1 year and between 10 and 15 mmHg in adults. The CSF space is a dynamic pressure system [7].

R. Kamel (✉)
Department of Otorhinolaryngology, Cairo University, Cairo, Egypt
e-mail: reda.kamel@kasralainy.edu.eg

H. Elbosraty
Department of Otorhinolaryngology, Cairo University, Cairo, Egypt

M. Hafez
Department of Neurosurgery, Cairo University, Cairo, Egypt

T. Kandil
Department of Otorhinolaryngology, Students Hospital, Cairo University, Cairo, Egypt

A. A. AlQahtani et al. (eds.), *CSF Rhinorrhea*, https://doi.org/10.1007/978-3-030-94781-1_2

2.4 Contents and Composition of CSF

The composition of CSF is strictly regulated [6] and is derived from blood plasma and is largely similar to it, except that CSF is nearly protein-free compared with plasma and has some different electrolyte levels [6, 8, 9]. CSF is mainly composed of water (99%), with the remaining 1% accounted for by proteins, ions, neurotransmitters, and glucose [10].

When compared to plasma, CSF has a higher concentration of sodium, chloride, and magnesium but a lower concentration of potassium and calcium. This difference is conferred by active transport from the interstitial compartment that is propagated by cytoplasmic carbonic anhydrases, which produce the H+, and HCO_3^- ions that are exchanged for Na^+ and Cl^- by basolateral transport proteins [11].

CSF contains approximately 0.3% plasma proteins, or approximately 15 to 40 mg/dL, depending on sampling site [12]. In general, globular proteins and albumin are in lower concentration in ventricular CSF compared to lumbar or cisternal fluid [13]. This continuous flow into the venous system dilutes the concentration of larger, lipid-insoluble molecules penetrating the brain and CSF [14]. CSF is normally free of red blood cells and at most contains only a few white blood cells. Any white blood cell count higher than this constitutes pleocytosis [15].

Unlike plasma, CSF has only trace amounts of cells, protein, and immunoglobulins [16]. Normal cell count of CSF is usually lower than 5 cells/mL [6]. Despite changes in blood composition and flow, the composition of CSF is kept constant. This provides a stable intraventricular environment, critical for maintaining normal neuronal function [7].

The composition of CSF shows a high dynamic range, and the levels of distinct proteins vary due to several influencing factors, such as site of production (brain or blood-derived), site of sampling (ventricular or lumbar), CSF flow rate (BCB function), diurnal fluctuations of CSF production rate, and finally, molecular size of blood-derived proteins (IgM vs. albumin) and circadian rhythm (glucose, prostaglandin D synthase). Alterations of lumbar CSF are mainly influenced by processes of the CNS located adjacent to the ventricular and spinal CSF space and less by pathologies in cortical areas remote from the ventricles [5].

2.5 Functions of CSF

The CSF protects the central nervous system (CNS) in different ways involving metabolic homeostasis, supply of nutrients, functioning as lymphatic system, and regulation of intracranial pressure. Moreover, CSF also plays a prominent role in brain development. It provides basic mechanical and immunological protection to the brain inside the skull [5]. CSF provides hydromechanical protection of the neuraxis through two mechanisms [6]. First, CSF acts as a shock absorber, cushioning the brain against the skull [7]. It protects the brain tissue from injury when jolted or hit, by providing a fluid buffer that acts as a shock absorber from mechanical injury [9, 17]. Second, CSF allows the brain and spinal cord to become buoyant, reducing the effective weight of the brain from its normal 1500 g to lesser 50 g. The reduction in weight lessens the force applied to the brain parenchyma and cerebral vessels during mechanical injury [7]. The actual mass of the human brain is about 1400–1500 g; however, the net weight of the brain suspended in CSF is equivalent to a mass of 25–50 g [17, 18]. The brain therefore exists in neutral buoyancy, which allows the brain to maintain its density without being impaired by its own weight, which would cut off blood supply and kill neurons in the lower sections without CSF [9].

The prevention of brain ischemia is aided by decreasing the amount of CSF in the limited space inside the skull. This decreases total intracranial pressure and facilitates blood perfusion. CSF also serves a vital function in cerebral autoregulation of cerebral blood flow [17].

Another function of CSF is to maintain homeostasis of the interstitial fluid of the brain. A stable environment for brain parenchyma is imperative for maintaining normal neuronal function. The major conduit of nutrient supply to the brain is the CP-CSF-ECSB (choroid plexus-CSF-extracellular space of the brain) connection [17]. Substrates needed by the brain are transported from the blood, through the CP, into the CSF, and then diffuse into the ECSB for transportation to their sites of action within the brain [16].

CSF allows for regulation of the distribution of substances between cells of the brain [7], and neuroendocrine factors, to which slight changes can cause problems or damage to the nervous system. For example, high glycerine concentration disrupts temperature and blood pressure control, and high CSF pH causes dizziness and syncope [15].

CSF also assists in the removal of waste products of brain metabolism, such as products of peroxidation, glycosylated proteins, excess neurotransmitters, debris from the lining of the ventricles, bacteria, viruses, and otherwise unnecessary molecules [6, 7, 16]. Accumulation of such unnecessary molecules, seen in aging and some neurodegenerative diseases, interferes with neuronal functioning of the brain. CSF is critical in the brain's lymphatic system. Metabolic waste products diffuse rapidly into CSF and are removed into the bloodstream as CSF is absorbed [19].

2.6 Secretion of CSF

CSF is predominantly, but not exclusively, secreted by the choroid plexuses located within the ventricles of the brain, with the two lateral ventricles [6]. Brain interstitial fluid, ependyma, and capillaries may also play a poorly defined role in CSF secretion [5, 7].

Sixty to seventy-five percent of CSF is produced by the choroid plexuses of the lateral ventricles and the tela choroidea of the third and fourth ventricles [7]. Its secretion varies between individuals with adult production, usually ranging between 400 and 600 mL/day [6]. CSF forms at a rate of about 0.3–0.4 mL/min; translating to 18–25 mL/h and 430–530 mL/day [11].

The constant secretion of CSF contributes to complete CSF renewal four to five times per 24-h period in the average young adult [1]. Reduction of CSF turnover may contribute to the accumulation of metabolites seen in aging and neurodegenerative diseases [6, 7].

The epithelial cells of the choroid plexus secrete cerebrospinal fluid (CSF), by a process that involves the movement of Na(+), Cl(−), and HCO(3)(−) from the blood to the ventricles of the brain. This creates the osmotic gradient, which drives the secretion of H(2)O. The unidirectional movement of the ions is achieved due to the polarity of the epithelium, i.e., the ion transport proteins in the blood-facing (basolateral) are different to those in the ventricular (apical) membranes [20].

The molecular constituents of CSF are mainly blood-derived (80%), while the remainder consists of brain-derived and intrathecally produced molecules (20%) [5].

The CSF space is separated from the vascular system by the blood–CSF barrier (BCB), whereas the blood–brain barrier (BBB), responsible for maintaining the homeostasis of the brain, is located between brain parenchyma and vascular system. Although both barriers have similar functions, they differ with regard to their morphologic and functional properties. Both barrier systems are permeable not only for small molecules, but also for macromolecules and circulating cells. The transport of molecules across the BBB and BCB is regulated by passive diffusion (e.g., albumin, immunoglobulins) and facilitated or active transport (e.g., glucose). The extracellular space volume, potassium buffering, CSF circulation, and interstitial fluid absorption are mainly regulated by aquaporin-4 channels, which are abundantly located at the blood–brain and brain–CSF interfaces [5].

Choroidal secretion of cerebrospinal fluid comprises two steps. The first step consists of passive filtration of plasma from choroidal capillaries to the choroidal interstitial compartment according to a pressure gradient. The second step consists of active transport from the interstitial compartment to the ventricular lumen across the choroidal epithelium, involving carbonic anhydrase and membrane ion carrier proteins [7].

The CP is a highly specialized simple cuboidal epithelium continuous with ependymal cells lining the ventricles of the brain. This simple cuboidal epithelium surrounds clusters of fenestrated capillaries allowing for the filtration of plasm [7]. Cells of the CP have dense microvilli present on their apical surface and are interconnected via tight junctions, creating a blood–CSF barrier that helps to control the composition of CSF [6]. Because there is no appreciable barrier between the CSF and the ECSB, the blood–CSF barrier also serves to regulate the environment of the brain [16]. Larger substances such as cells, protein, and glucose are not allowed passage, whereas ions and small molecules such as vitamins and nutrients are able to pass into the CSF relatively easily [21]. Water is allowed passage through the CP epithelium via epithelial AQP1 channels. Substances that may not pass through the blood–CSF barrier but are needed by the brain can be actively synthesized by or actively transported through the CP epithelial cells into the CSF. A 5 mV lumen positive voltage potential is present across CP epithelial cell membranes. This difference of electrical potential pulls sodium, chloride, and bicarbonate ions from the plasma into the CSF, creating an osmotic gradient, which then drives the movement of water into the CSF. No cells are able to pass through the blood–CSF barrier although small numbers of white blood cells are usually introduced to the CSF indirectly [7].

2.7 Mechanism of CSF Circulation

CSF circulates in a craniocaudal direction from ventricles to spinal subarachnoid space [5]. After production, CSF movement generally occurs through the ventricular system, assisted, in part, by ciliated ependyma which beat in synchrony [22]. Recent studies demonstrated that CSF movement is not presented as a circulation, but a permanent rhythmic systolic–diastolic pulsation in all directions. Such movement also represents the main force of substance distribution inside the CSF system. This distribution occurs in all directions, i.e., in the direction of the imagined circulation, as well as in the opposite direction [23].

CSF is secreted constantly with an unchanging composition, functioning to maintain a stable environment within the brain [7]. CSF is propelled along the neuroaxis from the site of secretion to the site of absorption mainly by the rhythmic systolic pulse wave within the choroidal arteries. Lesser determinants of CSF flow are frequency of respiration, posture, venous pressure of the jugular vein, physical effort of the subject, and time of day [16].

CSF flows throughout the ventricular system unidirectional in a rostral to caudal manner. CSF produced in the lateral ventricles would travel through the interventricular foramina to the third ventricle, through the cerebral aqueduct to the fourth ventricle, and then through the median aperture (also known as the foramen of Magendie) into the subarachnoid space at the base of the brain [6]. Once in the subarachnoid space, the CSF begins have a gentle multidirectional flow that creates an equalization of composition throughout the CS. CSF flows over the surface of the brain and down the length of spinal cord while in the subarachnoid space [7, 9, 16].

There is a connection from the subarachnoid space to the bony labyrinth of the inner ear making the cerebrospinal fluid continuous with the perilymph in 93% of people [7].

2.8 Absorption of CSF

From spinal subarachnoid space the CSF is removed via craniocaudal lymphatic routes and the venous system [5]. CSF leaves the subarachnoid space through arachnoid villi found along the superior sagittal venous sinus, intracranial venous sinuses, and around the roots of spinal nerves. Arachnoid villi are protrusions of arachnoid mater through the dura mater into the lumen of a venous sinus. A 3 to 5 mmHg pressure gradient between the subarachnoid space and venous sinus pulls CSF into the venous outflow system through the arachnoid villi [6].

Arachnoid granulations act as an avenue for CSF reabsorption into the blood circulation through a pressure-dependent gradient. The arachnoid granulations appear as outpouchings into the superior sagittal sinus (SSS) due to the pressure in the subarachnoid space being greater than the venous sinus pressure (NB: direct visualization of arachnoid granulations intraoperatively would reveal the inverse) [24].

There have been studies describing CSF reabsorption into the dural venous plexus. At birth, arachnoid granulations are not fully developed, and CSF absorption relies on the venous plexus of the inner surface of dura that is more robust in infants [25, 26].

CSF may also enter into the lymphatic system via the nasal cribriform plate or spinal nerve roots. Clearance of CSF is dependent upon the posture of the subject, pressure differentials, and pathophysiology [16].

Cranial and spinal arachnoid villi have been considered for a long time to be the predominant sites of CSF absorption into the venous outflow system. Experimental data suggest that cranial and spinal nerve sheaths, the cribriform plate, and the adventitia of cerebral arteries constitute substantial pathways of CSF drainage into the lymphatic outflow system [7].

2.9 The New Hypothesis of Production, Circulation, and Absorption of CSF

The classic hypothesis of CSF hydrodynamics presents the cerebrospinal fluid (CSF) as the "third circulation," which flows from the brain ventricles through the entire CSF system to the cortical subarachnoid space to eventually be passively absorbed into the SSS through arachnoid granulations. The choroid plexus represents a key organ in the classic CSF physiology and a powerful biological pump, which exclusively secretes CSF [6].

However, numerous evidence of a new hypothesis of CSF hydrodynamics demonstrate a significantly strong relationship between the CSF and interstitial fluid (IF). Moreover, CSF and IF are mainly produced and absorbed in the parenchymal capillaries of the brain and spinal cord. A considerable amount of CSF and IF is also absorbed by the lymphatic system, and CSF movement is not unidirectional flow. It is only local mixing and diffusion [27].

Recent studies presented arguments in favor of the thesis that the CPs are neither biological pumps nor the main site of CSF secretion; that they do not participate in regulation of ICP/CSF pressure; are not the reason for the existence of hydrostatic pressure gradient in the CSF system and that this gradient is not permanent (disappeared in the horizontal position); and that they do not generate imagined unidirectional CSF circulation, hydrocephalus development, and increased ICP/CSF pressure. The classic hypothesis cannot provide an explanation for these controversies but the recently formulated Bulat-Klarica-Orešković hypothesis can. According to this hypothesis, CSF production and absorption (CSF exchange) are constant and present everywhere in the CSF system, and although the CSF is partially produced by the CP, it is mainly formed as a consequence of water filtration between the capillaries and interstitial fluid. Accordingly, they postulated that CP, AV (arachnoid villi), and lymphatics become minor sites for CSF hydrodynamics [10, 23, 28, 29].

References

1. Hajdu SI. A note from history: discovery of the cerebrospinal fluid. Ann Clin Lab Sci. 2003;33:334–6.
2. Cushing H. Studies on the cerebro-spinal fluid: I. Introduction. J Med Res. 1914;31:1–9.
3. Dandy WE. Experimental hydrocephalus. Ann Surg. 1919;70:129–42.
4. Johanson CE, Duncan JA 3rd, Klinge PM, Brinker T, Stopa EG, Silverberg GD, et al. Multiplicity of cerebrospinal fluid functions: new challenges in health and disease. Cerebrospinal Fluid Res. 2008;5:10.
5. Tumani H, Huss A, Bachhuber F. The cerebrospinal fluid and barriers - anatomic and physiologic considerations. Handb Clin Neurol. 2017;146:21–32.
6. Spector R, Robert Snodgrass S, Johanson CE. A balanced view of the cerebrospinal fluid composition and functions: focus on adult humans. Exp Neurol. 2015;273:57–68.
7. Sakka L, Coll G, Chazal J. Anatomy and physiology of cerebrospinal fluid. Eur Ann Otorhinolaryngol Head Neck Dis. 2011;128(6):309–16.
8. Guyton AC, Hall JE. Textbook of medical physiology. 11th ed. W.B. Saunders; 2005. p. 764–7.

9. Saladin K. Anatomy and physiology. 6th ed. McGraw Hill; 2012. p. 519–20.
10. Bulat M, Klarica M. Recent insights into a new hydrodynamics of the cerebrospinal fluid. Brain Res Rev. 2011;65:99–112.
11. Brown PD, Davies SL, Speake T, Millar ID. Molecular mechanisms of cerebrospinal fluid production. Neuroscience. 2004;129:957–70.
12. Felgenhauer K. Protein size and CSF composition. Klin Wochenschr. 1974;52(24):1158–64.
13. Merril CR, Goldman D, Sedman SA, Ebert MH. Ultrasensitive stain for proteins in polyacrylamide gels shows regional variation in cerebrospinal fluid proteins. Science. 1981;211(4489):1437–8.
14. Saunders NR, Habgood MD, Dziegielewska KM. Barrier mechanisms in the brain, I. adult brain. Clin Exp Pharmacol Physiol. 1999;26:11–9.
15. Jurado R, Walker HK. Cerebrospinal fluid. In: Clinical methods: the history, physical, and laboratory examinations. 3rd ed. Butterworths; 1990.
16. Damkier HH, Brown PD, Praetorius J. Epithelial pathways in choroid plexus electrolyte transport. Physiology (Bethesda). 2010;25(4):239–49.
17. Wright BLC, Lai JTF, Sinclair AJ. Cerebrospinal fluid and lumbar puncture: a practical review. J Neurol. 2012;259(8):1530–45.
18. Noback C, Strominger NL, Demarest RJ, Ruggiero DA. The human nervous system. Humana Press; 2005. p. 93.
19. Ropper AH, Brown RH. Adams and victor's principles of neurology. 8th ed. McGraw-Hill Professional; 2005. p. 530.
20. Speake T, Whitwell C, Kajita H, Majid A, Brown PD. Mechanisms of CSF secretion by the choroid plexus. Microsc Res Tech. 2001;52(1):49–59.
21. Damkier HH, Brown PD, Praetorius J. Cerebrospinal fluid secretion by the choroid plexus. Physiol Rev. 2013;93(4):1847–92.
22. Roales-Buján R, Páez P, Guerra M, Rodríguez S, Vío K, Ho-Plagaro A, et al. Astrocytes acquire morphological and functional characteristics of ependymal cells following disruption of ependyma in hydrocephalus. Acta Neuropathol. 2012;124:531–46.
23. Orešković D, Radoš M, Klarica M. Role of choroid plexus in cerebrospinal fluid hydrodynamics. Neuroscience. 2017 Jun;23(354):69–87.
24. Brinker T, Stopa E, Morrison J, Klinge P. A new look at cerebrospinal fluid circulation. Fluids Barriers CNS. 2014;11:10. and Spector R, Robert Snodgrass S, Johanson CE. A balanced view of the cerebrospinal fluid composition and functions: focus on adult humans. Exp Neurol. 2015;273:57–68.
25. le Gros Clark WE. On the pacchionian bodies. J Anat. 1920;55:40–8.
26. Mack J, Squier W, Eastman JT. Anatomy and development of the meninges: implications for subdural collections and CSF circulation. Pediatr Radiol. 2009;39:200–10.
27. Miyajima M, Arai H. Evaluation of the production and absorption of cerebrospinal fluid. Neurol Med Chir (Tokyo). 2015;55(8):647–56.
28. Chikly B, Quaghebeur J. Reassessing cerebrospinal fluid (CSF) hydrodynamics: a literature review presenting a novel hypothesis for CSF physiology. J Bodyw Mov Ther. 2013;17(3):344–54.
29. Oresković D, Klarica M. The formation of cerebrospinal fluid: nearly a hundred years of interpretations and misinterpretations. Brain Res Rev. 2010;64:241–62.

3 Pathophysiology of Skull Base Defect and CSF Leak

Erin Reilly and Roy Casiano

3.1 Epidemiology of CSF Leaks

Cerebrospinal fluid rhinorrhea is the result of a pathologic communication between the subarachnoid space and the nasal cavity. This condition most often occurs secondary to an inciting event, but it can also develop unexpectedly. The epidemiology of CSF rhinorrhea has classically been reported in association with its etiology. An initial classification system described by Ommaya in 1968 divided CSF leaks into traumatic and non-traumatic origins [1]. Traumatic leaks were further subdivided into accidental and iatrogenic, and non-traumatic into high pressure (secondary to tumors or hydrocephalus) and normal pressure leaks (such as congenital). Schlosser et al. have more recently defined the five main causes of CSF leaks as: accidental trauma, surgical trauma, tumor related, congenital, and spontaneous [2]. The most common etiology overall is accidental trauma and accounts for 80% of all CSF leaks. Surgical or iatrogenic trauma is the second most common cause and is responsible for 16% of cases. Of note, this includes both otolaryngologic and neurosurgical procedures. The remaining 4% is of non-traumatic origin [3].

E. Reilly (✉)
Department of Otolaryngology, Saint Alphonsus Medical Center, Boise, ID, USA

R. Casiano
Department of Otolaryngology, University of Miami Miller School of Medicine, Miami, FL, USA

3.2 Etiology and Pathophysiology of CSF Leaks

3.2.1 Traumatic

Traumatic head injuries are the most common cause of CSF rhinorrhea. A closed head injury is complicated by a CSF leak in 1–3% of patients, which includes CSF otorrhea. This number increases to 5% if there is a CSF leak in the presence of a skull base fracture. The sphenoid (30%) and frontal sinuses (30%) are the most common sites of injury, followed by the ethmoid sinus (23%) [3]. The majority of these leaks occur as a result of blunt trauma, simply because of the higher incidence of blunt trauma overall compared to penetrating trauma. The exact mechanism of injury can range from a small bony fracture with laceration of the meningeal layers to significant comminution of the skull base. In contrast to the middle and posterior cranial fossae, a CSF leak from the anterior skull base is more frequent because of the firm adherence of the dura mater to the skull in this area. In addition, the horizontal cribriform plate is a thin and fragile bone that is covered only by an arachnoid layer, thus missing the protection of a true dural investment [4].

A. A. AlQahtani et al. (eds.), *CSF Rhinorrhea*, https://doi.org/10.1007/978-3-030-94781-1_3

3.2.2 Iatrogenic

CSF leak is a known complication of endoscopic sinus surgery, but the overall incidence is less than 1%. The ethmoid sinus or cribiform plate, in particular the posterior ethmoid roof near the anterior medial face of sphenoid, is the site of injury 80% of the time. A CSF leak of the frontal sinus occurs less frequently (8%) and is rarely encountered in the sphenoid sinus (4%) [3]. Iatrogenic trauma to the skull base is exacerbated by an inexperienced surgeon, impaired orientation, excessive inflammatory disease resulting in increased bleeding or loss of anatomical landmarks from previous surgery. Injury has been found to occur more commonly on the right side of the nasal cavity, due to the higher prevalence of right-handed surgeons and the tendency for the angle of surgical approach to drift medially [5]. Anatomical variations may also contribute to iatrogenic injuries, such as a lower cribiform height relative to the height of ethmoid roof (i.e. Keros classification), greater slope of the ethmoid roof in the sagittal plane or an excessive maxillary pneumatization causing a corresponding decrease in posterior ethmoid pneumatization [2, 6]. Iatrogenic injury of the skull base can also occur during neurosurgical procedures and is most common after a transsphenoidal hypophysectomy. In these cases, a CSF leak will occur if surgical manipulation disrupts the sellar diaphragm. The literature reports an intraoperative CSF leak rate ranging between 10% and 61% during sellar surgery [7].

3.2.3 Congenital

Congenital CSF leaks are the least frequent etiology encountered. Improper embryologic development of the anterior cranial fossa can cause lesions such as dermoids, gliomas, and cephaloceles, but these are infrequently associated with CSF rhinorrhea. Congenital cephaloceles are classified on the basis of location, and the basal subtype can occasionally present with a CSF leak. Examples of midline basal cephaloceles include transethmoidal, sphenoethmoidal, and sphenopharyngeal types. The basal variation comprises 10% of all cephaloceles and results from failed ossification of the skull base with extension of neural crest cells through the defect. Cephaloceles at the cribriform plate may be caused by aberrant development at a natural opening for an olfactory fili [8]. In contrast, sincipital (also known as frontoethmoidal) cephaloceles usually manifest as an external forehead or nasal mass because they are caused by failed detachment of the cutaneous ectoderm from the neuroectoderm of the anterior neuropore. During gestation, a transient dural diverticulum extends from the anterior cranial fossa to the skin through the fonticulus frontalis and prenasal space. The fonticulus frontalis temporarily separates the frontal and nasal bones, while the prenasal space is located between the nasal bones and cartilage. This dural diverticulum normally regresses between the fourth and seventh week of development and leaves a blind-ending sac called the foramen cecum. Any failure in this regression can cause an incomplete separation of the dura from the overlying skin, resulting in a cephalocele. There are three types of frontoethmoidal cephaloceles: frontonasal cephaloceles (40–60%), which protrude through the fonticulus frontalis into the glabella, nasoethmoidal cephaloceles (30%), which protrude through the foramen cecum into the nasal cavity, and naso-orbital cephaloceles, which protrude into the orbit through the lacrimal bone [9].

There is some debate surrounding CSF leaks in the sphenoid sinus with respect to a possible congenital origin. During embryogenesis, the sphenoid bone is formed from ossification and fusion of five cartilaginous areas that subsequently fuse into a single bone. In 1888, Sternberg described the development of a persistent lateral craniopharyngeal canal if there is incomplete fusion of the greater wing with the central cartilaginous precursors. It has been suggested that this preexisting embryologic skull base variant may predispose to CSF leaks later on in life. However, this theory has since been disproven as it ignores the known pattern of pneumatization of the sphenoid sinuses which are not present in this region at the time of birth. Furthermore, the location of Sternberg's canal has been described medial to the superior orbital fissure, and most spontaneous skull base defects within the sphenoid are within the lateral recess [10].

3.2.4 Neoplastic

Tumors most commonly lead to CSF leaks through direct tumor invasion across the skull base. This can occur from a primary brain tumor extending into the nasal cavity, or from a sinonasal mass that has spread intracranially. Rarely, tumors can indirectly lead to CSF leaks secondary to therapeutic treatments or by blocking CSF flow and causing hydrocephalus [11].

3.2.5 Spontaneous

Spontaneous CSF leaks are a distinct clinical entity defined as CSF rhinorrhea that occurs in the absence of any inciting event. However, we have recently discovered significant overlap in the demographic, clinical, and radiographic characteristics of patients with spontaneous CSF leak and idiopathic intracranial hypertension (IIH). 70% of patients with a spontaneous CSF leak meet the modified Dandy criteria used to diagnose IIH. For both conditions there is a female preponderance (70–80%) and a high incidence of comorbid obesity (80–90%) [12]. Elevated intracranial pressures have also been diagnosed via lumbar puncture both pre- and postoperatively [13, 14]. Nonetheless, the exact pathophysiology of both disease processes remains unknown. It is hypothesized that a constant pulsatile pressure exerted on the skull base at sites of inherent structural weakness results in gradual bony erosion. It has also been suggested that the floor of the middle cranial fossa harbors small arachnoid perforations or pits, and over time higher than normal forces can cause progressive thinning of the meninges with eventual rupture [15]. The cribiform plate and lateral recess of the sphenoid sinus are the most common sites affected, as they are regions of thin bone overlying a large pneumatized area. More specifically, the lateral lamella is the most frequent site of spontaneous CSF leaks. It is the thinnest bone of the skull base (<1 mm) and is located in the midline of the anterior cranial fossa, where CSF may preferentially gravitate. CSF leaks within the lateral recess of the sphenoid sinus have been thought to occur secondary to excessive pneumatization of the pterygoid process with attenuation of the sphenoid sinus roof.

References

1. Ommaya AK, Di Chiro G, Baldwin M, Pennybacker JB. Non-traumatic cerebrospinal fluid rhinorrhoea. J Neurol Neurosurg Psychiatry. 1968;31(3):214–25.
2. Schlosser RJ, Bolger WE. Nasal cerebrospinal fluid leaks: critical review and surgical considerations. Laryngoscope. 2004;114(2):255–65.
3. Prosser JD, Vender JR, Solares CA. Traumatic cerebrospinal fluid leaks. Otolaryngol Clin N Am. 2011;44(4):857–73.
4. Gonen L, Monteiro E, Klironomos G, Alghonaim Y, Vescan A, Zadeh G, Gentili F. Endoscopic endonasal repair of spontaneous and traumatic cerebrospinal fluid rhinorrhea: a review and local experience. Neurosurg Clin N Am. 2015;26(3):333–48.
5. Hosemann W, Draf C. Danger points, complications and medico-legal aspects in endoscopic sinus surgery. GMS Curr Top Otorhinolaryngol Head Neck Surg. 2013;12:Doc06.
6. Ledderose GJ, Stelter K, Betz CS, Englhard AS, Ledderose C, Leunig A. Cerebrospinal fluid leaks during endoscopic sinus surgery in thirty-two patients. Clin Otolaryngol. 2017;42(5):1105–8.
7. Jakimovski D, Bonci G, Attia M, Shao H, Hofstetter C, Tsiouris AJ, Anand VK, Schwartz TH. Incidence and significance of intraoperative cerebrospinal fluid leak in endoscopic pituitary surgery using intrathecal fluorescein. World Neurosurg. 2014;82(3):E513–23.
8. Kennedy DW, Hwang PH. Cerebrospinal fluid leaks and encephaloceles. In: Rhinology: diseases of the nose, sinuses and skull base. Thieme Publishers; 2012.
9. Van Wyhe RD, Chamata ES, Hollier LH. Midline craniofacial masses in children. Semin Plast Surg. 2016;30(4):176–80.
10. Baranano CF, Cure J, Palmer JN, Woodworth BA. Sternberg's canal: fact or fiction? Am J Rhinol Allergy. 2009;23(2):167–71.
11. Bedrosian JC, Anand VK, Schwartz TH. The endoscopic endonasal approach to repair of iatrogenic and noniatrogenic cerebrospinal fluid leaks and encephaloceles of the anterior cranial fossa. World Neurosurg. 2014;82(6):S86–94.

12. Wang EW, Vandergrift WA, Schlosser RJ. Spontaneous CSF leaks. Otolaryngol Clin N Am. 2011;44(4):845–56.
13. Chaaban MR, Illing E, Riley KO, Woodworth BA. Spontaneous cerebrospinal fluid leak repair: a five-year prospective evaluation. Laryngoscope. 2014;124(1):70–5.
14. Lobo BC, Baumanis MM, Nelson RF. Surgical repair of spontaneous cerebrospinal fluid (CSF) leaks: a systematic review. Laryngoscope Investig Otolaryngol. 2017;2(5):215–24.
15. Zocchi J, Pietrobon G, Lepera D, Gallo S, Russo F, Volpi L, Pellini R, Bignami M, Castelnuovo P. Spontaneous CSF leaks and IIH: a flawless connection? An experience with 167 patients. Laryngoscope. 2021;131(2):E401–7.

Part II

Clinical Presentation of CSF Rhinorrhea

4

Isaac L. Schmale, Samer Fakhri, and Martin J. Citardi

Key Points and High Risk Features

- Cerebrospinal fluid (CSF) rhinorrhea may be classified as traumatic (>90%) and nontraumatic (<10%).
- Approximately 80% of traumatic CSF leaks occur after accidental trauma, and the remaining 20% occur after neurosurgical and rhinologic procedures. Nontraumatic etiologies include idiopathic intracranial hypertension (IIH), neoplasms, and other causes of hydrocephalus.
- A detailed history and physical examination, which include a complete sinonasal evaluation, are necessary to rule out common conditions which may mimic CSF rhinorrhea.
- In a subset of patients with CSF rhinorrhea, clinical presentation is not straightforward, and missed or delayed diagnosis may occur. Clinicians must maintain a high degree of suspicion when common symptoms (namely rhinorrhea) do not closely match all of the features of common conditions (namely rhinitis).
- Clinical features of CSF rhinorrhea include:
  - Unilateral clear watery drainage
  - Drainage with a characteristic metallic or salty taste
  - Positional or exertional clear rhinorrhea
  - History of significant head trauma or sinus/skull base surgery
  - History of bacterial meningitis
  - Nasal drainage which does not respond appropriately to trial of rhinitis medication
  - Demographics: Female gender, middle aged, obesity
  - Signs or symptoms of intracranial hypertension: Papilledema, nonspecific positional headaches, double vision, balance dysfunction, pulsatile tinnitus (these signs and symptoms may be absent as an active CSF leak may reduce intracranial pressure sufficiently to avert the signs/symptoms of intracranial hypertension)
  - Both CT and MR imaging can show evidence of skull base defects, commonly at the lateral recess of the sphenoid or lateral lamella of the cribriform plate, the site of traumatic skull base disruption, and/or evidence of an empty sella.

I. L. Schmale
Department of Otolaryngology, University of Rochester Medical Center, Rochester, NY, USA

S. Fakhri
Department of Otolaryngolgology, Kelsey-Seybold Clinic, and Department of Otorhinolaryngology-Head and Neck Surgery, American University of Beirut, Beirut, Lebanon

M. J. Citardi (✉)
Department of Otorhinolaryngology, McGovern Medical School, The University of Texas Health Science Center, Houston, TX, USA
e-mail: Martin.J.Citardi@uth.tmc.edu

A. A. AlQahtani et al. (eds.), *CSF Rhinorrhea*, https://doi.org/10.1007/978-3-030-94781-1_4

4.1 Introduction

Cerebrospinal fluid (CSF) rhinorrhea results from a direct communication between the subarachnoid space and the paranasal sinuses. This communication may serve as a path for the spread of bacteria or other microorganisms that can cause intracranial infections, including bacterial meningitis. Additionally, skull base defects through which CSF drains can provide a route for the development of pneumocephalus, which may lead to brain compression. Although CSF rhinorrhea has a characteristic clinical presentation (namely unilateral watery rhinorrhea after a significant head trauma), its diagnosis and localization remain challenging in many patients. Several factors may make confirmation of CSF rhinorrhea difficult in specific settings. First, CSF rhinorrhea is relatively rare, while conditions such as allergic rhinitis, nonallergic rhinitis, and vasomotor rhinitis are relatively common. These conditions may mimic the signs and symptoms of CSF rhinorrhea or they may occur concurrently with CSF rhinorrhea. Second, CSF rhinorrhea is frequently intermittent. As such, confirmatory testing performed at a time when the CSF rhinorrhea is not active may lead to false negative results. Thus, a high degree of suspicion is required to make an accurate and timely diagnosis.

Table 4.1 Classification system for all causes of CSF rhinorrheax

I. Traumatic
A. Accidental
1. Immediate
2. Delayed
B. Surgical
1. Complication of neurosurgical procedures
a. Transsphenoidal hypophysectomy
b. Frontal craniotomy
c. Other skull base procedures
2. Complication of Rhinologic procedures
a. Sinus surgery
b. Septoplasty
c. Other combined skull base procedures
II. Nontraumatic
A. Elevated intracranial pressure
1. Intracranial neoplasm
2. Hydrocephalus
a. Noncommunicating
b. Obstructive
3. Idiopathic intracranial hypertension (IIH)
B. Normal intracranial pressure
1. Congenital anomaly
2. Skull base neoplasm
a. Nasopharyngeal carcinoma
b. Sinonasal tumors
3. Skull base erosive process
a. Sinus mucocele
b. Osteomyelitis
c. Granulomatous inflammatory processes, including granulomatosis with polyangiitis.
4. Idiopathic

4.2 Classification

Table 4.1 summarizes a classification system for all causes of CSF rhinorrhea. The importance of accurate classification was first recognized by Ommaya et al., who divided CSF rhinorrhea into traumatic and nontraumatic leaks [1]. The term "spontaneous" was felt to be inappropriate by these authors, who noted that after a thorough workup, a specific etiology can be found in most instances of the so-called spontaneous CSF rhinorrhea. Since most presentations of "spontaneous" CSF rhinorrhea have a specific etiology, this term is only appropriate in true idiopathic cases.

There is paucity of data about the incidence of CSF rhinorrhea. Only 4% of all CSF leaks are nontraumatic, and 16% occur as a direct result of intracranial and extracranial procedures [2]. Historically, approximately 80% of all cases of CSF rhinorrhea were related to accidental trauma, most frequently closed head injuries. However, CSF rhinorrhea is noted in only 2–3% of serious head trauma presentations [2]. A CSF leak is present in 12-30% of skull base fractures diagnosed on imaging [3]. The majority of traumatic CSF rhinorrhea presentations become clinically evident within 2 days and almost all manifest within 3 months after the traumatic event [4].

More recent data suggest that iatrogenic CSF leaks are more common than CSF leaks due to accidental trauma [5–8]. A 2007 survey of otolaryngologists showed that 25% of respondents had experienced an intraoperative CSF leak in the previous 5 years [9]. Overall, the rate of CSF leak due to endoscopic sinus surgery has been reported as 0.5% [10].

4.3 History

Specific aspects of a patient's clinical history should guide clinicians toward a diagnosis of CSF rhinorrhea (Fig. 4.1). Classically, a patient with active CSF rhinorrhea will endorse a history of unilateral watery, clear nasal discharge [11–13]. The discharge is frequently associated with a metallic or salty taste, although this is not always the case. Rhinorrhea caused by a CSF leak also tends to be positional, and patients may describe watery drainage that occurs when bending. Concomitant factors, such as a nasoseptal perforation, may lead to bilateral watery drainage. Rarely, a leak may originate from each side of an intact nasal septum through concurrent bilateral skull base defects. Additionally, if a skull base defect is posterior, the drainage may go posteriorly and only be felt in the throat or be mistakenly perceived as bilateral.

In the setting of rhinorrhea after trauma, the circumstances of the preceding traumatic event may raise suspicion for the presence of a skull base defect. Unilateral watery drainage that develops after a head injury or unilateral watery drainage noted after sinus surgery or skull base surgery should prompt further investigation to confirm and localize a potential CSF leak.

If a CSF leak involves the cribriform plate, then patients may report hyposmia, anosmia, and/or parosmias (although the vast majority of skull cribriform plate leaks do not have associated sense of smell complaints). Skull base neoplasms causing CSF leak are exceedingly rare and produce remarkably few symptoms, until the tumor becomes quite large and begins to damage or destroy adjacent structures and cranial nerves and other structures. Alternatively, skull base neoplasms that are responding to chemotherapy or radiation therapy treatment may shrink, and rarely, tumor shrinkage may lead to the development of a CSF leak as the tumor no longer is large enough to fill the skull base defect.

A detailed sinonasal history is important during the workup of patients with suspected CSF rhinorrhea. Inflammatory conditions such as chronic rhinosinusitis or allergic and nonallergic rhinitis may have fluctuating nasal symptoms which can mimic the complaints of a patient with an intermittent CSF leak [14, 15]. Additionally, some of these patients may have undergone previous sinus surgery, and thus CSF rhinorrhea may be a manifestation of unrecognized iatrogenic skull base injuries.

A detailed headache history must be explored. Some patients with idiopathic, nontraumatic CSF rhinorrhea can report non-specific, diffuse headaches that improve when the rhinorrhea occurs and worsens when the rhinorrhea stops. The pathophysiology of these headaches likely relates to variations in ICP. When the ICP is elevated, the headache occurs; however, with active CSF leak, the ICP tends to normalize and the headache improves. Alternatively, the headache may develop in the setting of low ICP due to CSF depletion [16]. Rarely, this occurs due to skull base defects; more commonly, CSF depletion results from dural defects along the spine.

Rarely, a chronic headache may result from an unrecognized intracranial neoplasm that is producing elevated ICP and/or hydrocephalus. Additionally, severe chronic headache may also occur due to low ICP caused by chronic CSF depletion through a high-volume leak. Patients with symptoms due to CSF depletion may report headaches which are made worse by sitting or standing upright and relieved by lying flat [16].

A history of bacterial meningitis, especially recurrent episodes of bacterial meningitis, strongly suggests a possible skull base defect that provides a route for the direct spread of bacteria from the paranasal sinuses to the intracranial space. Persistent rhinorrhea combined with a history of unexplained meningitis (isolated or recurrent) should raise the suspicion of a CSF leak and consideration of further confirmatory testing.

Certain clinical/demographic characteristics are associated with spontaneous CSF rhinorrhea. Among nontraumatic CSF rhinorrhea patients, from 77% to 87% of patients are female, typical age of presentation is between 41 and 65 years old, and the majority of patients in this population are obese (>30 kg/m^2) [11, 17, 18]. Overall the demographic pattern for spontaneous CSF

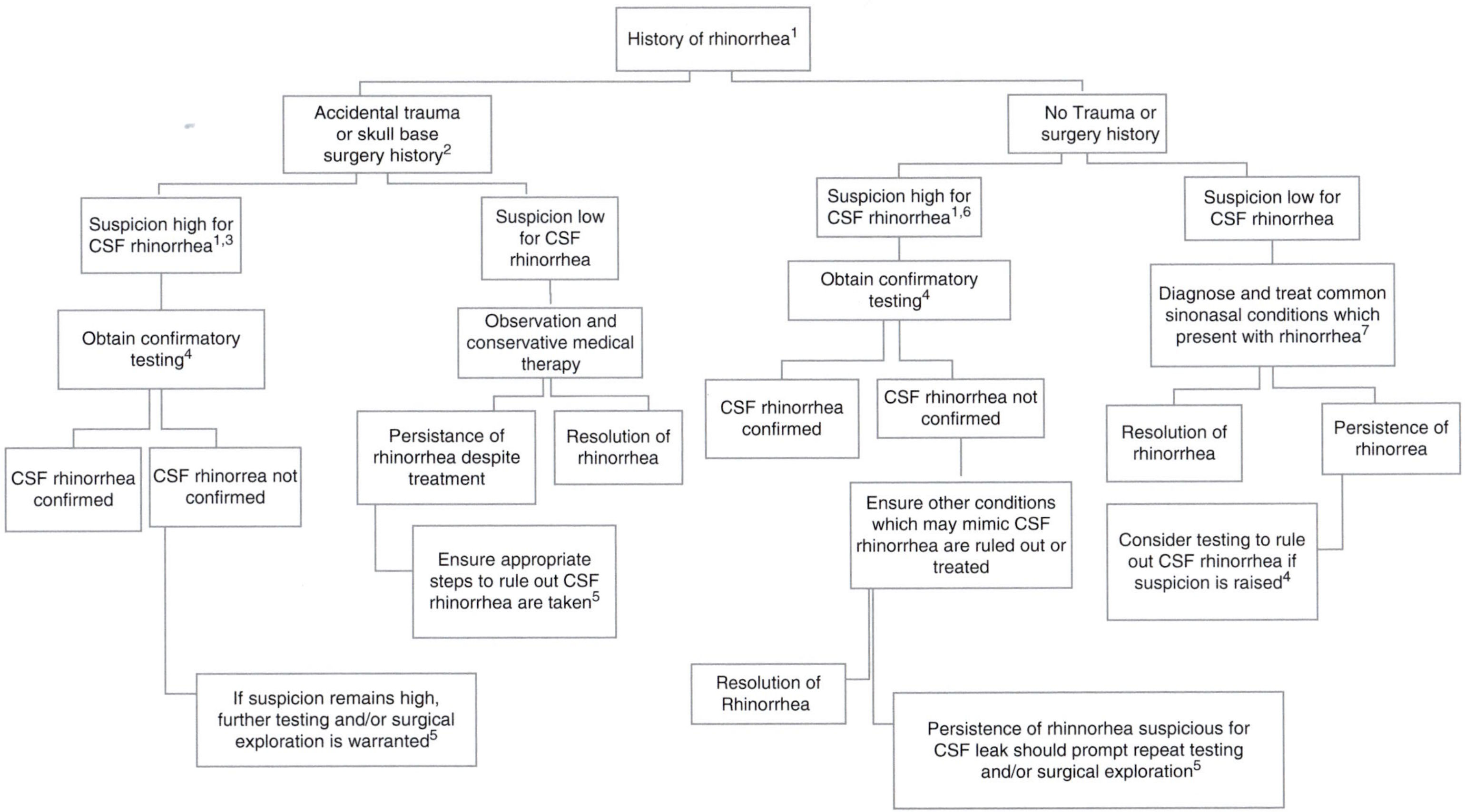

Fig. 4.1 CSF rhinorrhea clinical presentation algorithm. (1) High risk features for CSF rhinorrhea: clear, watery, unilateral, associated salty or metallic taste, positional or exertional exacerbations, history of meningitis and/or seizures. (2) Trauma or surgery history may be remote. (3) Imaging findings of skull base defects, meningoceles, empty sella, or fluid filled sphenoid on side of rhinorrhea should raise suspicion of CSF rhinorrhea. (4) Beta-2 transferrin testing should be obtained. If positive, the diagnosis of CSF rhinorrhea is confirmed. (5) Repeat beta-2 transferrin should be considered. Advanced imaging techniques such as CT cisternography and MR cisternography may be used; however, it must be remembered that both can be falsely negative if the CSF leak is not active or if it is very slow. Endoscopic surgical exploration can be aided with administration of intrathecal fluorescein at the time of the endoscopy. (6) Nasal drainage which does not respond appropriately to a trial of medication raises the possibility of a CSF leak. Clinical characteristics common to spontaneous CSF leak patients are female gender, middle-age, and obesity. Signs or symptoms of intracranial hypertension include papilledema, positional headaches, double vision, lateral rectus palsy, balance dysfunction, and pulsatile tinnitus. (7) Consider seasonal and perennial allergic rhinitis, nonallergic rhinitis, CRS, retained saline irrigations, or other conditions as history and physical suggest

leak populations mimics the idiopathic intracranial hypertension (IIH population) [19]. In fact, in 2006, Schlosser et al. demonstrated that 8 of 11 patients (73%) with apparent idiopathic CSF rhinorrhea strictly fulfilled the modified Dandy criteria to make the diagnosis of IIH [20].

CSF leaks that are seemingly idiopathic are frequently preceded by increases in intracranial pressure (ICP). If intracranial hypertension is the cause of CSF rhinorrhea, findings such as papilledema, double vision, balance dysfunction, and pulsatile tinnitus may be present. However, if a patient has an active leak, the drainage of CSF may be sufficient to prevent obvious clinical signs of intracranial hypertension. In a study by Aaron et al., patients with a spontaneous CSF leak were evaluated by ophthalmology preoperatively and 0/16 had papilledema, with 11/16 demonstrating CSF pressure of ≥35 after surgical repair [21]. Furthermore, in studies performed by Schlosser et al. and a subsequent study by Woodworth et al., 7/8 and 45/48 patients, respectively, had elevated ICP as measured by lumbar puncture post-endoscopic repair of spontaneous CSF leaks [22, 23]. For these reasons, some surgeons may routinely employ drugs such as acetazolamide (a carbonic anhydrase inhibitor that reduces ICP) postoperatively and/or include CSF diversions as part of the treatment. In contrast, other surgeons rarely rely upon these measures and report similarly good outcomes. Because (1) spontaneous CSF leaks are rarely preceded by the full set of signs and symptoms of elevated ICP, (2) surgeons report comparable closure rates regardless of attempts to reduce ICP, and (3) not all patients develop elevated ICP after successful CSF leak repair, the presumed ICP increase that preceded the CSF leak development must be transient or intermittent. Alternatively, ICP may reset after successful skull base repair.

4.4 Physical Exam

In a patient with suspected CSF rhinorrhea, the clinician should seek to demonstrate unilateral clear rhinorrhea by having the patient lean forward. This can take several seconds to several minutes. Importantly, even if the maneuver fails to elicit watery drainage, it should not be inferred that a CSF leak does not exist, especially if there is high clinical suspicion based on history and imaging findings.

When bloody nasal drainage is dropped on a piece of filter paper or paper towel a clear ring forms around the central bloody spot—demonstrating the "halo" sign. However, in the only study to date to analyze the halo sign for confirmation of CSF rhinorrhea, other clear fluids such as saline and tap water will also separate from blood to create a halo [24]. In practice, if collected drainage contains saliva, tears, or even normal nasal discharge, a falsely positive "halo" sign can be observed. Thus, a "halo" sign is not a reliable indicator for the presence of CSF.

The nasal exam with anterior rhinoscopy is usually non-specific and lacks adequate visualization of the most common areas of CSF leak. Nasal endoscopy may show glistening and/or increased moisture of the nasal mucosa at the site of the CSF leak (Fig. 4.2). A clear stream of fluid may represent an active CSF leak. In some patients, a small meningocele in the olfactory fossa may be seen. Even in those who have not had prior sinus surgery, a 3 mm or smaller telescope may be used to enter the sphenoid os (under ideal circumstances) and investigate the lateral recess for CSF leak or a meningocele.

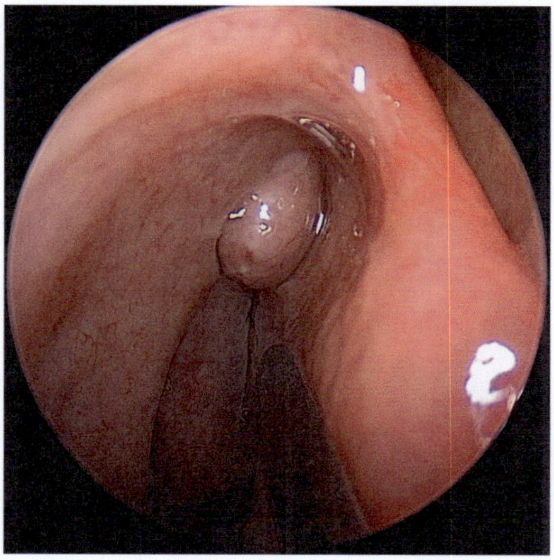

Fig. 4.2 Right nasal endoscopy demonstrating a small meningocele located in the superior aspect of the right middle meatus with associated clear glistening fluid

Additionally, anterior rhinoscopy together with endoscopy can provide evidence for the presence of other nasal conditions which may mimic CSF leak such as allergies, infection, and rhinosinusitis.

In patients with presumed idiopathic CSF rhinorrhea, the possibility of increased ICP and IIH should be carefully investigated. Patients with elevated ICP may have papilledema on fundoscopic exam when their leak is inactive. However, in a 2014 study, of 16 patients with elevated ICP who were treated for spontaneous CSF leaks, none had findings of papilledema preoperatively [21]. In addition, elevated ICP due to IIH has also been associated with abducens nerve palsy and as such these patients may have limitation of lateral gaze [25, 26].

4.5 Imaging Findings

CT and MRI imaging studies are complementary and can help localize skull base defects and concomitant pathology in most cases. CT scans allow visualization of bony details (Figs. 4.3 and 4.4), while MRI provides excellent soft tissue features (Fig. 4.3). With high-resolution CT (HRCT) scan, tri-planar views allow thorough evaluation of the integrity of the skull base and the location and configuration of the defects can be adequately assessed. Oakley et al. showed that among 14 studies evaluating the use of HRCT for localization of CSF leaks, 12 of them had sensitivities over 80% [27]. More recently, a 2019 systematic review showed that HRCT had a sensitivity of 58.8–100% at detecting the site of a CSF leak [28]. Zalpac et al. recommended HRCT in their algorithm for CSF leak localization citing an 87% accuracy rate and a substantially decreased cost [29]. Larger meningoceles or encephaloceles may also be seen on CT; however, MRI can help better define the nature and extent of intracranial contents associated with a skull base defect and better diagnose other conditions/pathologies (such as tumors and empty sella). The sensitivity for detection of CSF leak location on MRI varies from 11% to 100% in the published literature; however, when 3D techniques were used, the sensitivity increased to 75–100% [28]. When looking at studies utilizing MRI in comparison to HRCT, the sensitivities for CSF leak site identification were similar at 87–89% for MRI and 88–92% for HRCT [28]. Similarly, Mostafa and Khafagi showed that

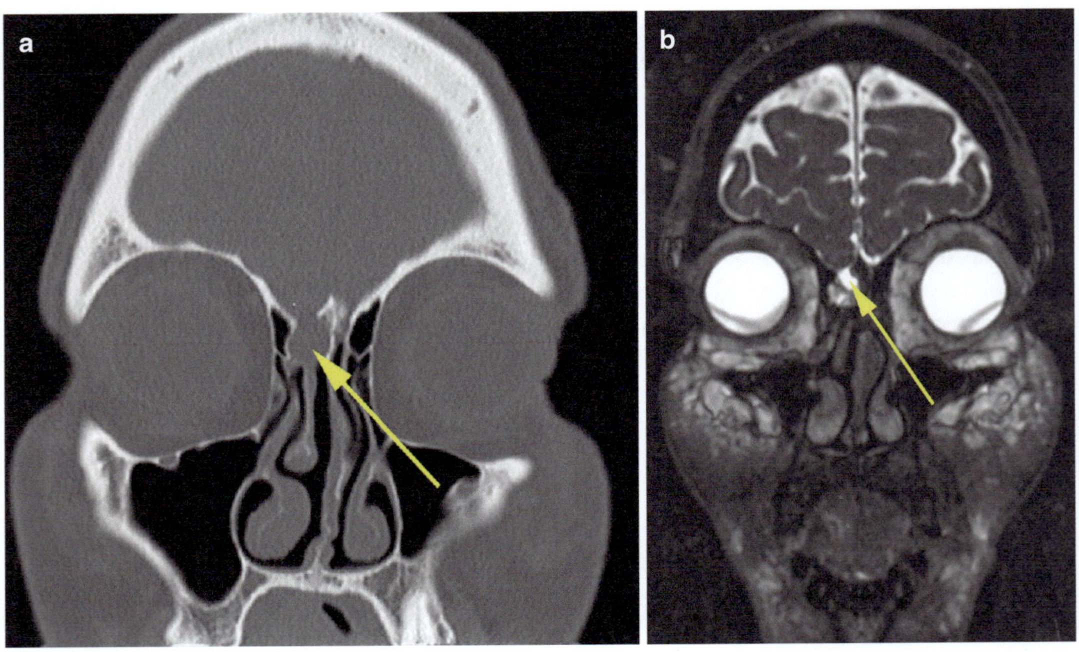

Fig. 4.3 Right ethmoid roof CSF leak due to a small meningocele (arrow) as seen on CT (**a**) and T-2 weighted MRI (**b**)

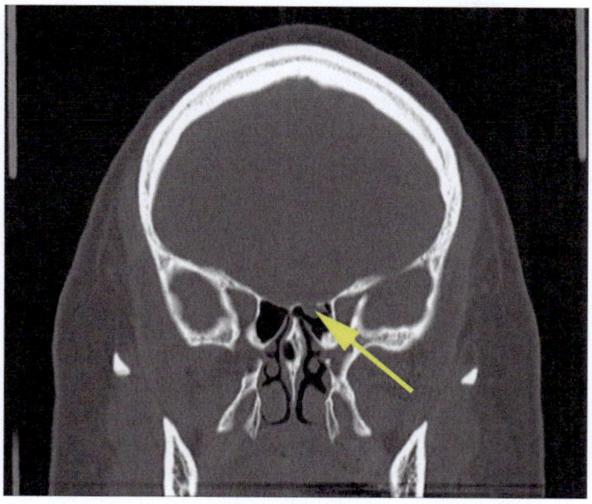

Fig. 4.4 Coronal CT demonstrating a left posterior ethmoid roof defect (arrow) after prior endoscopic sinus surgery

using superimposed HRCT and MRI images, the site of a CSF leak was accurately determined in 17 of 19 cases (89.5%) [30].

Given the cost and availability of CT imaging, HRCT remains first line for the localization/identification of CSF leaks. MRI plays a complementary role and may be most useful if HRCT is equivocal and/or if better detail of soft tissues is desired.

4.6 Differential Diagnosis

A wide range of rhinologic conditions may present with watery nasal drainage. These include inflammatory and non-inflammatory rhinitis, CSF otorrhea, ruptured cysts, and retained nasal irrigation liquid. Common inflammatory conditions, such as seasonal and perineal allergic rhinitis and less commonly chronic rhinosinusitis, can present with clear nasal drainage. Usually clinical features such as bilateral drainage, inciting factors (allergens, eating, cold weather, CRS exacerbation), and response to medical therapy are present.

CSF otorrhea may present as CSF rhinorrhea. In this setting, a skull base defect communicates between the middle ear space and the intracranial space. With an intact tympanic membrane, the CSF collects in the middle ear space and then drains down the Eustachian tube into the nasopharynx, where it may then present as watery nasal drainage. In a patient with a middle ear effusion and suspected or confirmed CSF rhinorrhea, investigations into a lateral skull base defect should be sought.

Patients who use sinonasal saline irrigations may note watery nasal drainage minutes to hours after completing an irrigation. When this problem occurs in the immediate postoperative period, it can be challenging to distinguish a true CSF leak and release of retained irrigation fluid. However, if irrigations are stopped, this will quickly eliminate any confusing drainage, but with a true CSF leak clear drainage will continue.

Occasionally, a sinus retention cyst may rupture and cause unilateral clear rhinorrhea. This typically happens after blunt head trauma or during a viral upper respiratory tract infection. This drainage usually quickly resolves. If imaging is performed, typically air fluid levels are seen in the involved sinus. A distinguishing characteristic of the cyst fluid from CSF is its yellow color that becomes evident upon contact with a white tissue or a white surface [31].

4.7 Conclusion

CSF rhinorrhea occurs when a skull base defect allows for the passage of CSF from the intracranial space to the nose and paranasal sinuses. CSF leaks can be categorized as traumatic and non-traumatic. Because the clinical presentation of CSF leaks can be variable, CSF leak diagnosis is often problematic. A detailed history and physical examination are essential to making an accurate and timely diagnosis. In patients with persistent rhinorrhea with key features (including unilaterality, intermittent nature made worse with exercise or straining, watery and clear drainage, salty/metallic taste), a CSF leak should be ruled out. Additionally, CSF rhinorrhea should be on the differential diagnosis list for any patient with persistent clear nasal drainage and a history of sinus/skull base surgery or bacterial meningitis. Specific imaging findings, including an empty sell or skull base defect, can raise suspicion of a

CSF leak. Demographic characteristics (female gender, middle age, and obesity) are also associated with CSF rhinorrhea. In patients with the appropriate clinical history and examination, confirmatory testing should be obtained to confirm or exclude the diagnosis of CSF rhinorrhea.

References

1. Ommaya AK, et al. Non-traumatic cerebrospinal fluid rhinorrhoea. J Neurol Neurosurg Psychiatry. 1968;31(3):214–25.
2. Loew F, et al. Traumatic, spontaneous and postoperative CSF rhinorrhea. Adv Tech Stand Neurosurg. 1984;11:169–207.
3. Dagi TF, George ED. Surgical management of cranial cerebrospinal fluid fistulas. In: Schmideck HH, Sweet WH, editors. Operative neurosurgical techniques. Philadelphia, PA: W.B. Saunders; 1995. p. 117–31.
4. Kerman M, Cirak B, Dagtekin A. Management of skull base fractures. Neurosurg Q. 2002;12(1):23–41.
5. Tabaee A, et al. The efficacy of computer assisted surgery in the endoscopic management of cerebrospinal fluid rhinorrhea. Otolaryngol Head Neck Surg. 2005;133(6):936–43.
6. Zuckerman JD, DelGaudio JM. Utility of preoperative high-resolution CT and intraoperative image guidance in identification of cerebrospinal fluid leaks for endoscopic repair. Am J Rhinol. 2008;22(2):151–4.
7. Banks CA, et al. Endoscopic closure of CSF rhinorrhea: 193 cases over 21 years. Otolaryngol Head Neck Surg. 2009;140(6):826–33.
8. Zweig JL, et al. Endoscopic repair of cerebrospinal fluid leaks to the sinonasal tract: predictors of success. Otolaryngol Head Neck Surg. 2000;123(3):195–201.
9. Platt MP, Shaye D, Parnes SM. Management of unexpected cerebrospinal fluid fistulae during endoscopic sinus surgery. Am J Rhinol. 2007;21(5):611–4.
10. Stankiewicz JA, et al. Complications in endoscopic sinus surgery for chronic rhinosinusitis: a 25-year experience. Laryngoscope. 2011;121(12):2684–701.
11. Chaaban MR, et al. Spontaneous cerebrospinal fluid leak repair: a five-year prospective evaluation. Laryngoscope. 2014;124(1):70–5.
12. Mathias T, et al. Contemporary approach to the diagnosis and management of cerebrospinal fluid rhinorrhea. Ochsner J. 2016;16(2):136–42.
13. Wang EW, et al. ICAR: endoscopic skull-base surgery. Int Forum Allergy Rhinol. 2019;9(S3):S145–s365.
14. Li M, et al. Delayed diagnosis and treatment of cerebrospinal fluid leakage in current practice. J Craniofac Surg. 2019;30(6):1657–61.
15. Ulrich MT, Loo LK, Ing MB. Recurrent CSF rhinorrhea misdiagnosed as chronic allergic rhinitis with subsequent development of bacterial meningitis. Case Rep Med. 2017;2017:9012579.
16. Spears RC. Low-pressure/spinal fluid leak headache. Curr Pain Headache Rep. 2014;18(6):425.
17. Lobo BC, Baumanis MM, Nelson RF. Surgical repair of spontaneous cerebrospinal fluid (CSF) leaks: a systematic review. Laryngoscope Investig Otolaryngol. 2017;2(5):215–24.
18. Marchiano E, et al. An analysis of patients treated for cerebrospinal fluid rhinorrhea in the United States from 2002 to 2010. J Neurol Surg B Skull Base. 2017;78(1):18–23.
19. Badia L, Loughran S, Lund V. Primary spontaneous cerebrospinal fluid rhinorrhea and obesity. Am J Rhinol. 2001;15(2):117–9.
20. Schlosser RJ, et al. Spontaneous cerebrospinal fluid leaks: a variant of benign intracranial hypertension. Ann Otol Rhinol Laryngol. 2006;115(7):495–500.
21. Aaron G, et al. Increased intracranial pressure in spontaneous CSF leak patients is not associated with papilledema. Otolaryngol Head Neck Surg. 2014;151(6):1061–6.
22. Schlosser RJ, et al. Cerebrospinal fluid pressure monitoring after repair of cerebrospinal fluid leaks. Otolaryngol Head Neck Surg. 2004;130(4):443–8.
23. Woodworth BA, et al. Spontaneous CSF leaks: a paradigm for definitive repair and management of intracranial hypertension. Otolaryngol Head Neck Surg. 2008;138(6):715–20.
24. Dula DJ, Fales W. The 'ring sign': is it a reliable indicator for cerebral spinal fluid? Ann Emerg Med. 1993;22(4):718–20.
25. Azarmina M, Azarmina H. The six syndromes of the sixth cranial nerve. J Ophthalmic Vis Res. 2013;8(2):160–71.
26. Krishna R, Kosmorsky GS, Wright KW. Pseudotumor cerebri sine papilledema with unilateral sixth nerve palsy. J Neuroophthalmol. 1998;18(1):53–5.
27. Oakley GM, et al. Diagnosis of cerebrospinal fluid rhinorrhea: an evidence-based review with recommendations. Int Forum Allergy Rhinol. 2016;6(1):8–16.
28. Eljazzar R, et al. Detection of cerebrospinal fluid leaks: is there a radiologic standard of care? A systematic review. World Neurosurg. 2019;127:307–15.
29. Zapalac JS, Marple BF, Schwade ND. Skull base cerebrospinal fluid fistulas: a comprehensive diagnostic algorithm. Otolaryngol Head Neck Surg. 2002;126(6):669–76.
30. Mostafa BE, Khafagi A. Combined HRCT and MRI in the detection of CSF rhinorrhea. Skull Base. 2004;14(3):157–62. Discussion 162
31. Hoang JK, Smith EC, Barboriak DP. Ruptured maxillary retention cyst: cause of unlateral rhinorrhea after trauma. Neuroradiology. 2009;30(6):1121–2.

5 Fluid Analysis in CSF Rhinorrhea

Saad Alsaleh, Sumaiya Muathen, and Amin Javer

5.1 Introduction

Cerebrospinal fluid (CSF) rhinorrhea is a condition that results from an abnormal communication between the central nervous system (CNS), specifically the subarachnoid space and the sinonasal cavity, that can become a conduit for free passage of intranasal microbial flora into the CNS with the potential for ascending contamination of the CSF [1]. It is a serious and potentially fatal condition that can still on occasion become a major challenge in its diagnosis and management. If left untreated, it may lead to ascending meningitis that develops in approximately 10–25% of patients and up to 10% of them can be fatal [1, 2].

The causes of CSF rhinorrhea can be divided into traumatic and nontraumatic (congenital or spontaneous) etiologies. Nonsurgical trauma is the etiology in 80% of cases, while iatrogenic trauma accounts as the cause in 16% of cases. Most traumatic CSF leaks present within the first 48 hours; however, a minority may be delayed for up to 3 months. Wound contracture, slow resolution of the edema, soft tissue or bony necrosis, and/or an increase in the intracranial pressure are some of the factors that may lead to a delay in the presentation of these cases. It is therefore essential to take a full and detailed history of prior trauma and surgical procedures in this group of patients [3, 4].

Nontraumatic CSF leaks account for approximately 4–10% of CSF rhinorrhea cases and can be challenging for the clinician to diagnose correctly. Nontraumatic CSF leaks are further subdivided into normal-pressure and high-pressure CSF leaks. Examples of high-pressures leaks include intracranial space-occupying lesions, hydrocephalus, and idiopathic intracranial hypertension (IIH). The causes of normal-pressure CSF leaks may include infections, encephalocele, cholesteatoma, arachnoid granulations, and empty sella syndrome. The latter was traditionally considered an idiopathic cause, but more recently has been shown to be associated with elevated intracranial pressure [3, 5, 6]. Spontaneous CSF rhinorrhea carries the highest recurrence rates ranging from 25% to 87%. This is most likely related to its etiology believed to be persistent or intermittent elevated intracranial pressure [7].

S. Alsaleh (✉)
Otolaryngology - Head and Neck Surgery Department, King Saud University, Riyadh, Saudi Arabia
e-mail: alssaad@ksu.edu.sa

S. Muathen
Rhinology and Endoscopic Skull Base Surgery Department, King Abdullah Medical City, Makkah, Saudi Arabia

A. Javer
St Paul's Sinus Centre, University of British Columbia, Vancouver, BC, Canada

A. A. AlQahtani et al. (eds.), *CSF Rhinorrhea*, https://doi.org/10.1007/978-3-030-94781-1_5

5.2 CSF Physiology

CSF is the end product of filtrated plasma, ependymal cells, and parenchymal capillaries at the choroid plexus that is located within the lateral ventricles. It circulates throughout the subdural space before it gets resorbed into the venous system. The main components that makeup CSF are water, various electrolytes, glucose, amino acids, and various proteins. CSF is colorless and lacks mononuclear, polymorphonuclear, or any other cell type [8, 9]. When the intracranial pressure becomes greater than central nervous system pressure, the arachnoid villi use one-way valves depending on hydrostatic pressure in a pulsatile manner to resorb the CSF [10]. The daily production rate of CSF is 400–600 ml which can increase significantly if there is a chronic loss of CSF volume. Normal intracranial pressure (ICP) level is in the range of 5–15 cm H2O which can be affected by a change in position. An ICP rate of greater than 20 cm H2O is considered elevated and requires a full evaluation [1].

5.3 CSF Rhinorrhea Diagnosis

Reliable diagnosis of CSF rhinorrhea in cases with suspicious nasal secretions is the cornerstone and first step in proper management. This is often problematic, especially in cases of subclinical CSF leaks [2]. Diagnosis of CSF rhinorrhea is usually made through a combination of a thorough clinical history and physical examinations followed by laboratory diagnostic procedures and imaging.

The central feature in the clinical history is unilateral rhinorrhea. This is usually described as watery, clear, and salty in taste. It often occurs intermittently but can be continuous and the amount of fluid leaking is as well variable. Although similar in presentation to perennial or seasonal allergic rhinoconjunctivitis, CSF rhinorrhea does not cause lacrimation, ocular or nasal pruritus, or sneezing. CSF rhinorrhea can be exacerbated by the Valsalva maneuver or by bending forward (teapot sign) and may present as postnasal drip when the patient lies supine (Fig. 5.1). It does not resolve with oral antihistamines, intranasal corticosteroids, antihistamines, or anticholinergics [11].

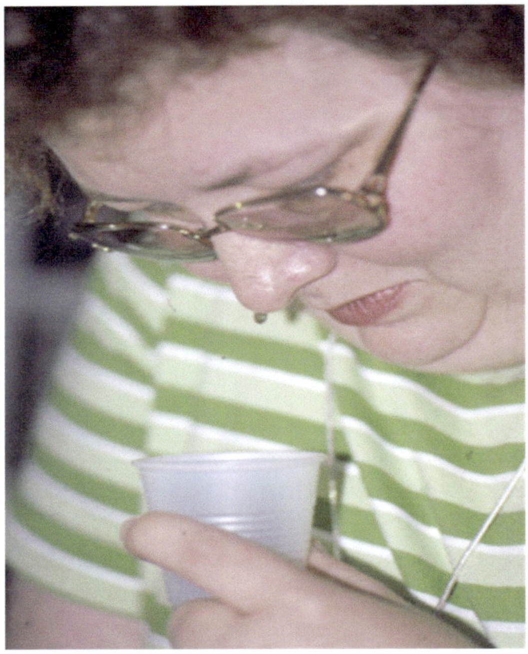

Fig. 5.1 CSF Rhinorrhea "teapot" sign

The initial step in the diagnostic approach to cases with CSF rhinorrhea would be the analysis of nasal secretions to detect the presence of CSF. This is done with the following tests:

5.4 Ring Sign

A ring or (halo) sign can often be appreciated when the CSF separates from blood over any white material like filter paper or other media. Blood remains in the center and CSF forms a clearer ring around it. Classically this sign has been used in patients with suspicious otorrhea or rhinorrhea after sustaining skull base trauma. Dula and Fales questioned the reliability of this sign and studied the occurrence of the ring sign by mixing different types of liquid media including CSF, normal saline, nasal secretion, and tap water with blood on different materials like coffee filters, bed linens, or paper towels. Each sample was examined by two emergency physicians who were blinded to the mixture. They found that mixtures of CSF and blood always produced a clinically evident ring sign if the CSF constitutes between 30% and 90% of the mixture. They also found this sign was not exclusive to CSF and could be seen consistently with tap water, saline, or rhinorrhea fluid mixed with blood [12].

Although this test is highly sensitive, the poor specificity seen above undermines its ability to be used as a confirmatory test for CSF rhinorrhea and should be abandoned.

5.5 Glucose Testing

Measurement of the concentration of glucose in CSF (glycorrhachia) was traditionally used to diagnose CSF in rhinorrhea as it can be done quickly and cheaply. The glucose concentration in CSF is approximately 60–70% of its concentration in blood ranging between 2.5 and 4.4 mmol/L. CSF glucose level can easily be affected by multiple factors such as CNS infections, hypo or hyperglycemia, and other systemic diseases [8, 9].

Little data is available regarding airway glucose levels in a normal state. Generally, in support of lung defense mechanisms against infection, there seems to be a low concentration of glucose in airway surface liquids. Hull et al. examined the nasal secretions of 17 normal children without CSF leak using glucose oxidase strips; 88% of them were found to have nasal secretions positive for the presence of glucose [13]. Metheny and colleagues, however, noted the presence of glucose in intubated ICU patients' broncho-tracheal secretions regardless of whether they had received enteral feeding or had a high blood glucose level [14]. The test was used as a simple bedside indicator for aspiration of enteral feeding [14, 15]. In another trial utilizing glucose oxidase strips, Philips et al. found that nasal glucose was undetectable in healthy volunteers but was detectable in half the volunteers who had acute viral rhinitis and in 90% of subjects with diabetes mellitus. Glucose was also found to be present in 51.6% of endotracheal secretions of intubated patients in the ICU, and this number was even higher in diabetic patients. In conclusion, it appears that normal airway secretions in healthy individuals do not contain glucose unless the patient has evidence of airway inflammation or hyperglycemia [16]. Accuracy of the glucose oxidase strip test was also compared to the β_2 transferrin assay in 19 CSF leak patients. Glucose strips test demonstrated 100% sensitivity, 45% specificity, 57% positive predictive value, and a 100% negative predictive value in diagnosing CSF rhinorrhea [17].

Examination of the glucose content in nasal secretion appears to be a highly sensitive test to detect CSF but with low specificity leading potentially to a large number of false positive results. To theoretically optimize the results, eliminating confounding factors such as airway inflammation, a high serum glucose level, and blood contamination of the sample is difficult especially in the setting of skull base trauma. Hence, this test should not be used routinely, and other, more accurate tests, should be relied upon as seen below.

5.6 Beta-2 Transferrin

In an effort to find a reliable test to confirm the presence of CSF in samples being tested, Meurman and Irjala were the first to demonstrate the presence of a β_2-fraction of transferrin among CSF glycoproteins in 1979 [18]. This β_2-isoform of transferrin is almost exclusively present in CSF and is thought to be the product of cerebral neuraminidase altering the β_1-isoform which is readily available in serum [19, 20]. Therefore, β_2-transferrin could serve as a reliable marker for CSF in any extracranial fluid being tested. However, it has also been demonstrated in low concentrations in the perilymph of cochlea [21] and aqueous and vitreous humor of the eye [22, 23].

Various methods of β_2-transferrin detection have been described, including isoelectric focusing [24, 25], silver staining [25], high-resolution immunofixation [20, 23, 25, 26], and sodium dodecyl sulfate–polyacrylamide gel electrophoresis (SDS-PAGE) with immunoblotting [27]. Unfortunately, these techniques are labor-intensive and require 2–4 h to perform in the laboratory [20, 28–30]. The cost of performing the test is around $ 50 [2].

β_2-transferrin assay (Fig. 5.2) is a non-invasive highly sensitive test that could help avoid conduction of further invasive and/or expensive investigations. The reported sensitivity ranged from 84% to 100% and specificity from 71% to 100% [17, 26, 27, 31]. Of note, the sensitivity of testing declines significantly if the sample is contaminated with blood and physicians should interpret the results in that situation with caution [26, 27]. Two-dimensional gel electrophoresis (2-DE), however, has been reported to maintain its sensitivity to detect β_2-transferrin despite gross blood contamination of samples [28].

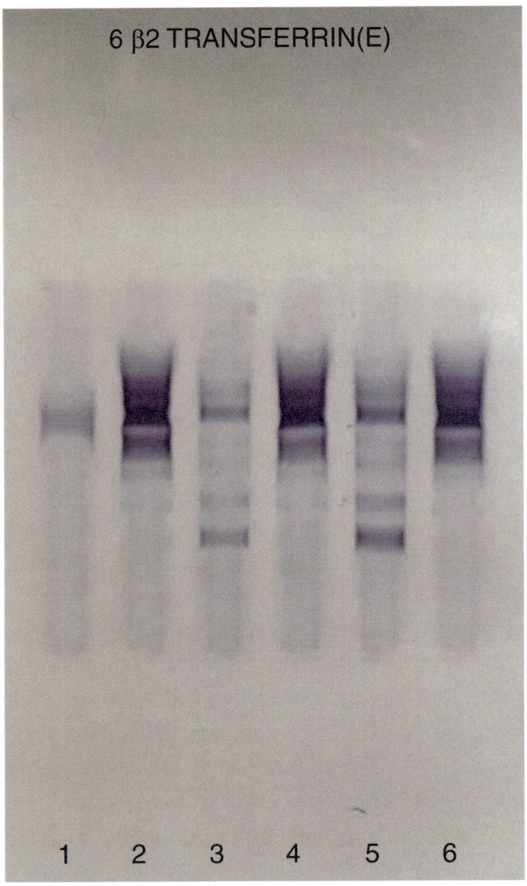

Fig. 5.2 β_2-transferrin gel electrophoresis image showing negative nasal sample in patient A (1), serum sample from patient A (2), positive control containing CSF (3), negative control containing serum (4), positive nasal sample containing CSF in patient B (5), serum sample from patient B (6). Photo credit/copyright: courtesy of Mari L DeMarco, Providence Health Care, 2019

With current electrophoretic techniques, the minimum required sample volume to detect β_2-transferrin is 2 μl [30]. However, it is generally recommended to collect at least 0.5 ml of fluid to account for possible contamination with other fluids [32]. Sample collection methods can be either by direct collection into a sterile container or by placing absorbent material (e.g. polyvinyl alcohol sponge or cotton pledget) in the nasal cavity for 30 min to 4 h, which is then centrifuged to obtain the sample [17, 27]. Other authors, however, expressed caution regarding the use of carrier material in sample collection for a β_2-transferrin assay. They state that it could potentially lead to specimen desiccation and protein adsorption which can result in test errors and false negative results [2, 33]. Clinical conditions that could also lead to false negative β_2-transferrin assay results would be central nervous system infections caused specifically by Streptococcus pneumoniae [34]. False positive results, however, can occur due to an abnormal presence of β_2-transferrin in the serum. This has been reported in patients with chronic liver disorders, neuropsychiatric disorders, hereditary disorders of glycoprotein metabolism (carbohydrate-deficient glycoprotein syndromes), or in the presence of genetic variants of transferrin that could be mistaken for the β_2-isoform [35–37]. Therefore, it is advisable to routinely analyze both the serum and nasal fluid of each individual patient for simultaneous comparison and to avoid false positive results [32, 33].

Another concern that physicians and patients share is the difficulty in collecting an adequate amount of fluid for analysis in cases of intermittent and low-flow CSF leaks. The patient is then obligated to collect the sample over days at home which can hypothetically lead to degradation of the protein content secondary to time and environmental factors. This belief, however, was challenged in two trials showing that β_2-transferrin can be detected in CSF samples stored in room temperature (25 °C) up to 14 days. Hence, refrigeration of the sample is not required provided that it is not exposed to temperatures above 25 °C [38, 39].

5.7 Beta-Trace Protein

Prostaglandin D2 synthase, commonly known as β-trace protein, was discovered in 1961 [40, 41]. Felgenhauer et al. later introduced it as a reliable marker for CSF rhinorrhea in 1987 [42]. It is the second most abundant protein in CSF after albumin and is produced mainly in the leptomeninges and choroid plexus [2, 43, 44]. High concentrations of β-trace protein were also found in the perilymph, urine, amniotic fluid, and seminal plasma [45–47]. Although not fully known, its physiological function has been investigated and a major role in regulating physiological sleep has been described [48, 49].

Although ubiquitous in many fluid compartments (including serum), β-trace protein possesses the highest CSF/serum ratio among all CSF proteins at 34:1 [50]. It has also been noted that it is absent in tear fluid and nasal secretion making it an ideal marker for the presence of CSF in rhinorrhea samples [51]. Immunoelectrophoretic techniques were initially used to quantify β-trace protein which required at least 3 h to perform in the laboratory [52]. This, however, was largely replaced with a less laborious automated nephelometry-based assay that shortened the analysis time to 15 minutes [51]. Another important advantage is the low cost of the test at $20 [2].

The minimum sample volume for a β-trace protein assay is reported to be around 5 μl and collection methods are quite similar to the β_2-transferrin assay techniques mentioned above [2, 27, 51, 52]. However, sample distortion has not been observed using carrier materials [2]. Blood contamination of the sample has less of an effect on the assay, compared to the β_2-transferrin assay, due to the predilution of samples [28, 53]. It has also been noted that β-trace protein is stable in room temperature for several days [52]. Excluding reports utilizing electrophoretic β-trace protein assays, multiple groups suggested different cut-off β-trace concentration values within nasal samples for the accurate diagnosis of CSF leaks and ranged between 0.496 and 6 mg/l. Using those values, the reported sensitivity ranged between 91 and 100% and specificity between 96% and 100% [29, 31, 51, 53–56]. As minor changes in cut-off values could lead to a negative impact on either the sensitivity or specificity of the assay, some groups have suggested adding the β-trace secretion to serum ratio to increase its diagnostic accuracy [31, 55, 57]. Markedly elevated levels of β-trace protein have been documented in the serum of renal failure patients which would eventually elevate the concentration of the protein in nasal secretions [58, 59]. The β-trace secretion to serum ratio could be utilized in that population of patients and avoid false positive results especially if the ratio is <1 [31]. However, a ratio ≥ 2 with a β-trace protein concentration of ≥ 0.7 mg/l in nasal secretion is highly suggestive of CSF rhinorrhea with a sensitivity of 98.3% and a specificity of 96% [55]. It is important to also note that bacterial meningitis could lower β-trace protein concentration in CSF, potentially leading to false negative assay results [2, 60].

The diagnostic accuracy of β-trace protein and β_2-transferrin assays has been compared in 5 different trials [2, 26, 28, 29, 57]. Both were reported to be highly sensitive and reliable tests; however, the majority favored the β-trace protein assay as the first line CSF leak screening test due to multiple advantages highlighted in Table 5.1.

5.8 Others

Transthyretin (prealbumin) has been investigated as a diagnostic marker for CSF. Poor diagnostic accuracy and reliability were demonstrated with

Table 5.1 Comparison between β2-transferrin and β-trace protein assays

	β_2-transferrin assay	β-trace protein assay
Methodology	Laborious manual procedure	Automated assay
Assay duration	2–4 h	15 min
Cost	$50	$20
False positive scenario(s)	• Chronic liver disorders • Hereditary glycoprotein metabolism disorders • Genetic variants of transferrin	Renal insufficiency
False negative scenario(s)	Strep. Pneumoniae meningitis	Bacterial meningitis

the usage of the prealbumin index and level compared to the β2-transferrin assay [17, 27]. However, a rapid (5 min) on-chip immunosubtraction assay of transthyretin has been proposed with a significant increase in test specificity but requires further trials [61].

Another promising and novel tool to distinguish CSF from other fluid types is the electronic nose. It is able to discriminate between vaporized liquids using organic semiconductors and analysis results are available within minutes. This technology has been shown to be rapid and highly accurate in detecting CSF, but its clinical applicability warrants further investigation [62–64].

5.9 Evidence-Based Practice

The approach to a patient with possible CSF rhinorrhea should start with confirming the presence of CSF in nasal discharge. Fluid analysis is a noninvasive cost-effective method that is incorporated as the first step in the diagnostic algorithm of clinically suspicious CSF leaks [65–68]. The β-trace protein and β_2-transferrin assays have proven to be of high reliability and accuracy in detecting the presence of CSF as mentioned above. Laboratory services to perform one or both tests should be available in any skull base surgery center to prevent any unnecessary delay in managing these cases. The ring sign, glucose, and prealbumin content of fluid have been shown to be inconsistent in the diagnosis of CSF leaks and should be abandoned. Localization of the CSF leakage site would be the next step in investigating these patients and will be covered elsewhere.

References

1. Mathias T, Levy J, Fatakia A, McCoul ED. Contemporary approach to the diagnosis and management of cerebrospinal fluid rhinorrhea. Ochsner J. 2016;16(2):136–42.
2. Meco C, Oberascher G, Arrer E, Moser G, Albegger K. β-Trace protein test: new guidelines for the reliable diagnosis of cerebrospinal fluid fistula. Otolaryngol Head Neck Surg. 2003;129(5):508–17.
3. Prosser JD, Vender JR, Solares CA. Traumatic cerebrospinal fluid leaks. Otolaryngol Clin N Am. 2011;44(4):857–73. vii.
4. Reddy M, Baugnon K. Imaging of cerebrospinal fluid rhinorrhea and otorrhea. Radiol Clin N Am. 2017;55(1):167–87.
5. Komotar RJ, Starke RM, Raper DM, Anand VK, Schwartz TH. Endoscopic endonasal versus open repair of anterior skull base CSF leak, meningocele, and encephalocele: a systematic review of outcomes. J Neurol Surg A Cent Eur Neurosurg. 2013;74(04):239–50.
6. Leng LZ, Brown S, Anand VK, Schwartz TH. "Gasket-seal" watertight closure in minimal-access endoscopic cranial base surgery. Operat Neurosurg. 2008;62(Suppl_5):ONS342-3.
7. Lieberman SM, Chen S, Jethanamest D, Casiano RR. Spontaneous CSF rhinorrhea: prevalence of multiple simultaneous skull base defects. Am J Rhinol Allergy. 2015;29(1):77–81.
8. Mundt LA, Shanahan K. Cerebrospinal fluid analysis. In: Graff's textbook of routine urinalysis and body fluids. Lippincott Williams & Wilkins; 2010. p. 237.
9. Roos K. Principles of neurologic infectious diseases. In: Principles of neurologic infectious diseases. McGraw Hill Professional; 2005. p. 4.
10. Wise SK, Schlosser RJ. Evaluation of spontaneous nasal cerebrospinal fluid leaks. Curr Opin Otolaryngol Head Neck Surg. 2007;15(1):28–34.
11. Rorie AC, Poole JA. Cerebrospinal fluid rhinorrhea. In: Rhinitis and related upper respiratory conditions. Springer; 2018. p. 115–21.
12. Dula DJ, Fales W. The 'ring sign': is it a reliable indicator for cerebral spinal fluid? Ann Emerg Med. 1993;22(4):718–20.
13. Hull HF, Morrow G. Glucorrhea revisited: prolonged promulgation of another plastic pearl. JAMA. 1975;234(10):1052–3.
14. Metheny NA, John RE, Clouse RE. Measurement of glucose in tracheobronchial secretions to

detect aspiration of enteral feedings. Heart Lung. 1998;27(5):285–92.

15. Winterbauer RH, Durning RB, Barron E, McFadden MC. Aspirated nasogastric feeding solution detected by glucose strips. Ann Intern Med. 1981;95(1):67–8.
16. Philips BJ, Meguer JX, Redman J, Baker EH. Factors determining the appearance of glucose in upper and lower respiratory tract secretions. Intensive Care Med. 2003;29(12):2204.
17. Warnecke A, Averbeck T, Wurster U, Harmening M, Lenarz T, Stöver T. Diagnostic relevance of β2-transferrin for the detection of cerebrospinal fluid fistulas. Arch Otolaryngol Head Neck Surg. 2004;130(10):1178–840.
18. Meurman OH, Irjala K, Suonpää J, Laurent B. A new method for the identification of cerebrospinal fluid leakage. Acta Otolaryngol. 1979;87(3–4):366–9.
19. Ryall RG, Peacock MK, Simpson DA. Usefulness of beta 2-transferrin assay in the detection of cerebrospinal fluid leaks following head injury. J Neurosurg. 1992;77(5):737–9.
20. Papadea C, Schlosser RJ. Rapid method for beta2-transferrin in cerebrospinal fluid leakage using an automated immunofixation electrophoresis system. Clin Chem. 2005;51(2):464–70.
21. Delaroche O, Bordure P, Lippert E, Sagniez M. Perilymph detection by beta 2-transferrin immunoblotting assay. Application to the diagnosis of perilymphatic fistulae. Clin Chim Acta. 1996;245(1):93–104.
22. Tripathi RC, Millard CB, Tripathi BJ, Noronha A. Tau fraction of transferrin is present in human aqueous humor and is not unique to cerebrospinal fluid. Exp Eye Res. 1990;50(5):541–7.
23. Zaret DL, Morrison N, Gulbranson R, Keren DF. Immunofixation to quantify beta 2-transferrin in cerebrospinal fluid to detect leakage of cerebrospinal fluid from skull injury. Clin Chem. 1992;38(9):1908–12.
24. Stibler H. The normal cerebrospinal fluid proteins identified by means of thin-layer isoelectric focusing and crossed immunoelectrofocusing. J Neurol Sci. 1978;36(2):273–88.
25. Roelandse FW, van der Zwart N, Didden JH, van Loon J, Souverijn JH. Detection of CSF leakage by isoelectric focusing on polyacrylamide gel, direct immunofixation of transferrins, and silver staining. Clin Chem. 1998;44(2):351–3.
26. McCudden CR, Senior BA, Hainsworth S, Oliveira W, Silverman LM, Bruns DE, et al. Evaluation of high resolution gel β(2)-transferrin for detection of cerebrospinal fluid leak. Clin Chem Lab Med. 2013;51(2):311–5.
27. Görögh T, Rudolph P, Meyer JE, Werner JA, Lippert BM, Maune S. Separation of beta2-transferrin by denaturing gel electrophoresis to detect cerebrospinal fluid in ear and nasal fluids. Clin Chem. 2005;51(9):1704–10.
28. Lescuyer P, Auer L, Converset V, Hochstrasser DF, Landis BN, Burkhard PR. Comparison of gel-based methods for the detection of cerebrospinal fluid rhinorrhea. Clin Chim Acta. 2012;413(13–14):1145–50.
29. Schnabel C, Di Martino E, Gilsbach JM, Riediger D, Gressner AM, Kunz D. Comparison of beta2-transferrin and beta-trace protein for detection of cerebrospinal fluid in nasal and ear fluids. Clin Chem. 2004;50(3):661–3.
30. Bachmann-Harildstad G. Diagnostic values of beta-2 transferrin and beta-trace protein as markers for cerebrospinal fluid fistula. Rhinology. 2008;46(2):82–5.
31. Risch L, Lisec I, Jutzi M, Podvinec M, Landolt H, Huber AR. Rapid, accurate and non-invasive detection of cerebrospinal fluid leakage using combined determination of beta-trace protein in secretion and serum. Clin Chim Acta. 2005;351(1–2):169–76.
32. Nandapalan V, Watson ID, Swift AC. Beta-2-transferrin and cerebrospinal fluid rhinorrhoea. Clin Otolaryngol Allied Sci. 1996;21(3):259–64.
33. Skedros DG, Cass SP, Hirsch BE, Kelly RH. Sources of error in use of beta-2 transferrin analysis for diagnosing perilymphatic and cerebral spinal fluid leaks. Otolaryngol Head Neck Surg. 1993;109(5):861–4.
34. Korem M, Ovadia H, Paldor I, Moses AE, Block C, Eliashar R, et al. False negative β-2 transferrin in the diagnosis of cerebrospinal fluid leak in the presence of Streptococcus pneumoniae. Laryngoscope. 2015;125(3):556–60.
35. Sloman AJ, Kelly RH. Transferrin allelic variants may cause false positives in the detection of cerebrospinal fluid fistulae. Clin Chem. 1993;39(7):1444–5.
36. Bell H, Tallaksen C, Sjåheim T, Weberg R, Raknerud N, Orjasaeter H, et al. Serum carbohydrate-deficient transferrin as a marker of alcohol consumption in patients with chronic liver diseases. Alcohol Clin Exp Res. 1993;17(2):246–52.
37. Stibler H. Carbohydrate-deficient transferrin in serum: a new marker of potentially harmful alcohol consumption reviewed. Clin Chem. 1991;37(12):2029–37.
38. Bleier BS, Debnath I, O'Connell BP, Vandergrift WA, Palmer JN, Schlosser RJ. Preliminary study on the stability of beta-2 transferrin in extracorporeal cerebrospinal fluid. Otolaryngol Head Neck Surg. 2011;144(1):101–3.
39. Zervos TM, Macki M, Cook B, Schultz LR, Rock JP, Craig JR. Beta-2 transferrin is detectable for 14 days whether refrigerated or stored at room temperature. Int Forum Allergy Rhinol. 2018;8(9):1052–5.
40. Clausen J. Proteins in normal cerebrospinal fluid not found in serum. Proc Soc Exp Biol Med. 1961;107:170–2.
41. Watanabe K, Urade Y, Mäder M, Murphy C, Hayaishi O. Identification of beta-trace as prostaglandin D synthase. Biochem Biophys Res Commun. 1994;203(2):1110–6.
42. Felgenhauer K, Schädlich HJ, Nekic M. Beta trace-protein as marker for cerebrospinal fluid fistula. Klin Wochenschr. 1987;65(16):764–8.

43. Blödorn B, Brück W, Tumani H, Michel U, Rieckmann P, Althans N, et al. Expression of the beta-trace protein in human pachymeninx as revealed by in situ hybridization and immunocytochemistry. J Neurosci Res. 1999;57(5):730–4.
44. Blödorn B, Mäder M, Urade Y, Hayaishi O, Felgenhauer K, Brück W. Choroid plexus: the major site of mRNA expression for the beta-trace protein (prostaglandin D synthase) in human brain. Neurosci Lett. 1996;209(2):117–20.
45. Michel O, Bamborschke S, Nekic M, Bachmann G. Beta-trace protein (prostaglandin D synthase) --a stable and reliable protein in perilymph. Ger Med Sci. 2005;3:Doc04.
46. Olsson JE. Correlation between the concentration of beta-trace protein and the number of spermatozoa in human semen. J Reprod Fertil. 1975;42(1):149–51.
47. Melegos DN, Diamandis EP, Oda H, Urade Y, Hayaishi O. Immunofluorometric assay of prostaglandin D synthase in human tissue extracts and fluids. Clin Chem. 1996;42(12):1984–91.
48. Urade Y, Hayaishi O. Prostaglandin D2 and sleep/wake regulation. Sleep Med Rev. 2011;15(6):411–8.
49. Urade Y, Hayaishi O. Prostaglandin D2 and sleep regulation. Biochim Biophys Acta. 1999;1436(3):606–15.
50. Reiber H. Dynamics of brain-derived proteins in cerebrospinal fluid. Clin Chim Acta. 2001;310(2):173–86.
51. Petereit HF, Bachmann G, Nekic M, Althaus H, Pukrop R. A new nephelometric assay for beta-trace protein (prostaglandin D synthase) as an indicator of liquorrhoea. J Neurol Neurosurg Psychiatry. 2001;71(3):347–51.
52. Bachmann G, Nekic M, Michel O. Clinical experience with beta-trace protein as a marker for cerebrospinal fluid. Ann Otol Rhinol Laryngol. 2000;109(12 Pt 1):1099–102.
53. Arrer E, Meco C, Oberascher G, Piotrowski W, Albegger K, Patsch W. beta-Trace protein as a marker for cerebrospinal fluid rhinorrhea. Clin Chem. 2002;48(6 Pt 1):939–41.
54. Sampaio MH, de Barros-Mazon S, Sakano E, Chone CT. Predictability of quantification of beta-trace protein for diagnosis of cerebrospinal fluid leak: cutoff determination in nasal fluids with two control groups. Am J Rhinol Allergy. 2009;23(6):585–90.
55. Bernasconi L, Pötzl T, Steuer C, Dellweg A, Metternich F, Huber AR. Retrospective validation of a β-trace protein interpretation algorithm for the diagnosis of cerebrospinal fluid leakage. Clin Chem Lab Med. 2017;55(4):554–60.
56. Morell-Garcia D, Bauça JM, Sastre MP, Yañez A, Llompart I. Sample-dependent diagnostic accuracy of prostaglandin D synthase in cerebrospinal fluid leak. Clin Biochem. 2017;50(1–2):27–31.
57. Kleine TO, Damm T, Althaus H. Quantification of beta-trace protein and detection of transferrin isoforms in mixtures of cerebrospinal fluid and blood serum as models of rhinorrhea and otorrhea diagnosis. Fresenius J Anal Chem. 2000;366(4):382–6.
58. Melegos DN, Grass L, Pierratos A, Diamandis EP. Highly elevated levels of prostaglandin D synthase in the serum of patients with renal failure. Urology. 1999;53(1):32–7.
59. Gerhardt T, Põge U, Stoffel-Wagner B, Klein B, Klehr HU, Sauerbruch T, et al. Serum levels of beta-trace protein and its association to diuresis in haemodialysis patients. Nephrol Dial Transplant. 2008;23(1):309–14.
60. Tumani H, Reiber H, Nau R, Prange HW, Kauffmann K, Mäder M, et al. Beta-trace protein concentration in cerebrospinal fluid is decreased in patients with bacterial meningitis. Neurosci Lett. 1998;242(1):5–8.
61. Apori AA, Brozynski MN, El-Sayed IH, Herr AE. Microfluidic validation of diagnostic protein markers for spontaneous cerebrospinal fluid rhinorrhea. J Proteome Res. 2013;12(3):1254–65.
62. Aronzon A, Hanson CW, Thaler ER. Differentiation between cerebrospinal fluid and serum with electronic nose. Otolaryngol Head Neck Surg. 2005;133(1):16–9.
63. Thaler ER. Candidate's thesis: the diagnostic utility of an electronic nose: rhinologic applications. Laryngoscope. 2002;112(9):1533–42.
64. Thaler ER, Bruney FC, Kennedy DW, Hanson CW. Use of an electronic nose to distinguish cerebrospinal fluid from serum. Arch Otolaryngol Head Neck Surg. 2000;126(1):71–4.
65. Zapalac JS, Marple BF, Schwade ND. Skull base cerebrospinal fluid fistulas: a comprehensive diagnostic algorithm. Otolaryngol Head Neck Surg. 2002;126(6):669–76.
66. Meco C, Oberascher G. Comprehensive algorithm for skull base dural lesion and cerebrospinal fluid fistula diagnosis. Laryngoscope. 2004;114(6):991–9.
67. Ziu M, Savage JG, Jimenez DF. Diagnosis and treatment of cerebrospinal fluid rhinorrhea following accidental traumatic anterior skull base fractures. Neurosurg Focus. 2012;32(6):E3.
68. Oakley GM, Alt JA, Schlosser RJ, Harvey RJ, Orlandi RR. Diagnosis of cerebrospinal fluid rhinorrhea: an evidence-based review with recommendations. Int Forum Allergy Rhinol. 2016;6(1):8–16.

Imaging in the Work-Up of CSF Leak

6

Roberto Maroldi and Giovanni Palumbo

6.1 Introduction

Cerebrospinal fluid (CSF) rhinorrhea is caused by the presence of both a dural and an osseous defect in the skull base, resulting in a communication between the intracranial cavity and either the nasal or the middle ear cavity [1].

Surgical localization can often be difficult, and the inability to accurately localize the skull base defect leads to increased rates of repair failure and complications, making pre-operative localization, through imaging, critical. The assessment of the location of the leakage is frequently a challenging diagnostic problem. This is due to the fact that the possible leaking sites are quite numerous and may occur in the anterior, middle, and posterior fossae. The fact that the leak may be found on the side opposite to the dripping nostril and the possible multiplicity of fistulae further complicate the matter [2].

The most common location of CSF leak, regardless of etiology, is the ethmoid bone, followed by the sphenoid bone [3]. As CSF leak into the middle ear can manifest with rhinorrhea, the tegmen tympani and tegmen antri should be included in the imaging field [4].

In the work-up of CSF rhinorrhea, either suspected or already clinically diagnosed, an imaging study of the skull base is mandatory. From a practical point of view the main goal of imaging is to identify the anatomic defect(s). In most cases, a well-performed radiological examination can provide additional information: a) localize the site(s) and assess the entity of the leak; b) check for sign of liquoral hypertension; c) evaluate related changes of brain and liquoral spaces (e.g., after a trauma); d) look for surgically relevant anatomic variants; e) aid in determining the underlying cause of the CSF leak. Ultimately, imaging is fundamental for proper treatment planning.

In order to acquire as much information as possible, it is up to the radiologist to perform a high-quality study—according to the patient's compliance. That means the radiologist must choose the best imagine technique and imaging protocol for every specific patient.

Three main imaging techniques are usually itemized in the scientific literature about CSF rhinorrhea: radionuclide cisternography, computed tomography (CT), and magnetic resonance (MR) [1–9]. Having to discuss the state of the art imaging for CSF rhinorrhea in 2020, we believe that only CT and MR are to be included, since the radionuclide cisternography is inaccurate, inappropriate and, ultimately, outdated [1, 9]. The one major issue, though, is that there is no imaging "gold standard" for the diagnosis of CSF skull base leaks. Actually, CT and MR are complementary rather than alternative techniques. In fact, while CT provides a detailed bony anatomy,

R. Maroldi (✉) · G. Palumbo
Department of Radiology, ASST Spedali Civili and University of Brescia, Brescia, Italy
e-mail: roberto.maroldi@unibs.it

A. A. AlQahtani et al. (eds.), *CSF Rhinorrhea*, https://doi.org/10.1007/978-3-030-94781-1_6

particularly skull base dehiscence and/or tiny fractures, it is MR that allows a better soft-tissue detail, including coexisting meningoencephalocele and incidental intracranial pathology [10]. Therefore, whenever possible, a complete first imaging examination should include both CT and the MR.

Finally, it should be underlined that performing a high-quality exam is critical but is just the first part of the job for the radiologist. In fact, then comes the analysis/interpretation of the images acquired. This requires a thorough understanding of the skull base anatomy as well as an ability to interpret high-resolution imaging.

6.2 CT

Non-contrast high-resolution computed tomography (HRCT) is an accessible, fast, noninvasive, easy to perform, and relatively economic imaging technique. It depicts the bone with fine detail, but it has low soft-tissue resolution.

CSF leakage is made possible by the presence of both a dural and an osseous defect. HRCT, due to intrinsic technical constraints, can clearly demonstrate only the osseous defect. It relies on indirect signs that combine the "defect" plus other findings indicating the existence of an active communication across the skull between the intra- and -extracranial content. These indirect signs include mucosal swelling, fluid levels within the paranasal sinuses, pneumocephalus, and meningoencephalocele (Fig. 6.1). The combination of the defect(s) and the indirect sign(s) leads to detection of the site of the leak. Therefore, a question arises as to whether a bony defect revealed by HRCT does correlate with the actual site of CSF leak (Fig. 6.2) [5]. In spite of these limitations, HRCT has demonstrated sensitivity and specificity up to 100%, for the detection of the leakage site. It should be noted, however, that the sensitivity and specificity values reported throughout the literature range from 37.5% to 100% and from 57% to 100%, respectively [3, 11]. Such heterogeneity may be attributed to two main factors: (a) different etiologies of CSF leak included in the studies and (b) the experience of radiologists, reflecting the learning curve.

Eventually, since the CSF leak is not directly imaged, HRCT findings need confirmation, either by contrast-enhanced CT cisternography (CTC) or MR or intraoperative localization through fluorescein.

Contrast-enhanced CT cisternography is a second level examination that relies on intrathecal injection of an iodinated contrast agent to highlight an active leakage of CSF. Intrathecal administration of iodinated nonionic low-osmolar contrast agent (e.g., iohexol, iopamidol) is approved by the Food and Drug Administration (FDA); nonetheless inherent risks of a lumbar puncture (bleeding, infection, spinal headache, neurologic injury) and potential adverse reaction to contrast material should never be overlooked. Approximately 3–10 mL of an iodinated nonionic low-osmolar contrast agent is administered by means of lumbar puncture. Then, the patient is placed in a Trendelenburg position to opacify the basal cisterns via gravity. Maneuvers that provoke an active leak, such as sneezing, laughing, head hanging, and Valsalva [12], may be performed prior to the CT scan. Both pre- and post-contrast images are acquired and subsequently compared in order to demonstrate the passage of the contrast agent through a defect of the skull base (Fig. 6.3a, b). Even if the CSF leak is not directly recorded while crossing the skull base, the accumulation of enhanced CSF within a sinus, the nasal cavity, or into the middle ear may be demonstrated through an increase in Hounsfield units of at least 50% after intrathecal contrast administration. A pre-cisternogram plain CT study is also useful as it permits to differentiate extracranial contrast agent accumulation from sclerotic sinus walls, benign high-attenuation inspissated sinus secretions, or blood [4]. The reported sensitivity of CTC for active leaks ranges from 85% to 92% but it has been reported as low as 33% in adverse conditions as the presence of low-flow fistula, hairlike communications, or inactive leaks [1, 3, 11], with an overall specificity of 94% [1]. A technical improvement of CTC could be provided by the use of dual-energy CT (DECT), a recently introduced CT scanner design whose main advantages are a better discrimination of iodine contrast (i.e., higher

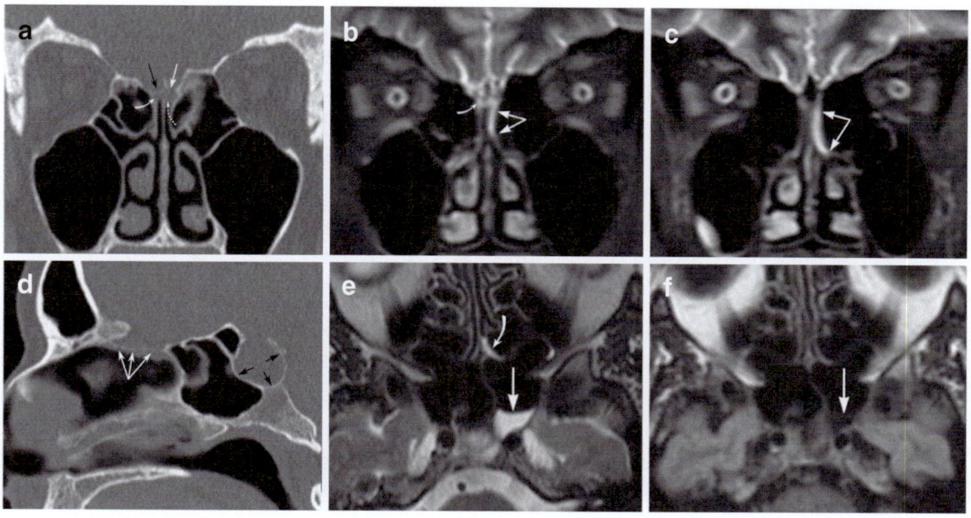

Fig. 6.1 Clear fluid loss from the left nostril in a 70 years old woman: suspected IIH (**a**) NECT coronal plane; (**b**) and (**c**) adjacent coronal MR STIR planes; (**d**) left parasagittal NECT plane; (**e**) and (**f**) axial T2w and FLAIR planes. In (**a**) both horizontal lamellae of the cribriform plate are abnormal: the right discontinuous (black arrow), the left unidentifiable (white straight arrow). Below both cribriform plates, a "mucosal thickening" lines the vault of the olfactory fissures (white curve arrows), larger on the left side (dashed curve arrow). In the parasagittal left NECT plane (**d**), the "thickened mucosa" extends all along the length of the olfactory fissure (white arrows), well below the floor of the olfactory fossa. The black arrows in D point to an enlarged sellar cavity. The two adjacent coronal STIR MR planes (**b**, **c**) show that the "mucosal thickening" corresponds to a hyperintense fluid signal located below the right (curved arrow) and left cribriform plates (white straight arrows). On the left, the hyperintense signal continues into a vertical "stripe" that follows the superior turbinate. This hyperintense stripe fills the left spheno-ethmoidal recess (white curved arrow in **e**). Within the sphenoid sinus the T2w axial plane shows an hyperintense fluid-air level (white arrow in **e**) that turns into no-signal in the corresponding FLAIR image (white arrow in **f**), indicating CSF fluid

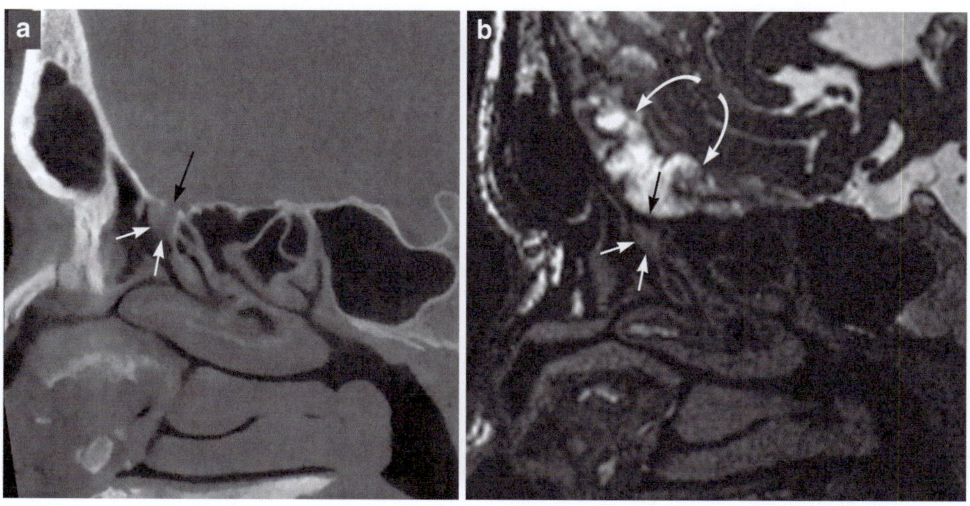

Fig. 6.2 Skull base trauma one year before: clear fluid from left nostril in a 42 years old man. (**a**) High-resolution sagittal CBCT (200 microns) and NCE-MR CISS (**b**). The CBCT shows a focal osseous defect of the ABS at the fronto-ethmoidal junction (black straight arrow) and a soft-tissue density projecting below the defect, into the upper frontal recess (white arrows). The NCE-MR shows a hypointense continuous line above the osseous defect (black arrow) demonstrating that the dura mater is intact. A fronto-basal post-traumatic malacia (curved white arrows in **b**) is present

sensitivity) and a lower radiation dose to the patient [13]. The first, and yet only, description of DECT applied to CT cisternography in a limited case series demonstrated promising results [14].

Overall, the use of CTC implies three potentially harmful drawbacks: (1) a high radiation dose related to multiple scans; (2) inherent risks related to lumbar puncture (bleeding, infection, spinal headache, neurologic injury); (3) a possible adverse reaction to intrathecal contrast material. Therefore, the decision to perform CTC should always be thoughtful.

When performing the CT scan (either HRCT or CTC), the scan protocol with the highest spatial resolution should always be used. Nowadays images with an isotropic voxel of 0.6 mm^3 can be obtained even with a low-end scanner, and they allow the identification of the osseous defect in most cases of CSF leak from the skull base. However, if the CT scan does not show any osseous defect but there is evidence (supported by clinical exams or by MR) of a CSF leak, the acquisition of a higher resolution CT scan with a cone-beam-CT (CBCT) should be considered (Fig. 6.4). CBCT is a peculiar type of X-ray tomographic scanner whose main advantages over CT are: (1) a higher spatial resolution with a voxel of 0.1 mm^3; (2) a lower radiation dose; (3) a lower metal artifacts; (4) relatively economic and small equipment. Though, it should be noted that it has some disadvantages: (1) a reduced field of view, i.e., the anterior skull base (ASB) and the temporal bone need to be scanned separately; (2) a longer time of acquisition (approximately 20 sec); (3) practically no soft-tissue resolution [15].

6.3 MR

Magnetic resonance (MR) offers noninvasive methods of directly imaging a CSF leak, thanks to the high contrast-to-noise ratio that allows to differentiate and characterize a wide range of soft tissues and fluids. Moreover, it does not require radiation exposure [9]. Nonetheless, MR imaging has some limitations: (a) safety concern linked to the use of a strong magnetic field; (b) a relatively long scan time; (c) a significant sensitivity to movements; (d) poor definition of bone structures. All these aspects underline that the selection and the compliance of the patient are important.

It should be noted, however, that the rapid technological improvements will make us reconsider in the near future many of present drawbacks [16–18].

Either using 1.5 or 3 Tesla MR equipment, the strategy of the imaging protocol is primarily aimed at highlighting the signal of CSF, within and outside the skull base while achieving the maximum spatial resolution. Furthermore, if a

Fig. 6.3 (**a**) This 47-year-old woman suffered several relapsing episodes of meningitis and underwent multiple lateral skull base approaches on the right side. In the left column (a1–a4) is the fusion of a non-contrast-enhanced MR cisternography (gray scale) with a superimposed CE-MR sequence (color-coded), which is also reported in the middle column (b1–b4). The right column shows the corresponding level of a post-lumbar puncture iodine-enhanced CT cisternography (CE-CTC) (c1–c4). Each row replicates the same axial adjacent planes, progressing from the Meckel's cave down to the soft palate. NCE-MR and CE-CTC demonstrate CSF leakage from the right Meckel's cave (mc). The CSF signal (yellow arrows) surrounds the parapharyngeal segment of the right internal carotid artery (ica, curved white arrow) draining from a leakage point in the floor of the right Meckel's cave, abnormally large. The peri-carotid parapharyngeal leak has a high signal on the NCE-MR and shows hyperdensity (iodine content) on the CE-CTC. Basilar artery, ba. (**b**) Four coronal MPR images at the same level of the skull base: SPACE-T2w (**a**), CE-MR (**b**), fusion of SPACE-T2w (gray scale) and superimposed CE-MR (color-coded) (**c**), color-coded iodine CT cisternography (**d**). The parapharyngeal segment of the right internal carotid artery (curved white arrows in **b** and **c**) is surrounded by CSF (yellow arrows and dots). The CSF appears bright in SPACE-T2w, dark in the CE-MR, green to yellow in the color-coded iodine CT cisternography

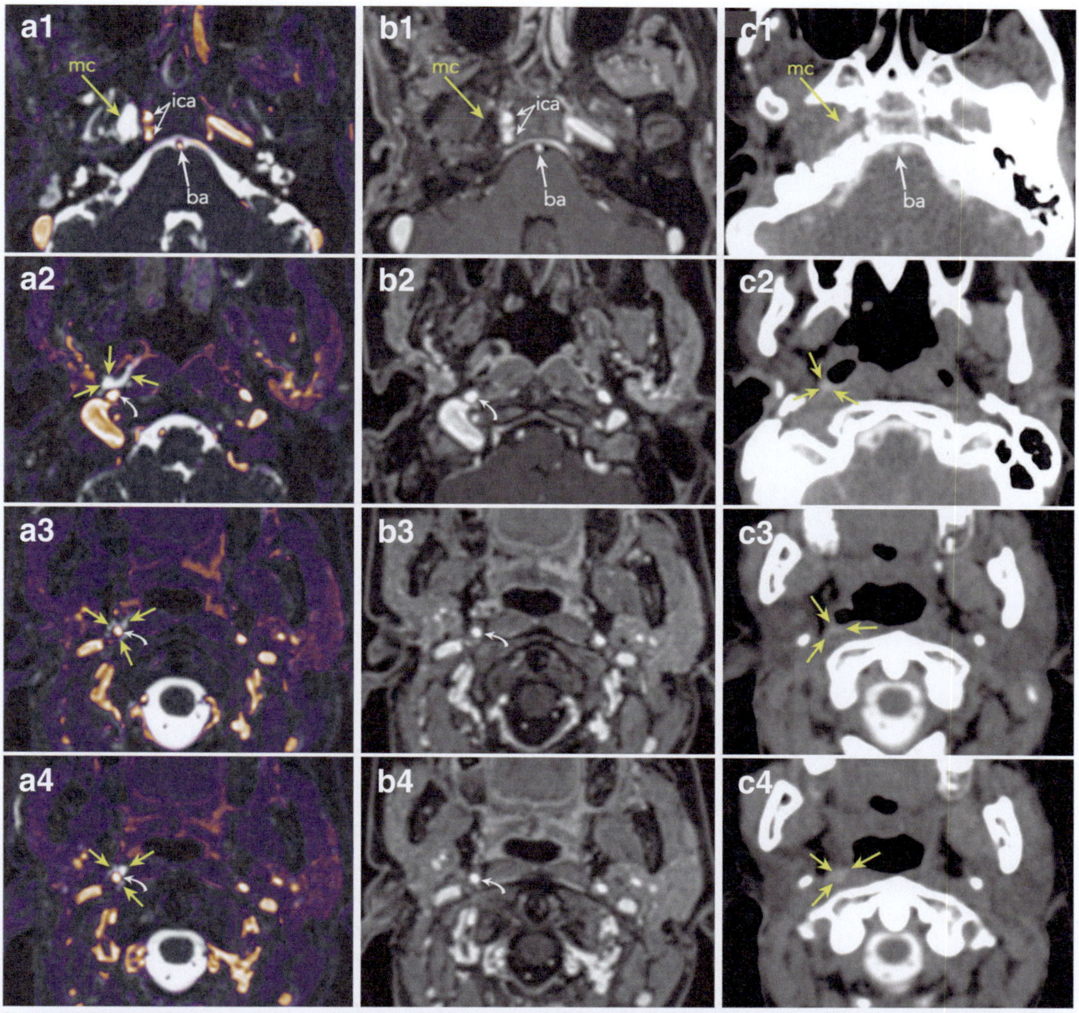
a1
mc
ica
ba
b1
mc
ica
ba
c1
mc
ba
a2
b2
c2
a3
b3
c3
a4
b4
c4

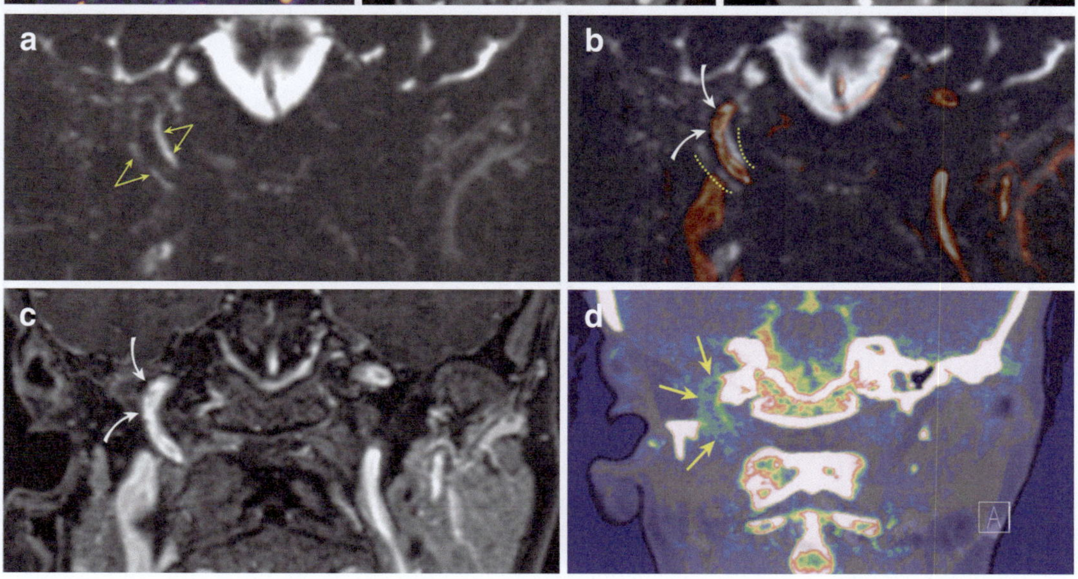
a
b
c
d
A

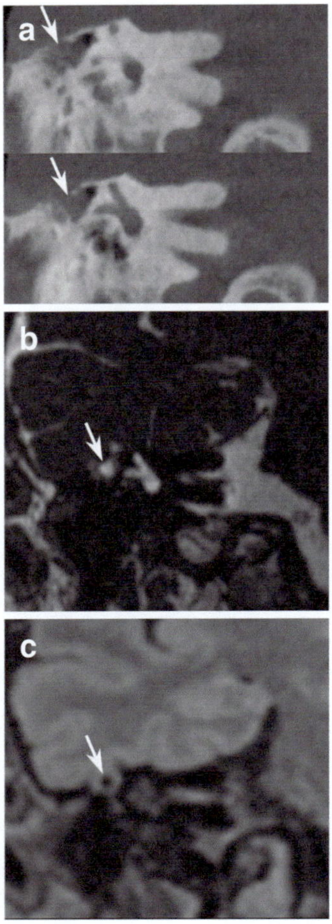

Fig. 6.4 Previous duraplasty for spontaneous CSF leak at cribriform plate. Persistent salty taste and no sign (neither radiologic nor endoscopic) of a leakage from the ASB floor. Two reformatted coronal CBCT adjacent slices (**a**), coronal CISS (**b**), reformatted coronal 3D-FLAIR (**c**). CBCT shows the dehiscence of the tegmen tympani (white arrows in **a**); MR demonstrates that the high T2w signal within the epitympanum (arrow in **b**) turns low intense-to-null signal in the FLAIR sequence (white arrow in **c**), indicating CSF

volumetric sequence has been acquired, additional planes can be computed from the original volume. In most MR equipment, a compromise between the volume covered and the spatial resolution is usually necessary. Otherwise, the sequence time may be excessively long, with more probable motion artifacts. As in most cases the focus is on the anterior skull base (ASB) floor, a direct sagittal volumetric acquisition is recommended. It entails some advantages: the volume needed to cover the width of the ASB floor is limited; the sagittal plane enables to explore the whole anterior–posterior extent of the ASB floor; the native sagittal plane is perpendicular to the floor and may demonstrate, simultaneously, the defect and the meningocele extending within a sinus cavities or within the nose.

Non contrast-enhanced magnetic resonance cisternography (NCE-MRC) relies on heavily T2-weighted 3D sequences (such as fast imaging with steady state acquisition, CISS, or sampling perfection with application optimized contrast using different flip angle evolutions, SPACE) to increase the conspicuity of contrast between CSF and the adjacent skull base while maintaining high spatial resolution [11, 19] (Fig. 6.5). In both sequences, the signal of brain parenchyma is suppressed (low signal), as well as the signal of the dura mater, normally seen as a continuous hypointense line; the CSF, instead, results hyperintense. In a positive study, a hyperintense CSF column is seen from the subarachnoid space communicating with the extracranial space with or without herniation of meninges and/or brain parenchyma. It should be noted, however, that tiny CSF leaks can be overlooked at NCE-MRC native images, resulting in false negative examination. Therefore, CISS/SPACE Maximum Intensity Projection (MIP) thin reconstructions should be considered, since they can make tiny leaks more evident.

If only an NCE-MRC is acquired, all conditions resulting in an increased thickness of the mucosa within the sinus cavities contacting the ASB floor (or retained fluid) may be misinterpreted as CSF. As for HRCT, these inflammatory conditions account for a relatively high incidence (42%) of false-positive results [9, 20]. For this reason, it should be recommended to integrate the protocol with a T2-weighted fluid attenuated inversion recovery (T2-FLAIR) sequence. If the suspected CSF tract appears hyperintense in NCE-MRC and shows a null signal in T2-FLAIR, the CSF content of the tract is confirmed (Fig. 6.6). The reported sensitivity of NCE-MRC varies from 74.7% to 100% [3], with accuracy ranging from 78% to 100% [4].

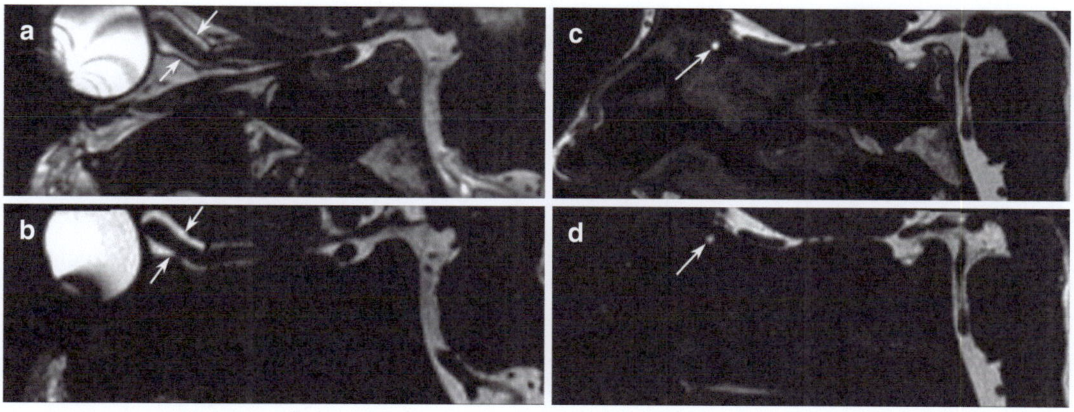

Fig. 6.5 Persistent headache in a 53 years old woman. CISS vs SPACE-T2w: parasagittal CISS (**a**) and SPACE-T2w (**b**) taken at the level of the right optic nerve. Midline sagittal CISS (**c**) and SPACE-T2w (**d**). In both sequences fluids are bright. While CISS preserves the overall anatomy, the SPACE-T2w retains only the fluids, suppressing the background anatomy

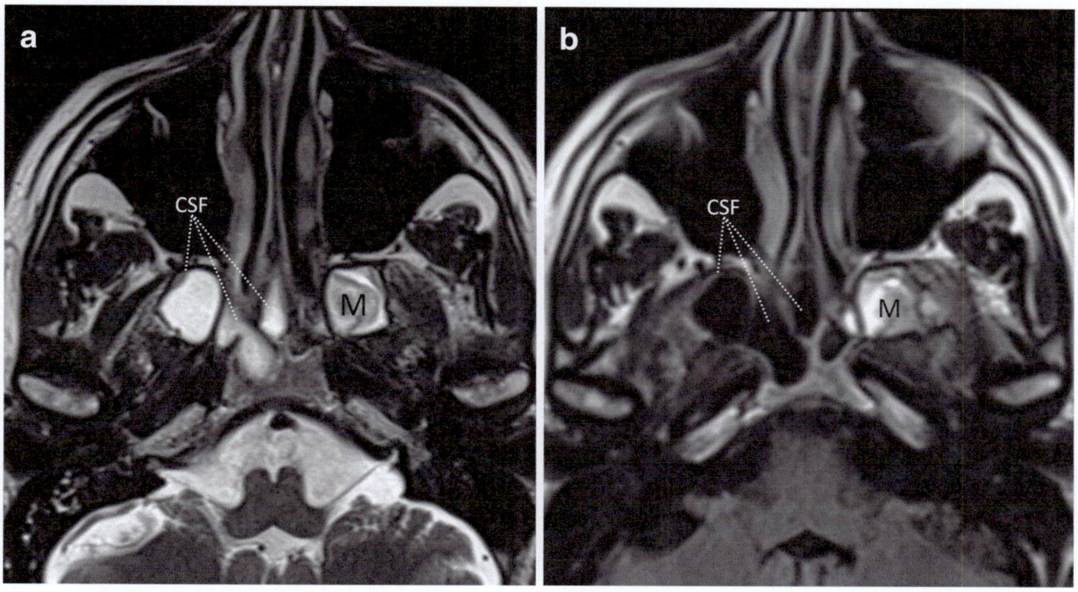

Fig. 6.6 Iatrogenic CSF leak post-septoplasty. Axial T2w (**a**) and FLAIR MR (**b**). In (**a**), hyperintense fluid fills both the right and left sphenoid sinuses (T2w sequence). The FLAIR image shows that the right sinus is filled by CSF (the signal turns null), while in the left sinus the mucous secretion remains with high signal (M)

Contrast-enhanced magnetic resonance cisternography (CE-MRC) is based on multi-planar T1-weighted sequences obtained before and after intrathecal gadolinium-based contrast agent (GBCA) administration through a lumbar puncture. The GBCA dose generally safely used in adults is 0.5–1.0 mL [11, 20], while in children the optimal dose is unclear in the literature [21]. Post-contrast images should be obtained in the second hour following intrathecal GBCA administration. Additional delayed (up to 24 h) post-contrast images should be obtained if no contrast is present within the middle or anterior cranial fossa. Maneuvers that can provoke an active leak just before post-contrast image acquisition can be helpful to image the leakage site. Similar to CTC, a positive study shows leakage of contrast agent through dural and adjacent osseous defects. CE-MRC has been reported to be up to 100% sensitive for high-flow leaks, and up to 60% to 70% sensitive for slow-flow leaks with an overall specificity range between 53% and 100% [1, 22].

Notably, intrathecal administration of GBCA is not approved, either by the FDA or by the European Medicines Agency (EMA). Its safety at low doses has been reported in several pilot studies in Europe [9, 11, 20, 23, 24], though this issue is controversial as rare cases of acute neurotoxic manifestations associated with intrathecal GBCA injection. These adverse events have been correlated mostly to high GBCA doses [23, 25, 26]. No long-term (up to 10 years in few cases) side effects related to low-dose intrathecal GBCA administration have been reported to date [22]. Different GBCA were also investigated, and the safest and the most recommended GBCA is the gadolinium diethylenetriamine penta-acetic acid (Gd-DTPA) [9, 20, 22]. According to the most recent evidence, administration of 0.5 mL Gd-DTPA seems to be safe in adult subjects with no history of allergic reaction to contrast agents [27]. However, long-term effects (i.e., more than 1 year) of intrathecal Gd-DTPA injection are not fully known yet, since there are no specific human studies analyzing the safety profile of Gd-DTPA when used in the intrathecal space [25, 28].

6.4 Traumatic (Accidental) CSF Leak

Skull base fractures are potentially devastating fractures of the craniofacial skeleton. These fractures involve one or more of the following bones: cribriform plate of the ethmoid bone, orbital plate of the frontal bone, sphenoid bone, occipital bone, or petrous or squamous temporal bone. Since the dura overlying the skull base is extremely adherent, even small fractures are associated with shear forces which can create tears in the meninges and thus predispose to CSF leaks (Fig. 6.7). In addition, encephaloceles or meningoencephaloceles can form in these skull base defects, potentially leading to a surgical emergency [29, 30].

The most common area involved in traumatic CSF fistula is the ethmoid-cribriform plate followed by the posterior wall of the frontal sinus, the orbital roof, the sphenoid sinus, and the temporal bone [1, 29].

Imaging findings in the acute setting include a non-displaced or comminuted fracture extending through the skull base and often the presence of pneumocephalus (Fig. 6.8). Skull base fractures may be difficult to detect on CT, particularly if linear and noncomminuted, and a thorough knowledge of skull base anatomy is necessary to avoid diagnosing "pseudofractures." As a matter of fact, small neural and vascular channels and foramina can mimic fracture lines. In addition, suture lines deserve special attention, because they can become diastatic and widened after skull base injury [31]. In dubious cases, three-dimensional volume rendering CT images are helpful in differentiating sutures from fractures [32]. Furthermore, HRCT may lead to false-positive results: congenital or acquired thinning or absence of portions of the bony skull base identified may not necessarily correspond to the site of CSF leak. In these cases, having an MRI may be crucial. In the diagnostic work-up of a post-traumatic CSF rhinorrhea, it is of critical importance not to forget the "bigger picture" of the skull base trauma. In this perspective, carotid CT-angiography is another essential pre-operative examination with the objective to rule out carotid pseudoaneurysms and carotid-cavernous fistulas [30].

6.5 Traumatic (Post-surgery) CSF Leak

In his century-old paper Mosher, speaking about the sinus surgery, said "Theoretically, the operation is easy. In practice, however, it has proved to be one of the easiest operations with which to kill a patient." Incidental CSF leak due to endonasal sinus surgery (ESS) is still observed, as a post-surgical complication, if not identified and corrected during surgery. Nevertheless, the improved technology, including dedicated surgical instru-

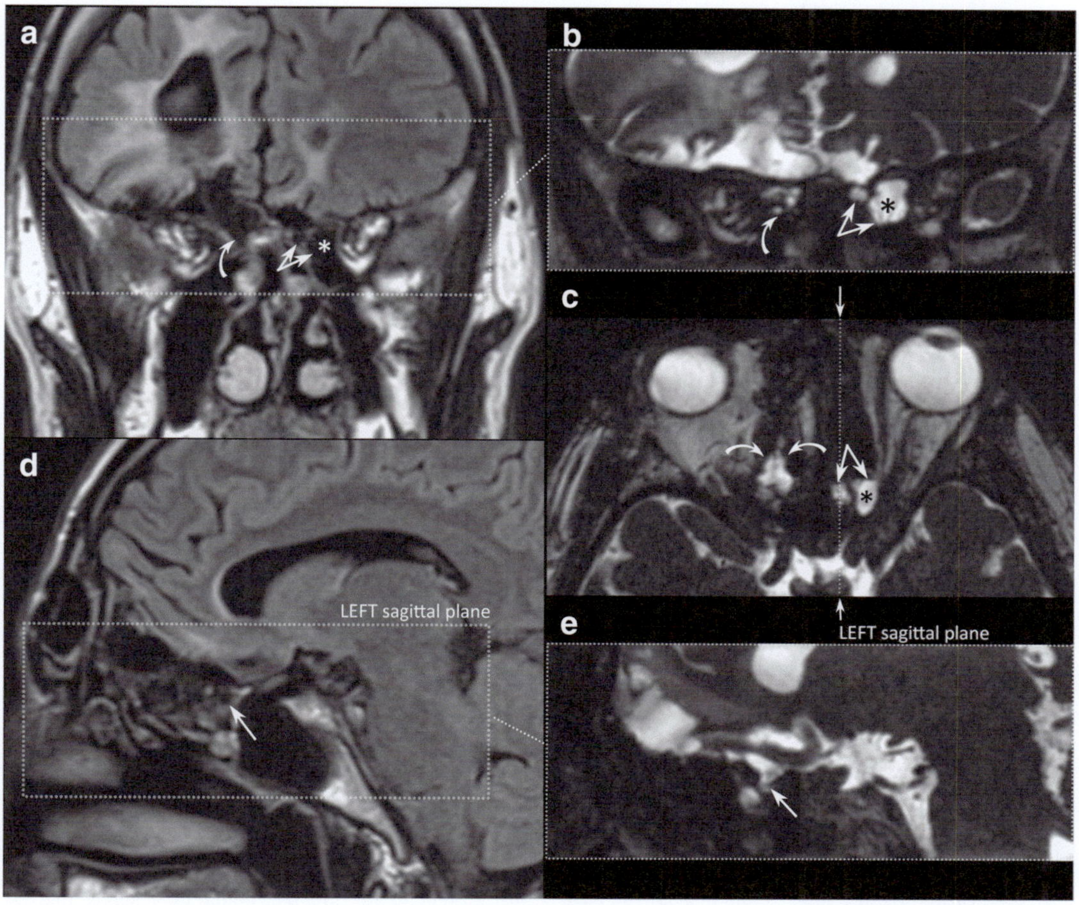

Fig. 6.7 CSF leak years after a complex craniofacial trauma. FLAIR (**a**) and CISS (**b**) in the same coronal plane, CISS (**c**) axial plane, FLAIR (**d**), and CISS (**e**) in the left parasagittal plane (indicated by the dotted line in (**c**). Bilateral multiple CSF collections are shown projecting through the ASB floor into posterior ethmoid cells (white arrows and black asterisk). The suppressed (null) signal in FLAIR images confirms that the high signal in CISS indicates CSF

ments, imaging studies, intraoperative image guidance navigation system, and the increased surgical experience and skills has allowed a progressive decrease of intraoperative CSF leaks [33]. The most common locations for iatrogenic injury to the skull base during ESS are the lateral lamella of the cribriform plate, the posterior fovea ethmoidalis, the frontal recess, and the sphenoid sinus [29]. When CSF rhinorrhea presents after surgical procedures (EES or other) and an imaging study is scheduled, the radiologist should be thoroughly informed about the surgical procedure details. Which means, as a first step, to distinguish between two main scenarios: (1) the onset of rhinorrhea after a surgical procedure that intentionally *violated* the skull base; (2) the onset of rhinorrhea after a surgical procedure that was not meant to address the skull base (Fig. 6.9a, b). Each scenario, then, requires a specific logical reasoning that, if correctly applied, facilitates the localization of the leakage point(s). As a second step, being aware of the type of surgical procedure will help the radiologist to correctly interpret the images.

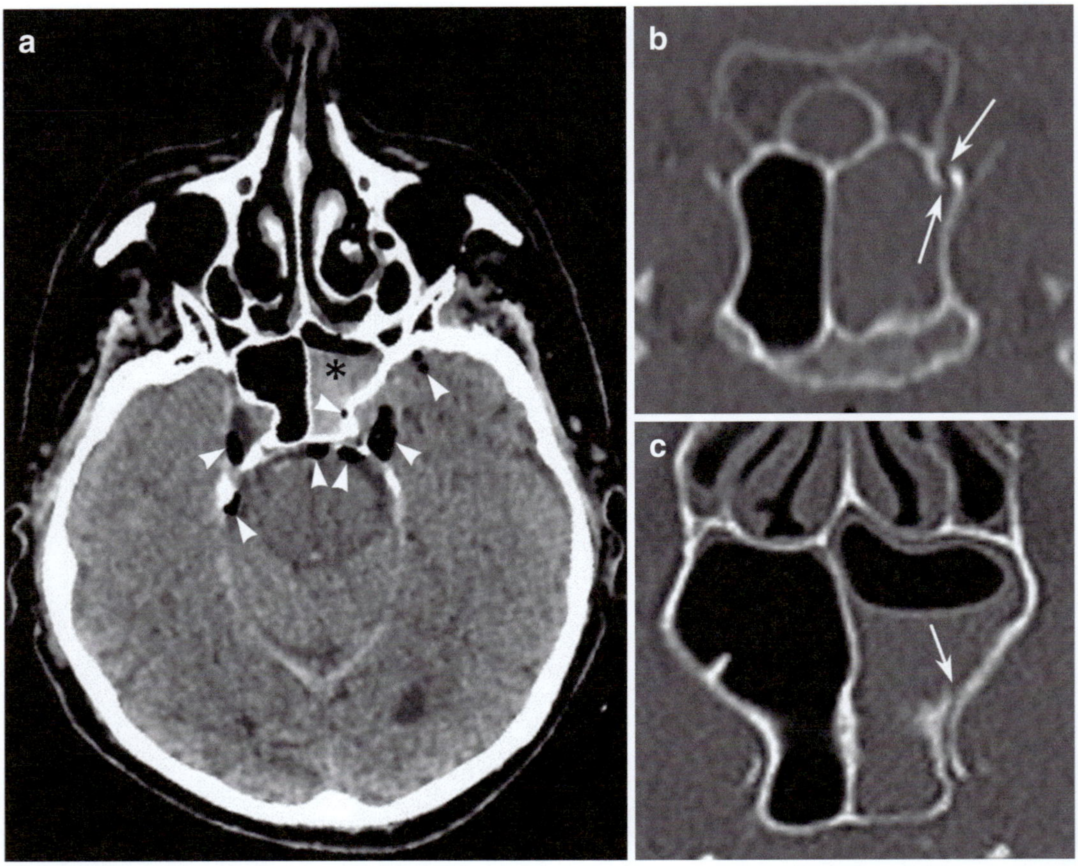

Fig. 6.8 Head trauma after falling from a chair. Emergency head NECT (axial plane, slice thickness 5 mm) (**a**). Head NECT acquired two days after, reconstructed (and zoomed-in) in the coronal (**b**) and axial (**c**) planes (slice thickness 0.5 mm, bone algorithm). The left sphenoid sinus is filled by a hyperdense fluid, consistent with blood (black asterisk in **a**). Multiple tiny air bubbles are present in the middle cranial fossa along the left greater sphenoid wing, along both the clinoid processes, in the perimesencephalic cistern and adjacent to the lateral wall of the left sphenoid sinus (white arrowhead in **a**). At this latter level, the thin slice NECT demonstrates the fracture point (white arrow in **b** and **c**)

6.6 Non-traumatic (Spontaneous) CSF Leak

CSF leaks that occur in the absence of a definable cause are labeled as spontaneous. However, according to the literature, the most likely etiology is idiopathic intracranial hypertension (IIH). In fact, most of the subjects presenting with spontaneous CSF rhinorrhea show clinical signs and radiographic features of chronically elevated intracranial pressure [1, 34]. A persistent elevation or a substantial fluctuation in intracranial pressure may lead to the development of prominent arachnoid villi, which act as minor CSF reservoirs. These prominent arachnoid granulations usually have no clinical significance, particularly when the underlying bone is solid. Conversely, when the underlying bone is pneumatized, a progressive thinning of the bone and eventual erosion and loss of dural integrity may lead to formation of a point of least resistance through which herniation of dura or brain tissue, and ultimately a CSF fistula, can develop (Fig. 6.10). As a matter of fact, patients with spontaneous CSF leaks have the highest rate (>50%) of meningoencephalocele formation among all types of CSF fistulas [7, 8].

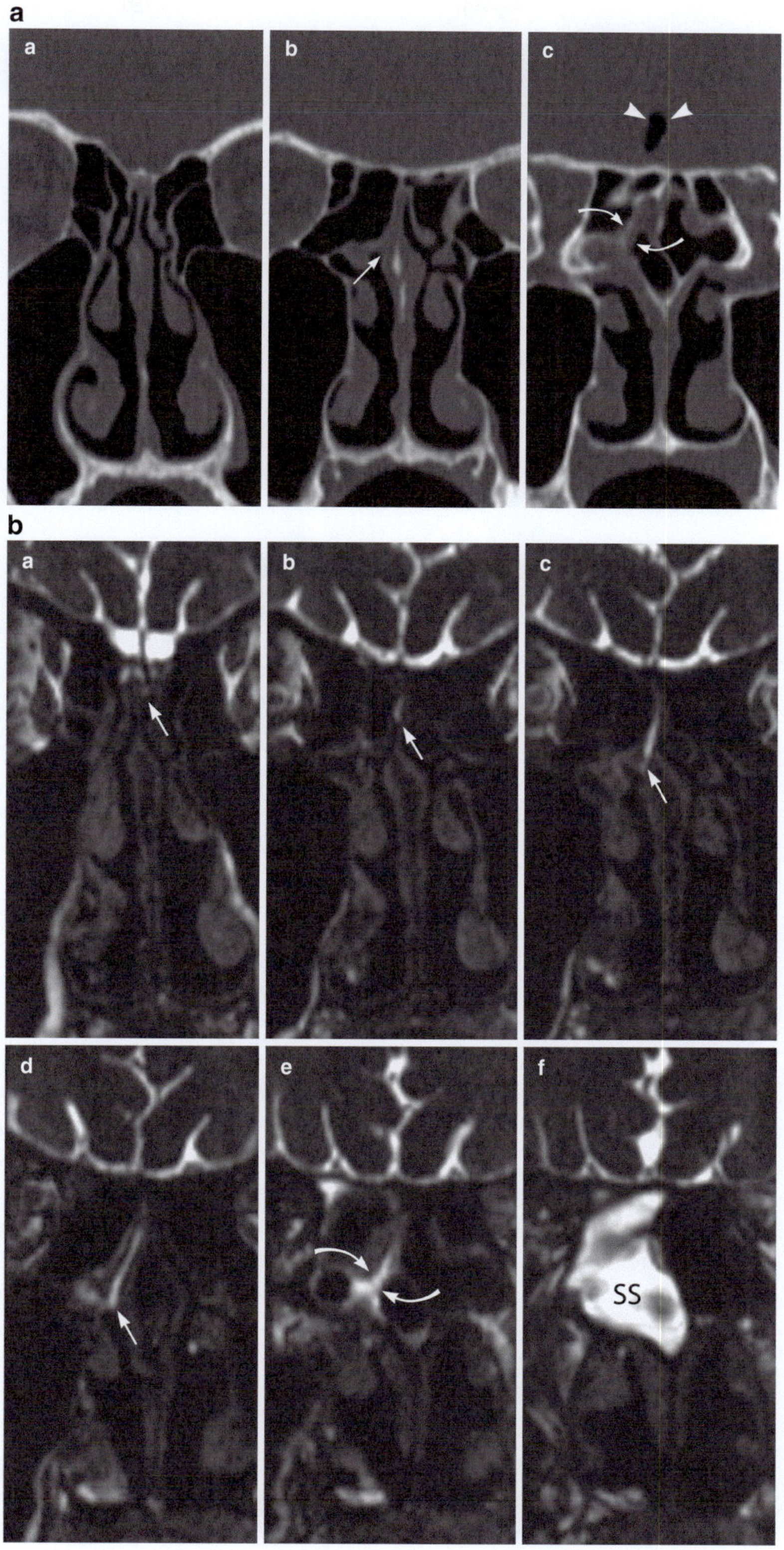

Fig. 6.9 (**a**) Onset of rhinorrhea post-septoplasty: CT. Coronal NECT progressing front-to-back (**a**–**c**). A focal "mucosal thickening" (straight arrow in **b**, curved arrows in **c**) is associated with intracranial air (arrowheads in **c**). The combination of the two findings confirms the suspect of CSF leakage. (**b**) Onset of rhinorrhea post-septoplasty: MR. Coronal NCE-MR CISS planes progressing front-to-back (from **a** to **f**) shows a hyperintense CSF "stripe" extending from the right olfactory recess along the superior turbinate (white arrows in **a**–**d**), reaching the spheno-ethmoidal recess (arrow in **e**), and collecting posteriorly into the right sphenoid sinus (SS)

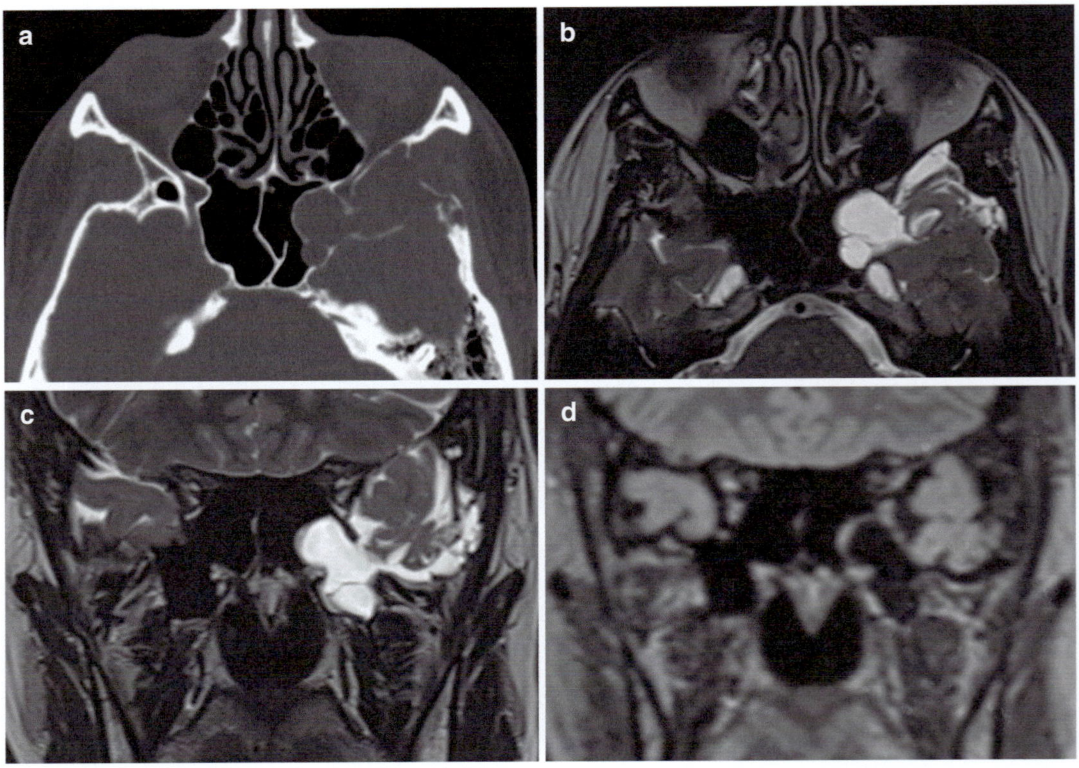

Fig. 6.10 Onset of visual impairment and heavy-head feeling: Gorham-Stout disease. Axial NECT (**a**) with corresponding axial T2w MR (**b**) and coronal T2w MR (**c**) with corresponding coronal FLAIR MR (**d**). Meningoencephalocele of the middle cerebral fossa extends into the left sphenoid sinus through a bone defect of the left sphenoid wing

Some patients with spontaneous CSF fistulas may not exhibit typical symptoms of IIH because they are actively leaking CSF and do not develop elevated intracranial pressure until after the CSF fistula is repaired. A circumstance which probably contributes to the long-term lack of surgical success in these patients [7, 34]. The pathogenesis of spontaneous CSF fistulas may also include other factors, such as osseous anatomic variations, aging, bone remodeling, recurrent infections, and low-grade inflammation, all of which may contribute to the development of multiple CSF fistulas that are either concomitantly or temporally separated [7, 35–37]. Among those anatomic variation is worth mention the Sternberg's (persistent lateral cranio-pharyngeal) canal, because of the confusing literature associated: the Sternberg's canal certainly predisposes the lateral sphenoid wall to the development of spontaneous CSF leaks, but it is not the primary cause [38]. Eventually, spontaneous CSF fistulas in the skull base are the result of a multifactorial process that involves both elevated intracranial pressure and an anatomic predisposition involving thinning of the cranial base. The most common sites for CSF leak in patients with spontaneous CSF rhinorrhea are the lateral recess of the sphenoid sinus (laterally to the foramen rotundum), the ethmoid roof or cribriform plate and, more rarely, the tegmen tympani and the roof of the Eustachian tube [1, 7, 8, 34, 39]. In addition, several patients (31%) have multiple skull base defects [8].

Although not highly specific, there are many imaging findings that are suggestive of IIH, especially when seen in combination, and can help a prompt additional work-up (Table 6.1). Overall, these findings reflect chronic changes that the increased pressure of the CSF produce, resulting not only in the progressive enlargement of CSF filled spaces (cisterns, optic nerve sheath) but also in the remodeling, thinning, and resorption of bony structures of the skull base or the calvaria [1, 8, 34, 40, 41] (Fig. 6.11). Recently, a significant relationship between the extrinsic stenosis of the transverse and sigmoid dural venous sinuses and IIH has been reported [42].

Table 6.1 Imaging findings suggestive of IIH

Intracranial CSF spaces	Empty sella, enlargement of Meckel's cave
Optic nerve	Optic nerve sheath enlargement and tortuosity Optic nerve-head protrusion with flattening of posterior globe Optic nerve-head edema with enhancement
Skull base and calvaria	Scalloping of inner table of calvarium Prominent arachnoid pits Multiple osseous defects along skull base Enlargement of skull base foramina
Dural sinuses	Stenosis of transverse and sigmoid dural venous sinuses

6.7 Non-traumatic (Pathology-Related) CSF Leak

Non-traumatic CSF rhinorrhea can be the symptomatic epiphenomenon of an underlying pathology. Tumors, mucoceles, osteonecrosis, or other erosive processes involving the skull base may be responsible for a CSF leak from the skull base. Tumors, particularly, can lead to CSF leaks either directly or indirectly. Direct tumor invasion across the anterior skull base can cause osteodural defects with significantly diseased or missing bone surrounding the defect. These tumors can be primary intracranial malignancies that extend down into the sinuses (Fig. 6.12), or they may be sinonasal primaries that extend intracranially. Conversely, tumors can indirectly lead to CSF leaks by obstructing CSF flow, resulting in an elevated ICP and hydrocephalus [12]. Interestingly, even the shrinkage of a neoplastic mass is reported to be a possible trigger for a CSF leakage. At first, tumor erosion into the dura and bone of the skull base creates a potential CSF fistula, held back by the tumor tissue itself. Next, rapid regression of tumor burden

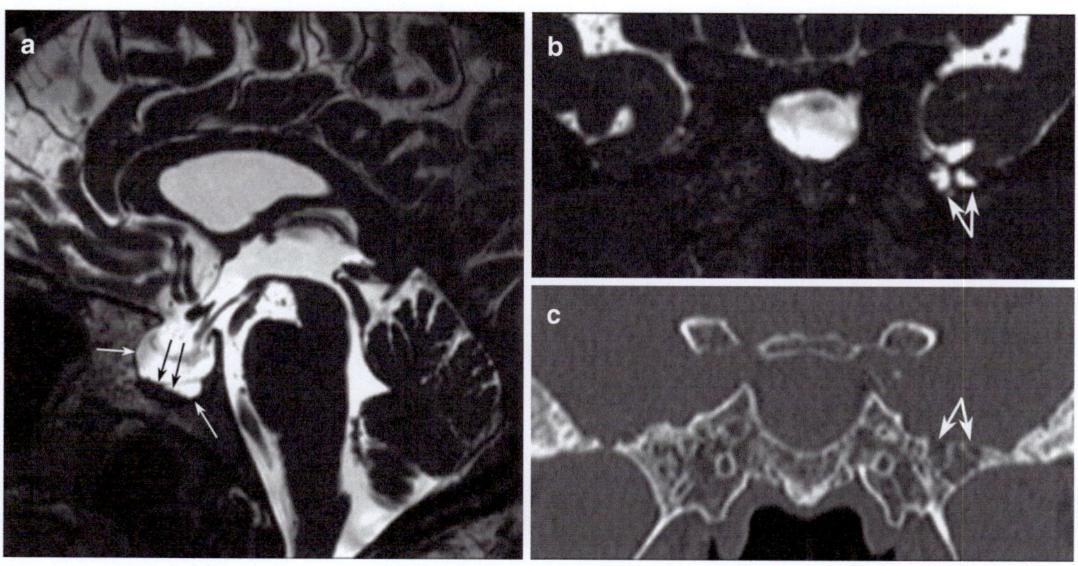

Fig. 6.11 Previous duraplasty for spontaneous CSF leak at the lamina cribra, persistent headache. Midline sagittal CISS NCE-MR (**a**), coronal CISS NCE-MR (**b**), and corresponding coronal NECT (**c**). The enlarged sella turcica (white arrows) is mostly filled by CSF, the pituitary gland (black arrows) being flattened against the sellar floor. The left greater sphenoid wing presents small bony defects, lobulated, CSF filled, consistent with aberrant arachnoid granulations, the so-called arachnoid pits (arrows in **b** and **c**)

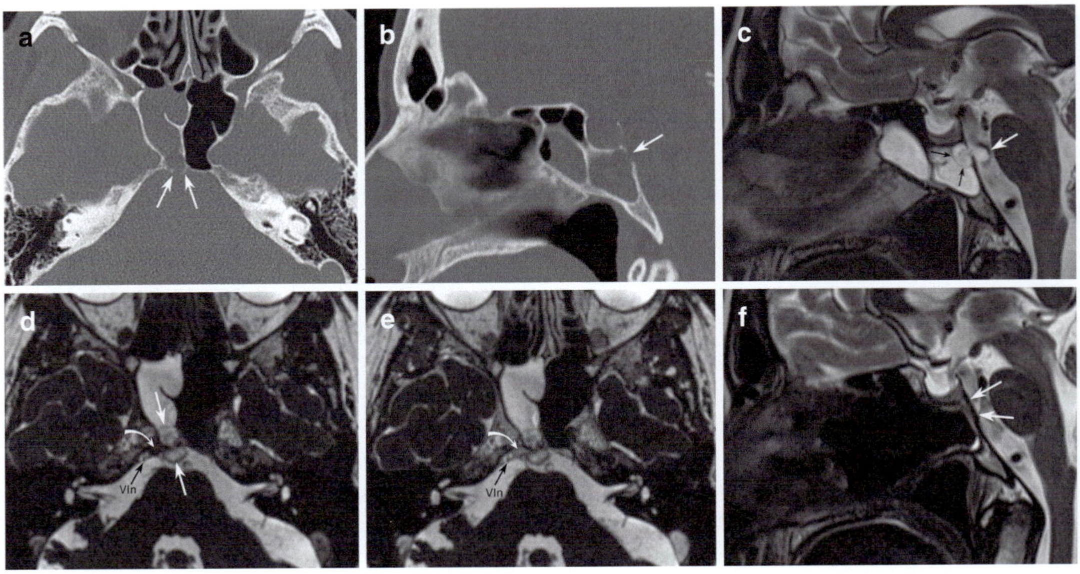

Fig. 6.12 Intermittent episodes of rhinorrhea for 2 years due to ecchordosis physaliphora. NECT in the axial (**a**) and sagittal planes (**b**); MR sagittal T2w (**c**), axial CISS before (**d**) and after (**e**) contrast agent administration. Sagittal T2w 1 year after duraplasty (**f**). CT demonstrates fluid filling the right sphenoid sinus with an air-fluid level. Focal bowing of the posterior wall of the sinus and irregular de-mineralization suggest a lesion originating from the sinus (white arrows in **a** and **b**). The sagittal T2w image identifies an hourglass "cystic" mass extending through the bone defect into the prepontine cistern (white arrow in **c**). A thin hypointense line delineates the intra-sinusal component of the lesion (black arrows in **c**). In the plain CISS sequence (**d**) the thin walls of the intra-sinusal and intracranial mass are demonstrated (opposed straight white arrows). Lateral to the lesion is a displaced basilar plexus (curved arrow) and the VI nerve at the Dorello's canal. In the post-contrast CISS (**e**) a small strip of the enhanced plexus (curved arrow) reaches the lateral surface of the lesion. Sagittal T2w acquired 1 year after endonasal resection and duraplasty (septal cartilage, fat from thigh, Hadad-Bassagasteguy flap) (white arrows in **f**)

(either spontaneous, apoplectic, or therapy-driven) uncovers the fistula site(s) clearing the path for CSF spillage [43].

6.8 Post-duraplasty Imaging

In the surgical management of CSF rhinorrhea both the endonasal and the open craniofacial approaches are currently used. Though, the endonasal approach has become the standard of care in the majority of anterior cranial fossa CSF leaks [44–46]. Small CSF leaks can also be closed by a "bath plug"-type closure, which involves a fat plug inlay followed by application of tissue sealant without a rigid buttress [47]. In cases with large intradural components, a proper reconstruction may be warranted. Duraplasty of the ASB can be constructed according to different techniques: (1) with a combination of intradural fat graft, inlay subdural collagen matrix, and/or the fascia lata with onlay vascularized naso-septal mucosal flap (NSF) [48] (2) with a multilayer reconstruction without the need of NSF [49] (3) with "gasket-seal" techniques, a single layer fascia lata buttressed by a bone inlay [50–52].

The NSF characteristically shows T2-isointense signal with C-shaped configuration, with full-thickness enhancement, immediately below the non-enhancing free grafts on both the coronal and sagittal projections (Fig. 6.13). The NSF tends to contract in size, appearing thinner at delayed post-operative imaging (from 3 to 6 months after the surgery). An apparent increase in thickness of the enhancement on the delayed scans may be explained by the presence of granulation tissue in the operative bed or, alternatively, by the increased mucosalization. Potential causes of flap failure are the vascular insufficiency (even if a small operative defect may not require a vascular flap

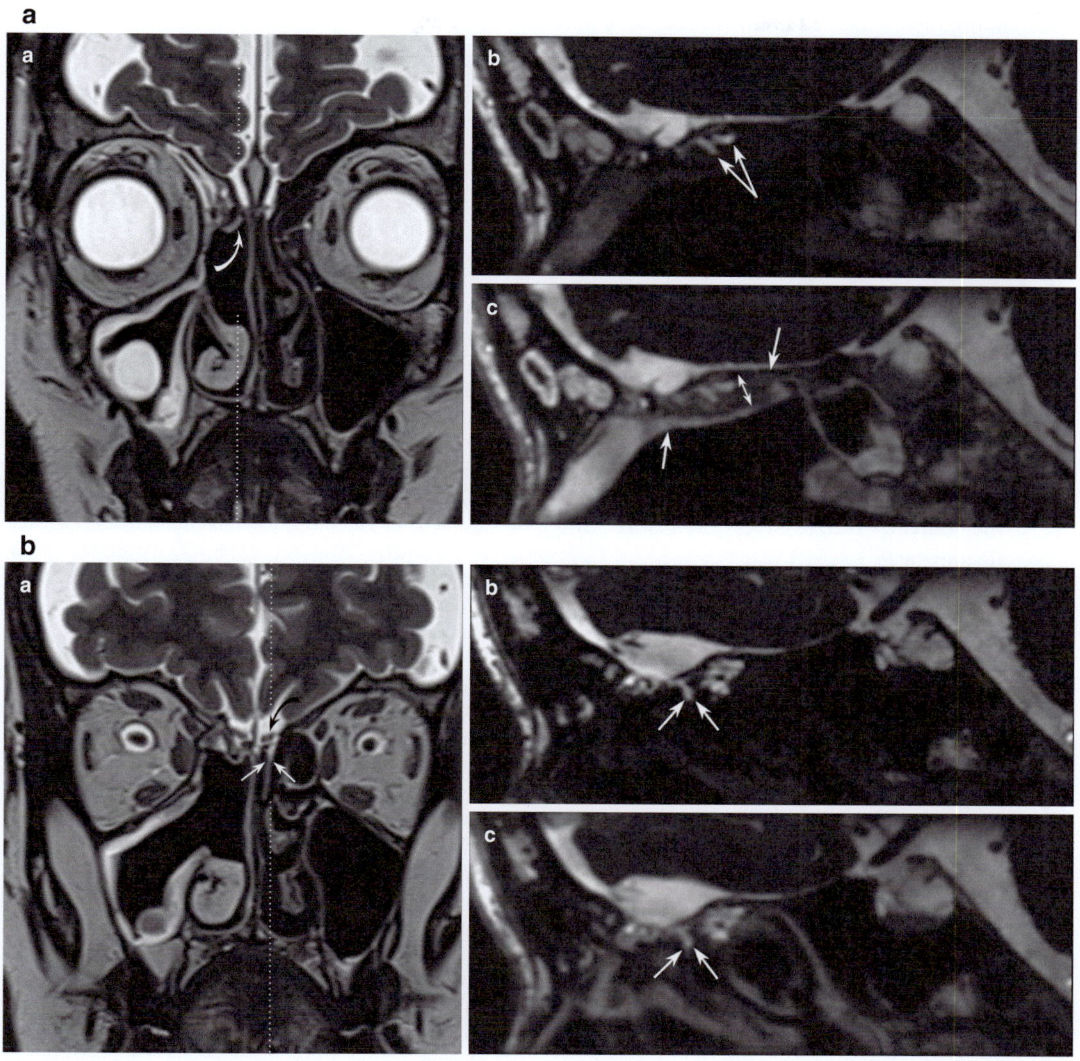

Fig. 6.13 (**a**) Female, 45 years old, persistent rhinoliquorrhea after duraplasty for CSF leak from the right fovea ethmoidalis. Coronal T2w (A) with sagittal CISS obtained before (B) and after (C) gadolinium through the plane of the dotted line in A. The coronal T2w shows the duraplasty (curved white arrow) on the roof of the right olfactory fossa occluding right frontal ostium. Two small meningoceles across the lamina cribra (white arrows in B) are more evident in the CISS without Gd; the naso-septal flap is nicely depicted in the CISS after Gd (white arrow in C). The two small meningoceles are encased between the dura mater (above) and the duraplasty (below). (**b**) Coronal T2W (A) with sagittal CISS obtained before (B) and after (C) gadolinium through the plane of the dotted line in A. The coronal T2w shows a hyperintense thigh column extending across the lamina cribra (white arrows); the sagittal CISS demonstrates that this T2-hyperintensity is self-contained and it is consistent with a small meningocele

for closure) and the flap migration or displacement from the operative defect [53].

The multilayer duraplasty is characterized by a multiple-layer sandwich of signals replacing the anterior skull base floor. On sagittal T2 sequences, triple layer duraplasty has a variable inner signal initially but a continuous and regular intracranial surface. Changes in thickness and signal are observed as the graft gradually integrates. In a few months, the thickness is reduced by about 50%. Over time, the 2 non-enhancing underlay layers are progressively surrounded by

2 enhancing layers located on the intracranial and nasal sides, respectively. On the nasal side, the enhancement is a result of various phases of tissue reorganization along the neo-nasal cavity roof. There, the overlay layer undergoes progressive necrosis. Therefore, it is progressively replaced by in-growth of the adjacent nasal mucosa. Mucosal edema, thin and smooth polypoid changes, hyperplastic scar, or granulation tissue may account for a very variable enhancement. The enhancement present at the intracranial side of the duraplasty is probably the result of increased vascularization of the integrating fascial graft. The fat grafts, which may be added within duraplasty to fill dead spaces and properly dress the defect, progressively reabsorb and nearly disappear at 1 year [54].

Skull base surgery has been greatly improved in recent years, especially by the development of new endoscopic reconstruction techniques. Though, post-operative complications continue to be a major concern, and post-operative imaging can be a valuable tool in their prompt identification. In this perspective, the radiologist should be aware of the normal post-operative changes, in order to recognize complications properly. Pneumocephalus, in particular, requires vigilant attention. In fact, although intracranial air is a relatively common (and benign) finding following both endoscopic and open procedures, it can be an indirect sign of CSF leak recurrence [55] and even constitute a surgical emergency [30, 54].

An early post-operative HRCT should always be performed to exclude acute intracranial complications such as tension pneumocephalus, hemorrhage, failure of the duraplasty, abscess [54]. MR instead, in combination with the endoscopy, should be the mainstay for the long-term follow-up.

References

1. Reddy M, Baugnon K. Imaging of cerebrospinal fluid rhinorrhea and otorrhea. Radiol Clin North Am [Internet]. 2017;55(1):167–87. https://doi.org/10.1016/j.rcl.2016.08.005.
2. Ommaya A, Di Chiro G, Baldwin M, Pennybacker J. Non-Taumatic cerebrospinal fluid rhinorrhoea. J Neurol Neurosurg Psychiatry. 1968;31(3):214–5.
3. Eljazzar R, Loewenstern J, Dai JB, Shrivastava RK, Iloreta AM. Detection of CSF leaks: is there a radiologic standard of care? A systematic review detection of CSF leaks: a systematic review. World Neurosurg [Internet]. 2019;127:307–15. https://doi.org/10.1016/j.wneu.2019.01.299.
4. Lloyd KM, DelGaudio JM, Hudgins PA. Imaging of skull base cerebrospinal fluid leaks in adults. Radiology. 2008;248(3):725–36.
5. Stone JA, Castillo M, Neelon B, Mukherji SK. Evaluation of CSF leaks: high-resolution CT compared with contrast- enhanced CT and radionuclide cisternography. Am J Neuroradiol. 1999;20(4):706–12.
6. Mathias T, Levy J, Fatakia A, McCoul ED. Contemporary approach to the diagnosis and management of cerebrospinal fluid rhinorrhea. Ochsner J [Internet]. 2016;16(2):136–42. Available from: https://www.ncbi.nlm.nih.gov/pubmed/27303222
7. Alonso RC, de la Peña MJ, Caicoya AG, Rodriguez MR, Moreno EA, de Vega Fernandez VM. Spontaneous skull base meningoencephaloceles and cerebrospinal fluid fistulas. Radiographics. 2013;33(2):553–70.
8. Wise SK, Schlosser RJ. Evaluation of spontaneous nasal cerebrospinal fluid leaks. Curr Opin Otolaryngol Head Neck Surg [Internet]. 2007;15(1):28–34. Available from: http://ovidsp.ovid.com/ovidweb.cgi?T=JS&PAGE=reference&D=emed8&NEWS=N&AN=2007025754
9. Algin O, Hakyemez B, Gokalp G, Ozcan T, Korfali E, Parlak M. The contribution of 3D-CISS and contrast-enhanced MR cisternography in detecting cerebrospinal fluid leak in patients with rhinorrhoea. Br J Radiol. 2010;83(987):225–32.
10. Prosser JD, Vender JR, Solares CA. Traumatic cerebrospinal fluid leaks. Otolaryngol Clin North Am [Internet]. 2011;44(4):857–73. Available from: http://www.sciencedirect.com/science/article/pii/S0030666511000983
11. Algin O, Turkbey B. Intrathecal gadolinium-enhanced MR cisternography: a comprehensive review. Am J Neuroradiol [Internet]. 2013;34(1):14–22. Available from: http://www.embase.com/search/results?subaction=viewrecord&from=export&id=L368319071%5Cn, http://www.ajnr.org/content/34/1/14.full.pdf+html%5Cn, http://dx.doi.org/10.3174/ajnr.A28%5Cn, http://sfx.library.uu.nl/utrecht?sid=EMBASE&issn=01956108&id=doi:10.3174%2Faj
12. Schlosser RJ, Bolger WE. Nasal cerebrospinal fluid leaks: critical review and surgical considerations. Laryngoscope [Internet]. 2004;114(2):255–65. Available from: http://ovidsp.ovid.com/ovidweb.cgi?T=JS&PAGE=reference&D=emed6&NEWS=N&AN=2004068325
13. Coursey CA, Nelson RC, Boll DT, Paulson EK, Ho LM, Neville AM, et al. Dual-energy multidetector CT:

how does it work, what can it tell us, and when can we use it in abdominopelvic imaging? Radiographics. 2010;30(4):1037–55.
14. Foust AM, Nguyen XV, Prevedello L, Bourekas EC, Boulter DJ. Dual-energy CT cisternography in the evaluation of CSF leaks: a novel approach. Radiol Case Reports [Internet]. 2018;13(1):237–40. https://doi.org/10.1016/j.radcr.2017.09.005.
15. Miracle AC, Mukherji SK. Conebeam CT of the head and neck, part 1: physical principles. Am J Neuroradiol. 2009;30(6):1088–95.
16. Eley KA, Mcintyre AG, Watt-Smith SR, Golding SJ. "Black bone" MRI: a partial flip angle technique for radiation reduction in craniofacial imaging. Br J Radiol. 2012;85(1011):272–8.
17. Eley KA, Watt-Smith SR, Golding SJ. "Black bone" MRI: a potential alternative to CT when imaging the head and neck: report of eight clinical cases and review of the Oxford experience. Br J Radiol. 2012;85(1019):1457–64.
18. Eley KA, Watt-Smith SR, Golding SJ. Three-dimensional reconstruction of the craniofacial skeleton with gradient echo magnetic resonance imaging ("black bone"): what is currently possible? J Craniofac Surg. 2017;28(2):463–7.
19. Eberhardt KEW, Tomandl BF, Romstöck J, Ganslandt O, Huk WJ. MR cisternography: a new method for the diagnosis of CSF-fistulas. Skull Base Surg [Internet]. 1999;9(Suppl. 2):11. Available from: http://www.embase.com/search/results?subaction=viewrecord&from=export&id=L128196783%5Cn, http://sfx.library.uu.nl/utrecht?sid=EMBASE&issn=09387994&id=doi:&atitle=MR+cisternography%3A+a+new+method+for+the+diagnosis+of+CSF+fistulae.&stitle=Eur+Radiol&title=Eu
20. Selcuk H, Albayram S, Ozer H, Ulus S, Sanus GZ, Kaynar MY, et al. Intrathecal gadolinium-enhanced MR cisternography in the evaluation of CSF leakage. Am J Neuroradiol. 2010;31(1):71–5.
21. Muñoz A, Hinojosa J, Esparza J. Cisternography and ventriculography gadopentate dimeglumine–enhanced MR imaging in pediatric patients: preliminary report. Am J Neuroradiol [Internet]. 2007;28(5):889–94. Available from: http://www.ajnr.org/content/28/5/889.abstract
22. Nacar Dogan S, Kizilkilic O, Kocak B, Isler C, Islak C, Kocer N. Intrathecal gadolinium-enhanced MR cisternography in patients with otorhinorrhea: 10-year experience of a tertiary referral center. Neuroradiology. 2018;60(5):471–7.
23. Arlt S, Cepek L, Rustenbeck HH, Prange H, Reimers CD. Gadolinium encephalopathy due to accidental intrathecal administration of gadopentetate dimeglumine [4]. J Neurol. 2007;254(6):810–2.
24. Aydin K, Terzibasioglu E, Sencer S, Sencer A, Suoglu Y, Karasu A, et al. Localization of cerebrospinal fluid leaks by gadolinium-enhanced magnetic resonance cisternography: a 5-year single-center experience. Neurosurgery [Internet]. 2008;62(3):584–9. https://doi.org/10.1227/01.neu.0000317306.39203.24.
25. Reeves C, Galang E, Padalia R, Tran N, Padalia D. Intrathecal injection of gadobutrol: a tale of caution. J Pain Palliat Care Pharmacother [Internet]. 2017;31(2):139–43. https://doi.org/10.1080/15360288.2017.1313353.
26. Li L, Gao FQ, Zhang B, Luo BN, Yang ZY, Zhao J. Overdosage of intrathecal gadolinium and neurological response. Clin Radiol. 2008;63(9):1063–8.
27. Edeklev CS, Halvorsen M, Løvland G, Vatnehol SAS, Gjertsen Ø, Nedregaard B, et al. Intrathecal use of gadobutrol for glymphatic MR imaging: prospective safety study of 100 patients. Am J Neuroradiol [Internet]. 2019;40(8):1257–64. Available from: http://www.ajnr.org/content/40/8/1257.abstract
28. Vanhee A, Paemeleire K, Casselman J, Vanopdenbosch L. MRI with intrathecal gadolinium to detect a CSF leak: feasibility and long term safety from an open label single Centre cohort study (P4.113). Neurol Int. 2016;86(16 Suppl):P4.113. Available from: http://n.neurology.org/content/86/16_Supplement/P4.113.abstract
29. Gray ST, Wu AW. Pathophysiology of iatrogenic and traumatic skull base injury. Compr Tech CSF Leak Repair Skull Base Reconstr. 2012;74:12–23.
30. Lin DT, Lin AC. Surgical treatment of traumatic injuries of the cranial base. Otolaryngol Clin North Am [Internet]. 2013;46(5):749–57. Available from: http://www.sciencedirect.com/science/article/pii/S0030666513000753
31. Baugnon KL, Hudgins PA. Skull base fractures and their complications. Neuroimaging Clin N Am [Internet]. 2014;24(3):439–65. https://doi.org/10.1016/j.nic.2014.03.001.
32. Idriz S, Patel JH, Ameli Renani S, Allan R, Vlahos I. CT of normal developmental and variant anatomy of the pediatric skull: distinguishing trauma from normality. Radiographics. 2015;35(5):1585–601.
33. Baban MIA, Hadi M, Gallo S, Zocchi J, Turri-Zanoni M, Castelnuovo P. Radiological and clinical interpretation of the patients with CSF leaks developed during or after endoscopic sinus surgery. Eur Arch Otorhinolaryngol. 2017;274(7):2827–35.
34. Wang EW, Vandergrift WA, Schlosser RJ. Spontaneous CSF leaks. Otolaryngol Clin North Am [Internet]. 2011;44(4):845–56. https://doi.org/10.1016/j.otc.2011.06.018.
35. Raghavan U, Majumdar S, Jones NS. Spontaneous CSF rhinorrhoea from separate defects of the anterior and middle cranial fossa. J Laryngol Otol [Internet]. 2002;116(7):546–7. Available from: https://www.cambridge.org/core/article/spontaneous-csf-rhinorrhoea-from-separate-defects-of-the-anterior-and-middle-cranial-fossa/32E776D3ECFD09DE77076AFF5DE65D0D
36. Quint DJ, Levy R, Cornett J, Donovan C, Markert J. Spontaneous CSF fistula through a congenitally fenestrated sphenoid bone. Am J Roentgenol

[Internet]. 1996;166(4):952–4. https://doi.org/10.2214/ajr.166.4.8610580.
37. Schick B, Brors D, Prescher A. Sternberg's canal - cause of congenital sphenoidal meningocele. Eur Arch Otorhinolaryngol. 2000;257(8):430–2.
38. Barañano CF, Curé J, Palmer JN, Woodworth BA. Sternberg's canal: fact or fiction? Am J Rhinol Allergy. 2009;23(2):167–71.
39. Woodworth BA, Prince A, Chiu AG, Cohen NA, Schlosser RJ, Bolger WE, et al. Spontaneous CSF leaks: a paradigm for definitive repair and management of intracranial hypertension. Otolaryngol Neck Surg [Internet]. 2008;138(6):715–20. https://doi.org/10.1016/j.otohns.2008.02.010.
40. Settecase F, Harnsberger HR, Michel MA, Chapman P, Glastonbury CM. Spontaneous lateral sphenoid cephaloceles: anatomic factors contributing to pathogenesis and proposed classification. Am J Neuroradiol. 2014;35(4):784–9.
41. Aaron GP, Illing E, Lambertsen Z, Ritter M, Middlebrooks EH, Cure J, et al. Enlargement of Meckel's cave in patients with spontaneous cerebrospinal fluid leaks. Int Forum Allergy Rhinol [Internet]. 2017;7(4):421–4. https://doi.org/10.1002/alr.21891.
42. Sundararajan SH, Ramos AD, Kishore V, Michael M, Doustaly R, DeRusso F, Patsalides A. Dural venous sinus stenosis: why distinguishing intrinsic-versus-extrinsic stenosis matters. Am J Neuroradiol. 2021; https://doi.org/10.3174/ajnr.A6890.
43. Priddy B, Hardesty DA, Beer-Furlan A, Otto B, Prevedello DM. Cerebrospinal fluid leak rhinorrhea after systemic erlotinib chemotherapy for metastatic lung cancer: a familiar problem from an unfamiliar culprit. World Neurosurg [Internet]. 2017;108:992.e11–4. Available from: http://www.sciencedirect.com/science/article/pii/S1878875017314936
44. Lanza DC, O'Brien DA, Kennedy DW. Endoscopic repair of cerebrospinal fluid fistulae and encephaloceles. Laryngoscope [Internet]. 1996;106(9):1119–25. https://doi.org/10.1097/00005537-199609000-00015.
45. Castelnuovo P, Dallan I, Battaglia P, Bignami M. Endoscopic endonasal skull base surgery: past, present and future. Eur Arch Otorhinolaryngol. 2010;267(5):649–63.
46. Martin TJ, Loehrl TA. Endoscopic CSF leak repair. Curr Opin Otolaryngol Head Neck Surg [Internet]. 2007;15(1):35–9. Available from: http://ovidsp.ovid.com/ovidweb.cgi?T=JS&PAGE=reference&D=emed8&NEWS=N&AN=2007025755
47. Wormald PJ, Mcdonogh M. The bath-plug closure of anterior skull base cerebrospinal fluid leaks. Am J Rhinol [Internet]. 2003;17(5):299–305. https://doi.org/10.1177/194589240301700508.
48. Kassam AB, Thomas A, Carrau RL, Snyderman CH, Vescan A, Prevedello D, et al. Endoscopic reconstruction of the cranial base using a pedicled nasoseptal flap. Neurosurgery. 2008;63(Suppl. 1):44–53.
49. Mattavelli D, Schreiber A, Ferrari M, Accorona R, Bolzoni Villaret A, Battaglia P, et al. Three-layer reconstruction with iliotibial tract after endoscopic resection of sinonasal tumors. World Neurosurg [Internet]. 2017;101:486–92. Available from: http://www.sciencedirect.com/science/article/pii/S1878875017302395
50. Leng LZ, Brown S, Anand VK, Schwartz TH. "Gasket-seal" watertight closure in minimal-access endoscopic cranial base surgery. Oper Neurosurg [Internet]. 2008;62(Suppl_5):ONS342-3. https://doi.org/10.1227/01.neu.0000326017.84315.1f.
51. Wessell A, Singh A, Litvack Z. One-piece modified gasket seal technique introduction background. J Neurol Surg B. 2013;74:305–10.
52. Zhao D, Tao S, Zhang D, Qin M, Bao Y, Wu A. "Five-layer gasket seal" watertight closure for reconstruction of the skull base in complex bilateral traumatic intraorbital meningoencephaloceles: a case report and literature review. Brain Inj [Internet]. 2018;32(6):804–7. https://doi.org/10.1080/02699052.2018.1440631.
53. Kang MD, Escott E, Thomas AJ, Carrau RL, Snyderman CH, Kassam AB, et al. The MR imaging appearance of the vascular pedicle nasoseptal flap. Am J Neuroradiol. 2009;30(4):781–6.
54. Maroldi R, Ravanelli M, Farina D, Facchetti L, Bertagna F, Lombardi D, et al. Post-treatment evaluation of paranasal sinuses after treatment of sinonasal neoplasms. Neuroimag Clin N Am [Internet]. 2015;25(4):667–85. https://doi.org/10.1016/j.nic.2015.07.009.
55. Banu MA, Szentirmai O, Mascarenhas L, Salek AA, Anand VK, Schwartz TH. Pneumocephalus patterns following endonasal endoscopic skull base surgery as predictors of postoperative CSF leaks. J Neurosurg JNS [Internet]. 2014;121(4):961–75. Available from: https://thejns.org/view/journals/j-neurosurg/121/4/article-p961.xml

Role of Fluorescein in the Diagnosis of CSF Leak

7

David Bedoya and Isam Alobid

First synthesized by Adolf von Baeyer in 1871, fluorescein is a recognized fluorophore—a substance able to absorb light, reach an excitation state, and finally return to a basal condition emitting light in a different wavelength than initially received. This process is perceived as an intense color when adequate light is presented. The fluorescence excitation spectrum of fluorescein can be found within wavelength light absorption at 494 nm and emission at 519 nm. It is well known as a green dye and available as sodium fluorescein in a single-use sachet or alkaline injectable solution of 2%, 5%, 10%, or 20% (Fig. 7.1). Fluorescein is used in ophthalmology as a topical medication for diagnostic purposes and intravenously for angiography in vascular disorders of the retina, in urology during intraoperative cystoscopy, and in heart surgery to localize muscular defects in ventricular muscle septal repair procedures.

The use of intrathecal dyes for the diagnosis and treatment of cerebrospinal fluid (CSF) rhinorrhea began with Fox in 1933 when he used indigo carmine for this purpose [1], and since then various colorants have been used, including methylene blue, sodium-24, and iofendylate. Although intrathecal fluorescein was first used by Kirchner and Proud in 1960 to identify the site of CSF leaks during extracranial approaches [2], an intranasal application was described in 1938 by Friedberg and Galloway [3]. In the resection of brain tumors like glioma, intraoperative fluorescence has renewed attention over fluorescein as a new application of this old dye to discriminate breakdown of the bloodbarrier due to their passive permeability of tissues, which could permit surgeons to discriminate tumor extension in a more precise way [4–7].

In patients with CSF rhinorrhea, ascending meningitis can be a catastrophic consequence [8], and even more today with the proven effectivity of endoscopic surgery to successfully close those skull base defects [9]. Fluorescein has been used for diagnosis and localization of skull base defects and for improving the results of surgical treatment, allowing to localize the defect intraoperatively and permitting obtaining a watertight closure of the defect. Fluorescein has shown a sensitivity of 92.9%, a specificity of 100%, and a negative and positive predictive values of 88.8% and 100%, respectively, when fluorescein coloration was used for the detection of intraoperative CSF leaks in a cohort of 419 patients and an improvement in watertight closure of the skull base defect [10, 11].

D. Bedoya · I. Alobid (✉)
Skull Base Unit, ENT Department, Hospital Clínic, Universitat de Barcelona, Barcelona, Spain
e-mail: Ialobid@clinic.cat

A. A. AlQahtani et al. (eds.), *CSF Rhinorrhea*, https://doi.org/10.1007/978-3-030-94781-1_7

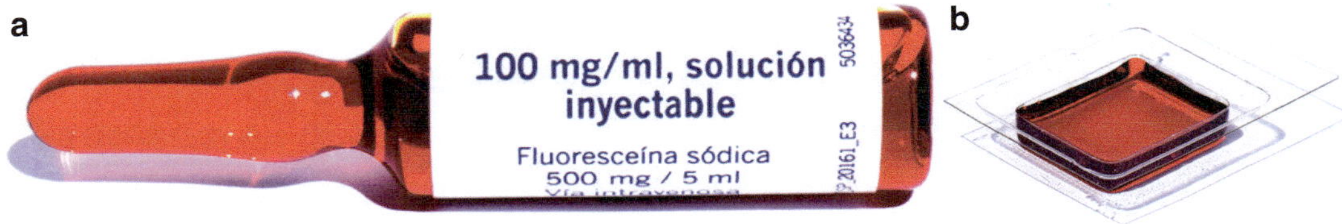

Fig. 7.1 (**a**) Sodium fluorescein is commercially available for intravenous application in ampoules of 10% or 20%. (**b**) In 10% concentration, fluorescein looks orange in color, it changes with dilution to yellow/green

7.1 Indications of Use

Management of CSF leaks and guaranteeing a watertight closure of the defect requires the surgeon to be able to differentiate a transparent liquid in a field with blood and secretions (Fig. 7.2), hence the importance of fluorescein as a tool to improve the diagnostic and therapeutic results in patients with CSF rhinorrhea.

Fluorescein can be used for diagnostic purposes in patients whose CSF leak is suspected, e.g., previous bacterial meningitis, unilateral runny nose, etc., or to improve the results of surgical management of the skull base defect. The main indications are described below:

- Diagnostic
  - Low-pressure fistula with hidden or intermittent CSF rhinorrhea, particularly in patients with spontaneous leak [12].
  - Detection of multiple skull base defects.
  - Patient with suspected CSF rhinorrhea originating from the middle ear and leaking through the Eustachian tube.
- Treatment (intraoperatively)
  - Surgical repair of skull base defects in patients with spontaneous CSF leaks, especially when multiple defects are suspected or when previous imaging techniques do not properly show the leakage site. In defects located in the cribriform area, fluorescein improves the ability to find the location intraoperatively of the defect independently of etiology [12] (Fig. 7.3).
  - During the skull base surgery, for watertight closure verification of reconstruction (Fig. 7.4).
  - In patients with pituitary tumors, when a not-to-reconstruct strategy is planned, due to small tumor size or absence of intraoperative leak, [13] fluorescein could be useful [14].

Any method that increases the ability of surgeons to detect CSF leaks during surgery is valuable. For tumor resection, fluorescein can be useful, although not absolutely indicated, to check the watertight closure of skull base defects intraoperatively. Seth et al. found similar results when the dye was not used [12], but Tabaee et al. found a low risk for postoperative CSF leaks in the absence of fluorescein leaks during surgery and, when intraoperative visualization of fluorescein occurred, an associated increase of risk in postoperative leaks [15]. The intraoperative detection of fluorescein can be present in 61% of pituitary surgeries [16] and can reduce postoperative CSF leaks to 2.8% in endoscopic skull base surgery for any indication because it improves the ability of the surgeon to detect small disruptions on arachnoids which, if they persist, will become CSF leaks [10]–a small volume of clear to transparent liquid in a zone with blood and secretion that can easily go unnoticed.

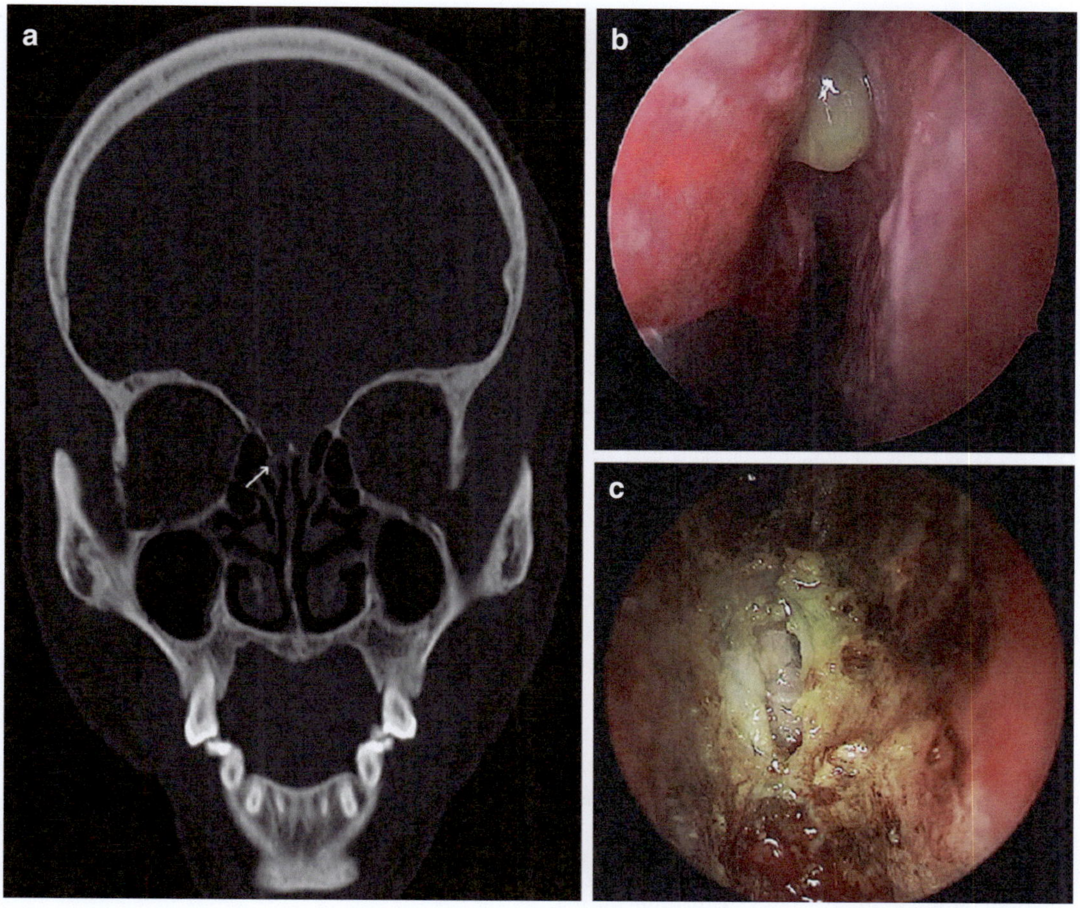

Fig. 7.2 Evaluation of a patient who consults for right CSF rhinorrhea, a right meningocele of the cribriform plate was found. (**a**) Computer tomography, white arrow shows the skull base defect. (**b**) Endoscopic evaluation with previous application of intrathecal fluorescein. (**c**) Skull base defect

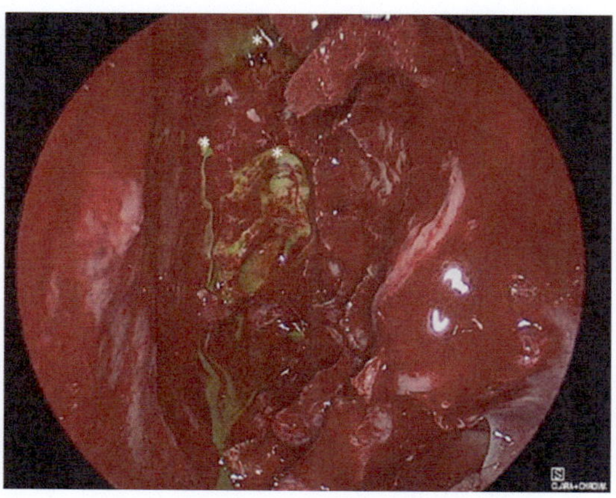

Fig. 7.3 Multiple defects (white asterisks) on a left cribriform plate found in a patient with CSF rhinorrhea during surgery, thanks to the visualization of fluorescein

7.2 Fluorescein and the Informed Consent

The most controversial topic in the intrathecal use of fluorescein is the off-label use of this diagnostic compound. In the USA, the Food and Drug Administration (FDA) does not have the intrathecal use of fluorescein as a permitted indication. However, that regulation does not extend to the practice of medicine, and off-label use of fluorescein can be considered [17–19]. It is very important to discuss with the patient about the off-label use and reports of neurological complication such as radicular symptoms, transient hemiparesis, seizures, and other less severe complaints

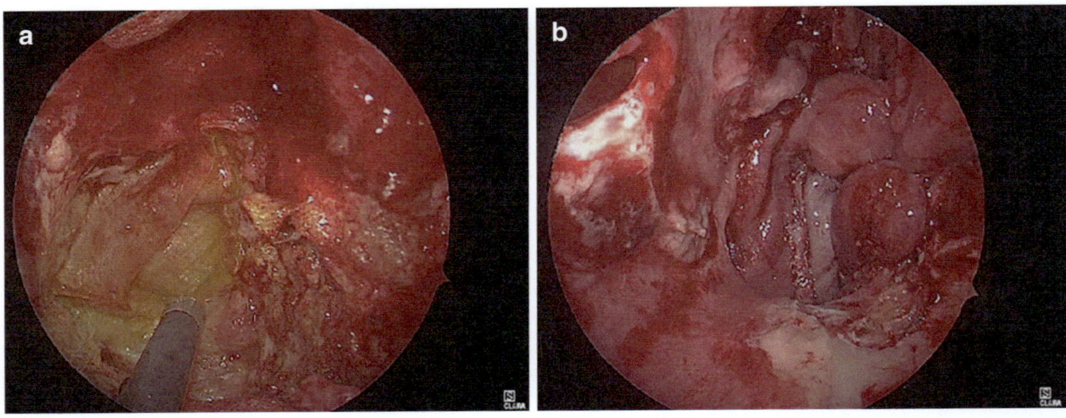

Fig. 7.4 Watertight confirmation of skull base defect reconstruction after nasoseptal flap and simultaneous inferior turbinate flap for a high flow CSF leak after a transclival approach. (**a**) During closure procedure. (**b**) At the end of the surgery

such as nausea and headache [12]. Conversely, the CSF leak also has potential complications, so the importance of closing the CSF leak must also be informed to the patient. It is important to inform about the lumbar puncture-related risks because, in some circumstances, the adverse events attributed to fluorescein could originate from complications of this procedure [20].

It is important to discuss with patients the potential failure of fluorescein visualization during surgery and the possibility of a new intervention. When fluorescein is not detected intraoperatively, there could be three times more risk of recurrence of CSF leak [12], although this does not necessarily imply a new surgery [10, 11].

7.3 Metabolism of Fluorescein

After intravenous administration, the fluorescein is rapidly metabolized. In this manner, 80–90% of fluorescein appears rapidly bound to plasma protein, and 10–20% remains as a free salt. A rapid conversion by the phase II reaction conjugates it with glucuronic acid, and 10 min after administration, the peak plasma concentration of sodium fluorescein declines and the glucuronate form increases [21]. Excretion is mainly renal in 48–72 h, and urine detection is possible for at least 24–36 h.

Intrathecal administration of fluorescein gets a rapid distribution in CSF due to the highly water solubility of the molecule [21]. The dye runs through the circulation of the CSF, including the ventricular system, and reaches the defect of the skull base, where it is expected to have its main output, and the rest is absorbed by the arachnoid granulations. The change in CSF color is maintained for 24 h in 80–91% of patients, in 36% at 48 h, and 26.1% more than 48 h [22, 23].

7.4 Intrathecal Use

7.4.1 Set-Up

Patients who will receive intrathecal fluorescein must be evaluated for current neurological states, including sensitivity and motricity of inferior extremities and ocular fundus, to determine the risk of potential complication and intracranial tension status [20]. The elements necessary to perform a lumbar puncture and dye administration are listed below:

- Sodium fluorescein: commercially available as injectable solution 10% or 25%
- Syringe, 10 mL
- Spinal needles, 20, 22, and/or 25 gauge
- Three-way stopcock
- Sterile dressing, gloves, and drapes
- Antiseptic solution

Although not available for intrathecal use, an ideal presentation for this purpose should be ampoules of fluorescein 5% (50 mg/1 mL) sterile and pyrogen-free, free of solid particles, iso-osmotic (292–297 mOsm/L), and a pH similar to the CSF (7.32) and, finally, without preservatives [24].

A traditional lumbar puncture technique at L3/L4 or L4/L5 space is performed by an adequately trained professional in an awake patient to evaluate possible complications. The patient is located seated or in the lateral position with the spine flexed maximally to open the interspinous spaces, a 24 gauge "pencil point" needle is used to diminish traumatic puncture due to blunt-type design. After the puncture, there must be a free flow of CSF to confirm the correct placement of CSF in the thecal space [25] (Fig. 7.5). If the patient has a lumbar drain, this route also can be used to administer the fluorescein.

A routine protocol is suggested to diminish the adverse effects of the procedure and get the best visualization of the dye through the defect in the skull base during surgery [26].

1. Premedication with systemic steroids to reduce the risk of chemical meningeal irritation, at doses of 0.1 mg/kg or 10 mg of intravenous dexamethasone [10, 20, 21, 26] and

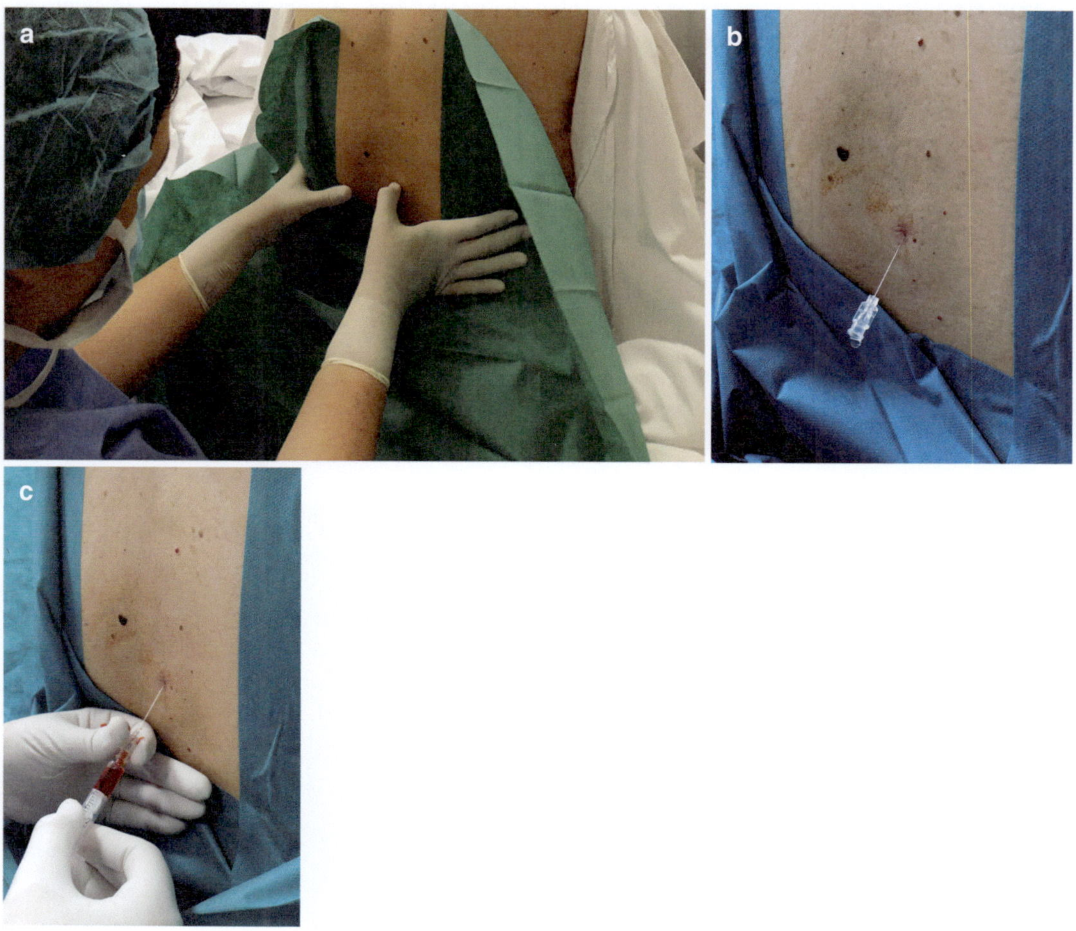

Fig. 7.5 Lumbar puncture technique for intrathecal administration. (**a**) L3/L4 or L4/L5 space is palpated, then an atraumatic puncture is recommended at this level, because the spaces are larger and in adults the spinal cord usually ends at L1/L2. (**b**) After the puncture, a "free flow" of the CSF leak is guaranteed to confirm the location in intrathecal space. (**c**) Slow administration of fluorescein

antihistamines, 50 mg of diphenhydramine (or dexchlorpheniramine 5 mg) [10, 20, 26]. The systemic steroid should be avoided in patients with Cushing's disease for postoperative monitoring.
2. Obtain 9 mL of CSF that will work as a diluent to return to the subarachnoid space mixed with fluorescein.
3. Administer fluorescein at the dosage described below. Slow intrathecal injection of CSF diluted with fluorescein is recommended from 10 to 30 min [12] or 0.1 mL/min [20].
4. Immediately after injection of the colorant, place the patient in the Trendelenburg position for 30 min to facilitate diffusion of the dye close to the skull base defect and away from the inferior roots in the spinal cord [21]. A dilution of 0.5 mL of 5% fluorescein diluted with 10 mL of distilled water to create a hypodense solution (1001) compared to CSF (density range 1004–1006) has been described to avoid this position [22, 23, 27].
5. In patients in whom the use of lumbar drainage is decided, CSF is obtained after drain placement, and drainage is closed after injection of fluorescein [15].
6. In cases of intraoperative use of intrathecal fluorescein, muscular relaxants should be avoided, if possible, to watch abnormal movements [20].

7.4.2 Dose

Since the beginning of its intrathecal use, the lowest possible dose of fluorescein has been recommended [28]. The original dosage was 1 mL of 5% fluorescein (50 mg of sodic fluorescein) diluted in 9 mL of CSF and injected into the lumbar subarachnoid space [2, 29]. Another way to dose it is 0.1 mg/kg to 50 mg or 0.1 mL/10 kg, maximal 1 mL [18].

A low dose has been suggested as secure and effective, including 0.2–0.5 mL of sodium fluorescein 5% (10–25 mg) or 0.25 mL of 10% (25 mg) solutions and also diluted to complete 10 mL of CSF [10, 21, 26, 30], administering 10 mg of intrathecal fluorescein diminishes the sensibility to detect CSF leaks during surgery [12]. In summary, the evidence shows that appropriate doses of intrathecal fluorescein range between 25 and 50 mg [29]. After the administration in the intrathecal space, fluorescein will be diluted with 100–150 mL of CSF, depending on the volume that each patient contains, this dilution modifies the color of the dye as we finally perceive in surgery (Fig. 7.6).

7.4.3 Timing

Some authors have reported the application of intrathecal fluorescein between 16 and 20 h

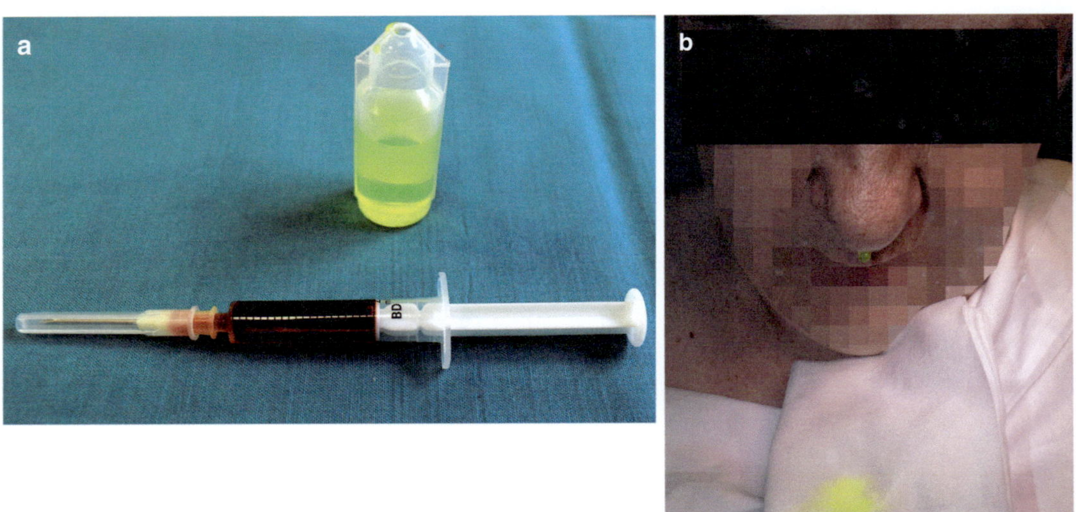

Fig. 7.6 Color changes in sodium fluorescein with different grades of concentration. (**a**) Dilution at 0.5% above and 10% below. (**b**) CSF rhinorrhea in a patient after intrathecal application of fluorescein

before nasal endoscopy or surgery [18]; more recent studies concluded that administration can be done 60 min before endoscopic evaluation or immediately before surgery, which allow the dye to disseminate throughout the CSF system and to be visualized in nose drippings through the skull base defect [12, 26]. If a hypodense solution is used, time can be as short as 10 min [22, 27].

7.4.4 Techniques to Improve Utilization

The use of intrathecal fluorescein, as described, usually leads to the correct visualization of the defect at the skull base, not only because of the color change but also because the slight increase in pressure that can occur changes an intermittent leak in to an active one, which is desirable in surgery to correct the defect. Nevertheless, some maneuvers can be useful to increase the visualization of the dye. In a diagnostic setting, the head can be located from a neutral position to flexion of the neck with the thorax and head down. It can also be useful to do Valsalva (intra-abdominal pressure augmented) [10] or Queckenstedt maneuvers (bilateral jugular vein compression), which increase the intracranial pressure and augment the flow of the CSF leak and, with it, the passage of the fluorescein to the nose.

7.4.5 What if Injected Pre-operatively but Not Visible?

The presence of fluorescein in the nasal cavity is strong evidence that a skull base defect exists. In some cases, it is not possible to find the typical yellow-green coloration after an adequate dose, administration and, time needed to find it in the nose. In those cases, the exposure of blue-light cobalt filter (465–495 nm) or ultraviolet/yellow light filter on the endoscope induces fluorescence of 520–530 nm, which can improve the localization of dye [26, 31]. Although the light modifications are not routinely required, it could be useful when the diagnosis is equivocal or fluorescein is difficult to visualize [10]. Simultaneous intravenous administration usually does not improve defect visualization [11, 26] and can increase the possibility of adverse events [21].

In patients with a history of meningitis, it is possible to find dural and/or arachnoid adhesions that restrict the diffusion of fluorescein to compartments delaying the course of the dye to the skull base defect [12]. In such cases, it could be prudent to wait for a more prolonged time before starting surgery or repeat the Trendelenburg maneuver to enhance the diffusion of the colorant. In all patients with lumbar subarachnoid drain, it is important to verify the closure of the system; otherwise, close it to avoid altering the CSF flow.

Finally, Trendelenburg and then Valsalva maneuver can be done, but if no fluorescein visualization is obtained, use neuronavigation and previous imaging check to try to find the skull base defect [11]. If the suspected CSF leak persists and no skull base defect is visible, it had been published to cover the most probable area (usually the cribriform plate) with a nasoseptal flap and recommend rigorous postoperative care and scheduling more frequent controls than usual.

7.4.6 Interpretation of False-Negative Results

Intrathecal fluorescein can be visualized during surgery in 80–96% of cases [11, 17], but it is important to remember that the absence of dye does not rule out the presence of a CSF leak [12]. In these cases, some situations may be occurring [10]:

- Tiny defects with intermittent closure with the brain;
- Transient CSF loss during lumbar subarachnoid placement, which can reduce the volume necessary below the level to reach the defect;
- Arachnoid scarring (i.e., prior meningitis);
- Severe lumbar stenosis;
- Short time from intrathecal injection;
- Low doses of fluorescein.

Raza et al., in their cohort of 419 patients, found 4.5% of false negatives, but no one developed a postoperative CSF leak [10]. This suggests that in patients with persistent absence of fluorescein visualization and despite that less than 25 mg was used, the probability of a CSF leak in the postoperative period could be lower. It could be explained by low pressure or irregular distribution of CSF or no active leak, but more studies are needed to clarify it.

7.4.7 Endoscopic Examination and Exploration of Potential Area

Nasal decongestion is highly recommended before doing an endoscopy evaluation of the nose in a patient with CSF rhinorrhea. After that, the schematic visualization of the nasal corridor should start through the floor until the cavum, to evaluate the nasopharyngeal orifice of the Eustachian tube for the possibility of a CSF leak originating in the middle ear. After that, a second evaluation should be orientated to the roof of the nasal cavity as possible, and the superior evaluation should be done carefully to find the CSF leak.

In the postoperative period of skull base tumor resection, a watertight test of reconstruction can be done, usually through an endoscopic evaluation on the fifth day and always on the bed of the patient to prevent efforts and temporary increments in intracranial pressure that can displace the flaps covering the defect (Fig. 7.7).

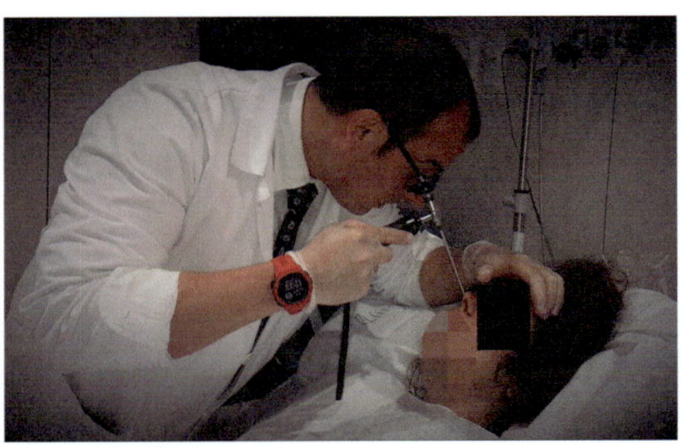

Fig. 7.7 Evaluation on the fifth postoperative day of a patient undergoing extended endonasal surgery to the skull base; the evaluation is performed in such a way that the patient remains in bed without making movements that could generate increases in intracranial pressure

7.5 Topical Fluorescein

In 2000, Jones et al. described the use of intranasal fluorescein in three patients to locate the defect at the skull base during surgery [32]. Saafan et al. validated it in 2006 in a study with 25 patients and used the dye during the pre-operative study as well as postoperative detection of a recurrence in patients with CSF rhinorrhea [33].

A change in the color of the fluorescein from yellow-brown to green or streaming of the fluorescein over the nasal mucosa and/or blood with the presence of CSF when the dye is directly applied in the suspected area can be expected [32]. Topical application of dye can be done after drying the area with suction and topical application of vasoconstrictor, then proceed to carefully place cotton pledgets impregnated with 1 mL of sodium fluorescein 5% or 10% in the middle meatus, the roof of the ethmoid plate, and spheno-ethmoidal recess; as described, the color change can be found at this moment. The patient may be asked to cough or strain while leaning forward or, in the case of intraoperative use, asking an anesthetist to induce a Valsalva maneuver in the patient to increase intracranial pressure.

Topical fluorescein could avoid complications associated with intrathecal use as a trauma for lumbar puncture and neural irritation for chemical effects of a high concentration of fluorescein. Liu Hai-sheng et al. did a study with 15 patients with CSF rhinorrhea and obtained successful diagnosis and treatment for 100% of patients [34]. Ozturk et al. published a study with 24 patients with only one failure to detect a second defect in sphenoid, even though this technique was used to correctly find the defects for the other patients [35]. In the same way, as described for intrathecal use, visualization can be enhanced with ultraviolet light, even for solutions as dilute as 1: 1,600,000 [28].

7.6 Pediatric Age Group and Use of Fluorescein

Intravenous use of fluorescein has not been studied in children, and dose-adaptation data are not available; therefore, efficacy and safety in this group have not been established. For intrathecal use, a dose of 0,1 mL/kg, with a maximum dose of 1 mL, of a hypodense solution (5% sodium fluorescein solution diluted in 10 mL of distilled sterilized water) has been used [23, 27].

7.7 Complications

The main limitation of intrathecal use of fluorescein is related to the adverse events reported almost from the first publications; however, this dye explains less than 0.1% of adverse events of all intrathecal medications uses [18]. Isolated reports assumed a chemical irritant direct effect from fluorescein [36]; furthermore, the majority of this complication could be related to incorrect dosage or timing of intrathecal administration. Meco and Oberascher reported a series of 900 cases without complications [37]; Felisati et al. summarized 1940 patients of different studies with intrathecal administration of 50 mg or less with four transient complications and two patients with simultaneous radiographic intrathecal contrast administration [17, 19]; Seth et al. reported use in 47 patients with no complications with 10 mg total dose [12]. Banu reported in a cohort of 50 patients one case (2.4%) of transient leg weakness following lumbar drain placement [11].

The following complications with the intrathecal use of fluorescein have been described:

- Headache, especially in patients with prolactin-secreting tumors [38]
- Nausea, vomiting, dizziness
- Hives, acute hypotension, anaphylaxis, and related anaphylactoid reaction.
- Lower-extremity weakness and numbness, opisthotonus, transient paraparesis, hemiparesis, myelopathy, seizures [39, 40]
- Cranial nerve palsies
- Neuropathic pain
- Pulmonary edema
- Death

Mechanisms of complications can be related to the method of administration, dose, formulations, or idiopathic [18]. In a canine model, Syms et al. found inflammatory changes expected with irritant material in the subarachnoid space in a dose-dependent manner [36]. An experimental study in a murine model suggested a potential effect of fluorescein to induce apoptosis, measured as NF-kB expression after direct exposition to dye [41]. Since the first reports of complications related to intrathecal fluorescein, it is common to find a different dose to that currently used or it happened in patients with previous seizures, trauma, cranial surgery, or repeated lumbar puncture [42].

Wolff et al. used intrathecal fluorescein for more than 25 years to localize skull base defect and reported 925 cases of suboccipitally administered fluorescein with 3 cases of epileptic crises and none with lumbar administration [31, 43]. Keerl et al. reported 420 intrathecal administration of fluorescein in 305 patients in different centers and reported to manufacturers and regulatory agencies: the results showed 7 major complications, all related to doses between 100 mg and 700 mg, at least more than double the dose that we consider appropriate today; furthermore, with none in the patients who received less than 50 mg, with the exception of two patients with grand mal seizures but with the simultaneous intrathecal application of contrast medium. The same study also found one death in a patient who received 5 mL of fluorescein, meaning they received between 500 and 1250 mg, if a concentration of 10% or 25% was used, which is an enormous dose compared with what is used today [18].

Guimaraes et al. published a study describing chemical and cytological changes with hypodense intrathecal fluorescein. They noticed changes in inflammatory cell count (neutrophils, lymphocytes, monocytes, eosinophils, and basophils) between 24 and 48 h, but no clinically related side effects, even in children [23]. In the same way, Demarco et al. did not find complications in a cohort of 20 patients with a hypodense solution [27]. Moseley et al. published a report of a case and survey reporting adverse effects of 625 intrathecal fluorescein applications and found 17 non-fatal major complications, including lower-extremity weakness, seizures, and decreased consciousness among others [44], but, again, doses between 5 and 250 mg of fluorescein were used, and in four cases without dilution before intrathecal application and their patients had previous cranial trauma and surgery and had suffered seizures before fluorescein administration [23]. Permanent spinal cord damage was reported with exposure to 700 mg of intrathecal fluorescein [18]. Seizures that occurred during intrathecal fluorescein can be successfully treated with benzodiazepines or barbiturates [39].

Placantonakis et al. published a study on 54 patients with symptoms attributable to lumbar puncture procedure drainage: malaise, headache, fever, nausea, and vomiting [26]. A series of 203 patients with endoscopic pituitary surgery found just two cases of hypotension and syncopal episodes [16]. Changes in the color of urine are frequent, and similar changes in tears can also occur [41].

Until now, the evidence and the routine use in clinical settings in different centers suggest that fluorescein could have a narrow toxic margin more than intrinsic neurological toxicity, and adverse effects are usually present when concentrations greater than 100 mg are administered in less than 10 min. Those complications are practically nonexistent when 50 mg or less are used [10, 17, 18].

Some patients have an increased risk for seizures, and special care should be taken into account in patients with previous hydrocephaly, spinal stenosis, neurological damage with brain edema or epilepsy, or those exposed to phenothiazine, tricyclic antidepressants, or benzodiazepines [20, 45]. Likewise, in all those patients with increased risk of related problems from a lumbar puncture (lumbar spine deformities or traumatic puncture) due to the risk of an epidural hematoma.

It is advisable to discuss with an anesthetist to avoid, if possible, using depolarizing muscle relaxants during general anesthesia to evaluate possible seizures during surgery [39]. Another unfavorable outcome related to intrathecal administration of fluorescein is the potential apparition of post lumbar puncture headache, defined as a positional headache arising within the first 7 days of the procedure. A recent study showed that intrathecal fluorescein administration is associated with 6.8% of positional headaches, which is less than that expected for lumbar puncture [18, 38]. Furthermore, blood contamination of intrathecal space can induce seizure-like activity, and therefore, it is important to keep adequate communication with the anesthetist and the other team members [20, 21, 39].

7.8 Conclusion

The use of intrathecal fluorescein in patients with CSF rhinorrhea at doses equal to or less than 50 mg diluted and slowly administered is a useful tool that facilitates the diagnosis and surgical treatment of defects of the skull base with an adequate safety profile, according to the evidence published in recent years.

References

1. Fox N. Cure in a case of cerebrospinal rhinorrhea. Archs Otolar. 1933;17:85–6.
2. Kirchner FR, Proud GO. Method for the identification and localization of cerebrospinal fluid, rhinorrhea and otorrhea. Trans Am Laryngol Rhinol Otol Soc. 1960;47:786–96.
3. Friedberg SA, Galloway TC. Spontaneous cerebrospinal fluid rhinorrhea. Ann Otol Rhinol Laryngol. 1938;47:792–4.
4. Hollon T, Stummer W, Orringer D, Suero Molina E. Surgical adjuncts to increase the extent of resection: intraoperative MRI, fluorescence, and Raman histology. Neurosurg Clin N Am. 2019;30(1): 65–74.
5. Neira JA, Ung TH, Sims JS, Malone HR, Chow DS, Samanamud JL, et al. Aggressive resection at the infiltrative margins of glioblastoma facilitated by intraoperative fluorescein guidance. J Neurosurg. 2016:1–12.
6. Stummer W, Suero Molina E. Fluorescence imaging/agents in tumor resection. Neurosurg Clin N Am. 2017;28(4):569–83.
7. Moore GE, Peyton WT, et al. The clinical use of fluorescein in neurosurgery; the localization of brain tumors. J Neurosurg. 1948;5(4):392–8.
8. Bernal-Sprekelsen M, Bleda-Vázquez C, Carrau RL. Ascending meningitis secondary to traumatic cerebrospinal fluid leaks. Am J Rhinol. 2000;14(4):257–9.
9. Bernal-Sprekelsen M, Alobid I, Mullol J, Trobat F, Tomás-Barberán M. Closure of cerebrospinal fluid

leaks prevents ascending bacterial meningitis. Rhinology. 2005;43(4):277–81.
10. Raza S, Banu M, Donaldson A, Patel K, Anand V, Schwartz T. Sensitivity and specificity of intrathecal fluorescein and white light excitation for detecting intraoperative cerebrospinal fluid leak in endoscopic skull base surgery: a prospective study. J Neurosurg. 2016;124(3):621–6.
11. Banu MA, Kim JH, Shin BJ, Woodworth GF, Anand VK, Schwartz TH. Low-dose intrathecal fluorescein and etiology-based graft choice in endoscopic endonasal closure of CSF leaks. Clin Neurol Neurosurg. 2014;116:28–34.
12. Seth R, Rajasekaran K, Benninger M, Batra P. The utility of intrathecal fluorescein in cerebrospinal fluid leak repair. Otol Head Neck Surg. 2010;143:626–32.
13. Cappabianca P, Cavallo LM, Esposito F, Valente V, De Divitiis E. Sellar repair in endoscopic endonasal transsphenoidal surgery: results of 170 cases. Neurosurgery. 2002;51:1365–71.
14. Doglietto F, Guerrini F, Maira G. Intrathecal fluorescein and sellar reconstruction in pituitary surgery: what might be truly useful? World Neurosurg. 2015;84(2):209–10.
15. Tabaee A, Placantonakis DG, Schwartz TH, Anand VK. Intrathecal fluorescein in endoscopic skull base surgery. Otolaryngol Head Neck Surg. 2007;137(2):316–20.
16. Jakimovski D, Bonc G, Attia M, Shao H, Hofstetter C, Tisouris A, Anand V, Schwartz. Incidence and significance of intraoperative cerebrospinal fluid leak in endoscopic pituitary surgery using intrathecal fluorescein. World Neurosurg. 2014;82(3-4):e513–23.
17. Felisati G, Bianchi A, Lozza P, Portaleone S. Italian multicentre study on intrathecal fluorescein for craniosinusal fistulae. Acta Otorhinolaryngol Ital. 2008;28:159–63.
18. Keerl R, Weber RK, Draf W, Wienke A, Schaefer SD. Use of sodium fluorescein solution for detection of cerebrospinal fluid fistulas: an analysis of 420 administrations and reported complications in Europe and the United States. Laryngoscope. 2004;114: 266–72.
19. Keerl R, Weber RK, Draf W, Radziwill R, Wienke A. Complications of lumbar administration of 5% sodium fluorescein solution for detection of cerebrospinal fluid fistula. Laryngorhinootologie. 2003;82(12):833–8.
20. Rodríguez M, Díaz C, Padilla M, Alcaraz A, Gonzalez P, Benitez M. Uso seguro de fluoresceína intratecal en la localización de las fístulas de líquido cefalorraquídeo: descripción de un caso e implementación de un algoritmo perioperatorio. Rev Esp Anestesiol Reanim. 2017;64(9):533–6.
21. Antunes P, Perdigao M. The use of intrathecal fluorescein in cerebrospinal fluid leak repair: management from an anesthesiologist's point – of - view. Acta Anaesthesiol Scand. 2016;60(9):1323–7.
22. Guimaraes R, Becker H. A new technique for the use of intrathecal fluorescein in the repair of cerebrospinal fluid rhinorrhea using a hypodense diluent. Rev Laryngol Otol Rhinol (Bord). 2001;122:191–3.
23. Guimarães RES, Stamm AEC, Giannetti AV, Crosara PFTB, Becker CG, Becker HMG. Chemical and cytological analysis of cerebral spinal fluid after intrathecal injection of hypodense fluorescein. Braz J Otorhinolaryngol. 2015;81:549–53.
24. Gil G, Bautista C, Oliveras M, Cabañas M, Hidalgo EG. Dosificación de fármacos en administración cerebroespinal. Farm Hosp. 2005;29:185–90.
25. Bateman N, Mason J, Jones NS. Use of fluorescein for detecting cerebrospinal fluid rhinorrhoea: a safe technique for intrathecal injection. ORL J Otorhinolaryngol Relat Spec. 1999;61(3):131–2.
26. Placantonakis DG, Tabaee A, Anand VK, Hiltzik D, Schwartz TH. Safety of low-dose intrathecal fluorescein in endoscopic cranial base surgery. Neurosurgery. 2007;61(Suppl 3):161–5.
27. Demarco RC, Tamashiro E, Valera FC, Anselmo-Lima WT. Use of a hypodense sodium fluorescein solution for the endoscopic repair of rhinogenic cerebrospinal fluid fistulae. Am J Rhinol. 2007;21(2):184–6.
28. Kirchner FR. Use of fluorescein for the diagnosis and localization of cerebrospinal fluid fistulas. Surg Forum. 1961;12:406–8.
29. Alobid I, Enseñat J, Rioja E, Enriquez K, Viscovich L, de Notaris M, Bernal-Sprekelsen M. Management of cerebrospinal fluid leaks according to size. Our experience. Acta Otorrinolaringol Esp. 2014;65(3): 162–9.
30. Javadi SA, Samimi H, Naderi F, Shirani M. The use of low- dose intrathecal fluorescein in endoscopic repair of cerebrospinal fluid rhinorrhea. Arch Iran Med. 2013;16(5):264–6.
31. Wolf G, Greistorfer K, Stammberger H. Endoscopic detection of cerebrospinal fluid fistulas with a fluorescence technique. Report of experiences with over 925 cases. Laryngorhinootologie. 1997;76:588–94.
32. Jones ME, Reino T, Gnoy A, Guillory S, Wackym P, Lawson W. Identification of intranasal cerebrospinal fluid leaks by topical application with fluorescein dye. Am J Rhinol. 2000;14:93–6.
33. Saafan M, Ragab S, Albirmawy O. Topical intranasal fluorescein: the missing partner in algorithms of cerebrospinal fluid fistula detection. Laryngoscope. 2006;116:1158–61.
34. Liu HS, Chen YT, Wang D, Liang H, Wang Y, Wang SJ, et al. The use of topical intranasal fluorescein in endoscopic endonasal repair of cerebrospinal fluid rhinorrhea. Surg Neurol. 2009;72(4):341–5.
35. Ozturk K, Karabagli H, Bulut S, Egilmez M, Duran M. Is the use of topical fluorescein helpful for management of CSF leakage? Laryngoscope. 2012;122(6):1215–8.
36. Syms CA 3rd, Syms MJ, Murphy TP, Massey SO. Cerebrospinal fluid fistulae in a canine model. Otolaryngol Head Neck Surg. 1997;117:542–6.
37. Meco C, Oberascher G. Comprehensive algorithm for skull base dural lesion and cerebrospinal fluid fistula diagnosis. Laryngoscope. 2004;114:991–9.

38. Zhang M, Azad TD, Singh H, Salam S, Jain S, Anand V, et al. Lumbar puncture for the injection of intrathecal fluorescein: should it be avoided in a subset of patients undergoing endoscopic endonasal resection of sellar and parasellar lesions? J Neurol Surg B Skull Base. 2018;79(6):554–8.
39. Jacob AK, Dilger JA, Hebl JR. Status epilepticus and intrathecal fluorescein: anesthesia providers beware. Anesth Analg. 2008;107(1):229–31.
40. Park K, Kim Y. A case of myelopathy after intrathecal injection of fluorescein. J Korean Neurosurg Soc. 2007;42:492–4.
41. Camlar M, Turk C, Oltulu F, Oren M, Buhur A, Yigitturk G, et al. How safe is the use of intrathecal fluorescein? An experimental study. Turk Neurosurg. 2019;29(4):549–54.
42. Mahaley MS Jr, Odom GL. Complication following intrathecal injection of fluorescein. Case report. J Neurosurg. 1966;25:298–9.
43. Stammberger H, Greistorfer K, Wolf G, Luxenberger W. Surgical occlusion of cerebrospinal fistulas of the anterior skull base using intrathecal sodium fluorescein. Laryngorhinootologie. 1997;76(10):595–607.
44. Moseley JI, Carton CA, Stern WE. Spectrum of complications in the use of intrathecal fluorescein. J Neurosurg. 1978;48:765–7.
45. Anari S, Waldron M, Carrie S. Delayed absence seizure: a complication of intrathecal fluorescein injection. A case report and literature review. Auris Nasus Larynx. 2007;34(4):515–8.

Diagnostic Algorithm for Cerebrospinal Fluid Leak

8

Lisa Caulley, Claire Hopkins, and Valerie J. Lund

8.1 Introduction

Cerebrospinal fluid (CSF) rhinorrhea results from disruption of the barriers between the CSF-containing subarachnoid spaces in the anterior or middle cranial fossae and the paranasal sinuses or nasal cavity [1, 2]. Identification of rhinorrhea as CSF can be challenging, as rhinorrhea, or discharge of fluid from the nasal cavity, is a common overlapping symptom in inflammatory and infectious rhinopathies [1, 3]. A fistula provides a pathway for pathogenic microorganisms to invade intracranially, a potentially devastating complication. A 10% risk of ascending meningitis per annum associated with CSF rhinorrhea makes accurate diagnosis of the fistula critical [4–6]. The diagnosis of CSF rhinorrhea is a two-step process to: (1) confirm the presence of a CSF leak through the objective evidence of extracranial CSF and (2) identify the position of the skull base defect, or defects, through which the CSF is draining. A thorough clinical, laboratory, and radiographic evaluation must be included in the diagnostic approach to confirm CSF rhinorrhea [7].

L. Caulley (✉)
Department of Otolaryngology - Head & Neck Surgery, University of Ottawa - L'Université d'Ottawa, Ottawa, Canada

Clinical Epidemiology Program and Center for Journalology, Ottawa Hospital Research Institute, Ottawa, Canada

Department of Epidemiology, Erasmus University Medical Center Rotterdam, Rotterdam, The Netherlands

C. Hopkins
Rhinology, King's College, London, UK

ENT Consultant, Guy's and St Thomas' Hospitals, London, UK

V. J. Lund
Emeritus Professor in Rhinology, UCL, London, UK

Honorary ENT Consultant, Royal National Throat, Nose and Ear Hospital, UCLH, London, UK
e-mail: v.lund@ucl.ac.uk

8.2 Differential Diagnosis

The nasal mucosa responds to the external environment in a limited number of ways, that is, through rhinorrhea, nasal obstruction, sneezing, pruritus, or bleeding [3]. As such, rhinorrhea is a non-specific finding with a broad differential of poorly understood and often overlapping pathologies that can make diagnosis of CSF challenging (Table 8.1).

Rhinitis is a common condition that may mimic the signs and symptoms of CSF rhinorrhea leading to its misdiagnosis or may occur simultaneously [1]. Rhinitis is defined as an inflammation of the lining of the nose and is characterized by nasal symptoms including anterior or posterior rhinorrhea, sneezing, nasal blockage, and nasal pruritus [8]. The presence of two nasal symptoms for at least 1 h daily for a minimum of 12 weeks per year is required for the

A. A. AlQahtani et al. (eds.), *CSF Rhinorrhea*, https://doi.org/10.1007/978-3-030-94781-1_8

Table 8.1 Differential diagnosis of rhinorrhea

Inflammatory
• Infectious
– Viral rhinitis
– Bacterial rhinitis
• Non-infectious
– Allergic rhinitis
Seasonal
Perennial
– Non-allergic rhinitis with eosinophilia
Non-Inflammatory
• Hormone-induced rhinitis
• Medication-induced rhinitis
• Occupation-induced rhinitis
• Vasomotor rhinitis
• Exercise-induced rhinitis
• Atrophic rhinitis
• Idiopathic rhinitis
Conditions that Mimic Rhinitis
• Foreign bodies
• Tumors
– Benign
– Malignant
• Choanal atresia
• Skull base defects
– Cerebrospinal fluid rhinorrhea
Spontaneous
Traumatic
Iatrogenic
Non-iatrogenic
Neoplasm
• Retained irrigation fluids

diagnosis of chronic rhinitis [9]. Chronic rhinitis is observed in infectious and inflammatory rhinopathies, including acute and chronic rhinosinusitis, allergic rhinitis, and non-allergic rhinitis.

8.2.1 Allergic Rhinitis

Allergic rhinitis, the most common form of non-infectious rhinitis, refers to inflammation of the nasal mucosa due to IgE-mediated reactions to extrinsic allergens [10]. In addition to bilateral clear rhinorrhea, allergic rhinitis can be differentiated from CSF rhinorrhea by the classic allergic profile of sneezing, nasal congestion, and pruritus of the nasal cavity and hard palate [8, 11]. Allergic rhinitis caused by intermittent aeroallergens, such as pollens from trees, grasses, and weeds, will characteristically lead to bilateral, clear rhinorrhea. By contrast, persistent allergic rhinitis, which is commonly triggered by dust mites, cockroaches, animal dander, and molds, is characterized by the cardinal symptom of nasal obstruction [12, 13]. Patients with allergic rhinitis may present with comorbid atopic conditions, including atopic dermatitis, conjunctivitis, and asthma. A family history of atopic diseases makes the diagnosis more likely and studies of parental involvement suggest a greater risk of atopic conditions when both parents are atopic than if one parent is atopic [14]. In vivo allergy testing, including skin prick and less commonly utilized intradermal tests, and in vitro allergy testing, such as radioallergosorbent tests (RAST), can assist in confirmation of an allergic etiology and can guide treatment [8, 15–18].

8.2.2 Non-Allergic Rhinitis

Chronic rhinitis in the absence of allergic disease is classified as non-allergic rhinitis and can be further subclassified as infectious, occupation-related, drug-induced, non-allergic rhinitis with eosinophilia syndrome, hormonal, or idiopathic rhinitis [8]. Over 200 million people worldwide suffer from non-allergic rhinitis and the prevalence of non-allergic rhinitis ranges from 28% to 60% among otorhinolaryngology and allergy clinic populations [9, 19–23]. As in allergic rhinitis, the nasal discharge can be profuse, watery, and is usually bilateral. Non-allergic rhinitis is diagnosed by means of a thorough clinical evaluation and appropriate testing to identify the underlying condition [19].

Viral and bacterial pathogens can activate an inflammatory process that can lead to rhinosinusitis.

Rhinorrhea secondary to rhinosinusitis presents in conjunction with nasal obstruction, facial pain or pressure, and smell dysfunction. The discharge is usually mucoid, mucopurulent, or frankly purulent though can be clear and usually bilateral, although it may be unilateral. Ensuing symptoms for 4 weeks or less should prompt consideration of an infectious etiology in the setting of acute rhinosinusitis, while symptoms that persist for 12 weeks or more are suggestive of chronic rhinosinusitis [8, 10, 24, 25].

Inhalant-induced rhinitis that arises following high-level or prolonged occupational exposure to airborne irritant chemicals is referred to as non-allergic occupational rhinitis or rhinopathy [9]. The incidence is estimated to be 5–15% [19]. Occupational-induced rhinitis has been observed in response to airborne allergens or irritants, including laboratory animal, wood dust, latex, grains, and chemicals, and demonstrate a temporal relationship with work environment exposure [8, 26–31]. Occupational-induced rhinitis should be differentiated from work-exacerbated rhinitis, which refers to pre-existing rhinitis exacerbated in the work environment [10, 31]. Again, while the discharge is usually watery, it is also bilateral.

Bilateral watery rhinorrhea in response to hot and spicy foods or alcoholic beverages is known as gustatory rhinitis. Gustatory rhinitis is produced by stimulation of muscarinic receptors in the nasal mucosa. The syndrome may respond to preprandial administration of ipratropium bromide [9, 32]. It is believed to be more common among the elderly and frequently overlaps with rhinitis of the elderly, a form of clear anterior rhinorrhea that affects elderly patients following age-related changes in the nose [9, 33].

Hormones of pregnancy, oral contraceptives, other estrogens, and even cyclical premenstrual hormonal changes have been found to contribute to rhinorrhea [19, 33]. Pregnancy-induced or gestational rhinitis presents in an estimated 1 in 5 pregnant women [33]. Increased circulating blood volume and estrogen may contribute to this effect by increasing histamine receptors in epithelial cells and the microvasculature, and exacerbating pre-existing rhinitis, however, the precise mechanism remains unclear [19, 23, 34–36]. Symptoms are transient and classically resolve within 2 weeks of delivery [23]. Hormonal imbalances of other metabolic disorders such as hypothyroidism and acromegaly have been suggested to cause or contribute to rhinitis, but the evidence for this association remains limited [33].

Several medications may induce rhinitis as an adverse effect of treatment [3, 8, 37]. Drug-induced rhinitis can result secondary to inflammation after ingestion or topical use of a medication [37]. For instance, non-steroidal anti-inflammatory drugs (NSAIDs) and aspirin induce a nasal inflammatory response via inhibition of cyclooxygenase-1 (COX-1) [37–39]. Neurogenic medication-induced rhinitis develops via neural stimulation of the nasal mucosa [37]. Alpha- and beta-adrenoceptor antagonists, such as guanethidine, methyldopa and beta-blockers, downregulate sympathetic tone and lead to nasal congestion and rhinorrhea [37, 40]. Overuse of topical nasal decongestants can result in persistent nasal congestion, rhinorrhea, and a characteristic beefy, red mucosa, known as rhinitis medicamentosa or rebound rhinitis [37, 41]. The pathophysiology of rhinitis medicamentosa remains unclear but is presumed to be caused by fatigue of the overstimulated alpha-adrenergic vasoconstrictor mechanisms and decreased sensitivity to endogenous catecholamines, resulting in reactive hyperemia and edema [37, 41–46]. Cocaine-induced rhinitis, resultant from one of the most commonly utilized intranasal illicit drugs, may result in prolonged vasoconstriction and rebound nasal mucosal edema and mucous production, similar to those seen in rhinitis medicamentosa [10, 47, 48].

Non-allergic rhinitis with eosinophilia (NARES) presents with perennial episodes of watery rhinorrhea, pruritus, epiphora, sneezing, and eosinophilia (5–20%) on nasal cytology in the setting of negative assessment for aeroallergen-specific IgE [9, 19]. The pathophysiology of the disease remains unclear but the prevalence of IgE-positive cells, eosinophils, and mast cells on histologic examination suggests an underlying local IgE-mediated process [19].

Idiopathic or vasomotor rhinitis refers to an upper respiratory hyper-responsiveness in the absence of identifiable trigger with no evidence of eosinophilia [8, 23]. There is a growing body of evidence to support avoidance of factors that may be exacerbating the rhinitis, such as cigarette smoke and other environmental triggers, as well as topical therapies, including intranasal steroids and intranasal ipratropium bromide to effectively reduce the rhinorrhea [49–54]. Paradoxically topical antihistamine nasal sprays have been found to be very effective for the overall treatment of vasomotor rhinitis, likely through anti-inflammatory mechanisms [50]. Three multicenter, placebo-controlled clinical trials have confirmed the efficacy of azelastine hydrochloride nasal spray, an intranasal antihistamine with inhibitory effects on chemical mediators of inflammation, to reduce vasomotor rhinitis symptoms [50, 55–57]. In a placebo-controlled study of levocabastine, a potent H_1-antagonist for vasomotor rhinitis, levocabastine was found to be superior to placebo for symptoms of nasal discharge and sneezing [50, 58].

8.2.3 Other Conditions Mimicking CSF Rhinorrhea

Unilateral rhinorrhea may be observed in asymmetrical pathologies, including nasal foreign bodies. In rare cases, sinonasal, orbital or brain tumor extension through the middle or anterior cranial fossa may lead to a CSF leak and associated central nervous system deficits [59].

Congenital choanal atresia occurs at an estimated frequency of 1 in 7000–8000 births [60]. It may be bilateral, presenting at birth as cyclical cyanosis that improves with crying. More commonly, it occurs unilaterally and may not become apparent until later in childhood at which time the obstruction can manifest as unilateral rhinorrhea from the obstructed nostril [61, 62]. Careful clinical assessment with endoscopy and imaging can diagnose these structural abnormalities.

Skull base defects in the middle cranial fossa can communicate with the middle ear space and mastoid behind an intact tympanic membrane. CSF that collects in the middle ear space can drain down the Eustachian tube into the nasal cavity. In this instance, CSF otorrhea may manifest as CSF rhinorrhea [1, 63].

Saline irrigations have been found to improve symptoms and quality of life in the management of chronic rhinitis. Nasal saline irrigations assist in restoring nasal and sinus physiology including improving muco-ciliary clearance; the disruption and removal of antigens, biofilms, and inflammatory mediators; and by direct protection of the sinonasal mucosa [25]. Intranasal saline irrigations can be retained in the paranasal sinuses after use, particularly after they have been surgically opened. Patients may note watery nasal drainage that occurs even hours after completing the irrigation upon moving the head. Retained saline irrigation can be challenging to distinguish from CSF rhinorrhea in the immediate postoperative period. However, a trial of discontinuation of saline irrigations will eliminate associated retained fluid and allow it to be distinguished from a true CSF leak.

8.3 Diagnostic Approach

Bilateral defects, anatomic abnormalities including septal perforations, and concomitant neuropathies can make it challenging to confirm and localize CSF rhinorrhea, and necessitate further investigations. A diagnostic algorithm for CSF rhinorrhea is outlined in Fig. 8.1 [7].

8.3.1 Clinical Evaluation

The diagnosis of CSF rhinorrhea begins with a directed history and physical exam. Rhinorrhea originating from a skull base defect is classically characterized as unilateral, dependent, clear rhinorrhea on endoscopy or a pulsatile mass. Patients may report observed rhinorrhea with positional variation, particularly when bending or lowering the head [1, 7]. Furthermore, CSF may be noted to have a salty or metallic taste by patients [1].

Skull base defects and their clinical consequences should be diagnosed and managed quickly and efficiently. A history of spontaneous or recurrent bacterial meningitis may suggest a possible skull base defect that places the central nervous system in contact with bacterial pathogens from the nasal cavity [1, 64]. A skull base defect at the level of the cribriform plate may

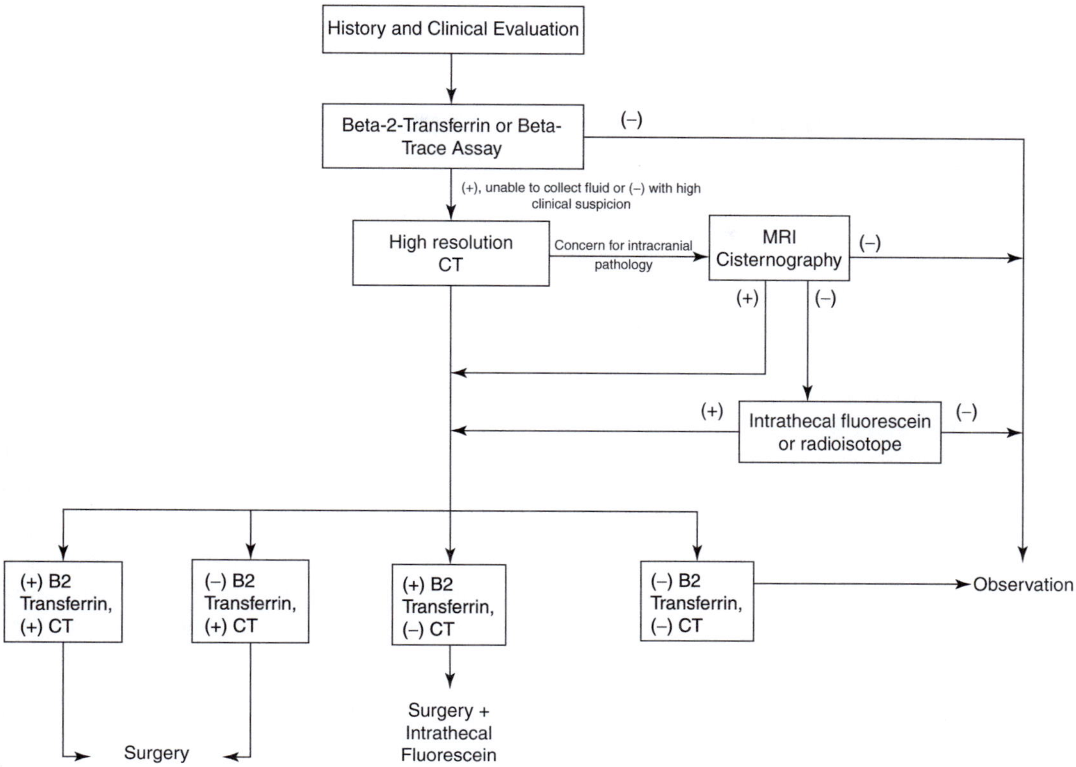

Fig. 8.1 Diagnostic algorithm for cerebrospinal fluid rhinorrhea. *CT* Computed tomography, *MRI* magnetic resonance imaging, *β-2* beta-2 transferrin

present as olfactory dysfunction, warranting careful clinical evaluation and magnetic resonance imaging of the olfactory fossa [1]. The presence of a meningocele or meningoencephalocele may produce unilateral nasal obstruction.

CSF leaks are classified based on their etiology: traumatic, iatrogenic, or spontaneous. An antecedent event of a head trauma, sinus, or skull base surgery in a patient with unilateral rhinorrhea should prompt consideration of a skull base defect [1]. CSF leaks are reported to occur in 2% to 20.8% of patients with traumatic basilar skull fractures [65]. In a review of 3402 patients who underwent endoscopic sinus surgery, CSF leak was reported in 19 (0.6%) patients [66].

Chronic headaches should be carefully investigated in the setting of clear, watery rhinorrhea for conditions that may result in increased intracranial pressure including idiopathic intracranial hypertension, hydrocephalus, intracranial neoplasms, and meningoceles. Evaluation and management of these intracranial pathologies is critical in the definitive treatment of CSF rhinorrhea. Idiopathic or benign intracranial hypertension is presumed to occur as a consequence of impaired CSF absorption, resulting in chronically elevated intracranial pressure. The disease occurs most commonly in obese middle-aged women and presents with signs and symptoms suggestive of increased intracranial pressure, including pressure headaches, pulsatile tinnitus, papilledema, and visual disturbances [67, 68]. Imaging studies generally show small ventricles and an empty sella [67]. Prolonged cerebrospinal fluid leaks can result in intracranial hypotension (<6 mm H_2O) resulting in descent of the brainstem, crowding of the posterior fossa, and stretching and impingement on cranial nerves. This can manifest clinically in patients as postural headaches, neck stiffness, cranial neuropathies, nausea, and emesis [69–71]. These cases may also have bilateral and/or multiple leak sites.

Clinical evaluation may provide useful insight into the source of the leak, associated pathology, and preoperative planning. On endoscopy, pulsatile, clear fluid may be visualized from a patent craniofacial fistula. The nasal cavity should be carefully inspected for any mass lesions that may be contributing to a CSF leak or that will need to be addressed for appropriate management of the CSF leak. Anatomical abnormalities, such as septal deviations, that may obstruct the nasal cavity and impede transnasal surgery should be noted. Although endoscopic examination of the nasal cavity frequently does not provide diagnostic certainty of a CSF leak, nasal examination can effectively eliminate alternative sources of clear rhinorrhea, such as inflammation of the sinonasal cavity and foreign bodies. Otoscopy should be performed to evaluate the ear for characteristic features of a middle ear effusion, such as an air-fluid level or opacification of the tympanic membrane. Any concerning findings on otoscopy warrant formal otologic diagnostic testing, including audiologic assessment.

8.3.2 Investigations

1. *The "halo" or "double-ring" sign* is a classic image in medicine and was taught as a method for determining whether bloody rhinorrhea contains CSF [72, 73]. This test is reliant upon the differing rates of separation of the components of CSF as they travel through a material [73]. The halo sign is consistently visible when CSF concentrations are 30% to 90% when mixed with blood [72]. However, the finding is not specific to CSF as blood mixed with other clear fluids can present in a similar configuration, limiting the utility of the test [2, 72]. As such, the clinical value of this sign remains controversial [72].
2. *Beta-2 (β-2) transferrin* is a highly reliable glycoprotein protein for human CSF and has become the gold standard in detection of CSF [3, 6, 59, 74, 75]. β-2 transferrin assays have a sensitivity of 87% to 100% and a specificity of 71% to 100% for CSF [6, 47, 74–82]. As such, it has been proposed that a negative β-2 transferrin test in a patient with a suspected CSF leak may be sufficient justification for not performing additional invasive procedures. β-trace protein is an alternative chemical marker that can be used in the detection of CSF. β-trace protein is produced by the meninges and choroid plexus and is released into CSF. It has 91% to 100% sensitivity and 86% to 100% specificity to detect CSF [1, 81–85]. β-2 transferrin and β-trace protein are limited by the prolonged analytical turnaround time for confirmation of the test [1]. Glucose testing of suspected CSF rhinorrhea has been found to be non-specific and insensitive and not routinely recommended in the diagnosis of CSF rhinorrhea [2, 86].
3. *High-resolution computed tomography (CT) scans*, that is, CT imaging with 1–2 mm axial sections and coronal and sagittal reconstructions of the paranasal sinuses, should be the first-line investigation for all patients with suspected or confirmed CSF rhinorrhea for diagnosis and surgical planning [87, 88]. High-resolution CT has a sensitivity of 87% to 92% and a specificity of 100% [2, 76, 88, 89]. Magnetic resonance (MR) cisternography has a sensitivity and specificity of 56% to 94% and 57% to 100%, respectively [2, 76, 88, 90–100]. At a cost of $504 United States Dollars (USD) per study, high-resolution CT is a more cost-effective localization tool compared to MR cisternography (with a cost of $913 USD) and should be used in the initial screen for CSF leak [2, 76]. In 45 clinically suspected CSF rhinorrhea patients, Shetty et al. [88] found that combined MR cisternography and plain high-resolution CT, with at least one study considered positive on the basis of detection of CSF leak, sensitivity was 95%, and specificity was 100%. CT cisternography is a valid option for CSF leak localiza-

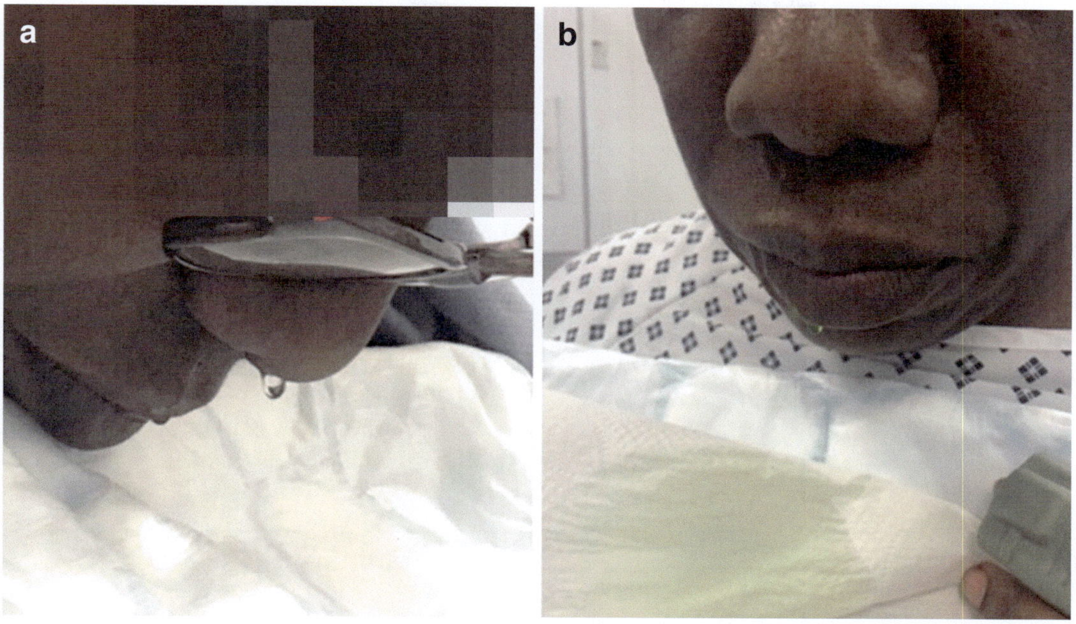

Fig. 8.2 Direct visualization of cerebrospinal fluid leak with the use of intrathecal fluorescein. (**a**) Clear rhinorrhea with dependent-positioning prior to intrathecal fluorescein injection; (**b**) fluorescein-stained cerebrospinal fluid visualized following intrathecal fluorescein injection

tion, with a sensitivity of 33% to 100% and a specificity of 94%. It remains more expensive ($1800 USD) to its counterparts suggesting high-resolution CT and/or MR cisternography should be considered first in the diagnostic workup of CSF rhinorrhea patients [2, 76, 89, 91, 93, 95, 98, 101, 102]. Both forms of cisternography require the leak to be active at the time of the imaging which is not always practical.

4. In patients with high clinical suspicion of CSF rhinorrhea, for instance, patients with recurrent meningitis, with negative radiographic findings, *diagnostic intrathecal assessments* can be considered to confirm the presence of CSF rhinorrhea. These studies have demonstrated utility in patients with CSF that is too slow or intermittent to produce a sufficient sample for cytologic testing [2]. An intrathecal agent, in the form of a radioactive tracer, injected intrathecally via lumbar puncture, while nasal pledgets are in place, or fluorescein dye [2]. Positive nasal pledgets for the intrathecal agent are confirmatory of a CSF leak and establish laterality of the fistula. Radionuclide cisternography has a sensitivity of 76% to 100% and a specificity of 100% [76, 89, 103]. However, as an invasive procedure at a cost of $2800 USD, repeating a β-2 transferrin can be considered before embarking on radionuclide cisternography [2, 76]. Intrathecal fluorescein is almost exclusively used in the intraoperative localization of CSF leaks when the source is unclear and as an adjunctive tool in their successful closure [104–106]. As CSF is translucent and the operative field is frequently blurred with blood and secretions, it may be difficult to recognize small CSF leaks [104–107]. Intrathecal fluorescein can provide direct endoscopic visualization of the CSF leak (Fig. 8.2). The protocol for intrathecal fluorescein use in this setting varies by hospital and department. Using a similar protocol to that described by Stammberger et al. [108] (Table 8.2), filtered fluorescein is diluted in the patient's own CSF and injected via lumbar puncture approximately 60 to 90 min before surgery while the patient remains in a reverse

Table 8.2 Protocol for intrathecal fluorescein use to minimize reaction

- Day before operation
  - Skin test patient with fluorescein (2% eye drop preparation)
- Day of operation
  - Ten milligrams intramuscularly of chlorpheniramine followed by (5 min later) intravenous dose of 0.25 mL of 10% fluorescein diluted to 0.5 mL with water for injection
  - Approximately 20 min later, an intrathecal injection of 0.2 mL of 10% of sterile and filtered fluorescein made up to 7.5 mL with CSF (25G spinal needle)
  - Patient then goes to the recovery area with the head of bed tipped down for approximately 1.5 h. Patient returns for normal general anesthetic for endoscopic sinus surgery

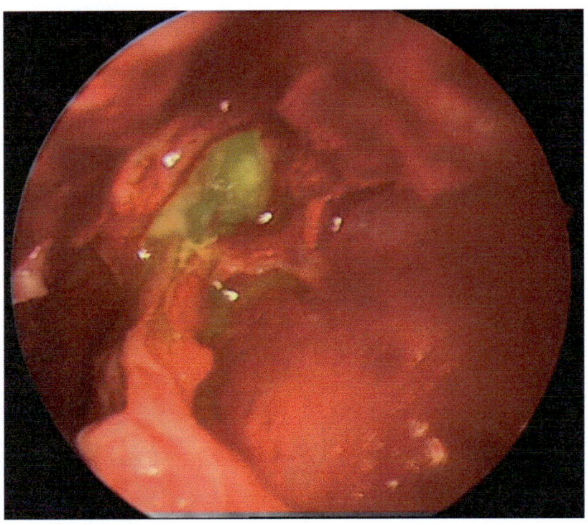

Fig. 8.3 A skull base defect localized intraoperatively after intrathecal fluorescein injection. The fluorescein-stained cerebrospinal fluid assists in diagnostic confirmation and successful closure of the defect

trendelenburg position [7, 59, 107, 108]. The nasal cavity, postnasal space, and middle ear should be carefully examined for the fluorescein dye to localize the source of the fistula. The fluorescent, green appearance of fluorescein often does not require visual augmentation intraoperatively (Fig. 8.3); however, a yellow light or blue light filter, sensitive to dilutions of up to 1 in ten million parts, can assist in localization of fluorescein-colored CSF [7, 59, 106, 109]. Intrathecal fluorescein use is generally considered safe when sterilized, filtered, and used in small concentrations, although maximum dose remains controversial [59, 107]. Reports have described complications, such as seizures, radicular symptoms, transient paresis, and death when inappropriate concentrations or types of fluorescein are utilized [59, 104, 107, 110–114]. It is important that the benefits and small but important risk of intrathecal fluorescein use are discussed with patients, and written consent obtained if appropriate. Intrathecal fluorescein has a sensitivity of 73% and specificity of 100% [2, 109]. However, its use in this setting remains off-label without clear guidelines [2].

8.4 Summary

Accurate confirmation of the presence of a CSF leak and localization of the skull base defect is essential for optimal management of CSF rhinorrhea. Initial evaluation relies on a thorough clinical history, physical examination, and endoscopic evaluation to rule out diseases that can mimic CSF rhinorrhea and identify the etiopathogenesis of the skull base defect. Cytologic studies are reliable as are specific markers in the initial screen of CSF rhinorrhea. High-resolution CT provides a detailed anatomical survey of the skull base to guide localization and surgical planning. MR cisternography is a useful tool for evaluation of intracranial pathology that should be addressed in the management of the CSF leak. As these tests are reliant on a constant flow of CSF for diagnosis, intrathecal agents can be considered in the diagnosis of intermittent or slow CSF leaks.

References

1. Citardi MJ, Fakhri S. Cerebrospinal fluid rhinorrhea. In: Cummings otolaryngology [Internet], vol. 6. Philadelphia: Elsevier Health Sciences; 2015. p. 803–15.
2. Oakley GM, Alt JA, Schlosser RJ, Harvey RJ, Orlandi RR. Diagnosis of cerebrospinal fluid rhinorrhea: an evidence-based review with recommendations. Int Forum Allergy Rhinol. 2016;6(1):8–16.
3. Knight A. The differential diagnosis of rhinorrhea. J Allergy Clin Immunol. 1995;95(5 Pt 2):1080–3.

4. Daudia A, Biswas D, Jones NS. Risk of meningitis with cerebrospinal fluid rhinorrhea. Ann Otol Rhinol Laryngol. 2007;116(12):902–5.
5. Eljamel MS, Foy PM, Swift AC, MacFarlane IA. Cerebrospinal fluid rhinorrhea occurring in long-term bromocriptine treatment for macroprolactinomas. Surg Neurol. 1992;38(4):321.
6. Nandapalan V, Watson ID, Swift AC. Beta-2-transferrin and cerebrospinal fluid rhinorrhoea. Clin Otolaryngol Allied Sci. 1996;21(3):259–64.
7. Lund VJ. Endoscopic management of cerebrospinal fluid leaks. Am J Rhinol. 2002;16(1):17–23.
8. Bousquet J, Khaltaev N, Cruz AA, Denburg J, Fokkens WJ, Togias A, et al. Allergic Rhinitis and its Impact on Asthma (ARIA) 2008 update (in collaboration with the World Health Organization, GA(2)LEN and AllerGen). Allergy. 2008;63(Suppl 86):8–160.
9. Hellings PW, Klimek L, Cingi C, Agache I, Akdis C, Bachert C, et al. Non-allergic rhinitis: position paper of the european academy of allergy and clinical immunology. Allergy. 2017;72(11):1657–65.
10. Wise SK, Lin SY, Toskala E, Orlandi RR, Akdis CA, Alt JA, et al. International consensus statement on allergy and rhinology: allergic rhinitis. Int Forum Allergy Rhinol. 2018;8(2):108–352.
11. Druce HM. Allergic and nonallergic rhinitis. In: Middleton EM, Yunginger JW, Busse WW, editors. Allergy: principles and practice. St. Louis, MO: Mosby Year-Book; 1998. p. 1005–16.
12. Wang DY, Raza MT, Gordon BR. Control of nasal obstruction in perennial allergic rhinitis. Curr Opin Allergy Clin Immunol. 2004;4(3):165–70.
13. Bousquet J, Van Cauwenberge P, Khaltaev N, Aria Workshop Group, World Health Organization. Allergic rhinitis and its impact on asthma. J Allergy Clin Immunol. 2001;108(5 Suppl):S147–334.
14. Torres-Borrego J, Molina-Teran AB, Montes-Mendoza C. Prevalence and associated factors of allergic rhinitis and atopic dermatitis in children. Allergol Immunopathol (Madr). 2008;36(2):90–100.
15. Wood RA, Phipatanakul W, Hamilton RG, Eggleston PA. A comparison of skin prick tests, intradermal skin tests, and RASTs in the diagnosis of cat allergy. J Allergy Clin Immunol. 1999;103(5 Pt 1):773–9.
16. Nelson HS, Oppenheimer J, Buchmeier A, Kordash TR, Freshwater LL. An assessment of the role of intradermal skin testing in the diagnosis of clinically relevant allergy to timothy grass. J Allergy Clin Immunol. 1996;97(6):1193–201.
17. Smart BA. Allergy testing using in vivo and in vitro techniques. Immunol Allergy Clin N Am. 1999;19(1):35–45.
18. Kim BJ, Mun SK. Objective measurements using the skin prick test in allergic rhinitis. Arch Otolaryngol Head Neck Surg. 2010;136(11):1104–6.
19. Joe SA, Liu JZ. Nonallergic rhinitis. In: Cummings otolaryngology [Internet], vol. 6. Philadelphia: Elsevier Health Sciences; 2015. p. 691–701.
20. Philip G, Togias AG, Nonallergic rhinitis. Pathophysiology and models for study. Eur Arch Otorhinolaryngol. 1995;252(Suppl 1):S27–32.
21. Georgitis JW. Prevalence and differential diagnosis of chronic rhinitis. Curr Allergy Asthma Rep. 2001;1(3):202–6.
22. Settipane RA, Charnock DR. Epidemiology of rhinitis: allergic and nonallergic. Clin Allergy Immunol. 2007;19:23–34.
23. Settipane RA, Kaliner MA. Chapter 14: nonallergic rhinitis. Am J Rhinol Allergy. 2013;27(3):48–51.
24. Fokkens WJ, Lund VJ, Mullol J, Bachert C, Alobaidi I, Baroody F, et al. EPOS 2012: European position paper on rhinosinusitis and nasal polyps 2012. A summary for otorhinolaryngologists. Rhinology. 2012;50(1):1–12.
25. Rosenfeld RM, Piccirillo JF, Chandrasekhar SS, Brook I, Ashok Kumar K, Kramper M, et al. Clinical practice guideline (update): adult sinusitis. Otolaryngol Head Neck Surg. 2015;152(2 Suppl):S1–S39.
26. Gautrin D, Desrosiers M, Castano R. Occupational rhinitis. Curr Opin Allergy Clin Immunol. 2006;6(2):77–84.
27. Heederik D, Venables KM, Malmberg P, Hollander A, Karlsson AS, Renstrom A, et al. Exposure-response relationships for work-related sensitization in workers exposed to rat urinary allergens: results from a pooled study. J Allergy Clin Immunol. 1999;103(4):678–84.
28. Bousquet J, Flahault A, Vandenplas O, Ameille J, Duron JJ, Pecquet C, et al. Natural rubber latex allergy among health care workers: a systematic review of the evidence. J Allergy Clin Immunol. 2006;118(2):447–54.
29. Gautrin D, Ghezzo H, Infante-Rivard C, Malo JL. Incidence and host determinants of work-related rhinoconjunctivitis in apprentice pastry-makers. Allergy. 2002;57(10):913–8.
30. Malo JL. Occupational rhinitis and asthma due to metal salts. Allergy. 2005;60(2):138–9.
31. EAACI Task Force on Occupational Rhinitis, Moscato G, Vandenplas O, Gerth Van Wijk R, Malo JL, Quirce S, et al. Occupational rhinitis. Allergy. 2008;63(8):969–80.
32. Raphael G, Raphael MH, Kaliner M. Gustatory rhinitis: a syndrome of food-induced rhinorrhea. J Allergy Clin Immunol. 1989;83(1):110–5.
33. Settipane RA. Other causes of rhinitis: mixed rhinitis, rhinitis medicamentosa, hormonal rhinitis, rhinitis of the elderly, and gustatory rhinitis. Immunol Allergy Clin N Am. 2011;31(3):457–67.
34. Caparroz FA, Gregorio LL, Bongiovanni G, Izu SC, Kosugi EM. Rhinitis and pregnancy: literature review. Braz J Otorhinolaryngol. 2016;82(1):105–11.
35. Incaudo GA, Takach P. The diagnosis and treatment of allergic rhinitis during pregnancy and lactation. Immunol Allergy Clin N Am. 2006;26(1):137–54.

36. Namazy JA, Schatz M. Diagnosing rhinitis during pregnancy. Curr Allergy Asthma Rep. 2014;14(9):458.
37. Varghese M, Glaum MC, Lockey RF. Drug-induced rhinitis. Clin Exp Allergy. 2010;40(3):381–4.
38. Szczeklik A, Nizankowska E. Clinical features and diagnosis of aspirin induced asthma. Thorax. 2000;55(Suppl 2):S42–4.
39. Szczeklik A, Sanak M, Niżankowska-Mogilnicka E, Kielbasa B. Aspirin intolerance and the cyclooxygenase-leukotriene pathways. Curr Opin Pulm Med. 2004;10(1):51–6.
40. Barnes PJ. Neurogenic inflammation in the airways. Respir Physiol. 2001;125(1–2):145–54.
41. Zucker SM, Barton BM, McCoul ED. Management of rhinitis medicamentosa: a systematic review. Otolaryngol Head Neck Surg. 2019;160(3):429–38.
42. Graf P. Adverse effects of benzalkonium chloride on the nasal mucosa: allergic rhinitis and rhinitis medicamentosa. Clin Ther. 1999;21(10):1749–55.
43. Mortuaire G, de Gabory L, Francois M, Masse G, Bloch F, Brion N, et al. Rebound congestion and rhinitis medicamentosa: nasal decongestants in clinical practice. Critical review of the literature by a medical panel. Eur Ann Otorhinolaryngol Head Neck Dis. 2013;130(3):137–44.
44. Passali D, Salerni L, Passali GC, Passali FM, Bellussi L. Nasal decongestants in the treatment of chronic nasal obstruction: efficacy and safety of use. Expert Opin Drug Saf. 2006;5(6):783–90.
45. Graf P. Rhinitis medicamentosa: a review of causes and treatment. Treat Respir Med. 2005;4(1):21–9.
46. Hall LJ, Jackson RT. Effects of alpha and beta adrenergic agonists on nasal blood flow. Ann Otol Rhinol Laryngol. 1968;77(6):1120–30.
47. Bateman N, Jones NS. Rhinorrhoea feigning cerebrospinal fluid leak: nine illustrative cases. J Laryngol Otol. 2000;114(6):462–4.
48. Wang SH, Wang HW, Wang JY. Effects of cocaine on human nasal mucosa. Eur Arch Otorhinolaryngol. 1993;250(4):245–8.
49. Hakansson K, von Buchwald C, Thomsen SF, Thyssen JP, Backer V, Linneberg A. Nonallergic rhinitis and its association with smoking and lower airway disease: a general population study. Am J Rhinol Allergy. 2011;25(1):25–9.
50. Lieberman P. The role of antihistamines in the treatment of vasomotor rhinitis. World Allergy Organ J. 2009;2(8):156–61.
51. Smith PK, Collins J. Olopatadine 0.6% nasal spray protects from vasomotor challenge in patients with severe vasomotor rhinitis. Am J Rhinol Allergy. 2011;25(4):e149–52.
52. Lieberman P, Meltzer EO, LaForce CF, Darter AL, Tort MJ. Two-week comparison study of olopatadine hydrochloride nasal spray 0.6% versus azelastine hydrochloride nasal spray 0.1% in patients with vasomotor rhinitis. Allergy Asthma Proc. 2011;32(2):151–8.
53. Meltzer EO. The treatment of vasomotor rhinitis with intranasal corticosteroids. World Allergy Organ J. 2009;2(8):166–79.
54. Naclerio R. Anticholinergic drugs in nonallergic rhinitis. World Allergy Organ J. 2009;2(8):162–5.
55. Banov CH, Lieberman P, Vasomotor Rhinitis Study Groups. Efficacy of azelastine nasal spray in the treatment of vasomotor (perennial nonallergic) rhinitis. Ann Allergy Asthma Immunol. 2001;86(1):28–35.
56. Gehanno P, Deschamps E, Garay E, Baehre M, Garay RP. Vasomotor rhinitis: clinical efficacy of azelastine nasal spray in comparison with placebo. ORL J Otorhinolaryngol Relat Spec. 2001;63(2):76–81.
57. Lieberman P, Kaliner MA, Wheeler WJ. Open-label evaluation of azelastine nasal spray in patients with seasonal allergic rhinitis and nonallergic vasomotor rhinitis. Curr Med Res Opin. 2005;21(4):611–8.
58. van de Heyning PH, van Haesendonck J, Creten W, Rombaut N. Effect of topical levocabastine on allergic and non-allergic perennial rhinitis. A double-blind study, levocabastine vs. placebo, followed by an open, prospective, single-blind study on beclomethasone. Allergy. 1988;43(5):386–91.
59. Lund VJ, Stammberger H, Nicolai P, Castelnuovo P, Beal T, Beham A, et al. European position paper on endoscopic management of tumours of the nose, paranasal sinuses and skull base. Rhinol Suppl. 2010;22:1–143.
60. Menasse-Palmer L, Bogdanow A, Marion RW. Choanal atresia. Pediatr Rev. 1995;16(12):475–6.
61. Samadi DS, Shah UK, Handler SD. Choanal atresia: a twenty-year review of medical comorbidities and surgical outcomes. Laryngoscope. 2003;113(2):254–8.
62. Teissier N, Kaguelidou F, Couloigner V, Francois M, Van Den Abbeele T. Predictive factors for success after transnasal endoscopic treatment of choanal atresia. Arch Otolaryngol Head Neck Surg. 2008;134(1):57–61.
63. Kirtane MV, Gautham K, Upadhyaya SR. Endoscopic CSF rhinorrhea closure: our experience in 267 cases. Otolaryngol Head Neck Surg. 2005;132(2):208–12.
64. Tebruegge M, Curtis N. Epidemiology, etiology, pathogenesis, and diagnosis of recurrent bacterial meningitis. Clin Microbiol Rev. 2008;21(3):519–37.
65. Buchanan RJ, Brant A, Marshall LR. Traumatic cerebrospinal fluid fistulas. In: Winn H, editor. Youmans neurological surgery. 5th ed. Philadelphia: Saunders; 2004. p. 5265–72.
66. Stankiewicz JA, Lal D, Connor M, Welch K. Complications in endoscopic sinus surgery for chronic rhinosinusitis: a 25-year experience. Laryngoscope. 2011;121(12):2684–701.
67. Schlosser RJ, Woodworth BA, Wilensky EM, Grady MS, Bolger WE. Spontaneous cerebrospinal fluid leaks: a variant of benign intracranial hypertension. Ann Otol Rhinol Laryngol. 2006;115(7):495–500.
68. Badia L, Loughran S, Lund V. Primary spontaneous cerebrospinal fluid rhinorrhea and obesity. Am J Rhinol. 2001;15(2):117–9.

69. Lay CM. Low cerebrospinal fluid pressure headache. Curr Treat Options Neurol. 2002;4(5):357–63.
70. Mokri B. Spontaneous low pressure, low CSF volume headaches: spontaneous CSF leaks. Headache. 2013;53(7):1034–53.
71. Scott S, Davenport R. Low pressure headaches caused by spontaneous intracranial hypotension. BMJ. 2014;349:g6219.
72. Dula DJ, Fales W. The 'ring sign': is it a reliable indicator for cerebral spinal fluid? Ann Emerg Med. 1993;22(4):718–20.
73. Sunder R, Tyler K. Basal skull fracture and the halo sign. CMAJ. 2013;185(5):416.
74. Meurman OH, Irjala K, Suonpaa J, Laurent B. A new method for the identification of cerebrospinal fluid leakage. Acta Otolaryngol. 1979;87(3–4):366–9.
75. Oberascher G, Arrer E. Efficiency of various methods of identifying cerebrospinal fluid in Oto- and rhinorrhea. ORL J Otorhinolaryngol Relat Spec. 1986;48(6):320–5.
76. Zapalac JS, Marple BF, Schwade ND. Skull base cerebrospinal fluid fistulas: a comprehensive diagnostic algorithm. Otolaryngol Head Neck Surg. 2002;126(6):669–76.
77. Marshall AH, Jones NS, Robertson IJ. An algorithm for the management of CSF rhinorrhoea illustrated by 36 cases. Rhinology. 1999;37(4):182–5.
78. Normansell DE, Stacy EK, Booker CF, Butler TZ. Detection of beta-2 transferrin in otorrhea and rhinorrhea in a routine clinical laboratory setting. Clin Diagn Lab Immunol. 1994;1(1):68–70.
79. Gorogh T, Rudolph P, Meyer JE, Werner JA, Lippert BM, Maune S. Separation of beta2-transferrin by denaturing gel electrophoresis to detect cerebrospinal fluid in ear and nasal fluids. Clin Chem. 2005;51(9):1704–10.
80. Warnecke A, Averbeck T, Wurster U, Harmening M, Lenarz T, Stover T. Diagnostic relevance of beta2-transferrin for the detection of cerebrospinal fluid fistulas. Arch Otolaryngol Head Neck Surg. 2004;130(10):1178–84.
81. Arrer E, Meco C, Oberascher G, Piotrowski W, Albegger K, Patsch W. beta-Trace protein as a marker for cerebrospinal fluid rhinorrhea. Clin Chem. 2002;48(6 Pt 1):939–41.
82. McCudden CR, Senior BA, Hainsworth S, Oliveira W, Silverman LM, Bruns DE, et al. Evaluation of high resolution gel beta(2)-transferrin for detection of cerebrospinal fluid leak. Clin Chem Lab Med. 2013;51(2):311–5.
83. Bachmann G, Nekic M, Michel O. Clinical experience with beta-trace protein as a marker for cerebrospinal fluid. Ann Otol Rhinol Laryngol. 2000;109(12 Pt 1):1099–102.
84. Petereit HF, Bachmann G, Nekic M, Althaus H, Pukrop R. A new nephelometric assay for beta-trace protein (prostaglandin D synthase) as an indicator of liquorrhea. J Neurol Neurosurg Psychiatry. 2001;71(3):347–51.
85. Schnabel C, Di Martino E, Gilsbach JM, Riediger D, Gressner AM, Kunz D. Comparison of beta2-transferrin and beta-trace protein for detection of cerebrospinal fluid in nasal and ear fluids. Clin Chem. 2004;50(3):661–3.
86. Chan DT, Poon WS, Ip CP, Chiu PW, goh KY. How useful is glucose detection in diagnosing cerebrospinal fluid leak? The rational use of CT and Beta-2 transferrin assay in detection of cerebrospinal fluid fistula. Asian J Surg. 2004;27(1):39–42.
87. Alobaidi I, Ensenat J, Rioja E, Enriquez K, Viscovich L, de Notaris M, et al. Management of cerebrospinal fluid leaks according to size. Our experience. Acta Otorrinolaringol Esp. 2014;65(3):162–9.
88. Shetty PG, Shroff MM, Sahani DV, Kirtane MV. Evaluation of high-resolution CT and MR cisternography in the diagnosis of cerebrospinal fluid fistula. AJNR Am J Neuroradiol. 1998;19(4):633–9.
89. Stone JA, Castillo M, Neelon B, Mukherji SK. Evaluation of CSF leaks: high-resolution CT compared with contrast-enhanced CT and radionuclide cisternography. AJNR Am J Neuroradiol. 1999;20(4):706–12.
90. Algin O, Hakyemez B, Gokalp G, Ozcan T, Korfali E, Parlak M. The contribution of 3D-CISS and contrast-enhanced MR cisternography in detecting cerebrospinal fluid leak in patients with rhinorrhoea. Br J Radiol. 2010;83(987):225–32.
91. Mostafa BE, Khafagi A. Combined HRCT and MRI in the detection of CSF rhinorrhea. Skull Base. 2004;14(3):157–62. Discussion 62.
92. Sillers MJ, Morgan CE, el Gammal T. Magnetic resonance cisternography and thin coronal computerized tomography in the evaluation of cerebrospinal fluid rhinorrhea. Am J Rhinol. 1997;11(5):387–92.
93. Tahir MZ, Khan MB, Bashir MU, Akhtar S, Bari E. Cerebrospinal fluid rhinorrhea: an institutional perspective from Pakistan. Surg Neurol Int. 2011;2:174.
94. Tuntiyatorn L, Laothamatas J. Evaluation of MR cisternography in diagnosis of cerebrospinal fluid fistula. J Med Assoc Thail. 2004;87(12):1471–6.
95. Goel G, Ravishankar S, Jayakumar PN, Vasudev MK, Shivshankar JJ, Rose D, et al. Intrathecal gadolinium-enhanced magnetic resonance cisternography in cerebrospinal fluid rhinorrhea: road ahead? J Neurotrauma. 2007;24(10):1570–5.
96. Gupta V, Goyal M, Mishra N, Gaikwad S, Sharma A. MR evaluation of CSF fistulae. Acta Radiol. 1997;38(4 Pt 1):603–9.
97. Rajeswaran R, Chandrasekharan A, Mohanty S, Murali K, Joseph S. Role of MR cisternography in the diagnosis of cerebrospinal fluid rhinorrhoea with diagnostic nasal endoscopy and surgical correlation. Indian J Radiol Imag. 2006;16(3):315–20.
98. Eberhardt KE, Hollenbach HP, Deimling M, Tomandl BF, Huk WJ. MR cisternography: a new method for the diagnosis of CSF fistulae. Eur Radiol. 1997;7(9):1485–91.

99. Ecin G, Oner AY, Tokgoz N, Ucar M, Aykol S, Tali T. T2-weighted vs. intrathecal contrast-enhanced MR cisternography in the evaluation of CSF rhinorrhea. Acta Radiol. 2013;54(6):698–701.
100. El Gammal T, Sobol W, Wadlington VR, Sillers MJ, Crews C, Fisher WS 3rd, et al. Cerebrospinal fluid fistula: detection with MR cisternography. AJNR Am J Neuroradiol. 1998;19(4):627–31.
101. Ozgen T, Tekkok IH, Cila A, Erzen C. CT cisternography in evaluation of cerebrospinal fluid rhinorrhea. Neuroradiology. 1990;32(6):481–4.
102. Payne RJ, Frenkiel S, Glikstein R, Mohr G. Role of computed tomographic cisternography in the management of cerebrospinal fluid rhinorrhea. J Otolaryngol. 2003;32(2):93–100.
103. Flynn BM, Butler SP, Quinn RJ, McLaughlin AF, Bautovich GJ, Morris JG. Radionuclide cisternography in the diagnosis and management of cerebrospinal fluid leaks: the test of choice. Med J Aust. 1987;146(2):82–4.
104. Messerklinger W. Nasal endoscopy: demonstration, localization and differential diagnosis of nasal liquorrhea. HNO. 1972;20(9):268–70.
105. Stammberger H, Greistorfer K, Wolf G, Luxenberger W. Surgical occlusion of cerebrospinal fistulas of the anterior skull base using intrathecal sodium fluorescein. Laryngo Rhino Otologie. 1997;76(10):595–607.
106. Wolf G, Greistorfer K, Stammberger H. Endoscopic detection of cerebrospinal fluid fistulas with a fluorescence technique. Report of experiences with over 925 cases. Laryngo Rhino Otologie. 1997;76(10):588–94.
107. Placantonakis DG, Tabaee A, Anand VK, Hiltzik D, Schwartz TH. Safety of low-dose intrathecal fluorescein in endoscopic cranial base surgery. Neurosurgery. 2007;61(3 Suppl):161–5. Discussion 5–6.
108. Stammberger H. Special problems. In: Hawke M, editor. Functional endoscopic sinus surgery: the Messerklinger technique. Philadelphia: BC Decker; 1991.
109. Seth R, Rajasekaran K, Benninger MS, Batra PS. The utility of intrathecal fluorescein in cerebrospinal fluid leak repair. Otolaryngol Head Neck Surg. 2010;143(5):626–32.
110. Keerl R, Weber RK, Draf W, Wienke A, Schaefer SD. Use of sodium fluorescein solution for detection of cerebrospinal fluid fistulas: an analysis of 420 administrations and reported complications in Europe and the United States. Laryngoscope. 2004;114(2):266–72.
111. Locatelli D, Rampa F, Acchiardi I, Bignami M, De Bernardi F, Castelnuovo P. Endoscopic endonasal approaches for repair of cerebrospinal fluid leaks: nine-year experience. Neurosurgery. 2006;58(4 Suppl 2):ONS-246-56. Discussion ONS-56-7.
112. Mahaley MS Jr, Odom GL. Complication following intrathecal injection of fluorescein. J Neurosurg. 1966;25(3):298–9.
113. Moseley JI, Carton CA, Stern WE. Spectrum of complications in the use of intrathecal fluorescein. J Neurosurg. 1978;48(5):765–7.
114. Wallace JD, Weintraub MI, Mattson RH, Rosnagle R. Status epilepticus as a complication of intrathecal fluorescein. Case report. J Neurosurg. 1972;36(5):659–60.

Part III

9 Conservative Management of CSF Leak

Camila Dassi, Manuel Bernal-Sprekelsen, and Richard Douglas

9.1 Introduction

Transnasal endoscopic surgery has revolutionized the management of cerebrospinal fluid (CSF) leaks over the last three decades. Surgery for this indication has evolved from neurosurgical open repairs, necessitating craniotomy and brain retraction that may produce significant morbidity and mixed results, to transnasal endoscopic repairs that are highly effective and almost free of complications.

As the barrier to perform transnasal endoscopic repairs has become lower, so has the role of conservative management of CSF leaks become relatively less. This chapter will briefly discuss the current state of nonsurgical management of CSF leaks. We feel that there are two clinical scenarios where medical management may have a significant role to play: low volume leaks immediately after nonsurgical head trauma, and as an adjuvant to surgical therapy when high flow leaks are being closed without a certainty of success [1].

CSF leakage resulting in intermittent or continuous watery rhinorrhea is usually associated with a bony skull base defect and disruption of the layers of the arachnoid, dura, and sinonasal mucosa [2]. CSF leaks are uncommon but may be associated with life-threatening complications such as meningitis, pneumocephalus, or intracranial abscess formation. Accordingly, each patient with a CSF leak requires careful and timely assessment and treatment (Fig. 9.1).

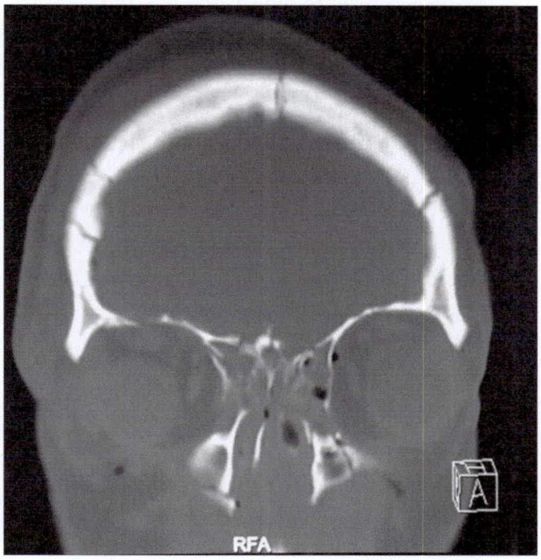

Fig. 9.1 A coronal CT of a patient with multiple fractures of the skull and clear rhinorrhea. It would be reasonable to treat the CSF leak conservatively in the early post-injury period

Identifying the underlying etiology and pathophysiology of CSF leaks is the key to accomplishing a successful outcome [3]. CSF leaks can be characterized into traumatic (including surgical and accidental trauma) and nontraumatic. The

C. Dassi · R. Douglas (✉)
Department of Surgery, The University of Auckland, Auckland, New Zealand

M. Bernal-Sprekelsen
University of Valencia Medical School, Valencia, Spain
e-mail: mbernal@clinic.cat

A. A. AlQahtani et al. (eds.), *CSF Rhinorrhea*, https://doi.org/10.1007/978-3-030-94781-1_9

nontraumatic group can be sub-classified into being associated with either normal or high intracranial pressure [4, 5]. Tumors, CSF obstruction, congenital lesions, benign intracranial hypertension (BIH) resulting in spontaneous CSF leak and hydrocephalus are the main etiologies.

When investigating the cause of clear rhinorrhea, beta-2 transferrin or beta-trace positivity on a sample of nasal fluid has both high sensitivity and specificity for confirming that the rhinorrhea is caused by CSF leakage. Thin slice CT scanning is generally the most helpful initial radiological investigation [6, 7]. MR scans are frequently required to determine the nature of the soft tissue around the site of leakage, as well as the presence of any other intracranial pathology: T2-weighted MR sequences are particularly helpful as they differentiate fluid from soft tissue so clearly.

Once a CSF leak has been confirmed and localized, the optimal management will be based on a number of variables. Except for those caused by blunt trauma, CSF leaks are usually managed surgically in order to avoid potentially severe complications [4, 8].

9.2 Indications of Conservative Management

Among all CSF leaks, more than 90% result from traumatic etiologies (80% nonsurgical and around 20% surgical). More than half of the nonsurgical traumatic leaks occur within the first 2 days after the injury, 70% within the first 7 days, and nearly all occur within the first 90 days [5, 9]. Some series have suggested that up to 30% of the patients with skull base fractures will develop a CSF leak during the first 3 months [10]. The sphenoid sinus (30%), frontal sinus (30%), and ethmoid/cribriform plate (23%) are the most common sites of CSF rhinorrhea following trauma [4, 5].

Traditionally, cases of CSF leak caused by trauma have been treated conservatively with a spontaneous closure rate after 1 week of up to 85% of cases [11]. Based on this observation, a trial of conservative management is generally recommended unless there is a very high flow leak, neurological deterioration, or other intracranial pathology [4]. Prompt surgical intervention is usually advised in cases of penetrating trauma, depressed skull base fractures, and impacted foreign bodies [10, 12].

Conservative management consists of a period of nonsurgical treatment that aims to reduce intracranial pressure (ICP) to decrease the flow of CSF through the dural defect. The measures include bed rest, head elevation to 30°, blood pressure control, and avoidance of nose blowing, coughing, straining, and vomiting [6].

It is usual for trials of conservative management to not last for not more than about a week at most due to an increasing risk of meningitis after the first week if closure is not achieved.

9.3 Modalities of Conservative Management

9.3.1 Pharmaceutical Treatment

Stool softeners, anti-emetics, and antitussives can be used during conservative treatment to reduce oscillations in the intracranial pressure associated with Valsalva maneuvers [5, 10].

9.3.1.1 Antibiotics

Randomized controlled trials have shown no clear reduction of meningitis risk by the prescribing of prophylactic antibiotics for patients with active CSF leaks [5, 11, 13]. Further, in a recent Cochrane review, no significant differences were found between antibiotic prophylaxis groups and control groups regarding meningitis rates, overall mortality, meningitis-related mortality, and the necessity of surgical repair in patients with CSF leakage [14].

Moreover, even when a conservative treatment is chosen in cases of traumatic CSF leak, the use of prophylactic antibiotics is not supported by the available data [14]. Therefore, antibiotic prophylaxis to prevent ascending bacterial meningitis in the presence of CSF leak is reserved for high-risk cases such as those associated with acute rhinosinusitis or contaminated wounds [5].

9.3.1.2 Acetazolamide

Acetazolamide is a diuretic that reduces the rate of production of CSF by the choroid plexus by up to half [15]. The inhibition of the carbonic anhydrase enzyme, which normally catalyzes the conversion of H_2O and CO_2 to HCO_3^- and H^+, is the primary mechanism of action of this drug [15].

Acetazolamide has a major role in cases of spontaneous CSF leak associated with elevated ICP [16, 17]. Once the leak has been repaired, a percentage of patients may then develop symptoms due to a postoperative elevation in ICP. Postsurgical long-term therapy can be prescribed in order to achieve better management of the ICP and the symptoms related to it. Some severe cases require ventriculoperitoneal shunting [16].

Regarding traumatic CSF leaks, acetazolamide has been used as an adjunct to decrease the volume of CSF. However, there is a lack of scientific evidence that supports its efficacy to improve the rates of spontaneous closure of the defect during the conservative management [16].

Acetazolamide therapy inevitably results in a metabolic acidosis, with an associated hypokalemia [16, 18]. Accordingly, it is suggested that patients on this medication have their plasma electrolyte levels checked periodically. Common side effects related to acetazolamide therapy include fatigue, abdominal pain, nausea, vomiting, and paresthesiae [15]. Further, care should be taken on the administration of acetazolamide in patients with impaired renal or hepatic function. Drug interactions with certain antibiotics, sodium bicarbonate, amphetamines, and salicylates have been documented [19].

9.3.2 Lumbar Drain

If low flow post-traumatic leaks do not stop spontaneously within a couple of days, then insertion of a lumbar drain and controlled drainage of CSF (5–10 mL/h) may be helpful. Recently, a study showed that insertion of a lumbar drain 48 h after injury had a positive impact on decreasing the amount of days with active leak compared to the non-drained group [10]. Subsequently, however, there was no significant difference in recurrence of leakage and incidence of meningitis between the two groups.

Lumbar drains in the context of a CSF leak are a two edged sword. Optimal drainage decreases CSF pressure and reduces flow across the dural opening to encourage its closure. However, with excessive drainage the flow can be reversed, exposing the patient to the risks of pneumocephalus and contamination of the meningeal space with nasal bacteria [20]. Lumbar drains require continuous monitoring by experienced nurses in a neurosurgical intensive care ward. Continuous sampling and protein and glucose measurements, cell count, and cultures of the CSF are required to detect meningitis quickly should it develops [5]. Complications related to the lumbar drain include headaches, pneumocephalus, cerebral herniation, meningitis, seizures, and stroke [10].

There are a few absolute contraindications of lumbar drain placement such as the presence of infected skin over the puncture site and radiological evidence of divergent pressures between the supratentorial and infratentorial compartments. Among the relative contraindications, ICP, brain abscess, and coagulopathy are the most important ones [21].

9.3.3 Immunization

The risk for an individual patient with a CSF leak of developing ascending meningitis is difficult to determine as it depends on the etiology and flow of the leak. Some authors believe that the overall risk of developing meningitis in patients with persistent spontaneous CSF leak is as high as 19%, [22] and this risk may even be higher in cases of post-traumatic CSF leaks [23].

The potential for immunization against the most common bacterial pathogens of meningitis is a relatively recent advance in the management of CSF leaks [13]. Vaccines for the three most common pathogens associated with bacterial meningitis (*Streptococcus pneumoniae, Haemophilus influenzae,* and *Neisseria meningitidis*) [24] are given commonly as part of the immunization program for children, the elderly, or patients with co-morbidities in most developed countries. However, there have been limited published data regarding the use of vaccination specifically in the presence of a CSF leak [13]. Considering the high risk of meningitis and its potential sequela, it is reasonable to administer prophylaxis against meningitis pathogens in patients with proven CSF leaks [6].

9.3.3.1 Pneumococcal Vaccine

Several different types of pneumococcal vaccine are currently available in majority of the countries: 23-valent polysaccharide unconjugated vaccine (PPSV23) and a 7, 10, and 13 valent conjugated vaccines [25].

Pediatric Recommendations

The Advisory Committee on Immunization Practices (ACIP) recommends the routine use of the 13-valent vaccine (PCV13) for all children aged less than 6 years and for children aged 6–18 years with immunocompromising conditions, including CSF leak [25].

Adult Recommendations

Regarding adults, the ACIP recommends PPSV23 vaccination among all adults aged ≥65 years and for adults at high risk aged 19–64 years at the time of diagnosis of the high-risk condition. Extended protection might be given through use of both pneumococcal vaccines (PPSV23 and PCV13) [26].

9.3.3.2 Meningococcal and Haemophilus Vaccine

The impact of immunization with *N. meningitis* and *H. influenzae* on the prevalence of meningitis associated with CSF leak is not well documented. However, taking into account the safety of those vaccines and the potentially fatal outcomes of bacterial meningitis it is prudent to encourage the immunization for both pathogens in all patients with a CSF leak [13].

9.4 Risk of Meningitis During Conservative Treatment

The risk of ascending meningitis is one of the biggest concerns related to CSF leak and its repair. During the first 24 h after injury, the risk of meningitis is estimated in 0.6%, rising to 5–11% seven days and to 55–88% after that period [6].

After a traumatic CSF leak, the cumulative risk of suffering bacterial meningitis has been estimated to be more than 85% over a 10-year period. The recurrence of CSF leakage after initial spontaneous cessation was 7% and meningitis was recurrent in 30.6% [27]. Less common complications, such as pneumocephalus and intracranial abscesses, can occur in patients with CSF leak [16, 22].

The rate of meningitis reflects a number of different factors including the duration of the CSF leak, the location of the defect on the skull base, and the presence of acute rhinosinusitis. It has been showed that post-traumatic CSF leaks that last more than a week are related to an increased risk of meningitis [5]. Further, there is a significantly increased incidence of ascending meningitis noted during the long-term follow-up of patients managed conservatively, even when leak cessation is achieved within the first 7 days after trauma [5, 23, 28]. Bacterial meningitis remains a risk up to 20 years after traumatic CSF leaks [29]. Close observation of clinical signs and symptoms of meningitis such as fever, altered mental status, headache, and nuchal rigidity must be prioritized during the watchful period. In case of suspected meningitis, empiric antimicrobial therapy should be started once blood cultures have been obtained and prior to head CT. Following this, a head CT scan should be performed to exclude other intracranial complications and, if there is no contraindication, a lumbar puncture for CSF sampling should be done [30].

9.5 Indications of Surgical Intervention

Surgical closure provides the most definitive treatment for CSF leaks. With the advances in minimally invasive endoscopic approaches leading to improved success rates and reduced surgical morbidity, conservative treatment of CSF leaks is reserved for very specific cases and should be interrupted after three to 7 days if there is no cessation of the leakage [6, 9, 23]. Some authors advocated that an early endoscopic repair, even in traumatic cases, should be considered as the optimal strategy to decrease the overall risk of meningitis [6].

Some other relative indications of surgical intervention in traumatic CSF leak include concomitant intracranial injuries that require surgery, fractures associated with defects more than 10 mm or with encephaloceles/meningoceles, and fractures with delayed onset presentation of CSF leak or associated with meningitis (after at least 7 days of the resolution of the infection) [6].

Iatrogenic CSF leaks that are recognized intraoperatively should be promptly repaired. In cases where the CSF leak is diagnosed postoperatively, the surgical repair should be done as soon as possible. It is also reasonable to start conservative measures, especially avoidance of nose blowing, coughing, and sneezing to prevent pneumocephalus, until the definitive treatment of the CSF leak is accomplished [5].

Small skull base defects, usually related to a low CSF flow, have been satisfactorily repaired using free grafts which in some cases can be used in association with different types of avascular materials. For larger defects, multilayered reconstruction often involving vascularized flaps is strongly recommended [31–33].

References

1. Mirza S, Thaper A, McClelland L, Jones NS. Sinonasal cerebrospinal fluid leaks: management of 97 patients over 10 years. Laryngoscope. 2005;115(10):1774–7.
2. Alobid I, Enseñat J, Rioja E, Enriquez K, Viscovich L, de Notaris M, et al. Management of cerebrospinal fluid leaks according to size. Our experience. Acta Otorrinolaringol Esp. 2014;65(3):162–9.
3. DeConde AS, Suh JD, Ramakrishnan VR. Treatment of cerebrospinal fluid rhinorrhea. Curr Opin Otolaryngol Head Neck Surg. 2015;23(1):59–64.
4. Banks CA, Palmer JN, Chiu AG, O'Malley BW, Woodworth BA, Kennedy DW. Endoscopic closure of CSF rhinorrhea: 193 cases over 21 years. Otolaryngol Head Neck Surg. 2009;140(6):826–33.
5. Prosser JD, Vender JR, Solares CA. Traumatic cerebrospinal fluid leaks. Otolaryngol Clin N Am. 2011;44(4):857–73.
6. Phang SY, Whitehouse K, Lee L, Khalil H, McArdle P, Whitfield PC. Management of CSF leak in base of skull fractures in adults. Br J Neurosurg. 2016;30(6):596–604.
7. Oakley GM, Alt JA, Schlosser RJ, Harvey RJ, Orlandi RR. Diagnosis of cerebrospinal fluid rhinorrhea: an evidence-based review with recommendations. Int Forum Allergy Rhinol. 2016;6(1):8–16.
8. Woodworth BA, Prince A, Chiu AG, Cohen NA, Schlosser RJ, Bolger WE, et al. Spontaneous CSF leaks: a paradigm for definitive repair and management of intracranial hypertension. Otolaryngol Head Neck Surg. 2008;138(6):715–20.
9. Oh J-W, Kim S-H, Whang K. Traumatic cerebrospinal fluid leak: diagnosis and management. Korean J Neurotrauma. 2017;13(2):63–7.
10. Albu S, Florian IS, Bolboaca SD. The benefit of early lumbar drain insertion in reducing the length of CSF leak in traumatic rhinorrhea. Clin Neurol Neurosurg. 2016;142:43–7.
11. Bell RB, Dierks EJ, Homer L, Potter BE. Management of cerebrospinal fluid leak associated with craniomaxillofacial trauma. J Oral Maxillofac Surg. 2004;62(6):676–84.
12. Yilmazlar S, Arslan E, Kocaeli H, Dogan S, Aksoy K, Korfali E, et al. Cerebrospinal fluid leakage complicating skull base fractures: analysis of 81 cases. Neurosurg Rev. 2006;29(1):64–71.
13. Rimmer J, Belk C, Lund VJ, Swift A, White P. Immunisations and antibiotics in patients with anterior skull base cerebrospinal fluid leaks. J Laryngol Otol. 2014;128(7):626–9.
14. Ratilal BO, Costa J, Pappamikail L, Sampaio C. Antibiotic prophylaxis for preventing meningitis in patients with basilar skull fractures. Cochrane Database Syst Rev. 2015;(4):CD004884.
15. Uldall M, Botfield H, Jansen-Olesen I, Sinclair A, Jensen R. Acetazolamide lowers intracranial pressure and modulates the cerebrospinal fluid secretion pathway in healthy rats. Neurosci Lett. 2017;03(645):33–9.
16. Tilak AM, Koehn H, Mattos J, Payne SC. Preoperative management of spontaneous cerebrospinal fluid rhinorrhea with acetazolamide: acetazolamide for spontaneous CSF leaks. Int Forum Allergy Rhinol. 2019;9(3):265–9.
17. Schlosser RJ, Wilensky EM, Grady MS, Palmer JN, Kennedy DW, Bolger WE. Cerebrospinal fluid pressure monitoring after repair of cerebrospinal fluid leaks. Otolaryngol Head Neck Surg. 2004;130(4):443–8.
18. Schlosser RJ, Bolger WE. Nasal cerebrospinal fluid leaks: critical review and surgical considerations. Laryngoscope. 2004;114(2):255–65.
19. Saito H, Ogasawara K, Suzuki T, Kuroda H, Kobayashi M, Yoshida K, et al. Adverse effects of intravenous acetazolamide administration for evaluation of cerebrovascular reactivity using brain perfusion single-photon emission computed tomography in patients

with major cerebral artery steno-occlusive diseases. Neurol Med Chir (Tokyo). 2011;51(7):479–83.
20. Pepper J-P, Lin EM, Sullivan SE, Marentette LJ. Perioperative lumbar drain placement: an independent predictor of tension pneumocephalus and intracranial complications following anterior skull base surgery. Laryngoscope. 2011;121(3):468–73.
21. Tuettenberg J, Czabanka M, Horn P, Woitzik J, Barth M, Thomé C, et al. Clinical evaluation of the safety and efficacy of lumbar cerebrospinal fluid drainage for the treatment of refractory increased intracranial pressure. J Neurosurg. 2009;110(6):1200–8.
22. Daudia A, Biswas D, Jones NS. Risk of meningitis with cerebrospinal fluid rhinorrhea. Ann Otol Rhinol Laryngol. 2007;116(12):902–5.
23. Bernal-Sprekelsen M, Bleda-Vázquez C, Carrau RL. Ascending meningitis secondary to traumatic cerebrospinal fluid leaks. Am J Rhinol. 2000;14(4):257–9.
24. Brodie HA. Prophylactic antibiotics for posttraumatic cerebrospinal fluid fistulae. A meta-analysis. Arch Otolaryngol Head Neck Surg. 1997;123(7):749–52.
25. Centers for Disease Control and Prevention (CDC). Use of 13-valent pneumococcal conjugate vaccine and 23-valent pneumococcal polysaccharide vaccine among children aged 6-18 years with immunocompromising conditions: recommendations of the Advisory Committee on Immunization Practices (ACIP). MMWR Morb Mortal Wkly Rep. 2013;62(25):521–4.
26. Centers for Disease Control and Prevention (CDC). Use of 13-valent pneumococcal conjugate vaccine and 23-valent pneumococcal polysaccharide vaccine for adults with immunocompromising conditions: recommendations of the advisory committee on immunization practices (ACIP). MMWR Morb Mortal Wkly Rep. 2012;61(40):816–9.
27. Eljamel MS, Foy PM. Acute traumatic CSF fistulae: the risk of intracranial infection. Br J Neurosurg. 1990;4(5):381–5.
28. Bernal-Sprekelsen M, Alobid I, Mullol J, Trobat F, Tomás-Barberán M. Closure of cerebrospinal fluid leaks prevents ascending bacterial meningitis. Rhinology. 2005;43(4):277–81.
29. Schick B, Weber R, Kahle G, Draf W, Lackmann GM. Late manifestations of traumatic lesions of the anterior skull base. Skull Base Surg. 1997;7(2):77–83.
30. Tohge R, Takahashi M. Cerebrospinal fluid rhinorrhea and subsequent bacterial meningitis due to an atypical clival fracture. Intern Med. 2017;56(14):1911–4.
31. Thorp BD, Sreenath SB, Ebert CS, Zanation AM. Endoscopic skull base reconstruction: a review and clinical case series of 152 vascularized flaps used for surgical skull base defects in the setting of intraoperative cerebrospinal fluid leak. Neurosurg Focus. 2014;37(4):E4.
32. Archer JB, Sun H, Bonney PA, Zhao YD, Hiebert JC, Sanclement JA, et al. Extensive traumatic anterior skull base fractures with cerebrospinal fluid leak: classification and repair techniques using combined vascularized tissue flaps. J Neurosurg. 2016;124(3):647–56.
33. Hadad G, Bassagasteguy L, Carrau RL, Mataza JC, Kassam A, Snyderman CH, et al. A novel reconstructive technique after endoscopic expanded endonasal approaches: vascular pedicle nasoseptal flap. Laryngoscope. 2006;116(10):1882–6.

Traumatic CSF Leaks 10

Corinna G. Levine, Mohammad H. Al-Bar, and Adam J. Folbe

10.1 Introduction

Among the etiologies of cerebrospinal fluid (CSF) leak, trauma accounts for at least 95% of reported leaks [1, 2] A CSF leak develops only in areas where both a dural defect and a bony defect result from the trauma. Most injuries that cause fractures in the skull base bone do not result in a CSF leak [3, 4]. However, traumatic head injury is more likely to cause CSF leak in the anterior cranial fossa where the dura is more firmly attached to the skull base bone than in middle and posterior cranial fossa [5].

The presenting symptoms of a posttraumatic CSF leak include rhinorrhea, headache, hyposmia, and meningitis. A radiologic sign of a possible CSF leak could be pneumocephalus (Fig. 10.1). The timing of presentation of a CSF leak after trauma can be as early as 2 days or as late as several months. About half of the patients will present within 2 days of the injury, and 70% will present within the first 2 weeks [3]. The exact nature of early versus late presentations of a CSF leak is not well understood. Early leaks are often result from a direct fracture of the skull base and concomitant tear in the underlying dura. A late leak may be caused by the same damage, but the presentation can be delayed secondary to intranasal tissue edema that eventually resolves, a blood clot that gets absorbed, or a loss of tissue from the wound edges that eventually allows the fluid to leak [6, 7].

10.2 Causes of Traumatic CSF Leak

- The majority of CSF leaks are traumatic in nature. Injuries to the base of skull can be the result of accidental injury or intraoperative (iatrogenic) injury. The type of trauma can be helpful in determining the most likely location of CSF fistula (Fig. 10.2). While most CSF leaks present at the time of or soon after the injury, this presentation can be delayed. Thus, for patients presenting with clear rhinorrhea, it is important to review any recent traumatic and surgical history.

C. G. Levine (✉)
Rhinology and Skull Base Surgery, Department of Otolaryngology, University of Miami Miller School of Medicine, Miami, FL, USA
e-mail: cxl861@med.miami.edu

M. H. Al-Bar
Otolaryngology Department, King Fahd Hospital, Imam Abdulrahman Bin Faisal University, Al Khobar, Saudi Arabia

A. J. Folbe
Rhinology and Endoscopic Skull Base Surgery, Department of Otolaryngology Head and Neck Surgery, Oakland University William Beaumont School of Medicine, Royal Oak, MI, USA

A. A. AlQahtani et al. (eds.), *CSF Rhinorrhea*, https://doi.org/10.1007/978-3-030-94781-1_10

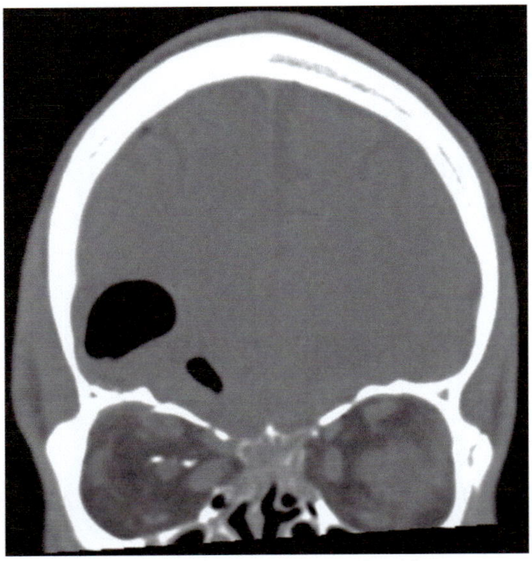

Fig. 10.1 Pneumocephalus in posttraumatic CSF leak

10.2.1 Accidental Injury

The most common causes of accidental traumatic injury resulting in CSF leak include motor vehicle accidents, falls, and assaults. These injuries can result in penetrating trauma with large disruptions in the skull base and CSF fistulas 8–9% of the time [8, 9]. More often, accidental injury results in closed head injuries or non-penetrating trauma, which make up the most common cause of traumatic CSF leak [10]. Up to 2% of all closed head trauma and 10–30% of adult skull base fractures result in traumatic CSF leak [3]. While penetrating trauma can occur in any location, non-penetrating trauma is most likely seen in the frontal sinuses and the cribriform plate [11]. Conservative management can be effective in a majority of skull base fractures [12].

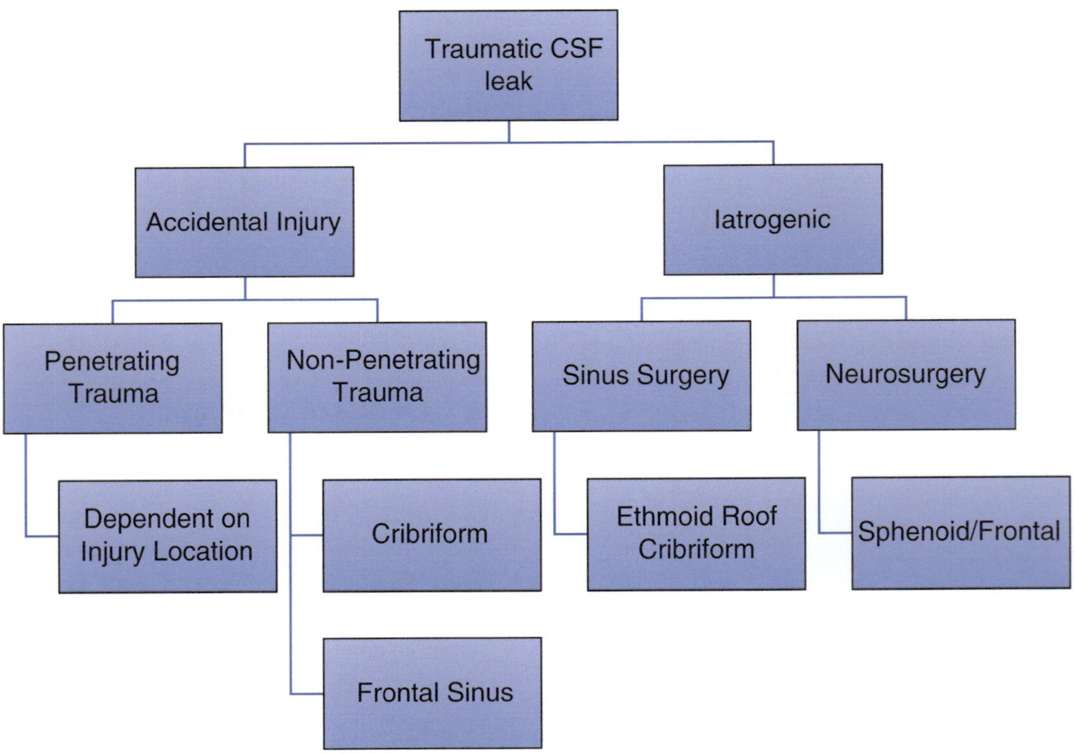

Fig. 10.2 Most likely site of skull base injury by traumatic etiology

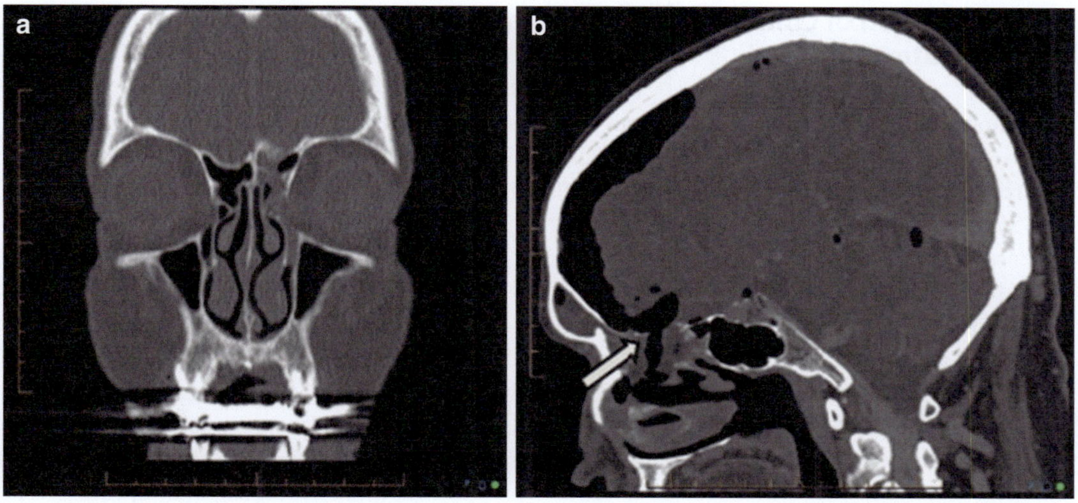

Fig. 10.3 Endoscopic balloon skull base trauma. (**a**) coronal CT view; (**b**) saggital CT view; arrow indicates site of ballon injury penetrating the skull base

10.2.2 Iatrogenic Injury

The number of traumatic CSF leaks resulting from iatrogenic injury appears to be rising and is becoming a more common cause of CSF leak [7]. Prior studies reporting that nearly 80% of traumatic CSF leaks resulted from non-surgical trauma [13], but recently several studies indicate that the proportion of traumatic CSF leaks resulting from iatrogenic injury is increasing [14]. The authors speculate that a main reason for change is likely the increasing volume of endoscopic sinus and skull base surgery. The field of endoscopic surgery is growing. With improvements in endoscopic techniques and new instrumentation, many more providers are opting to utilize endoscopic approaches and in some cases they have replaced open procedures at the standard first-line approach [15, 16]. While the incidence of injury during sinus surgery is rare, between 0.17% and 0.5% [17–19], the shear number of surgeries performed is high.

Traditionally, most injuries after sinus surgery occur in the ethmoid roof and the cribriform region [14]. Ethmoid roof injuries frequently occur at the junction of the ethmoid and sphenoid skull base where the angle of the skull base slopes inferiorly. Injuries to the cribriform often occur on the side of the surgeons dominant hand in the lateral lamella where the bone is thin and the surgeons hand will tend to move more medially when the patient's head is not well positioned. However, with the increase in sinus balloon use [20], we are beginning to see new injuries to the anterior skull base that do not always follow the historical pattern [21] (Sinus balloon injury Fig. 10.3).

Iatrogenic CSF rhinorrhea can also result after neurosurgical procedures. In particular, CSF leak occurs after approaching tumors of the skull base either endoscopically or via open approaches. Pituitary tumors are among the most common surgically resected tumors. In the last decade, transsphenoidal approaches have surpassed other options as the most common surgical approach to pituitary tumors [22]. Thus, it is not surprising that iatrogenic sphenoid CSF leak after transsphenoidal pituitary surgery (0–15% occurrence) [23] is the most common site of iatrogenic CSF leak after neurosurgical procedures.

10.3 Duration of Conservative Treatment

Many non-penetrating traumatic CSF leaks will resolve with conservative management. The literature supports spontaneous resolution of 50–85% of posttraumatic CSF leaks with 7 days of conservative management [3, 24, 25]. In contrast, the resolution of iatrogenic CSF leaks is much more variable with reports as low as 2% [26]. One reason for this difference may be related to the size of the defect and the amount of dural and meningeal disruption. Non-penetrating trauma often results in bony fracture lines at points of skull base weakness. In contrast, iatrogenic injury can range from small bony cracks to large defects involving dura and brain parenchyma [1].

10.3.1 Conservative Management

Conservative non-surgical management uses strict precautions designed to reduce a patients' tendency to increase their intracranial pressure and minimize stress on the site of healing. Patients are traditionally placed on bed rest with the head of the bed elevated to ≥30° to reduce pressure increases with standard movement. Additionally activities leading to increased intracranial pressure and valsalva are restricted/minimized. These include (Table 10.1) nose blowing, yawning, use of straws, sneezing, and coughing with the mouth open, avoiding straining with bowel movements (routine stool softeners), and ceasing use of incentive spirometry. Several studies have examined the frequency of CSF leak resolution with conservative medical management and report that 68–85% of patients have resolution of their CSF leak [24, 27]. The duration of conservative management recommended varies significantly from 3 days [28] to 7–10 days [3, 24, 29]. However, there is general agreement that after 7–10 days of conservative treatment additional interventional measures must be considered given at least eightfold increased risk of meningitis [27, 30, 31].

Table 10.1 Conservative CSF leak treatment

Bed rest
Head of bed ≥30°
Minimize increases of intracranial pressure
Minimize Valsalva

10.3.2 Lumbar Drain

Lumbar drain has been reported to be useful when strict conservative management fails [24, 32] and some practitioners use it as part of their initial non-surgical treatment algorithm. The goal of CSF leak drainage is reduction of pressure in the fistula without causing pneumocephalus or CSF hypovolemia. The usual recommendation is for drainage of 10–15 mL per hour [28]. The duration of CSF drainage varies widely from 3 to 10 days [24, 33–35].

In some studies the lumbar drain conservative CSF leak management has been reported to raise the success of non-surgical repair to near 90% [24]. A 2001 survey of otolaryngologists managing CSF leaks found that the majority utilized lumbar drains in their management [36]. A paucity of evidence exists to form clear recommendations on the use of drains after traumatic CSF leak and before surgical repair [37]. In contrast, there is a growing body of literature on the use of lumbar drains after skull base surgery, but many of the results are conflicting even among high level studies: A recent meta-analysis by D'Anza et al. [38] indicates there is no difference in the postoperative CSF leak rate after skull base surgery with or without a lumbar drain. In contrast, Zwagerman et al. [33] published a randomized trial of over 150 endoscopic skull base surgery patients treated with and without a lumbar drain after surgery, indicating that those who had a lumbar drain at their institution were threefold less likely to develop a CSF leak.

10.3.3 Acetazolamide

Acetazolamide is a carbonic anhydrase inhibitor that reduces CSF production by up to 48% [39].

Acetazolamide is often used in the management of spontaneous CSF leaks. Less is known about its role in traumatic CSF leaks. Gosal et al. conducted a single center randomized study of traumatic CSF leak patients treated with conservative management. Half the patients were given acetazolamide and the other half were not. Duration of leak was 5 days in the acetazolamide treated group and 4 days in the control group [40]. The adequacy of randomization is unclear from the manuscript, which may impact the significance of the results. While more work needs to be done investigating the role of acetazolamide, this initial study does not indicate significant benefit by adding acetazolamide in traumatic CSF leak patients.

10.3.4 Inappropriate for Conservative Treatment

Certain patients are not appropriate for conservative treatment. Those patients with penetrating injury, intracranial hematoma, traumatic meningocele or encephalocele, significant pneumocephalus, and large defects (Fig. 10.4) with low potential for healing should not be treated with conservative management and require prompt surgical intervention [2].

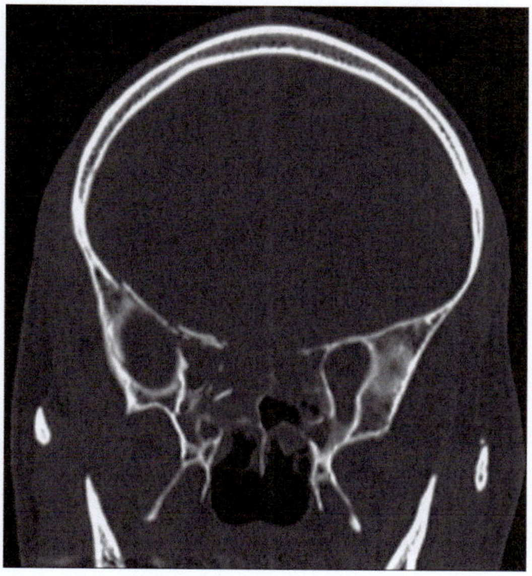

Fig. 10.4 Coronal CT of large skull base fracture

10.4 Management of ICU Patients with Skull Base Fracture

CSF leak caused by blunt trauma responds well to conservative treatment such as bed rest, head elevation, avoids straining, and/or lumber drain [6, 7, 27]. In those ICU patients with low level of consciousness who have the potential for a CSF leak, but without overt signs of skull base defect or CSF leak on examination, it may be reasonable to observe them. Reports of spontaneous resolution with conservative measures may be as high as 85% [41]. In patients with meningitis, providers need to have a high leve of suspicion of an undiagnosed CSF leak. The role of antibiotic prophylaxis in these patients is not clear and is discussed below. ICU patients with known and persistent CSF leak, despite conservative management, or with delayed discovery of a CSF leak the chance of spontaneous cessation is low and the risk of meningitis is increased. Thus, in this group operative intervention is usually required to address the CSF leak [42–44].

10.5 Risk of Meningitis

The risk of meningitis in skull base fracture and CSF leak is well known [45]. The risk increases when the onset of CSF leak after injury is delayed or with prolonged CSF leak duration. Studies report that the risk in the first day is 0.62% and can increase significantly in the first week and by over tenfold (8%) per week for the first 2 weeks [46, 47]. In nearly 20% of patients the first sign of a CSF leak is meningitis. It remains a major complication of skull base fracture and subsequent CSF leak with a mortality rate of 10%. In skull base fractures, delayed meningitis indicates a persistent communication (fistula) between the nasal cavity and the brain; hence, the need for surgical repair of defect in most cases. This persistence might be related to infection, posttraumatic hydrocephalus, and increase in intracranial pressure. In some instances, meningitis by itself can cause inflammation leading to healing of the dura and closure of the defect. Another significant factor that may contribute to increased risk of meningitis is the mechanism of injury. Penetrating injury has a significant higher risk of contamination, infection, meningitis, and brain abscess [8]. Iatrogenic CSF leak has a lower incidence of meningitis. Pathogens commonly isolated in meningitis among all types of CSF leaks include Streptococcus pneumoniae and Haemophilus influenza. In traumatic CSF leaks, there is not clear evidence of a single organism, but staph aureus appears to be one of the more common organisms.

10.6 Prophylactic Antibiotics

Prophylactic antibiotics treatment for CSF leaks remains an area of discussion. There is some controversy about the effectiveness of prophylactic antibiotics in the literature. In a number of systemic review articles and Cochrane systemic reviews, the studies report no significant decrease in risk of developing meningitis with usage of prophylactic antibiotics [25, 48–50]. Additionally, most evidence from randomized controled trials and other research literatures does not support the routine use of prophylactic antibiotics. These studies found no significant reduction in the risk of meningitis using prophylactic antibiotics for CSF leaks or in the immediate period after base of skull fractures [25, 48, 49, 51]. However, a few studies and review articles reported that the use of prophylactic antibiotic may decrease the risk of meningitis from 10% to 2.5% [52] and from 20% to 10% [47]. Perioperative antibiotics directed toward gram negative bacteria are used by some practitioners, particularly in situations where patients have nasal packing or a concurrent lumbar drain in place [14].

10.7 Recognition of Intraoperative Iatrogenic CSF Leak

The most important step in identifying a CSF leak is having a clinical suspicion. Most iatrogenic CSF leaks are present and recognizable at the time of surgery. A small portion is present in delayed fashion days to weeks or months after surgery as edema resolves.

10.7.1 Risk Assessment and Prevention

Certain features put patients at increased risk of iatrogenic CSF leak. Patients who have inadvertent injury to the skull base during sinus surgery are more likely to have a lower cribriform height relative to their ethmoid roof and greater slope of the skull base in either the coronal or sagittal planes [53, 54]. Skull base asymmetry, Onodi cells, and scarring are other features that should be noted prior to surgery. Patients with these features need to be identified preoperatively and extra care taken in these locations. This begins with the systematic assessment of imaging prior to surgery. All patients being taken for endoscopic sinus and skull base surgery should have commuted tomography images in coronal, sagittal, and axial views. The authors teach trainees the use of the "CLOSE" System [55] as a methodical means of reviewing preoperative imaging and areas of greatest risk of injury.

In addition to reviewing imaging anatomy in transsphenoidal pituitary surgery, other features have been shown to be associated with intraoperative and postoperative CSF leak including body mass index, hydrocephalus, suprasellar tumor extension, and craniopharyngioma [56, 57].

Intraoperatively many surgeons choose to use image guidance. The use of image guidance may be helpful, but has not been proven to prevent iatrogenic skull base injury [58–60]. Other important principals of prevention during surgery include proper patient positioning, systematic identification of anatomic landmarks, and good hemostasis.

10.7.2 Identification

The entirety of the exposed skull base should be carefully inspected prior to completing any sinus surgery. Particular attention must be paid to areas of anatomic propensity for injury as seen on preoperative imaging. Good hemostasis enables complete evaluation of these anatomic areas. Many iatrogenic leaks are identifiable during the surgery as a persistent leak of clear fluid in an area of disrupted skull base bone. The dura defect may or may not be fully visible. In the case of suspected CSF leak, the authors have the anesthetist perform a valsalva to 40 mmHG to evaluate the area of concern under high pressure.

If a CSF leak is identified, it is imperative to carefully assess the area of leak in order to determine size and depth, proximity to surrounding structures, signs of intracranial bleeding, and assess the integrity of the remaining skull base. If possible the defect should be repaired during the same surgery (see "Timing of Surgical Intervention" below). If it is not feasible to repair the injury at the time of surgery or there is high suspicion of an injury that could not be identified, then postoperative imaging is warranted to define the area of defect and evaluate for pneumocephalus or intracranial bleeding.

Imaging after injury is essential for localizing the injury site and defining injury extent. Imaging should also be used to rule out other significant complications necessitating immediate repair, such as severe pneumocephalus or intracranial hemorrhage. Finally, imaging can be used to help plan for operative repair. In a recent article, Oakley et al. performed an evidence based review on diagnosing CSF leaks. In cases where the skull base injury may not be obvious, a high resolution CT scan and intrathecal flourescene have a high success rate in identifying the location of the leak [47] (see Chap. 20 for more details).

10.8 Timing of Surgical Intervention of Iatrogenic CSF Leak

The timing of surgical intervention for iatrogenic CSF leak depends significantly on the timing of CSF leak recognition:

10.8.1 Intraoperatively

CSF leaks recognized at the time of surgery should be repaired during the same surgery. Immediate treatment minimizes the risk of infection and optimizes patient care (see Chap. 20 for details on repair options).

10.8.2 Delayed Recognition

CSF leaks that present after completion of surgical intervention should be treated as related to surgery until proven otherwise. These patients should be examined immediately and appropriate imaging performed (see Chap. 20). Large defects require immediate surgical intervention. For small defects, it may be reasonable to trial several days to a week of conservative treatment which has been reported successful in certain situations such as after pituitary surgery where reconstruction was performed despite the lack of an active leak intraoperatively [61]. Outside of these specific situations, the authors believe that iatrogenic CSF leaks that present in a delayed fashion are less likely to resolve with conservative treatment alone and require surgical intervention.

10.9 Special Considerations

10.9.1 CSF Otorhinorrhea

In rare cases patients with a normal endoscopic sinus exam and intact anterior skull base on imaging will present with reports of clear rhinorrhea and salty post-nasal drainage. It is important to remember that middle and posterior cranial fossa injury can also occur through sphenoid bone injury and temporal bone fractures. In these instances the CSF leak is actually coming from the middle ear space and exiting from the Eustachian tube. It is also possible that a temporal bone fracture can track from the greater wing of the sphenoid into the sphenoid sinus [62]. Management of these CSF leaks is outside the scope of this text, but it is important this possibility is recognized and investigated thoroughly.

10.9.2 Positive Pressure Ventilation

The use of positive pressure ventilation in patients with skull base defects or patients with recent repairs of skull base defects is not well studied. There is an increasing number of patients on positive pressure masks for treatment of obstructive sleep apnea. Some posttraumatic CSF leak patients may present with significant pneumocephalus and headaches if they start using CPAP machines.

The timing of resuming positive pressure ventilation in the postoperative period is somewhat controversial. In a recent study by Choi et al., the authors surveyed members of the North American Skull Base Society, about their recommendations on the timing of CPAP after surgery. The results of the surveyed showed that there is variability among the, and most patients started CPAP about 14–21 days after surgery [49].

References

1. Schlosser RJ, Bolger WE. Nasal cerebrospinal fluid leaks: critical review and surgical considerations. Laryngoscope. 2004;114(2):255–65.
2. Oh JW, Kim SH, Whang K. Traumatic cerebrospinal fluid leak: diagnosis and management. Korean J Neurotrauma. 2017;13(2):63–7.
3. Yilmazlar S, Arslan E, Kocaeli H, et al. Cerebrospinal fluid leakage complicating skull base fractures: analysis of 81 cases. Neurosurg Rev. 2006;29(1):64–71.
4. Fain J, Chabannes J, Peri G, Jourde J. Frontobasal injuries and csf fistulas. Attempt at an anatomoclinical classification. Therapeutic incidence. Neurochirurgie. 1975;21(6):493–506.
5. Abuabara A. Cerebrospinal fluid rhinorrhoea: diagnosis and management. Med Oral Patol Oral Cir Bucal. 2007;12(5):E397–400.
6. McCormack B, Cooper PR, Persky M, Rothstein S. Extracranial repair of cerebrospinal fluid fistulas: technique and results in 37 patients. Neurosurgery. 1990;27(3):412–7.
7. Hegazy HM, Carrau RL, Snyderman CH, Kassam A, Zweig J. Transnasal endoscopic repair of cerebrospinal fluid rhinorrhea: a meta-analysis. Laryngoscope. 2000;110(7):1166–72.
8. Aarabi B. Causes of infections in penetrating head wounds in the Iran-Iraq War. Neurosurgery. 1989;25(6):923–6.
9. Meirowsky AM, Caveness WF, Dillon JD, et al. Cerebrospinal fluid fistulas complicating missile wounds of the brain. J Neurosurg. 1981;54(1):44–8.
10. Zlab MK, Moore GF, Daly DT, Yonkers AJ. Cerebrospinal fluid rhinorrhea: a review of the literature. Ear Nose Throat J. 1992;71(7):314–7.
11. Choi D, Spann R. Traumatic cerebrospinal fluid leakage: risk factors and the use of prophylactic antibiotics. Br J Neurosurg. 1996;10(6):571–5.
12. Sivanandapanicker J, Nagar M, Kutty R, et al. Analysis and clinical importance of skull base fractures in adult patients with traumatic brain injury. J Neurosci Rural Pract. 2018;9(3):370–5.
13. Loew F, Pertuiset B, Chaumier EE, Jaksche H. Traumatic, spontaneous and postoperative CSF rhinorrhea. Adv Tech Stand Neurosurg. 1984;11:169–207.
14. Psaltis AJ, Schlosser RJ, Banks CA, Yawn J, Soler ZM. A systematic review of the endoscopic repair of cerebrospinal fluid leaks. Otolaryngol Head Neck Surg. 2012;147(2):196–203.
15. Kennedy DW. Technical innovations and the evolution of endoscopic sinus surgery. Ann Otol Rhinol Laryngol Suppl. 2006;196:3–12.
16. Govindaraj S, Adappa ND, Kennedy DW. Endoscopic sinus surgery: evolution and technical innovations. J Laryngol Otol. 2010;124(3):242–50.
17. Kennedy DW, Shaman P, Han W, Selman H, Deems DA, Lanza DC. Complications of ethmoidectomy: a survey of fellows of the American Academy of Otolaryngology-Head and Neck Surgery. Otolaryngol Head Neck Surg. 1994;111(5):589–99.
18. Ramakrishnan VR, Kingdom TT, Nayak JV, Hwang PH, Orlandi RR. Nationwide incidence of major complications in endoscopic sinus surgery. Int Forum Allergy Rhinol. 2012;2(1):34–9.
19. Bumm K, Heupel J, Bozzato A, Iro H, Hornung J. Localization and infliction pattern of iatrogenic skull base defects following endoscopic sinus surgery at a teaching hospital. Auris Nasus Larynx. 2009;36(6):671–6.
20. Chaaban MR, Baillargeon JG, Baillargeon G, Resto V, Kuo YF. Use of balloon sinuplasty in patients with chronic rhinosinusitis in the United States. Int Forum Allergy Rhinol. 2017;7(6):600–8.
21. Alam ES, Hadley JA, Justice JM, Casiano RR. Significant orbital and intracranial complications from balloon sinus dilation as a stand-alone and powered dissector-assisted procedure. Laryngoscope. 2018;128(11):2455–9.
22. Lobo B, Heng A, Barkhoudarian G, Griffiths CF, Kelly DF. The expanding role of the endonasal endoscopic approach in pituitary and skull base surgery: a 2014 perspective. Surg Neurol Int. 2015;6:82.
23. Kerr JT, Chu FW, Bayles SW. Cerebrospinal fluid rhinorrhea: diagnosis and management. Otolaryngol Clin N Am. 2005;38(4):597–611.
24. Bell RB, Dierks EJ, Homer L, Potter BE. Management of cerebrospinal fluid leak associated with craniomaxillofacial trauma. J Oral Maxillofac Surg. 2004;62(6):676–84.
25. Friedman JA, Ebersold MJ, Quast LM. Persistent posttraumatic cerebrospinal fluid leakage. Neurosurg Focus. 2000;9(1):e1.

26. Savva A, Taylor MJ, Beatty CW. Management of cerebrospinal fluid leaks involving the temporal bone: report on 92 patients. Laryngoscope. 2003;113(1):50–6.
27. Mincy JE. Posttraumatic cerebrospinal fluid fistula of the frontal fossa. J Trauma. 1966;6(5):618–22.
28. Dalgic A, Okay HO, Gezici AR, Daglioglu E, Akdag R, Ergungor MF. An effective and less invasive treatment of post-traumatic cerebrospinal fluid fistula: closed lumbar drainage system. Minim Invasive Neurosurg. 2008;51(3):154–7.
29. Arnold MA, Tatum SA 3rd. Frontal sinus fractures: evolving clinical considerations and surgical approaches. Craniomaxillofac Trauma Reconstr. 2019;12(2):85–94.
30. Leech PJ, Paterson A. Conservative and operative management for cerebrospinal-fluid leakage after closed head injury. Lancet. 1973;1(7811):1013–6.
31. Brodie HA. Prophylactic antibiotics for post-traumatic cerebrospinal fluid fistulae. A meta-analysis. Arch Otolaryngol Head Neck Surg. 1997;123(7):749–52.
32. Ziu M, Savage JG, Jimenez DF. Diagnosis and treatment of cerebrospinal fluid rhinorrhea following accidental traumatic anterior skull base fractures. Neurosurg Focus. 2012;32(6):E3.
33. Zwagerman NT, Wang EW, Shin SS, et al. Does lumbar drainage reduce postoperative cerebrospinal fluid leak after endoscopic endonasal skull base surgery? A prospective, randomized controlled trial. J Neurosurg. 2018;1-7
34. Albu S, Florian IS, Bolboaca SD. The benefit of early lumbar drain insertion in reducing the length of CSF leak in traumatic rhinorrhea. Clin Neurol Neurosurg. 2016;142:43–7.
35. Friedman JA, Ebersold MJ, Quast LM. Post-traumatic cerebrospinal fluid leakage. World J Surg. 2001;25(8):1062–6.
36. Senior BA, Jafri K, Benninger M. Safety and efficacy of endoscopic repair of CSF leaks and encephaloceles: a survey of the members of the American Rhinologic Society. Am J Rhinol. 2001;15(1):21–5.
37. Mourad M, Inman JC, Chan DM, Ducic Y. Contemporary trends in the management of post-traumatic cerebrospinal fluid leaks. Craniomaxillofac Trauma Reconstr. 2018;11(1):71–7.
38. D'Anza B, Tien D, Stokken JK, Recinos PF, Woodard TR, Sindwani R. Role of lumbar drains in contemporary endonasal skull base surgery: meta-analysis and systematic review. Am J Rhinol Allergy. 2016;30(6):430–5.
39. Carrion E, Hertzog JH, Medlock MD, Hauser GJ, Dalton HJ. Use of acetazolamide to decrease cerebrospinal fluid production in chronically ventilated patients with ventriculopleural shunts. Arch Dis Child. 2001;84(1):68–71.
40. Gosal JS, Gurmey T, Kursa GK, Salunke P, Gupta SK. Is acetazolamide really useful in the management of traumatic cerebrospinal fluid rhinorrhea? Neurol India. 2015;63(2):197–201.
41. Phang SY, Whitehouse K, Lee L, Khalil H, McArdle P, Whitfield PC. Management of CSF leak in base of skull fractures in adults. Br J Neurosurg. 2016;30(6):596–604.
42. Manelfe C, Cellerier P, Sobel D, Prevost C, Bonafe A. Cerebrospinal fluid rhinorrhea: evaluation with metrizamide cisternography. AJR Am J Roentgenol. 1982;138(3):471–6.
43. Talamonti G, Fontana R, Villa F, et al. "High risk" anterior basal skull fractures. Surgical treatment of 64 consecutive cases. J Neurosurg Sci. 1995;39(3):191–7.
44. Eljamel MS, Foy PM. Post-traumatic CSF fistulae, the case for surgical repair. Br J Neurosurg. 1990;4(6):479–83.
45. Jones NS, Becker DG. Advances in the management of CSF leaks. BMJ. 2001;322(7279):122–3.
46. Lin DT, Lin AC. Surgical treatment of traumatic injuries of the cranial base. Otolaryngol Clin N Am. 2013;46(5):749–57.
47. Brodie HA, Thompson TC. Management of complications from 820 temporal bone fractures. Am J Otol. 1997;18(2):188–97.
48. Ratilal BO, Costa J, Sampaio C, Pappamikail L. Antibiotic prophylaxis for preventing meningitis in patients with basilar skull fractures. Cochrane Database Syst Rev. 2011;(8):CD004884.
49. Ratilal BO, Costa J, Pappamikail L, Sampaio C. Antibiotic prophylaxis for preventing meningitis in patients with basilar skull fractures. Cochrane Database Syst Rev. 2015;(4):CD004884.
50. Villalobos T, Arango C, Kubilis P, Rathore M. Antibiotic prophylaxis after basilar skull fractures: a meta-analysis. Clin Infect Dis. 1998;27(2):364–9.
51. Ratilal B, Costa J, Sampaio C. Antibiotic prophylaxis for preventing meningitis in patients with basilar skull fractures. Cochrane Database Syst Rev. 2006;(1):CD004884.
52. Bernal-Sprekelsen M, Bleda-Vazquez C, Carrau RL. Ascending meningitis secondary to traumatic cerebrospinal fluid leaks. Am J Rhinol. 2000;14(4):257–9.
53. Heaton CM, Goldberg AN, Pletcher SD, Glastonbury CM. Sinus anatomy associated with inadvertent cerebrospinal fluid leak during functional endoscopic sinus surgery. Laryngoscope. 2012;122(7):1446–9.
54. Baban MIA, Hadi M, Gallo S, Zocchi J, Turri-Zanoni M, Castelnuovo P. Radiological and clinical interpretation of the patients with CSF leaks developed during or after endoscopic sinus surgery. Eur Arch Otorhinolaryngol. 2017;274(7):2827–35.
55. O'Brien WT Sr, Hamelin S, Weitzel EK. The preoperative sinus CT: avoiding a "CLOSE" call with surgical complications. Radiology. 2016;281(1):10–21.
56. Patel PN, Stafford AM, Patrinely JR, et al. Risk factors for intraoperative and postoperative cerebrospinal fluid leaks in endoscopic transsphenoidal sellar surgery. Otolaryngol Head Neck Surg. 2018;158(5):952–60.

57. Dlouhy BJ, Madhavan K, Clinger JD, et al. Elevated body mass index and risk of postoperative CSF leak following transsphenoidal surgery. J Neurosurg. 2012;116(6):1311–7.
58. Smith RR, Ragput A. Mucosal tears on endoscopic insufflation resulting in perforation: an interesting presentation of collagenous colitis. J Am Coll Surg. 2007;205(5):725.
59. Ramakrishnan VR, Kingdom TT. Does image-guided surgery reduce complications? Otolaryngol Clin N Am. 2015;48(5):851–9.
60. Dalgorf DM, Sacks R, Wormald PJ, et al. Image-guided surgery influences perioperative morbidity from endoscopic sinus surgery: a systematic review and meta-analysis. Otolaryngol Head Neck Surg. 2013;149(1):17–29.
61. Sanders-Taylor C, Anaizi A, Kosty J, Zimmer LA, Theodosopoulos PV. Sellar reconstruction and rates of delayed cerebrospinal fluid leak after endoscopic pituitary surgery. J Neurol Surg B Skull Base. 2015;76(4):281–5.
62. Gray ST, Wu AW. Pathophysiology of iatrogenic and traumatic skull base injury. Adv Otorhinolaryngol. 2013;74:12–23.

11 Spontaneous CSF Leak

Mohammed H. K. Hassab, Ahmed A. Ibrahim, and Mohamed Eid

Cerebrospinal fluid (CSF) leak occurring in a patient without a clear triggering factor such as accidental trauma, surgery, tumor, or congenital malformation is labeled spontaneous. Typically, these leaks occur in areas where the anterior or middle skull base and the dura are breached into the nasal cavity or the paranasal sinuses. Furthermore, spontaneous leaks can occur in the lateral skull base where the bone and dura are breached over the temporal bone. This chapter will focus on spontaneous CSF leaks due to defects in the anterior and middle skull base and presenting with CSF rhinorrhea. It will review the proposed pathophysiology for this disease as well as its relation to elevated intracranial pressure (ICP) and idiopathic intracranial hypertension (IIH). The clinical presentation and diagnostic evaluation of patients with spontaneous CSF rhinorrhea will be discussed. Further, the management strategy of this condition will be outlined especially measures to reduce ICP following surgical repair.

Supplementary Information The online version contains supplementary material available at [https://doi.org/10.1007/978-3-030-94781-1_11].

M. H. K. Hassab (✉) · A. A. Ibrahim
Department of Otorhinolaryngology, Alexandria Faculty of Medicine, Alexandria, Egypt

M. Eid
Department of Radiology, Alexandria Faculty of Medicine, Alexandria, Egypt

11.1 Incidence and Demographics

In early reported series of CSF leaks in the 1990s, spontaneous CSF leaks accounted for 3–5% of all leaks. However, in series reported in the 2000s, spontaneous CSF leaks accounted for 14–46% of all leaks which may indicate either a rise in the incidence of the disease and/or increased diagnosis and management of patients with this condition by otolaryngologists [1–3].

Typically, spontaneous CSF leak occurs in middle-aged overweight or obese women. In most reported case series of this disease, women were affected more than man comprising 77–85% of all patients. The average age of patients, across different studies, varied between 50 and 61 years. The majority of patients had an elevated body mass index (BMI) [4–6]. Woodworth et al. [5] found that 82% of patients in their series had an elevated BMI averaging 36.2. Seth et al. [4] and Schlosser et al. [6] found similar level of obesity in their series of patients with spontaneous CSF leaks.

11.2 Pathophysiology of Spontaneous CSF Leak

The exact pathophysiology of spontaneous CSF leak is still a matter of debate; however, a lot of evidence points that it is likely a variant of idiopathic intracranial hypertension (IIH) [5–7].

A. A. AlQahtani et al. (eds.), *CSF Rhinorrhea*, https://doi.org/10.1007/978-3-030-94781-1_11

11.3 Idiopathic Intracranial Hypertension (IIH)

This disease has been previously known as pseudotumor cerebri syndrome, meningeal hydrops, and benign intracranial hypertension. It is defined as an elevation in CSF pressure with normal brain parenchyma, absence of ventriculomegaly, and no identifiable cause [7, 8].

Patients classically present with severe headaches, papilledema, and vision loss, which may progress to blindness in advanced or rapidly progressive cases. Actually, visual loss represents the major morbidity associated with IIH. Lesser described, but relatively common symptoms are dizziness and/or tinnitus [1, 8].

Over 80% of patients presenting with IIH are women of childbearing age. Ninety percent are obese. Although the overall incidence of IIH is estimated at 0.9 per 100,000, this rate increases 20-fold to 19 per 100,000 when only considering overweight women [9, 10]. IIH incidence may be increasing proportionately to the obesity epidemic occurring globally. Nonobese patients, males, older adults, and children can also be diagnosed but may present with different symptoms and have worse outcomes [11]. Interestingly, studies have shown that men with IIH are more likely to have obstructive sleep apnea (OSA) and twice as likely to develop severe visual loss [12].

11.4 Pathophysiology of IIH

CSF is produced in the choroid plexus within the lateral, third, and fourth ventricles at a rate of 0.35 mL/min and flows from the ventricular system into the subarachnoid space. CSF absorption occurs at the arachnoid villi along the cerebral convexities. These arachnoid villi project into the dural sinuses and act as one-way valves that typically require a pressure gradient of 1.5 to 7 cm H_2O that promote anterograde flow of CSF into the low-pressure vascular dural sinuses. Normal CSF pressure in the lumbar cistern, when measured in the lateral decubitus position, is between 5 and 15 cm H_2O. Several factors affect CSF pressure including time of the day, age, activity level as well as the cardiopulmonary cycles [13].

.Most investigators agree that *cerebral venous hypertension* is the primary factor underlying IIH, which in turn leads to dysfunctional arachnoid granulations, impaired CSF absorption, and elevated intracranial pressures (ICP) [8, 14]. The pathophysiology behind the *cerebral venous hypertension*, however, remains controversial. Excluding an identifiable/treatable cause such as cerebral venous thrombosis, tumors, trauma, hemorrhage, and infection, *cerebral venous hypertension* and *IIH* are proposed to arise from one of the two mechanisms:

- *Truncal Obesity*: Adipose accumulation around the abdominal compartment is thought to compress this space and its contents, which in turn raises central venous pressure, cerebral venous pressure, and ICP. Cohort studies of patients undergoing gastric bypass have demonstrated normalization of ICPs with diminishing abdominal girth [15, 16].
- *Dural Venous Sinus Stenosis*: The prevailing theory suggests that IIH may arise via stenosis of the dural venous sinuses. Several investigators have demonstrated transverse sinus stenosis on magnetic resonance venography (MRV) in a majority of IIH patients (Fig. 11.1). Intramural manometry has also demonstrated

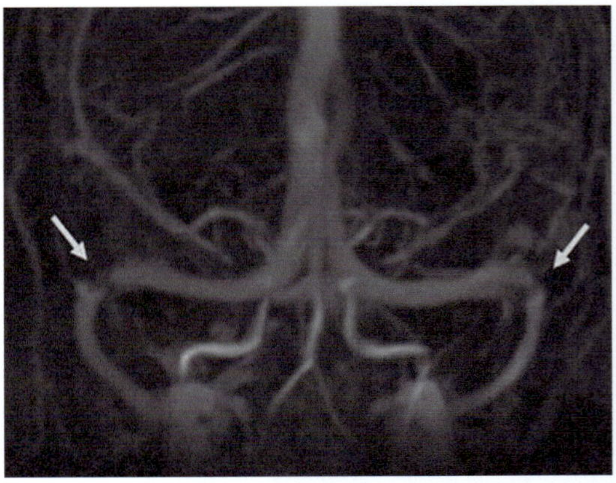

Fig. 11.1 3D-MRV sequence showing bilateral stenoses at the junction of the transverse and the sigmoid sinuses (white arrows) in a patient with IIH

pressure gradients across stenotic sinuses that normalize when stented [17, 18]. Opponents of this theory argue that elevated ICP may be the cause of venous sinus stenosis/compression rather than the effect, as stenosis is known to resolve following lumbar puncture [14, 19].

11.5 Relationship Between Spontaneous CSF Leak and IIH

Most of the patients with spontaneous CSF rhinorrhea show clinical signs and radiographic features of increased intracranial pressure (ICP) such as empty sella syndrome (80%), arachnoid pits (63%), and a thinned and broadly attenuated skull base. In their study, Psaltis et al. [20] found that patients with spontaneous CSF rhinorrhea had thinner skull bases in the region of the ethmoidal roof, lateral lamella, and anterior face of the sella compared with patients with traumatic leaks and non-leaking controls. CSF pressure monitoring, using lumbar drain pressures, shows in most cases of spontaneous CSF leak undergoing surgical repair an average pressure of 25–27 cm H_2O that is well above the normal range of 10–15 cm H_2O pressure [4, 7]. Interestingly, Schlosser et al. [7] noticed that the age, gender, and BMI trends in patients with spontaneous CSF leak closely resemble those seen in patients with IIH. In their series of patients with spontaneous CSF leaks, 72% of patients met the modified Dandy criteria for IIH. These include symptoms of elevated ICP, CSF opening pressure >25 cm H_2O, absence of localizing or focal neurologic signs, normal CSF composition with exclusion of cerebral venous thrombosis (by CT or MRI). This led the authors to speculate that many spontaneous CSF leaks may be an end result of IIH. They suggest that dural pulsations generated from elevated ICP exert direct pressure on the bony skull base. This continued pressure will result in erosion of the thinnest areas of the skull base with herniation of the brain and meninges and CSF leakage. They presume that elevated ICP and a thinned broadly attenuated skull base (often secondary to hyperpneumatization) are important predisposing factors for spontaneous CSF leaks [1, 7].

11.6 Clinical Picture

Clear watery usually unilateral rhinorrhea developing without an inciting event is the main presentation of this condition. In most cases, putting the head in a dependent position will make the watery leak obvious. Difficulty in sleeping in the supine position and persistent cough because of aspiration are common complaints in these patients. History of meningitis and/or seizures may be present. A salty taste of the trickling fluid is confirmed in the majority of patients. Secondary symptoms related to elevated ICP may be found in this group of patients such as headache, visual disturbances, tinnitus, and dizziness and may persist even after surgical repair [1].

11.7 Diagnostic Approach

The diagnosis of a spontaneous CSF leak is achieved through combining the clinical picture, endoscopic picture with identification of beta trace protein/beta2 transferrin in nasal secretions together with performing imaging studies. Besides confirming the nature of leaking fluid, this will identify the site of the leak in the skull base. Ophthalmological evaluation with fundus examination is essential to detect papilledema, visual field defects, and other ophthalmological signs of elevated ICP.

11.8 Imaging Studies in Spontaneous CSF Rhinorrhea

CSF rhinorrhea occurs when there is a communication between the subarachnoid space and the sinonasal (or middle ear) cavity through an osteodural defect in the skull base. Imaging studies are critical for the accurate identification of the site and size of this osteodural defect. This would enable planning of the appropriate management to prevent further rhinorrhea and other potential complications. Imaging studies are also essential for ruling out secondary causes such as tumors or congenital lesions. Furthermore, they outline radiologic findings of elevated ICP and/or IIH if present.

Non-contrast enhanced high-resolution computed tomography (HRCT) and magnetic resonance cisternography (MRC) are the main imaging techniques utilized in the investigation of a clinically suspected spontaneous CSF rhinorrhea. They do not depend on the presence of active CSF leakage. They are also less expensive, non-invasive (no lumbar puncture or intrathecal contrast injection) and have shorter examination times and higher compliance rates [21, 22].

Plain HRCT is usually the initial radiologic investigation of choice. It has reported 92% sensitivity and 100% specificity in detecting bony defects in the skull base. MRC provides important *complementary information* to the HRCT (Fig. 11.2). It is non-invasive and can demonstrate the CSF leak without the disadvantages of ionizing radiation and lumbar puncture. It is performed heavily utilizing T2-weighted images with fat suppression highlighting the bright CSF

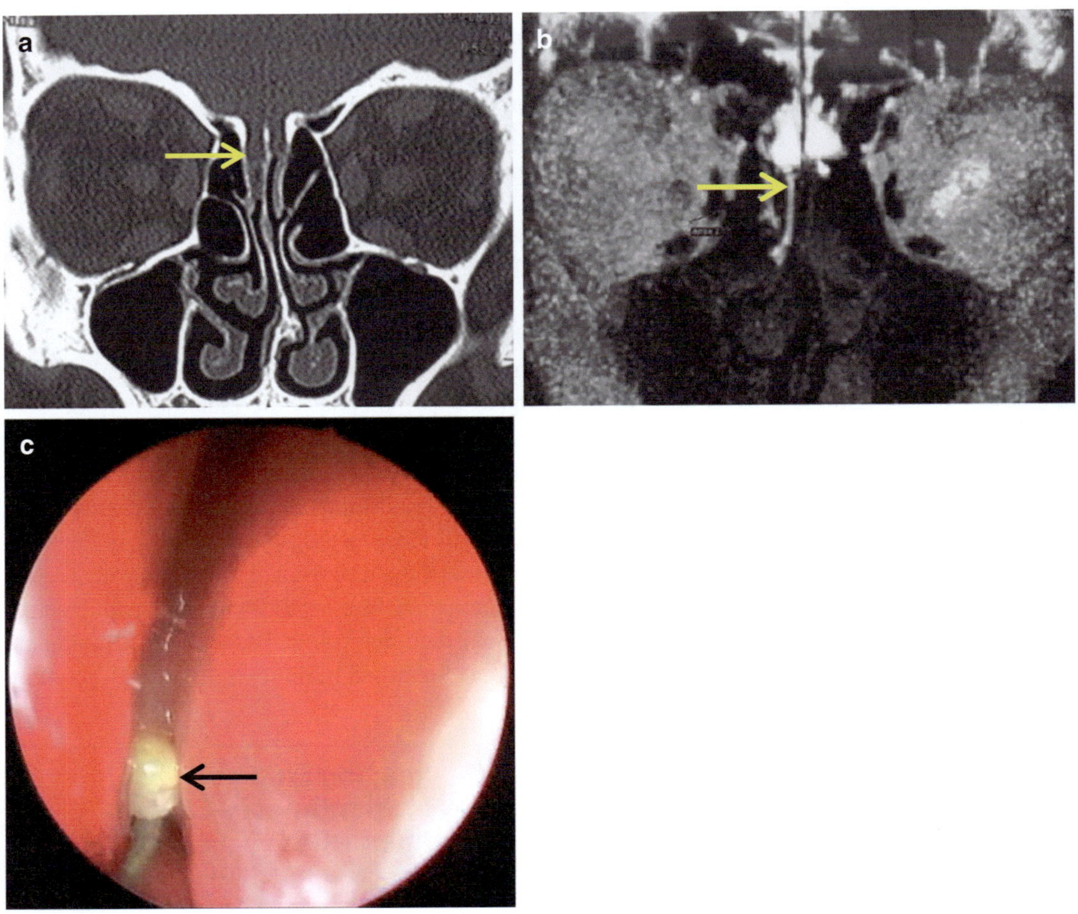

Fig. 11.2 (**a**) Coronal high-resolution CT shows a tiny right cribriform plate defect, with opacification of the underlying olfactory recess (yellow arrow) suggestive of a meningocele. (**b**) Coronal 3D T2 MRI (MR cisternography) sequence of the same patient shows the CSF-like signal (yellow arrow) confirming the meningocele and CSF leak. (**c**) Endoscopic picture of the right olfactory cleft of the same patient at the time of surgical exploration showing a very small meningocele stained with fluorescein (black arrow)

signal against a dark background of soft tissue and bone structures. These 3D sequences are acquired in the coronal plane and can be reformatted in multiple planes [1, 21, 22].

11.9 Radiologic Findings in Spontaneous CSF Rhinorrhea

11.9.1 Skull Base Osteodural Defect

HRCT in spontaneous CSF rhinorrhea will show a skull base defect with opacification or mucosal thickening of the adjacent sinus or air cells. The most common location for this defect varies by case series but generally involves the cribriform plate, ethmoidal roof, and lateral wall of the sphenoid. Central sphenoid, frontal sinus, and the clivus are relatively rare locations for spontaneous CSF leaks [4, 5, 23]. Occasionally, multiple bony defects are present in the same patient and this possibility should always be considered whenever managing patients with spontaneous CSF leak as its reported incidence varies between 3% and 16% in patients with spontaneous leaks (Fig. 11.3) [4, 5]. MRC will show a contiguous high T2 weighted signal CSF column communicating between the subarachnoid space and the sinonasal cavity via the skull base.

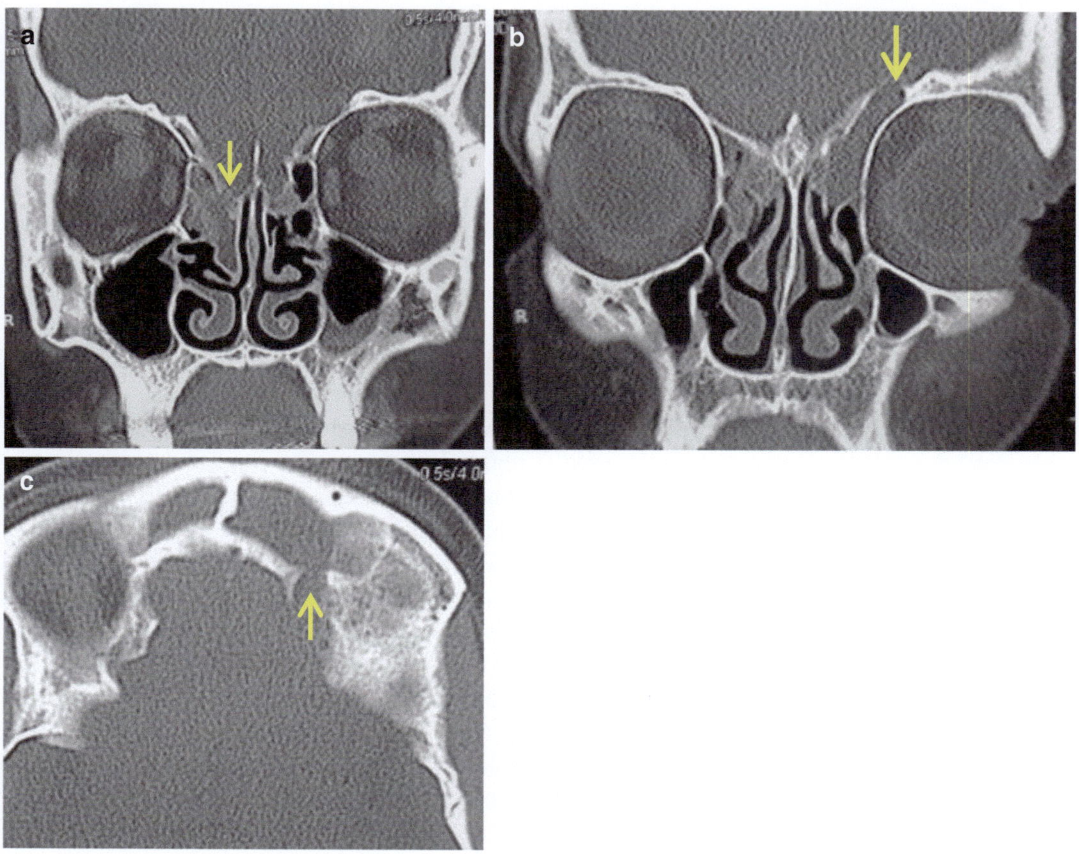

Fig. 11.3 (**a**) Coronal high-resolution CT shows a bony defect (yellow arrow) of the right lateral lamella with opacified underlying ethmoidal air cells. Also note the widened optic nerve sheaths. Coronal (**b**) and axial (**c**) high-resolution CT of the same patient show a second bony defect (yellow arrow) at the postero-superior wall of the left frontal sinus

11.9.2 Meningocele/Meningoencephalocele

Besides the bony defect, the majority of patients will have herniation of meninges and/or brain parenchyma extracranially forming a meningocele or a meningoencephalocele. MRC will accurately show the nature of the herniating tissues [1, 21, 22].

11.9.3 Signs of Increased ICP

Patients with spontaneous CSF rhinorrhea will commonly have radiologic evidence of elevated ICP (Fig. 11.4). The most common sign is an empty sella turcica. Patients with IIH will show additional signs of elevated ICP such as prominent arachnoid pits, dilated optic nerve sheaths, dilated Meckel's caves, posterior globe flattening or stenosis of cerebral venous sinuses, and a thinned and broadly attenuated skull base [1, 21, 22].

11.10 Treatment of Spontaneous CSF Rhinorrhea

Effective management is essential in patients with spontaneous CSF fistulas to prevent meningitis, encephalitis, pneumocephalus, brain abscess, and other potential complications. If left untreated, 10% of patients may develop meningitis each year, and as many as 40% may develop meningitis in the long term [22]. Some spontaneous CSF fistulas may resolve spontaneously or with a trial of conservative measures including acetazolamide therapy. Interestingly, in a study by Tilak AM et al. [24] a trial of acetazolamide therapy (250 mg twice daily) as an initial option in their study which included 16 patients resulted in resolution of the spontaneous CSF leak in five patients (31.3%). Those five patients had an average BMI < 39.15. This suggests a relationship between the effectiveness of acetazolamide and the BMI. Accordingly, they recommend a treatment trial with acetazolamide 250 mg BID for 30 days in patients with BMI less than 39.15 [24].

The endoscopic surgical repair of spontaneous CSF fistulae is the mainstay of treatment. It is safe, effective, and entails minimal morbidity when compared to a neurosurgical craniotomy approach. Accordingly, it is considered to be the standard of care for most cases. Details of surgical repair of different types of CSF leak are covered elsewhere in this book. However, there are essential considerations in the management plan of patients with spontaneous CSF leaks that are imperative for success. First, it is critical to understand the role of elevated ICP in the operative and perioperative planning. Failure to consider this role may account for higher possibility of failure of the repair or recurrence of the CSF leak. Another critical consideration is that in many instances in this group of patients, the defect is very small and may not be obvious on the preoperative CT or at the time of surgical exploration. In other instances, more than one defect may exist in the same patient. Hence, the real challenge here will be the accurate identification of the skull base defect at the time of surgery and exploring the possibility of coexistent multiple defects. Accordingly, our surgical technique typically starts with performance of a lumbar puncture and intrathecal injection of fluorescein. This indeed helps to accurately localize the skull base defect or defects intraoperatively and demonstrates the adequacy of the repair. Whether to use lumbar drains or not is controversial. Using lumbar drains is attended with potential complications that include persistent lumbar leakage after removal, over drainage, and retained catheters, pneumocephalus, brain herniation [25, 26]. Up to the present time there are no evidence-based studies that favor their use in this group of patients, hence their judicious use is recommended. Occasionally, a decision to insert a lumbar drain is considered in patients with obviously high flow leaks to facilitate the repair and allow graft placement at the time of surgery and to reduce the pressure at the repair site during the early healing phase. In regard the repair technique, and because of the elevated ICP, we prefer underlay repair whenever feasible. This will depend upon the site and size of the skull

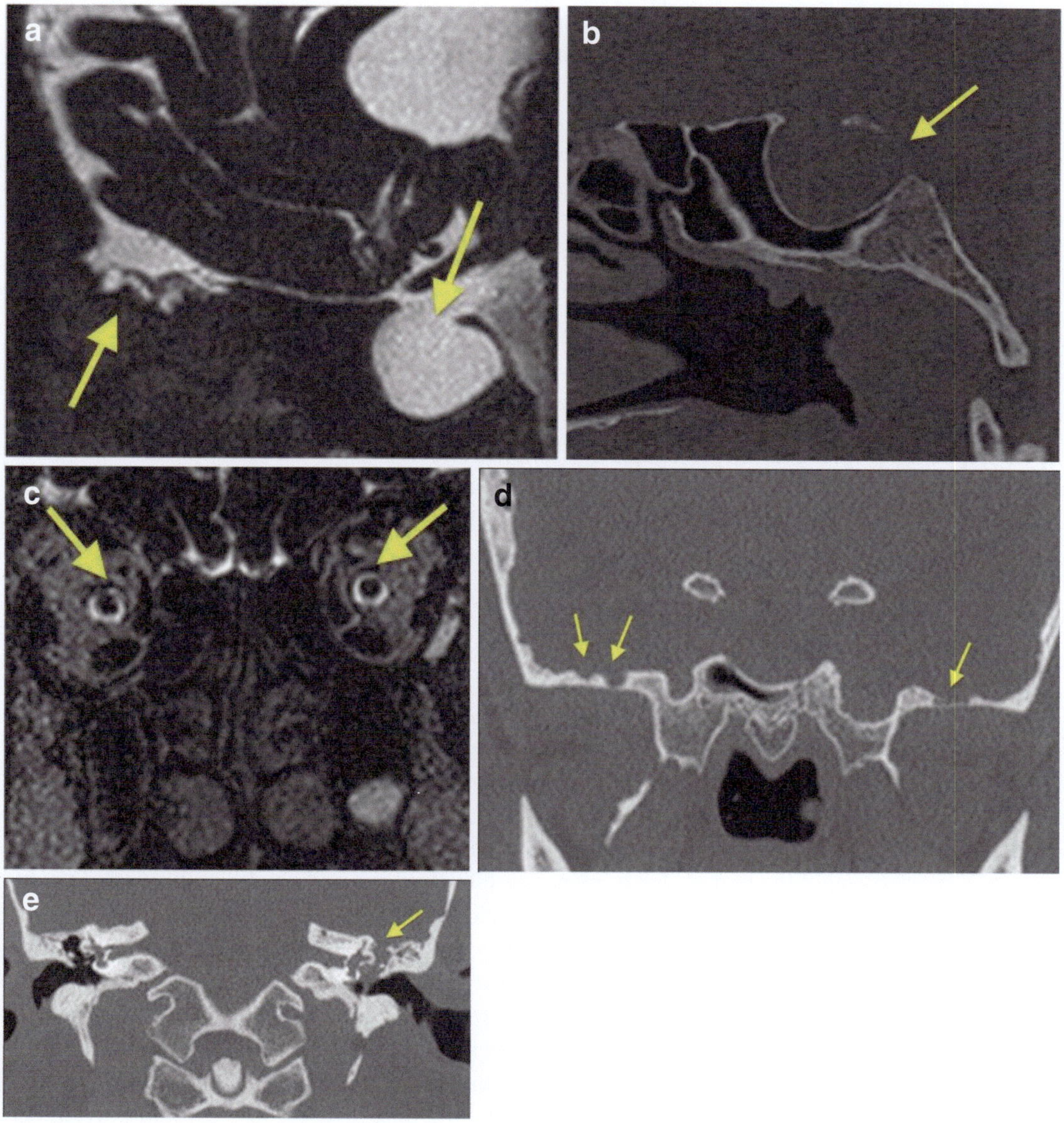

Fig. 11.4 (**a**) Sagittal reformat of 3D T2 MRI (MR cisternography) sequence shows ballooned "empty" sella turcica, as well as multiple dilated CSF sheaths around the olfactory rootlets. Findings suggestive of IIH. (**b**) Sagittal reformat of high-resolution CT shows empty sella with marked rarefaction of the dorsum sellae (yellow arrow). (**c**) Coronal 3D T2 MRI (MR cisternography) sequence shows dilated optic nerve sheaths (yellow arrows): optic hydrops, in favor of IIH. (**d**, **e**) Coronal high-resolution CT showing multiple herniation arachnoid pits of the floor of the middle cranial fossa (yellow arrows in **d**), and a defect of the left tegmen tympani (yellow arrow in **e**) that showed a meningocele in MR cisternography (not shown), both in keeping with IIH

base defect. So for defects in the ethmoidal roof, underlay repair can be carried out with ease. Here, grafting material including, cartilage or bone, can be placed in the defect in an underlay fashion. This is followed by placement of overlay mucosal grafts (usually free, less commonly pedicled) to cover the defect area. Conversely, for very small defects (<3 mm) and for defects in the cribriform plate where the bone surrounding the defect area is very thin and the dura is adherent, placement of an underlay graft is quite difficult and the use of overlay technique is more practical (video). In all instances, the mucosal grafts are secured into position with gelfoam and/or oxidized cellulose. Nasal packing is inserted to support the repair and typically removed on the third to fifth postoperative day.

11.11 Outcome of Surgical Repair and Postoperative Management

Spontaneous CSF leaks that are associated with elevated ICP have the highest failure/recurrence rate (25%–87%) after surgical repair compared with that for other types of CSF leaks (less than 10%) [1]. Short-term and long-term recurrences of spontaneous CSF leaks are believed to result from lack of management of elevated ICP in this group of patients. However, Soler and Schlosser [1] in a systematic review and meta-analysis of studies reporting success rate after surgical repair have found that the success rate for surgical repair of spontaneous CSF leaks has increased over time reaching 91.1%. This probably reflects a better understanding of the importance of management of the elevated ICP in this group of patients. Chaaban et al. [27] found that the CSF pressure significantly rises following surgical repair of the skull base defect. Teachey et al. [28] in their study, which included a prospective case series and a systematic review of published series, showed that intervention for managing this elevated ICP improves success rate after surgical repair. Successful primary repair was 92.82% in patient cohorts where ICP evaluation and intervention with acetazolamide or CSF shunt systems were performed, but was significantly decreased to 81.87% in series with no active management of elevated ICP.

The diagnosis of elevated ICP can be made directly via lumbar puncture or indirectly based on the presence of papilledema or radiologic evidence of increased ICP. The diagnosis of elevated ICP via lumbar puncture is based on an elevated opening pressure. However, if the CSF is already leaking, this opening pressure will be unreliable. Accordingly, some surgeons monitor continuously the CSF pressure following the surgical repair till it reaches a steady state [29, 30]. Other surgeons perform a separate lumbar puncture in the postoperative period to obtain a reliable opening pressure reading. Soler and Schlosser [1] consider a patient to have elevated ICP if there are radiologic signs of increased ICP, especially an empty sella. Also, they suspect an obese patient to have elevated ICP, even if radiologic findings are normal.

Postoperatively, in patients with elevated ICP, it is critical to decrease this pressure with medical, nutritional, or surgical means. These patients should be referred to an ophthalmologist to assess and manage papilledema, if present. They should also be subjected to other measures to decrease the elevated ICP. The first of these measures is keeping them on long-term *acetazolamide therapy*. As a carbonic anhydrase inhibitor, Acetazolamide reduces CSF production, thereby reduces CSF pressure. The usual dose of this drug is 500 twice a day [1, 27]. However, side effects such as numbness, paresthesias, altered taste, and lethargy have been associated with the use of this drug and can be problematic in some patients. The effect of other drugs on ICP has been investigated with variable results. Steroids have been used for IIH with demonstrated efficacy. However, the symptoms typically recur following tapering of the dose, which combined with the possibility of weight gain in obese patients, makes this a less favorable treatment. Other medications with some reported benefit include furosemide, bendroflumethiazide, and topiramate; however, the mainstay of medical therapy in patients with IIH has been acetazolamide [27]. The second measure is *weight loss*. Soler and Schlosser [1] consider weight loss to be the most important medical treatment for IIH. Studies consistently report improvement in ICP following low calorie diets. Sinclair et al. [31] in their cohort prospective study on 25 women with IIH put on low calorie diet (425 Kcal/day) for 3 months had a mean decrease in ICP of 8 cm H_2O. Accordingly, weight loss via diet modification and exercise is very much encouraged in this group of patients. Further, and as mentioned earlier in this chapter, CSF pressures were also found to be substantially reduced following bariatric surgery [15, 16]. Assessment of patients for the presence of *OSA* is another essential step. Because many of the patients with this disease are obese, OSA is another frequently encountered comorbidity, particularly in men. Fleischman et al. [32] found in their study that patients with spontaneous CSF rhinorrhea were more likely than their nonspontaneous counterparts to have a diagnosis of OSA (30.0% vs.14.3%). It has been shown that during apneic episodes, the ICP rises transiently. This would aggravate the dural pulsations that predispose to spontaneous CSF leak. Although there is no conclusive evidence that suggests treating OSA reduces CSF pressures, observational studies have reported that nocturnal oxygenation improves the signs and symptoms of idiopathic intracranial hypertension in men. So patients with positive history and clinical picture of OSA should be referred for polysomnography and managed accordingly. At the present time, there is no evidence-based information in regard when it is safe to restart OSA patient on CPAP after surgical repair [26]. Fleischman et al. [32] recommend cessation of CPAP during an active CSF leak, as well as for 6 weeks after repair, as it poses significant risk for breakdown of the repair site and development of pneumocephalus.

Permanent CSF diversion techniques such as lumboperitoneal or ventriculoperitoneal shunts may be considered in select patients with evidence of elevated ICP. At this point in time, there is no definitive protocol to determine which patients require this procedure. Soler and Schlosser [1] suggested that permanent CSF diversion techniques may be considered in patients who have failed multiple technically adequate endoscopic repairs or developed new leaks at different sites. Chaaban et al. [27] measured the CSF pressure in their study patients after surgical repair on postoperative day 2 before and after administration of acetazolamide. Based on this study, they recommend permanent CSF diversion for patients with starting pressures >35 cm H_2O, poor responses to acetazolamide (generally <10 cm H_2O change and pressure remaining >25 cm H_2O), and multiple skull base defects/CSF leak sites.

References

1. Soler ZM, Schlosser RJ. Spontaneous cerebrospinal fluid leak and management of intracranial pressure. Adv Otorhinolaryngol. 2013;74:92–103.
2. Lanza DC, O'Brien DA, Kennedy DW. Endoscopic repair of cerebrospinal fluid fistulae and encephaloceles. Laryngoscope. 1996;106:1119–25.
3. Carrau RL, Snyderman CH, Kassam AB. The management of cerebrospinal fluid leaks in patients at risk for high- pressure hydrocephalus. Laryngoscope. 2005;115:205–12.
4. Seth R, Rajasekaran K, Luong A, Benninger MS, Batra PS. Spontaneous CSF leaks: factors predicative of additional interventions. Laryngoscope. 2010;120:2141–6.
5. Woodworth BA, Prince A, Chiu AG, et al. Spontaneous CSF leaks: a paradigm for definitive repair and management of intracranial hypertension. Otolaryngol Head Neck Surg. 2008;138:715–20.
6. Schlosser RJ, Bolger WE. Spontaneous nasal cerebrospinal fluid leak and empty Sella syndrome: a clinical association. Am J Rhinol. 2003;17:91–6.
7. Schlosser RJ, Woodworth BA, Wilensky EM, Grady MS, Bolger WE. Spontaneous cerebrospinal fluid leaks: a variant of benign intracranial hypertension. Ann Otol Rhinol Laryngol. 2006;115:495–500.
8. Stevens SM, Rizk HG, Golnik K, Andaluz N, Samy RN, Meyer TA, Lambert PR. Idiopathic intracranial hypertension: contemporary review and implications for the otolaryngologist. Laryngoscope. 2018;128(1):248–56.
9. Wall M. Idiopathic intracranial hypertension (pseudotumor cerebri). Curr Neurol Neurosci Rep. 2008;8:87–93.
10. Jindal M, Hiam L, Raman A, Rejali D. Idiopathic intracranial hypertension in otolaryngology. Euro Arch Otorhinolaryngol. 2009;266:803–6.
11. Lee MW, Vedanarayanan VV. Cerebrospinal fluid opening pressure in children: experience in a controlled setting. Pediatr Neurol. 2011;45:238–40.
12. Bruce BB, Kedar S, Van Stavern GP, et al. Idiopathic intracranial hypertension in men. Neurology. 2009;72:304–9.
13. Yang Z, Wang B, Wang C, Liu P. Primary spontaneous cerebrospinal fluid rhinorrhea: a symptom of idiopathic intracranial hypertension? J Neurosurg. 2011;115(1):165–70.
14. De Simone R, Ranieri A, Bonavita V. Advancement in idiopathic intracranial hypertension pathogenesis: focus on sinus venous stenosis. Neurol Sci. 2010;31(Suppl 1):33–9.

15. Michaelides EM, Sismanis A, Sugerman HJ, Felton WL III. Pulsatile tinnitus in patients with morbid obesity: the effectiveness of weight reduction surgery. Am J Otol. 2000;21:682–5.
16. Handley JD, Baruah BP, Williams DM, Horner M, Barry J, Stephens JW. Bariatric surgery as a treatment for idiopathic intracranial hypertension: a systematic review. Surg Obes Relat Dis. 2015;11:1396–403.
17. Farb RI, Vanek I, Scott JN, et al. Idiopathic intracranial hypertension: the prevalence and morphology of sinovenous stenosis. Neurology. 2003;60:1418–24.
18. Ahmed RM, Wilkinson M, Parker GD, et al. Transverse sinus stenting for idiopathic intracranial hypertension: a review of 52 patients and of model predictions. Am J Neuroradiol. 2011;32:1408–14.
19. Higgins JN, Pickard JD. Lateral sinus stenosis in idiopathic intracranial hypertension resolving after CSF diversion. Neurology. 2004;62:1907–8.
20. Psaltis AJ, Overton LJ, Thomas WW, Fox NF, Banks CA, Schlosser RJ. Differences in skull base thickness in patients with spontaneous cerebrospinal fluid leaks. Am J Rhinol Allergy. 2014;28:e73–9.
21. Choong CC, Venkatesh SK, Phadke RV. Spontaneous cerebrospinal fluid rhinorrhea: computed tomography and magnetic resonance imaging findings. Singap Med J. 2013;54(3):176–81.
22. Alonso RC, de la Peña MJ, Caicoya AG, Rodriguez MR, Moreno EA, de Vega Fernandez VM. Spontaneous skull base meningoencephaloceles and cerebrospinal fluid fistulas. Radiographics. 2013;33(2):553–70.
23. Van Zele T, Kitice A, Vellutini E, Balsalobre L, Stamm A. Primary spontaneous cerebrospinal fluid leaks located at the clivus. Allergy Rhinol (Providence). 2013;4(2):100–4.
24. Tilak AM, Koehn H, Mattos J, Payne SC. Preoperative management of spontaneous cerebrospinal fluid rhinorrhea with acetazolamide. Int Forum Allergy Rhinol. 2019;9(3):265–9.
25. Lobo BC, Baumanis MM, Nelson RF. Surgical repair of spontaneous cerebrospinal fluid (CSF) leaks: a systematic review. Laryngoscope Investig Otolaryngol. 2017;2(5):215–24.
26. Oakley GM, Orlandi RR, Woodworth BA, Batra PS, Alt JA. Management of cerebrospinal fluid rhinorrhea: an evidence-based review with recommendations. Int Forum Allergy Rhinol. 2016;6(1):17–24.
27. Chaaban MR, Illing E, Riley KO, Woodworth BA. Acetazolamide for high intracranial pressure cerebrospinal fluid leaks. Int Forum Allergy Rhinol. 2013;3(9):718–21.
28. Teachey W, Grayson J, Cho DY, Riley KO, Woodworth BA. Intervention for elevated intracranial pressure improves success rate after repair of spontaneous cerebrospinal fluid leaks. Laryngoscope. 2017;127(9):2011–6.
29. Schlosser RJ, Wilensky EM, Grady MS, Palmer JN, Kennedy DW, Bolger WE. Cerebrospinal fluid pressure monitoring after repair of cerebrospinal fluid leaks. Otolaryngol Head Neck Surg. 2004;130:443–8.
30. Xie YJ, Shargorodsky J, Lane AP, Ishii M, Solomon D, Moghekar A, Gallia GL, Reh DD. Perioperative continuous cerebrospinal fluid pressure monitoring in patients with spontaneous cerebrospinal fluid leaks. Int Forum Allergy Rhinol. 2015;5(1):71–7.
31. Sinclair AJ, Burdon MA, Nightingale PG, et al. Low energy diet and intracranial pressure in women with idiopathic intracranial hypertension: prospective cohort study. BMJ. 2010;340:c2701.
32. Fleischman GM, Ambrose EC, Rawal RB, Huang BY, Ebert CS Jr, Rodriguez KD, Zanation AM, Senior BA. Obstructive sleep apnea in patients undergoing endoscopic surgical repair of cerebrospinal fluid rhinorrhea. Laryngoscope. 2014;124:2645–50.

12 Multidisciplinary Approach to CSF Leak

Katie Phillps, Peter H. Hwang, and Zara M. Patel

12.1 Multidisciplinary Approach to the Cerebrospinal Fluid Leak

Cerebrospinal fluid (CSF) rhinorrhea can have multiple possible etiologies. Broadly, CSF rhinorrhea is often classified into four categories: congenital, traumatic, neoplastic, or spontaneous. Based on the cause, presentation, location of the leak, and clinical status of the patient, a multidisciplinary team is often required for treatment and optimal long term success.

In today's era of endoscopic approaches, surgical repair of an anterior skull base CSF leak is approximately 90% effective with long term follow-up [1–4], yet there is a specific subgroup of patients that has a lower rate of success. In patients who have spontaneous CSF rhinorrhea, thought to be a sequela of idiopathic intracranial hypertension (IIH) [5], recurrence of CSF leak is more common. A wide range of recurrence rates (25–87%) has been published [6], although more recent series report recurrence rates at the lower end of this range (25–30%) [7, 8]. However, when patients with spontaneous CSF leak are treated by a multidisciplinary team in an effort to identify and treat the underlying increased intracranial pressure, success rates of over 90% [9, 10] have been published, matching the success rates of repair for other etiologies of CSF leak.

IIH, previously referred to as benign intracranial hypertension or pseudotumor cerebri, is an idiopathic disease process where the patient exhibits signs and symptoms of increased intracranial pressure without evidence of an intracranial lesion on imaging. The incidence is approximately one to three per 100,000 people and is most common in obese, middle-aged women [11]. Patients may report headache and visual disturbance or may have no symptoms other than spontaneous CSF rhinorrhea. When the leak site is repaired, some patients may then go on to develop symptoms as intracranial pressure increases, as the pressure release of the leak site has been closed off [12, 13]. Described below are specific multidisciplinary teams that may be of use to patients with spontaneous CSF rhinorrhea thought to be secondary to increased intracranial hypertension.

12.2 Otolaryngology/Head and Neck Surgery

Patients with spontaneous CSF rhinorrhea often present to or are referred most commonly to an otolaryngologist. These patients may present with a variety of complaints including rhinorrhea, nasal obstruction, post-nasal drip, taste

K. Phillps
University of Cincinatti, Cincinatti, OH, USA

P. H. Hwang · Z. M. Patel (✉)
Department of Otolaryngology - Head and Neck Surgery, Stanford University, Stanford, CA, USA
e-mail: hwangph@stanford.edu; zmpatel@stanford.edu

A. A. AlQahtani et al. (eds.), *CSF Rhinorrhea*, https://doi.org/10.1007/978-3-030-94781-1_12

changes including a metallic or salty taste, pulsatile tinnitus, headaches, balance problems, visual disturbance, or history of meningitis. The otolaryngologist must then obtain a comprehensive history and exam which includes an endoscopic nasal exam. If clinical suspicion for an anterior skull base CSF leak arises, a diagnostic work-up, as previously detailed in this book, includes establishing that the rhinorrhea is CSF via beta-2 transferrin laboratory testing, imaging to detect the location of the leak, and further delineation of the etiology of the CSF leak. If there is no obvious history of trauma, skull base mass, or concern for congenital etiology, then the diagnosis is often classified into the spontaneous CSF rhinorrhea category and further diagnostic work-up to confirm this presumed diagnosis is recommended.

Although thin cut CT is the best first imaging study to obtain to pinpoint the site of leak given the bony detail provided by CT, magnetic resonance imaging (MRI) can then also be obtained if there is a need to further characterize the CSF leak as soft tissue is often better captured on MRI. MRI can be helpful to identify if there is brain parenchyma herniating through the skull base defect, to ascertain if CSF is in the nasal cavity, often using a fast spin-echo sequence with fat suppression and image reversal [14], and to look for radiographic findings which are commonly associated with IIH including empty expanded sella (Fig. 12.1) and encephaloceles in other locations. Likewise, CT can also identify other commonly associated IIH findings including broadly attenuated skull base, arachnoid pits, and other skull base defects. Empty sella syndrome is highly correlated with IIH and can be associated with endocrine abnormalities which may warrant endocrine consultation [15]. If there is an intermittent leak and the site cannot be found by using the above imaging techniques, CT or MR cisternogram can be used as adjunct options to locate the precise site of leakage.

After a diagnostic work-up confirms an anterior skull base CSF leak, endoscopic repair is indicated, using a variety of techniques described elsewhere in this book depending on the location of the leak. The decision for perioperative lumbar drain is currently debated in the literature. A survey in 2001 of the American Rhinologic Society found that approximately 67% of those surveyed said they used a perioperative lumbar drain when repairing anterior skull base CSF leaks [16]. In recent years, however, there has been a general shift in practice, trending away from the routine placement of lumbar drains. Those in favor highlight the importance of perioperative lumbar drain for assistance in intraoperative localization of CSF leak especially in those with a questionable diagnosis and keeping intracranial pressures low post-operatively to protect the integrity of the graft [12, 13]. However, risks associated with lumbar drains include infection, dislodgement, post-spinal headaches, pneumocephalus, brainstem herniation, and retained catheters. The added risks of lumbar drain placement, in combination with evidence showing that there is no difference in rate of recurrence whether or not a drain is used, are cited as reasons to discourage perioperative lumbar drain [17]. The authors of this chapter do not routinely place lumbar drains for repair of CSF leaks, unless there is a need for use of intraoperative intrathecal fluorescein to try and locate a leak which has failed to show itself on all above-mentioned imaging exams.

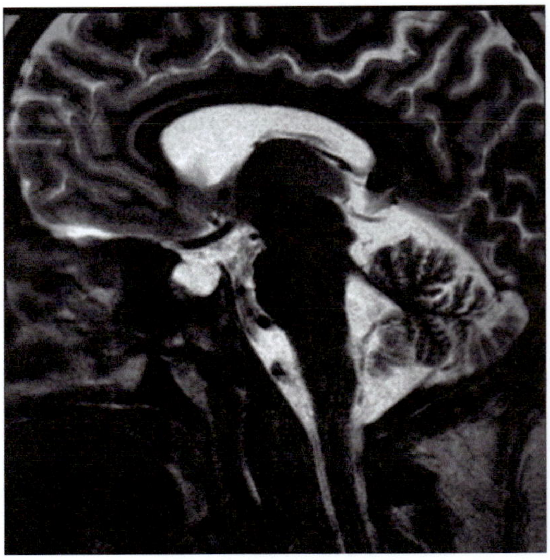

Fig. 12.1 Sagittal inversion recovery MRI demonstrating a flattened pituitary gland commonly seen in patients with IIH. Provided by Mary Beth Cunnane, MD

Patients with spontaneous CSF rhinorrhea were classically described as having normal

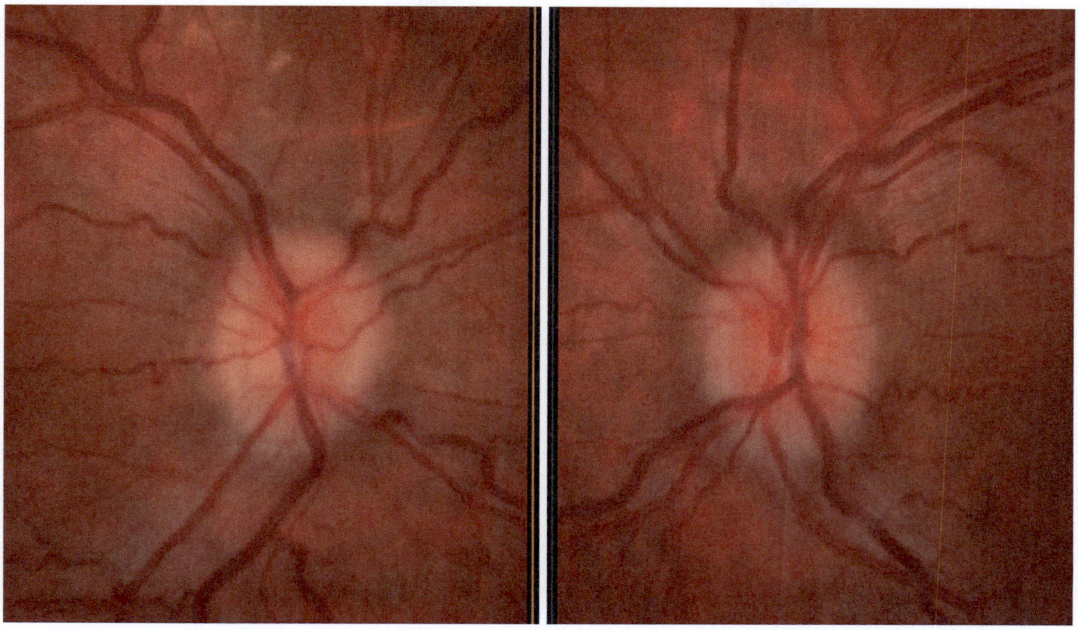

Fig. 12.2 Color fundus photo demonstrating bilateral disk edema. Provided by Edith Reshef, MD

intracranial pressure (ICP) [18]. However, further study of this population, particularly obese middle-aged women, has revealed that while these patients may have normal intracranial pressure at the time of repair, they may actually have underlying IIH, revealed only post-operatively after the leak site has closed [13]. The hypothesized mechanism relates to termination of the "pressure-valve" release effect of CSF leakage with surgical closure, followed by an increase in the pressure within the subarachnoid space, possibly leading to IIH symptomatology.

Follow-up is critically important after repair to both assess the graft site and to debride as necessary to ensure appropriate healing while taking care to not disturb the repair. As time elapses after surgery, it then becomes necessary to monitor for symptom recurrence, if rhinorrhea itself recurs, or if patients note new symptoms consistent with IIH. This is often the time to obtain consultations with other specialties depending on the clinical scenario. The authors preference is to obtain a pre-operative ophthalmology consultation if the patient reports visual changes recognizing no evidence of IIH may be present in the setting of an active leak and visual changes may be a result of etiologies beyond IIH. Post-operatively, the authors consider either referral to ophthalmology and neurology to assess for elevated intracranial pressure (Fig. 12.2) or start patients on a trial of acetazolamide depending on the individual clinical scenario.

12.3 Neurosurgery

Patients with CSF rhinorrhea may also first present to a neurosurgeon and should be worked up in a similar manner to the method previously described. The neurosurgeon may therefore be a co-surgeon with an otolaryngologist to primarily repair the anterior skull base CSF leak or may be involved in any potential perioperative lumbar drain placement and management, depending on the method and relationship at each specific institution, and who the patient was first referred to.

After repair, further treatment of IIH should be initiated if patients are noted to have perioperative increased intracranial pressure, develop recurrent symptoms consistent with IIH, or develop a secondary CSF leak either at the primary location or a secondary location along the skull base. A trial of acetazolamide and weight loss should first be initiated, but if symptoms are refractory or severe, more invasive means may be trialed. Options include bariatric surgery to optimize weight loss, serial lumbar punctures, cerebrospinal fluid diversion, optic nerve sheath fenestration or decompression or venous sinus stenting. Which intervention is most appropriate to treat the patient is based on the presenting symptoms and clinical status of the patient and is best decided with a multidisciplinary discussion. A recent systematic review of surgical interventions for IIH including optic nerve sheath fenestration, cerebrospinal fluid diversion, and dural venous sinus stenting found similar visual outcomes across all interventions and improved headache outcomes with cerebrospinal fluid diversions and endovascular stenting [19].

Cerebrospinal fluid diversion is most commonly done via a lumboperitoneal shunt (LPS) or a ventriculoperitoneal shunt (VPS). Multiple case series have found that visual and headache outcomes are similar for the two types of shunts, but that patients who receive the VPS have fewer complications and fewer revisions relative to the LPS group [19, 20]. The disadvantage of a VPS can be the technically challenging placement in an IIH patient due to the relatively smaller ventricles and excessive abdominal fat. A lumbopleural shunt is another variation of a CSF fluid diversion which has been described in the literature, although the safety profile, efficacy, and need for revision are not well understood [21]. Ultimately, the selection of CSF diversion technique is often dictated by the surgeon's expertise.

Alternatively, a relatively new option for patients with IIH refractory to medical management is placement of a venous sinus stent. It has been reported that 30–93% of IIH patients have a focal stenosis in their dural sinus outflow tract [22–24] (Fig. 12.3), therefore affording a focal site to target with an endovascular stent if the cerebral venous pressure gradient is ≥8 mmHg across the stenosis [25]. Stenosis often occurs in the lateral sinuses and upper sigmoid sinus and is thought to be caused by hypertrophied arachnoid granulations. Outcomes of venous sinus stent placement have been relatively positive, with improvement in papilledema noted in approximately 90% of patients, improvement in visual acuity in 78–85% of patients, and improvement in headaches in approximately 80% of patients [19, 25]. The reported major complication rate is low (1.5%) but includes subdural hematoma, subarachnoid hemorrhage, and intracerebral bleeding. Minor complication rate was 4.9% and included retroperitoneal hemorrhage, femoral pseudoaneurysm, neck hematoma, femoral vein thrombosis, and transient hearing loss. Overall treatment failure, defined as need to convert to another treatment modality was 2.4% [25]. After placement of stents, patients are treated with a dual-antiplatelet therapy including aspirin and clopidogrel over the next 3 months at minimum. Therefore pre-operative counseling regarding the bleeding risks associated with these medications is also necessary.

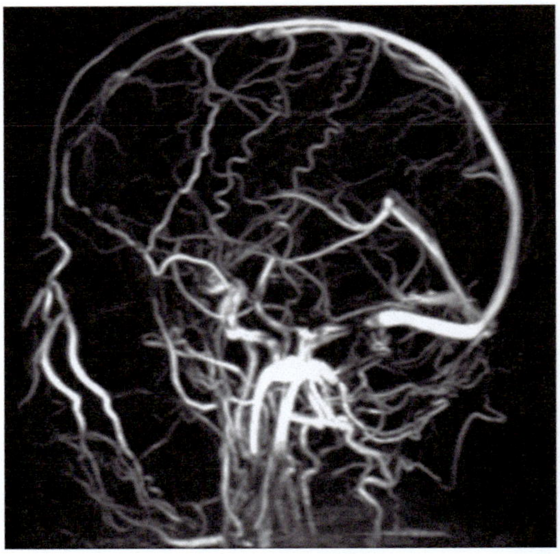

Fig. 12.3 Magnetic resonance venography (MRV) demonstrating severe narrowing of the right transverse sinus common in patients with IIH. Provided by Mary Beth Cunnane, MD

12.4 Neurology

Pre-operative consultation with the neurology service is recommended for any patient with spontaneous anterior skull base CSF leak who reports other signs or symptoms consistent with IIH. The neurologist, often in conjunction with the primary care doctor and the ophthalmologist, will provide long term follow-up for IIH patients and is crucial in determining when further treatment and interventions are necessary.

Often patients are initially started on acetazolamide, a carbonic anhydrase inhibitor which is thought to decrease CSF production from the choroid plexus, thereby decreasing the intracranial pressure. The most commonly reported side effects of acetazolamide therapy include myopia, paresthesia, loss of appetite, metabolic acidosis, and electrolyte imbalance [26]. It is therefore recommended that patients be monitored for adverse effects and have electrolyte levels checked periodically. Prior groups have proposed either 500 mg twice daily or once nightly of the sustained release form of acetazolamide, although, notably, the dosage recommendations are not evidence based [13]. The medication is purposely dosed at night to have the highest effect during REM sleep when the intracranial pressure is known to peak. A recent prospective trial of patients with recent CSF leak repair found that administration of acetazolamide significantly decreased intracranial pressure 21.9 ± 7.5 cm H_2O in the 4–6 h time frame after administration [27]. Although a recent Cochrane review of treatment for IIH found there was not enough evidence in the literature to support recommending acetazolamide for the treatment of IIH [28], acetazolamide is still considered by many to be the first-line medication treatment for IIH and is often the first step trialed in conjunction with weight loss before more invasive interventions are considered.

12.5 Ophthalmology

Patients with spontaneous CSF rhinorrhea may also present with visual disturbance. If patients report visual changes, pre-operative consultation with ophthalmology is recommended. Ophthalmology work-up may include perimetry, optical coherence tomography, ocular sonography, or MRI. Optical coherence tomography helps to characterize papilledema by evaluating the retinal nerve fiber layer thickness (Figs. 12.4, 12.5, and 12.6). Ocular sonography is a non-invasive way to detect increased intracranial pressure by measuring the optic nerve sheath diameter. MRI is useful to assess whether neuro-imaging ocular findings typically associated with IIH are present including prominent subarachnoid space around the optic nerves, vertical tortuosity of the optic nerves, flattening of the posterior sclera, and enhancement of the intra-ocular optic nerve (Fig. 12.7). Likewise, after surgical repair of the CSF leak, follow-up with ophthalmology is warranted to follow the patient's exam. In post-operative patients who have undergone leak repair but then report recurrence of pre-operative

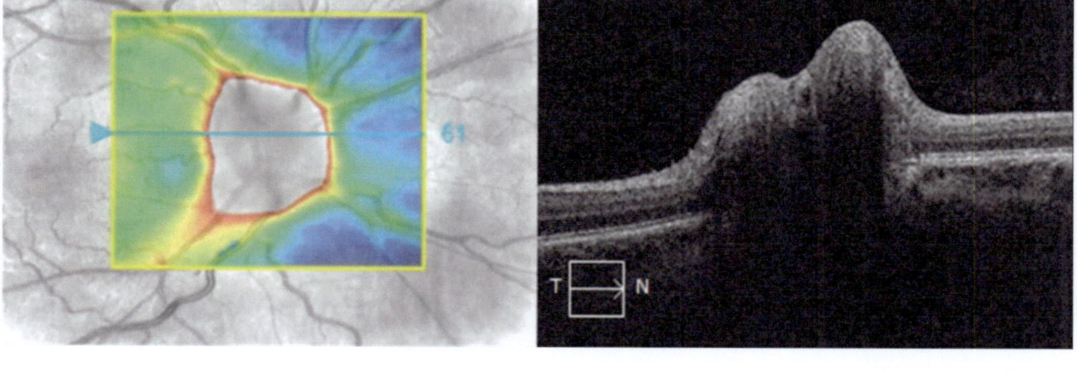

Fig. 12.4 Optic coherence tomography (OCT) cross section of the right optic nerve head demonstrating elevation of the nerve fiber layer. Provided by Edith Reshef, MD

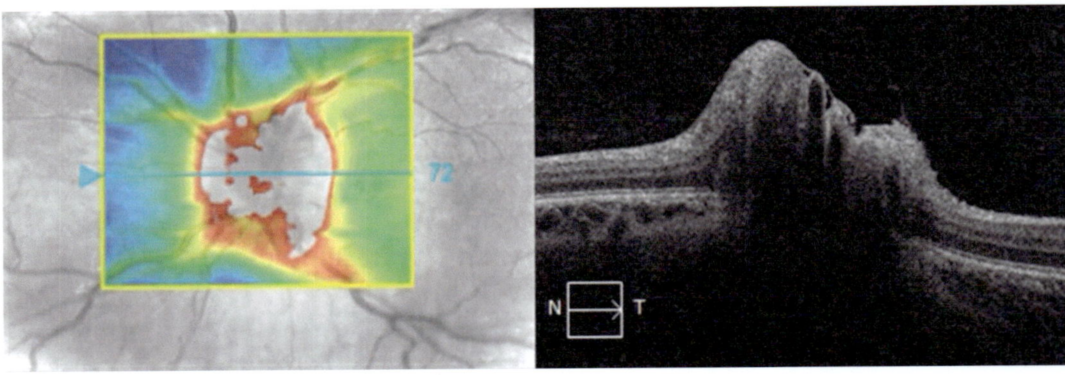

Fig. 12.5 Optic coherence tomography (OCT) cross section of the left optic nerve head demonstrating elevation of the nerve fiber layer. Provided by Edith Reshef, MD

symptoms or new symptoms, such as visual changes, headaches, pulsatile tinnitus or rhinorrhea, ophthalmology consultation is again useful to assess for papilledema as a non-invasive way to evaluate for return of increased intracranial pressure.

For patients who develop signs and symptoms consistent with IIH after repair of anterior skull base CSF leaks, further multidisciplinary consultation and treatment is necessary. For patients with acute visual loss or severe visual disturbance despite medical therapy, optic nerve sheath fenestration or optic nerve decompression is then often recommended.

Optic nerve sheath fenestration aids in reducing CSF pressure exerted on the retrolaminar optic nerve with the purpose of preventing further visual loss and possibly improving vision, decreasing intracranial pressure, and improving headache symptoms. Optic nerve sheath fenestration is often done unilaterally, even if bilateral papilledema is present, to preclude the possible complication of bilateral blindness. Yet, despite unilateral surgery, improvements can be noted bilaterally. Various surgical approaches have been described, with the medial transconjunctival access being the most commonly used today. A recent meta-analysis found that in patients undergoing optic nerve sheath fenestration, visual acuity improved in 59% of patients, vision stabilized in 95% of patients, visual fields improved in 68% of patients, papilledema improved in 80% of patients, and headache improved in 44% of patients. Minor complications, such as diplopia and anisocoria, occurred at a rate of 16.4%, while major complications, including central retinal artery occlusion, acute angle-closure glaucoma, infection and iatrogenic traumatic optic neuropathy, occurred at a rate of 1.5% [29].

Alternatively, endoscopic endonasal optic nerve decompression without sheath fenestration has been proposed as a less invasive means to treat IIH patients with visual disturbance who have been refractory to medical management (Fig. 12.8). This procedure is done by a rhinologist. While visual and headache outcomes are less robust than with complete fenestration [30], the endonasal approach is less invasive. Relative to the medial transconjunctival approach, which involves disrupting the medial rectus muscle, the endoscopic endonasal approach has less morbidity. Thus, some have proposed endonasal optic nerve decompression as an initial procedure to assess if symptoms can be ameliorated. If symptoms progress or do not improve after a decompression, the patient can then move forward with the optic nerve sheath fenestration. The mechanism regarding how the optic nerve decompression without the sheath fenestration assists in decreasing intracranial pressure is not completely understood. More research is needed before the endoscopic endonasal orbital nerve decompression is included in the standard treatment protocol for patients with IIH.

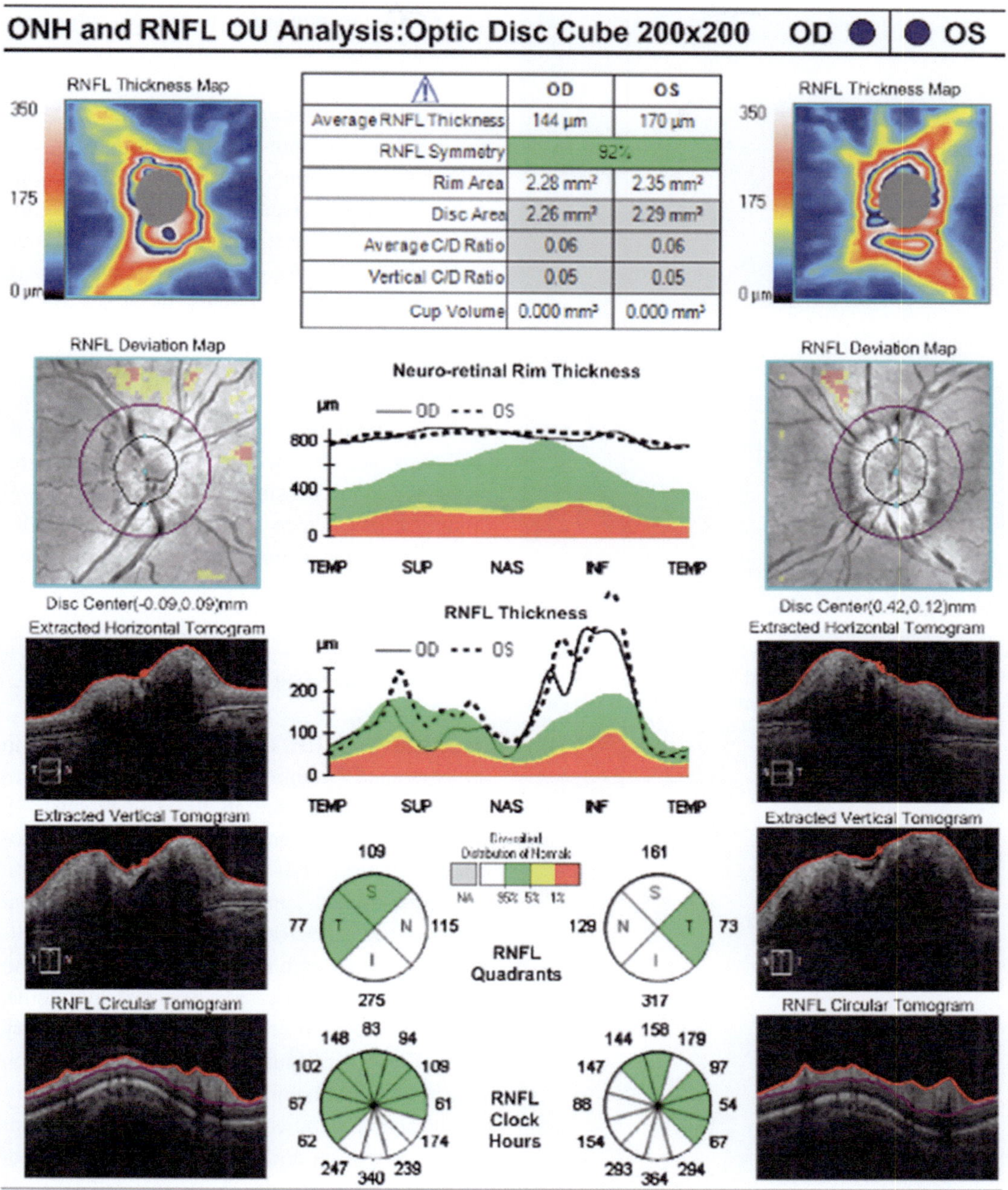

Fig. 12.6 Retinal nerve fiber layer (RNFL) analysis by OCT demonstrating increased RNFL thickness due to edema. Provided by Edith Reshef, MD

12.6 Bariatric Surgery

Patients with spontaneous anterior skull base CSF leaks who meet the criteria for IIH may ultimately be best served with bariatric surgery, although they must first have their CSF leak repaired and undergo conservative treatment for IIH before bariatric surgery should be considered. The etiology of IIH is not well understood, but obesity is a well-known associated factor and is thought to be part of the underlying pathophysiology of the disease. Bariatric surgery has been shown to have

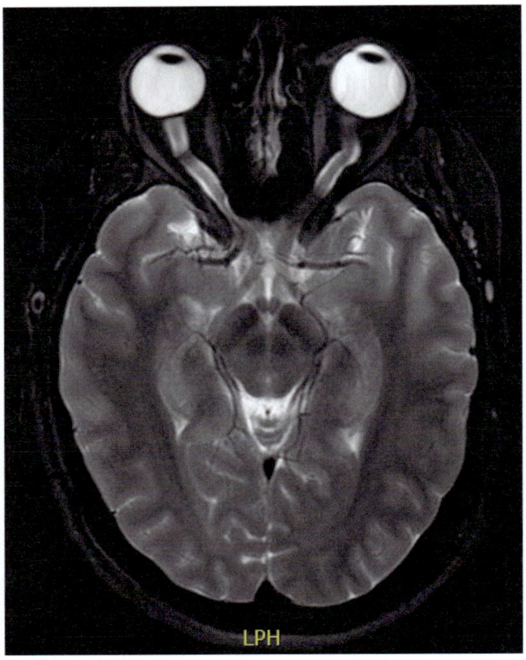

Fig. 12.7 Axial T2 weighted MRI demonstrating fattening of the posterior globes and prominence of CSF in the optic nerve sheaths commonly seen in patients IIH. Provided by Mary Beth Cunnane, MD

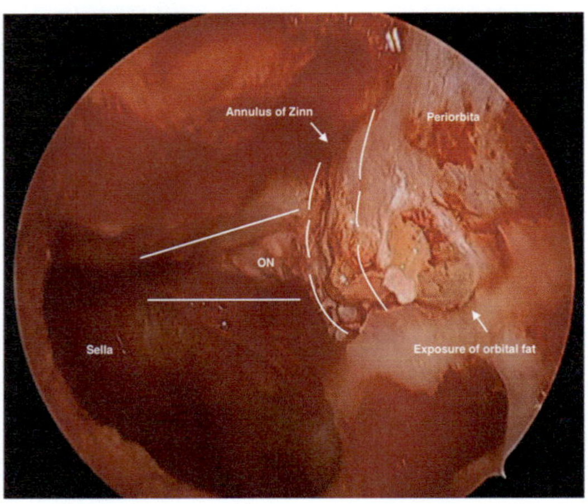

Fig. 12.8 Optic nerve decompression which shows a left orbit and optic nerve decompression highlighting the sella, annulus of zinn, optic nerve, and exposure of periorbital and orbital fat

significant and long lasting weight loss effects which have benefits in many disease processes. Patients with IIH who undergo bariatric surgery have a 20–35% weight reduction at 2–3 years of follow-up and maintain 14–37% greater weight loss relative to non-surgical controls who have pursued lifestyle modifications [31].

In a review of multiple cases series of patients with IIH who underwent bariatric surgery, 92% had resolution of pre-operative symptoms, and 97% had resolution of papilledema, 92% had improvement in visual field deficits, with the remaining 8% reporting stabilization of their visual fields [32]. Another systematic review of IIH patients who underwent bariatric surgery found that the post-operative lumbar pressure opening pressure decreased by an average of 18.9 cm H_2O along with improvement in pre-operative symptoms [33]. Bariatric surgery complications include nutritional deficiencies as well as a myriad of possible abdominal and bowel complications, which should be discussed with the patient prior to making the decision to proceed with bariatric surgery.

12.7 Endocrine

In patients with IIH, an empty sella turcica with an associated flattening of the pituitary gland is radiographically present in 70% of patients [34], although not all of these patients will have endocrine abnormalities. The most common endocrine-related complaints include menstrual irregularities, galactorrhea, hirsutism, and sterility. For patients with radiographic findings of an empty sella and endocrine-associated symptoms, further work-up of the hypothalamic pituitary adrenal axis is warranted. Endocrine consultation with accurate dynamic hormone testing to identify hormonal deficiencies is necessary, both for precise diagnosis and treatment in the form of hormone replacement. This constellation of imaging findings, symptoms, and hormonal imbalance constitutes primary empty sella syndrome [15].

For patients with IIH and primary empty sella syndrome, weight loss is advocated and has shown to be effective in improving symptoms [35]. If patients do require hormone replacement and are candidates for bariatric surgery, there should be a pre-operative discussion between the endocrinologist, the bariatric surgeon, and a nutritionist, as the risk of malabsorption syndrome after bariatric surgery can pose risks to adequate hormone replacement [15]. If the risks of malabsorption are too high or could not be tolerated, other means of treating IIH should be considered.

12.8 Sleep Medicine

As already mentioned above, obesity is an associated factor in spontaneous anterior skull base CSF leaks from IIH, and therefore these patients are also at risk for obstructive sleep apnea (OSA) [36]. Patients with OSA are typically treated with continuous positive airway pressure (CPAP), which can lead to a dilemma post-operatively regarding whether CPAP should be used. The advantage of using CPAP includes avoiding hypoxic nocturnal episodes, which can themselves lead to further elevation of intracranial pressure that exerts more pressure on the graft site. Alternatively, withholding CPAP prevents possible positive pressure-induced pneumocephalus, disruption of the graft site, and potential meningitis. An additional consideration is whether or not the patient has received post-operative nasal packing, which may impede the effectiveness of CPAP.

Surgeons of the North American Skull Base Society were surveyed regarding when they would recommend resuming CPAP to their patients after skull base repair. In the presence of a CSF leak and repair, the mean duration for resumption of CPAP was 14.3 days for small leaks and 20.7 days for larger leaks [37]. Researches at the University of Pittsburg Medical Center reported outcomes in their skull base surgical patients with and without OSA and found that patients with OSA were more likely to require oxygen post-operatively when their CPAP was held, yet there was no significant increase in risk of serious respiratory complications despite the post-operative hypoxemia. However, when patients who did not carry a formal OSA diagnosis but were suspected to have OSA were examined, it was found that this group of patients did have an increased risk for serious respiratory complications. This effect was attributed to a lack of attentiveness in regard to these patients' respiratory status post-operatively, given the lack of OSA diagnosis [38]. Conversely, when 17,777 patients who underwent transsphenoidal pituitary surgery were examined, it was found that patients with OSA had increased risk of hypoxemia and subsequent tracheostomy, but were not at increased risk for other complications [39].

Given the potential risks for using CPAP immediately post-operatively, there seems to be a general consensus to hold CPAP in the immediate post-operative setting but there is not clear evidence regarding when the optimal time to restart a patient's CPAP would be to reduce serious respiratory complications and prevent further increased intracranial pressure exacerbation. Currently there is a paucity of evidence to provide guidance in these issues and contemporary practice is often dictated by surgeon experience and local practice patterns.

12.9 Conclusion

Anterior skull base CSF leak repair often has a high success rate when treating patients with traumatic, congenital, or neoplastic CSF leaks. When repairing patients with spontaneous CSF leaks, the success rates were historically lower as the underlying etiology of these leaks was not yet recognized. With the recognition that spontaneous skull base CSF leaks are due to the idiopathic intracranial hypertension disease process, and with a multidisciplinary approach to treatment, success rates are now similar to the other etiologies of skull base CSF leak (Fig. 12.9). The coordination of otolaryngologists, neurologists, neurosurgeons, ophthalmologists, endocrinologists, bariatric surgeons, and sleep physicians, along with the primary care physician, provides a multifaceted approach to help these complex patients achieve improved outcomes in vision, headache, quality of life, and skull base repair.

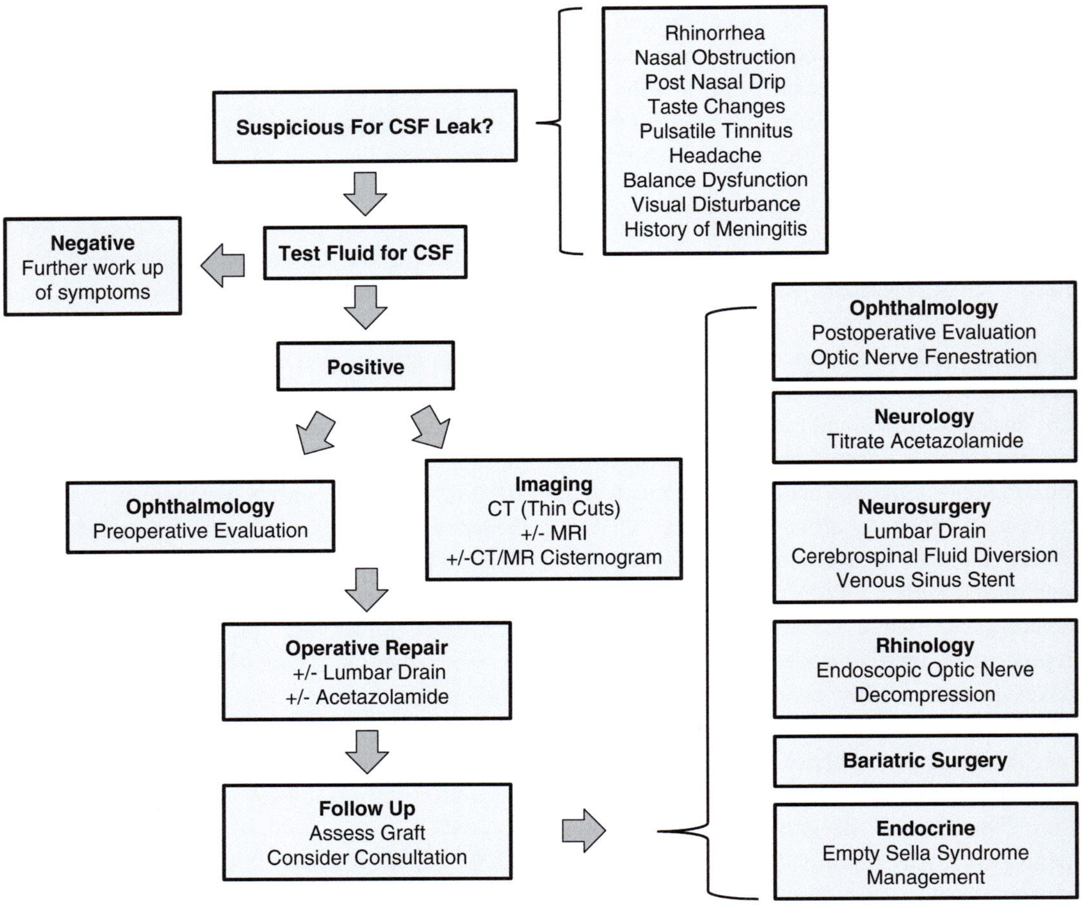

Fig. 12.9 Algorithm for multidisciplinary approach to an anterior skull base CSF leak

References

1. Mattox DE, Kennedy DW. Endoscopic management of cerebrospinal fluid leaks and cephaloceles. Laryngoscope. 1990;100:857–62.
2. Gassner HG, Ponikau JU, Sherris DA, et al. CSF rhinorrhea:95 consecutive surgical cases with long term follow-up at the Mayo clinic. Am J Rhinol. 1999;13:439–47.
3. Schick B, Ibing R, Brors D, et al. Long-term study of endonasal duraplasty and review of the literature. Ann Otol Rhinol Laryngol. 2001;110:142–7.
4. Banks CA, Palmer JN, Chiu AG, O'Malley BW Jr, Woodworth BA, Kennedy DW. Endoscopic closure of CSF rhinorrhea: 193 cases over 21 years. Otolaryngol Head Neck Surg. 2009;140(6):826–33.
5. Bidot S, Levy JM, Saindane AM, Oyesiku NM, newman NJ, Biousse V. Do most patients with a spontaneous cerebrospinal fluid leak have idiopathic intracranial hypertension? J Neuroophthalmol. 2019;39(4):487–95.
6. Hubbard JL, McDonald TJ, Pearson BW, Laws ER. Spontaneous cerebrospinal fluid rhinorrhea: evolving concepts in diagnosis and surgical management based on the Mayo Clinic experience from 1970 through 1981. Neurosurgery. 1985;16(3):314–21.
7. Gendeh BS, Mazita A, Selladural BM, et al. Endonasal endoscopic repair of anterior skull base fistulas: the Kuala Lumpur experience. J Laryngol Otol. 2005;119:866–74.
8. Dunn CJ, Alaani A, Johnson AP. Study on spontaneous cerebrospinal fluid rhinorrhea: its etiology and management. J Laryngol Otol. 2005;119:12–5.
9. Teachey W, Grayson J, Cho DY, Riley KO, Woodworth BA. Intervention for elevated intracranial pressure improves success rate after repair of spontaneous cerebrospinal fluid leaks. Laryngoscope. 2017;127(9):2011–6.

10. Woodworth BA, Prince A, Chiu AG, et al. Spontaneous CSF leaks: a paradigm for definitive repair and management of intracranial hypertension. Otolaryngol Head Neck Surg. 2008;138(6):715–20.
11. Radhakrishnan K, Ahlskog JE, Garrity JA, Kurland LT. Idiopathic intracranial hypertension. Mayo Clin Proc. 1994;69(2):169–80.
12. Wise SK, Schlosser RJ. Evaluation of spontaneous nasal cerebrospinal fluid leaks. Curr Opin Otolaryngol Head Neck Surg. 2007;15(1):28–34.
13. Schlosser RJ, Wilensky EM, Grady MS, et al. Cerebrospinal fluid pressure monitoring after repair of cerebrospinal fluid leaks. Otolaryngol Head Neck Surg. 2004;130:443–8.
14. Eljamel MS, Pidgeon CN, Toland J, Phillips JK, O'Dwyer AA. MRI cisternography and the localization of CSF fistulae. Br J Neurosurg. 1994;8(4):433–7.
15. Chiloiro S, Giampietro A, Bianchi A, et al. Diagnosis of endocrine disease: primary empty sella: a comprehensive review. Eur J Endocrinol. 2017;117(6):275–85.
16. Senior BA, Jafri K, Benninger M. Safety and efficacy of endoscopic repair of CSF leaks and encephaloceles: a survey of the members of the American Rhinologic Society. Am J Rhinol. 2001;15(1):21–5.
17. Jiang ZY, McLean C, Perez C, Barnett S, Friedman D, Tajudeen BA, Batra PS. Surgical outcomes and postoperative management in spontaneous cerebrospinal fluid rhinorrhea. J Neurol Surg B Skull Base. 2018;79(2):193–9.
18. Ommaya AK, DiChiro G, Baldwin M, Pennybacker JP. Nontraumatic cerebrospinal fluid rhinorrhea. J Neurol Neurosurg Psychiatry. 1968;31:214–5.
19. Lai LT, Danesh-Meyer HV, Kaye A. Visual outcomes and headache following interventions for idiopathic intracranial hypertension. J Clin Neurosci. 2014;21(10):1670–8.
20. Tarnaris A, Toma AK, Watkins LD, Kitchen ND. Is there a difference in outcomes of patients with idiopathic intracranial hypertension with the choice of cerebrospinal fluid diversion site: a single centre experience. Clin Neurol Neurosurg. 2011;113(6):477–9.
21. Alkosha HM, Zidan AS. Role of lumbopleural shunt in management of idiopathic intracranial hypertension. World Neurosurg. 2016;88:113–8.
22. Farb RA, Vanek I, Scott JN, Mikulis DJ, Willinsky RA, Tomlinson G, terBrugge KG. Idiopathic intracranial hypertension: the prevalence and morphology of sinovenous stenosis. Neurology. 2003;60(9):1418–24.
23. Higgins JN, Gillard JH, Owler BK, Harness K, Pickard JD. MR venography in idiopathic intracranial hypertension: unappreciated and misunderstood. J Neurol Neurosurg Psychiatry. 2004;75(4):621–15.
24. Johnston I, Kollar C, Dunkley S, Assaad N, Parker G. Cranial venous outflow obstruction in the pseudotumor syndrome: incidence, nature and relevance. J Clin Neurosci. 2002;9(3):273–8.
25. Leishangthem L, SirDeshpande P, Dua D, Satti SR. Dural venous sinus stenting for idiopathic intracranial hypertension: an updated review. J Neuroradiol. 2019;46(2):148–54.
26. Bagnato F, Good J. The use of antiepileptics in migraine prophylaxis. Headache. 2006;56(3): 603–15.
27. Chaaban MR, Illing E, Riley KO, Woodworth BA. Acetazolamide for high intracranial pressure cerebrospinal fluid leaks. Int Forum Allergy Rhinol. 2013;3(9):718–21.
28. Piper RJ, Kalyvas AV, Young AM, Hughes MA, Jamjoom AA, fouyas IP. Interventions for idiopathic intracranial hypertension. Cochrane Database Syst Rev. 2015;7(8):CD003434.
29. Satti SR, Leishangthem L, Chaudry MI. Meta-analysis of CSF diversion procedures and dural venous sinus stenting in the setting of medically refractory idiopathic intracranial hypertension. AJNR Am J Neuroradiol. 2015;36(10):1899–904.
30. Tarrats L, Hernandez G, Busquests JM, Portela JC, Serrano LA, Gonzalez-Sepulveda L, Sanchez-Perez JR. Outcomes of endoscopic optic nerve decompression in patients with idiopathic intracranial hypertension. Int Forum Allergy Rhinol. 2017;7(6):615–23.
31. American College of Cardiology/American Heart Association Task Force on Practice Guidelines OEP. Executive summary: guidelines for the management of overweight and obesity in adults: a report of the American College of Cardiology/American Heart Association Task Force on Practice Guidelines and the Obesity Society published by the Obesity Society and American College of Cardiology/American Heart Association Task Force on Practice Guidelines. Obesity. 2013;22(Suppl 2):S5–S39.
32. Fridley J, Foroozan R, Sherman V, Brandt ML, Yoshor D. Bariatric surgery for the treatment of idiopathic intracranial hypertension. J Neurosurg. 2011;114(1):34–9.
33. Handley JD, Baruah BP, Williams DM, Horner M, Barry J, Stephens JW. Bariatric surgery as a treatment for idiopathic intracranial hypertension: a systematic review. Surg Obes Relat Dis. 2015;11(6):1396–403.
34. Brodsky MC, Vaphiades M. Magnetic resonance imaging in pseudotumor cerebri. Ophthalmology. 1998;105(9):1686–93.
35. Sugerman HJ, Felton WL, Salvant JB, Sismanis A, Kellum JM. Effects of surgically induced weight loss on idiopathic intracranial hypertension in morbid obesity. Neurology. 1995;45(9):1655–9.
36. Bakhsheshian J, Hwang MS, Friedman M. Association between obstructive sleep apnea and spontaneous cerebrospinal fluid leaks: a systematic review and meta-analysis. JAMA Otolaryngol Head Neck Surg. 2015;141:733–8.

37. Choi DL, Reddy K, Weitzel EK, Rotenberg BW, Vescan A, Algird A, Sommer D. Postoperative continuous positive airway pressure use and nasal saline rinses after endonasal endoscopic skull base surgery in patients with obstructive sleep apnea: a practice pattern survey. Am J Rhinol Allergy. 2019;33(1):51–5.
38. Huyett P, Soose RJ, Schell AE, Fernandez-Miranda JC, Gardner PA, Synderman CH, Wang EW. Risk of postoperative complications in patients with obstructive sleep apnea following skull base surgery. Otolaryngol Head Neck Surg. 2018;158(6):1140–7.
39. Chung SY, Sylvester MJ, Patel VR, Zaki M, Baredes S, Liu JK, Eloy JA. Impact of obstructive sleep apnea in transsphenoidal pituitary surgery: an analysis of inpatient data. Laryngoscope. 2018;128(5):1027–32.

Part IV

History of Surgical Approaches and Techniques for Skull Base Reconstruction

13

Mario Turri-Zanoni, Giorgio Sileo, and Iacopo Dallan

13.1 Historical Background

Endonasal surgery dates back to the times of Hippocrates, who described different methods to remove nasal polyps such as the "sponge method" and, for larger ones, by fashioning a loop around the base of the polyps and removing them through the nasopharynx; afterwards the nasal cavities were filled with stents soaked with oil, honey, and copper powder [1]. In 1806, Bozzini was the first to report the use of a primitive light conducting device to examine the nasal cavities and in 1879 Nitze-Lieter developed a light-carrying cystoscope, the forerunner of all modern rigid endoscopes, which was then modified and used a year later by Zaufal to visualize the Eustachian tube orifice [1]. Hirschmann performed in 1902 the endoscopic evaluation of the maxillary sinus, while the evaluation of the ethmoid sinuses was described a year later and it is considered to be the first case of endoscopic sinus surgery for chronic inflammation [2]. In 1912, Mosher described the open intranasal ethmoidectomy and, a few years later, he wrote about it: "It has been said that the ethmoidal operation is the easiest in surgery. So, it is to the operator who lacks a surgical conscience. Theoretically, the operation is easy, in practice it has proved to be one of the easiest operations with which to kill a patient" [3]. This emphasizes the rudimentary state of endonasal surgery at that time.

Similarly, the concept to separate the intracranial compartment from the nasal cavities was introduced only in the past century. In 1926 Walter Dandy performed one of the first successful surgical closures of a cerebrospinal fluid (CSF) leak through a frontal craniotomy and, some years later, in 1941, he described his transcranial approach to orbital tumors, the first report of surgery for anterior skull base tumors [4]. A few years later, Dohlman et al. reported an extracranial approach (naso-orbital incision) to close an ethmoidal roof defect using a nasoseptal mucosa flap [5], whereas in 1952 Hirsch firstly used an exclusive endonasal approach (transseptal-transsphenoidal) for skull base reconstruction at the sphenoid sinus level,

M. Turri-Zanoni (✉)
Division of Otorhinolaryngology, Department of Biotechnology and Life Sciences, University of Insubria, Varese, Italy

Head and Neck Surgery and Forensic Dissection Research Center (HNS and FDRc), Department of Biotechnology and Life Sciences, University of Insubria, Varese, Italy

G. Sileo
Division of Otorhinolaryngology, Department of Biotechnology and Life Sciences, University of Insubria, Varese, Italy

I. Dallan
Head and Neck Surgery and Forensic Dissection Research Center (HNS and FDRc), Department of Biotechnology and Life Sciences, University of Insubria, Varese, Italy

First ENT Unit, Azienda Ospedaliero-Universitaria Pisana, Pisa, Italy

A. A. AlQahtani et al. (eds.), *CSF Rhinorrhea*, https://doi.org/10.1007/978-3-030-94781-1_13

employing a mucosal perichondrial flap harvested from the nasal septum [6].

Reports of endoscopic surgery seemed to fade in favor of open procedures because of problems with illumination and instrumentation, until 1950s when Hopkins's rod lens system was developed. Since its introduction and first applications by Messerklinger in the 1970s, endonasal endoscopic surgery has spread all over the world, thanks to the contribution of pioneering surgeons such as Stammberger, Wigand, Kennedy, Draf, Lund, and others; although, in that years, skull base surgery was still performed by external transcranial approaches. Gradually, the endoscopic techniques, initially used only for chronic inflammatory disease of the sinuses, were adapted and expanded for other pathologies affecting the paranasal sinuses and skull base, firstly non-neoplastic conditions.

In the early 1980s, Wigand et al. dealt with minor CSF leaks encountered during endoscopic ethmoidectomies [7]. Ten years later, Mattox et al. were the first to describe an endoscopic management of CSF leaks and encephalocele; afterwards, Lanza et al. demonstrated that the endoscopic endonasal approach might be safe and effective: indeed, between 1991 and 1995, they performed endoscopic reconstruction of skull base defects in 36 patients, with a success rate of 94.4% [8, 9].

The increasing ability to repair the skull base defect through an endoscopic endonasal approach represented a step forward, deeply inspiring surgeons in an effort to manage skull base tumors in a minimally invasive way. Initially, the endoscopic management of intranasal and skull base neoplasms was confined to benign small lesions. In 1992, Waitz et al. proved that, even with large lesions, a successful and safe endoscopic removal of inverted papillomas was feasible: they reported on a series of 51 patients, 35 of which were treated endoscopically, whereas 16 underwent an extranasal approach [10]. Likewise, treatment of fibro-osseous lesions has been described [11]. In the same years, endoscopic trans-sphenoidal approaches for the management of pituitary tumors were also developed, besides angled endoscopes allowed a more thorough inspection of the sella [12, 13]. With endoscopic techniques, the integrity of the facial skeleton is maintained and external incisions are avoided, although concerns persisted regarding the oncological safety when performing endoscopic cancers removal. Some years later, in the late 1990s, few pioneering authors postulated, in carefully selected cases, the possibility of endoscopic endonasal management of malignant tumors of the sinonasal tract. The dogma of "en bloc" resection [14, 15] was gradually put aside and replaced with the concept of "disassembling" of the tumor: between 1989 and 1999 Stammberger et al. treated 43 patients with skull base tumors endoscopically, reaching overall control rates similar to those obtained with external approaches [16]. In the same years, May et al. introduced the four-hands surgical technique, which enabled to perform expanded endonasal approaches by using more surgical instruments in a single nasal cavity with the cooperation of two working surgeons [17]. In this regard, pioneering case-series demonstrated the feasibility of endoscopic accessibility even to remote regions of the skull base, thus allowing possible endoscopic treatment of relatively large skull base tumors [14].

Increasing with experience in endoscopic surgery, it appeared clear that the efficacy of any surgical skull base procedure was directly determined by the ability to repair the possible resulting skull base defect, which has been a major challenge over the past decades. While reconstruction procedures in craniofacial surgery were already consolidated, including pericranial flaps and galeal-pericranial flaps, which have received the widest consent, the endoscopic endonasal skull base reconstruction techniques have been developed in recent years. Early endoscopic endonasal reconstructive techniques were based on experience with the repair of defects following spontaneous CSF leaks and those resulting from accidental or iatrogenic trauma. Over time, multiple reports have validated that small skull base defects can be reconstructed via endoscopic endonasal surgery using a wide variety of free grafting techniques, with a success rate of 96% [18].

The simplest reconstruction technique, which was described for managing small defects of the olfactory cleft, was the *overlay technique*. In this case, the recipient site should be stripped of its mucosal layer in the area to be covered by a graft, which is usually either mucoperichondrial or mucoperiosteal harvested from the ipsilateral or contralateral nasal cavity, put in place with the mucosa side facing the nasal cavity [18]. If used, fibrin glue is placed along the graft margins but, preferably, not under it. Afterwards, the *underlay technique* has been introduced, where the graft is placed between the dura and the bone of the skull base, and it is recommended to create the underlay graft larger than the dural defect to compensate for shrinking of the graft during healing [18]. The combination of underlay and overlay grafts in association with intracranial intradural grafts represents the *multilayer technique*: in this case, it is recommended not to bury any nasal mucosa under the graft or flap in order to avoid the formation of mucocele. The basic principle of multilayered reconstruction is to re-establish the single tissue barriers. The technique usually involves the application of three layers: the first is usually made up of autologous fascia (iliotibial tract or temporal fascia) or dural substitutes, placed *intracranially intradurally,* to serve as a guide for fibroblast migration; it must be one-third larger than the dural defect; the second *intracranial-extradural* layer guarantees the plasty with greater stability; the third layer, *extracranial-intranasal* (overlay), facilitates the sealing capacity of the plasty by guiding the repair mechanisms of the nasal mucosa [19]. This latter layer can be made of fascia or free mucosal grafts harvested from nasal septum or turbinate. Healing and re-epithelization is much more rapid when mucoperiosteum is used as a third layer (overlay), rather than fascia lata, which can sometimes become necrotic even after 1 or 2 months. The "fat plug" technique is a variant of the multilayer technique in which a fat lobule is used as intracranial intradural graft, it was described for the first time by Wormald et al: they introduced a fat plug with a vicryl suture into the intradural space, thus sealing successfully the skull base defect in six patients [20].

Despite the advances obtained, in the early 2000s, when dealing with large skull base defects produced by expanded endonasal approaches, especially when placed in the middle or posterior cranial base, the reconstruction still represented a challenge because of the size of the defects, the lack of supporting structures, and the effects of gravity. The introduction in 2006 of the nasoseptal flap by Hadad and Bassagasteguy (HBF) has completely revolutionized the surgery in this field [21]. The flap is supplied by posterior nasoseptal arteries and can be designed according to the size and shape of the anticipated defect, although it is best to overestimate the size and then trim the flap if needed. The HBF had a profound impact on the advancement and acceptance of expanded endonasal approaches because the incidence of post-surgical CSF leaks dramatically decreased to <5%, thus allowing further expansion of endoscopic skull base procedures. The HBF has become a mainstay reconstructive option after expanded endonasal approaches due to its versatility, wide arc of rotation, generous size, and relative ease of harvesting. After that, many other pedicled vascularized flaps have been developed for the reconstruction of skull base defects resulting from endoscopic expanded approaches, with a further decrease in cerebrospinal fluid leak incidence, even when dealing with middle and posterior skull base defects. Figure 13.1 shows the evolution of the skull base reconstruction techniques from the beginning of the nineteenth century to the introduction of the HBF.

A recent refinement of the multilayer repair was the introduction of the "Gasket-seal closure" technique in 2008, which represented a practical and effective method to manage skull base defects placed at the sphenoethmoidal-planum and clivus level (middle and posterior cranial fossae), where dural undermining is more risky due to the proximity of neurovascular structures such as cranial nerves, carotid artery and basilar tip [22]. Leng et al. described this technique in treating 10 patients and none of them showed postoperative CSF leakage after 12 months of follow-up [22]. This method provides a really watertight closure because the graft is placed on the dural defect and its central portion is pushed inside the defect, using shaped fragment of septal or conchal cartilage, which is fixed beyond the dural border to

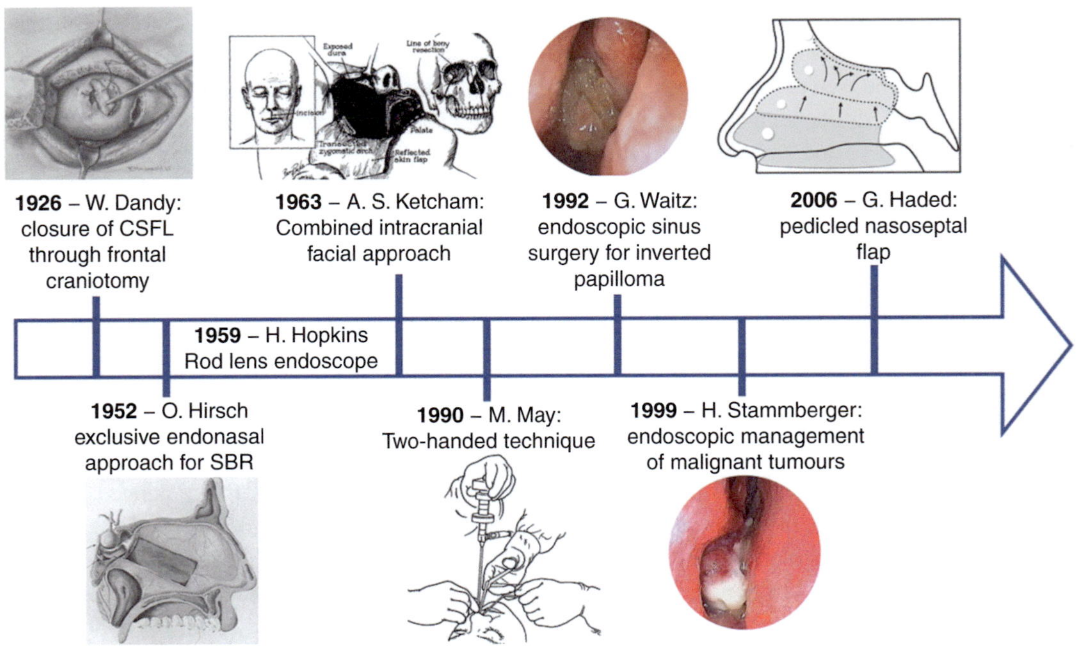

Fig. 13.1 Evolution of the skull base reconstruction techniques from the beginning of nineteenth century to date

seal the closure [22]. The combined use of a gasket-seal closure and a vascularized pedicle nasoseptal flap multilayered reconstruction technique for high-flow cerebrospinal fluid leaks after endonasal endoscopic skull base surgery represented a further step forward in minimizing postoperative CSF leak rates and improving mucosal healing of the nasal cavities after surgery [23]. Nowadays, the progressive refinements in surgical instrumentation, the increasing surgical experience, and confidence demonstrated that endoscopic surgery is an effective and reliable treatment for the management of skull base defects.

13.2 Evolution of Materials and Techniques for Skull Base Repair

The materials used for the repair of skull base defects are different and there has been an evolution of the heterologous or autologous tissues which have been employed over the years. The process of wound healing after dura repair using a degradable transplant is believed to occur by endogenous tissue (fibroblast migration from dura borders) replacing the graft, resulting ultimately in a thick scar. Collagen grafts are extremely effective in this context. Non-degradable materials, however, cannot be replaced by endogenous tissue due to their resistance against enzymatic and cellular processes; when they are biocompatible, they become covered with a thin layer of tissue during the healing process [24]. This is why it is stated that the ideal material for duraplasty should be:

- autologous, in order to avoid all potential risks of heterogeneous grafts;
- free of biological hazards in order to avoid HIV infection, hepatitis, and other transmittable diseases;
- able to facilitate fibroblastic migration and connective tissue deposition;
- capable of guaranteeing a good cost-effectiveness ratio.

13.2.1 Heterologous Materials

Synthetic materials, like Gore-Tex® patches, are episodically mentioned in literature. However, contact with brain surface or other neurologically sensitive structures should be strictly avoided. Other materials, such as bovine or human lyophilized dura, have been used in the past, but since there has been evidence of prion-associated diseases, they should no longer be used in routine [25]. Collagen membrane made of bovine (Achilles) tendon (DuraGen®—Integra Life Sciences, Plainsboro, NJ) has to be combined with other modalities of reconstruction because it lacks sufficient strength to provide a watertight seal. In 2005, Kassam et al. described a technique that involves a first layer of DuraGen, placed subdurally through the dural defect, a second layer of acellular dermis (Alloderm; Life-Cell Corporation, Branchburg, NJ) external to the dura, then fat graft stabilized with fibrin glue and a balloon stent [26]. Another option is Biodesign® (Cook Biomedical, West Lafayette, IN), a resorbable biomaterial derived from the extracellular matrix of porcine small intestine submucosa: Illing et al. in 2013 reported its effective and safe use for skull base reconstruction in 155 patients, obtaining a success rate of 100% after 77 weeks of follow-up [27].

13.2.2 Autologous Grafts

- *Fascia lata or iliotibial tract*, a much-preferred autologous grafting material with good healing properties. It is easy to harvest and large grafts can be obtained. It can be used in association with other grafts, whether free or pedicled. In 2017, Mattavelli et al. reported an overall CSF leak rate of 5.8% in 186 patients who underwent a three-layer reconstruction with iliotibial tract after transnasal craniectomy [19]. According to the authors it is a feasible, reproducible, and safe option for reconstruction of anterior skull base defects, especially when vascularized flaps are not available [19]. Figure 13.2 shows the harvesting of fascia lata and its placing to cover a skull base defect in a multilayer fashion.
- *Fascia temporalis,* it is easier to harvest but is thinner and weaker than the fascia lata, and only smaller grafts can be obtained.
- *Mucoperiosteum/mucoperichondrium*, harvested from septum or turbinates.
- *Cartilage*, it can be harvested from the nasal septum, the ear concha, or tragus, but in experimental studies performed by Schick et al. in 2003, no evidence of cellular migration was found into its surface [24]. For this reason, according to Draf et al., in case of use of cartilage graft it is recommendable to leave additional perichondrium or periostium attached to it in order to allow cellular migration [28].
- *Bone*, it can be harvested from the nasal septum or turbinates, but it can be dislocated or even extruded, especially after radiotherapy.
- *Fat*, it can be used as an obliteration material, possibly in combination with fascia, in cases of hypo-pneumatized sinuses. Some further applications are to stabilize the overlay graft or, taken in small pieces, as "cushion-like device" between grafts in the multilayer duraplasty.

13.2.3 Pedicled Flaps

- *Hadad-Bassagasteguy Flap (HBF):* is a vascular pedicle flap supplied by the nasoseptal artery, which arises from the posterior nasal artery, one of the terminal branches of the maxillary artery [21]. The posterior nasoseptal arteries supply the entire length of the nasal septum and anastomose with the ethmoidal arteries superiorly, the greater palatine artery inferiorly, and the anterior facial artery anteriorly. This rich vascular pedicle ensures versatility, wide arc of rotation, generous size, and relative ease of harvesting; therefore, it has become a mainstay reconstructive option after expanded endonasal

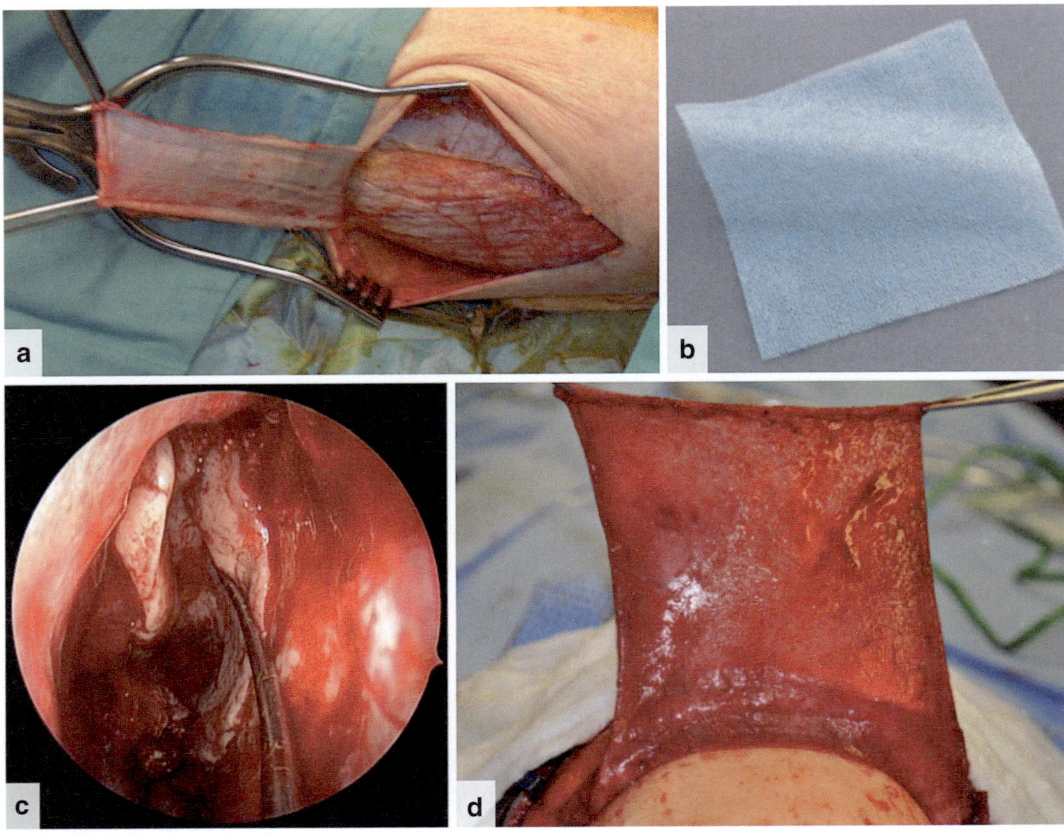

Fig. 13.2 Materials used for skull base reconstruction. Fascia lata (**a**), synthetic dural substitute (**b**), Hadad-Bassagasteguy flap in right nasal fossa (**c**), pericranial flap (**d**)

approaches. Its introduction has led to a significant decrease in post-surgical cerebrospinal fluid leaks (<5%), thus allowing the expansion of endoscopic skull base procedures [29]. In 2006, Hadad et al. made a retrospective review of 43 patients underwent endonasal skull base surgery and reconstruction with this flap: no infectious or wound complications were noticed and only two patients (5%) had cerebrospinal fluid leaks [21]. This pedicled flap is recommended for reconstruction of large dural defects of the anterior, middle, clival, and parasellar skull base [21]. If the anticipated defect is large and a single unilateral flap would inadequately close it, a bilateral nasoseptal flap can be used: when planum sphenoidale, sella, cavernous sinus, and clivus are opened in patients with well pneumatized sphenoid sinus a contralateral flap is designed to complement the first flap and cover the defect. This flap is called the "Janus flap" because, once in place, it looks like the two heads of the Roman god Janus [30].

- *Posterior Pedicle Inferior Turbinate Flap (PPITF)*: In 2007, Fortes et al. developed a flap of the inferior turbinate mucoperiosteum pedicled on the inferior turbinate artery, which was used to treat four patients who had undergone an extended endonasal approach [31]. It has a good arch of rotation and it is based on the inferior turbinate artery, a terminal branch of the postero-lateral nasal artery, which is a terminal branch of the sphenopalatine artery. It represents a reliable alternative for the reconstruction of moderate size skull base defects of the posterior fossa and clivus, especially in patients with prior posterior septectomy or wide sphenoidotomies [31].
- *Posterior-Pedicled Middle Turbinate Flap (PPMTF)*. Described by Prevedello et al. in 2009 in six fresh cadaveric heads, the PPMTF

was able to cover defect of the planum and fovea ethmoidalis with a mean surface area of 5.6 cm^2 [32]. Two years later, Simal et al. reported adequate reconstruction in a series of ten cases who underwent endonasal endoscopic approach [33]. The PPMTF is suitable for the reconstruction of small defects after sellar, transtuberculum/transplanum, or unilateral transcribriform approaches. Its blood supply is mainly provided by the middle turbinate branch of the sphenopalatine artery that runs through the posterior attachment and constitutes its pedicle [32]. It can be challenging to harvest because of the anatomical variations of the middle turbinate that can be found in 25% of patients [34].

- *Septal Flip Flap (SFF)*: In 2016, Battaglia et al. described in four patients the use of a flap from the contralateral nasal septum based on the septal branches of the anterior and posterior ethmoidal arteries, obtaining successful skull base reconstruction in all cases without intra- or postoperative complications. Moreover, postoperative nasal crusting was significantly reduced with faster healing of the surgical cavity [35]. Three years later, Bozkurt et al. noticed no flap loss or necrosis in 24 patients who underwent skull base reconstruction with septal flip-flap following resection of sinonasal cancers [36]. Their retrospective review showed that the SFF can be easily harvested and, thanks to its rich blood supply, allows rapid healing over a previously irradiated wound bed [36].
- *Temporo-Parietal Fascia Flap (TPFF).* The transpterygoid transposition of the TPFF into the nasal cavity through a temporal-infratemporal soft tissue tunnel and a transpterygoid window was firstly described by Fortes et al. in 2007 [37]. The flap was used successfully for the reconstruction of large skull base defects in two patients who had undergone preoperative radiotherapy [37]. The TPFF is thin and pliable and because of its large surface area (17 × 14 cm) it can be used for the reconstruction of several defects including intraoral defects, oronasal fistulas, and large defects of the anterior, middle, clival, and parasellar skull base, particularly in patients with a history of posterior septectomy or previous radiotherapy. It is a pedicled flap based on the anterior branch of the superficial temporal artery, which is one of the terminal branches of the external carotid artery. According to Bolzoni-Villaret et al. when local flaps are not available, for oncologic reasons or previous surgery, the TPFF provides healthy and well-vascularized tissue to protect critical structures or irradiated denuded bone [38].
- *Trans-Frontal Pericranial and Galeopericranial Flap*: Since the introduction of craniofacial surgery in 1963 by Ketcham et al., the galeopericranial flap was widely used for anterior cranial base reconstruction [39]. Between 1987 and 1997, Cantù et al. performed 168 craniofacial resections using the pedicled pericranial flap as a reconstruction because it is adaptable, thin, and easily to harvest [40]. The pericranial flap was moved into the cranium and sutured to six small holes made on the bone edges, two in the residual sphenoid roof and four laterally in the orbital roofs [40]. Pericranial and galeopericranial flaps are based on the supraorbital and supratrochlear arteries, which yield a very large surface area [41]. Their use after endoscopic skull base procedures requires the introduction of the externally harvested flap into the nasal cavities through a bony window at the nasion. Castelnuovo et al. described a case series of 18 patients submitted to combined cranio-endoscopic resection of sinonasal cancers, where the pericranial flap harvested from a transcranial approach was successfully used to reconstruct the skull base decfect [42]. The pericranial flap can be harvested via a standard coronal incision or using an endoscopic assisted technique. In 2009 Zanation et al. demonstrated the feasibility of an endoscopic harvesting of the pericranial flap for endonasal skull base reconstruction: this flap was firstly used in cadaveric models, then applied in a 79-year-old female who had undergone endoscopic skull base and dural resection of an esthesioneuroblastoma [43]. The patients had an excellent healing and no evidence of postoperative cerebrospinal fluid leak [43].

- *Oliver Pedicled Palatal Flap (OPPF)*: In 2009, Oliver et al. investigated the feasibility in cadaveric models of novel modifications of the known island palatal flap, including the release of the descending palatine vessels (DPV) and transposition of the flap into the nasal cavity, to allow for pedicled reconstruction of skull base defects after endoscopic endonasal approaches [44]. The OPPF is an excellent alternative when previous expanded endonasal approaches and/or open skull base surgical procedures have eliminated all other reconstructive options [44]. Differently from the HBF, the OPFF can be harvested and transposed into the nasal cavity after the surgical resection [44]. A potential complication is the possibility of oronasal fistula which can be avoided by preserving the nasal floor mucosa overlying the palatal defect.

13.2.4 Free Revascularized Flaps

In case of large and multi-compartmental defects of the skull base, involving multiple cranial fossa or after previous treatment such as surgery or radiotherapy, the previously described surgical techniques including grafts and pedicled flaps are not able to obtain a watertight skull base closure [45]. In such cases, free revascularized flaps should be harvested. Once the pedicle is isolated and cut, it is transferred at a distance and revascularized with micro-anastomosis of the pedicle with the receiver site. The facial, superficial temporal, and external carotid arteries are the preferable recipient arteries, whereas the primary recipient veins are usually the external jugular and facial veins [45]. They can be fascia-muscle-cutaneous, generally employed for soft tissue reconstruction, such as the radial forearm flap, the anterolateral thigh (ALT) flap, the latissimus dorsi flap, and the rectus abdominis myocutaneous (RAM) flap. Otherwise, they can be osteo-muscle-cutaneous, generally for combined bone reconstruction, like the fibular flap, the scapular flap, and the iliac crest flap. In 2016, Cherubino et al. published a retrospective review of ten patients, affected by locally advanced malignant tumor, who underwent cranio-orbital reconstruction using a chimeric ALT flap [46]. After a mean follow-up of 12.4 months, three patients died of the disease, two were alive with disease, while five patients (50%) were currently alive without evidence of disease. Only one ALT flap had a serious venous congestion that occurred 48 h postoperatively and required surgical revision, the other flaps survived without any partial or total necrosis. No complications, such as postoperative CSF leaks and infections, were observed in this cohort, thus demonstrating that the chimeric ALT flap is reliable and adequate for a patient-tailored three-dimensional reconstruction and able to resist to the postoperative adjuvant treatments [46].

13.3 Future Directions

Endoscopic endonasal skull base reconstruction has been demonstrated to be an effective, safe, and reliable approach in most cases of skull base defects, regardless of the size of the defect (Fig. 13.3) [47].

One of the main liabilities of the endoscopic technique, however, in contrast with microscopic procedures, is the lack of binocular vision and consequently of third dimension that is the reason why surgeons seek sensorial and tactile feedback during manipulation of instruments by constantly moving the scopes in and out or from side to side. Recently introduced HD stereoscopes produce a three-dimensional (3-D) image of the surgical field, with natural binocular ability to perceive depth, volume, and distance accurately. Castelnuovo et al. compared the 3D technology with the high definition 2D scopes in four patients who underwent endoscopic endonasal skull base reconstruction [48]. The 3D endoscopic skull base reconstruction obtained primary closure without complications in all cases and, according to the subjective opinion of such experienced endosurgeons, improved depth perception, distance and size estimation, ability to identify specific anatomic structures, and hand–eye coordination. The main drawbacks detected were inferior sharpness, contrast, and lighting

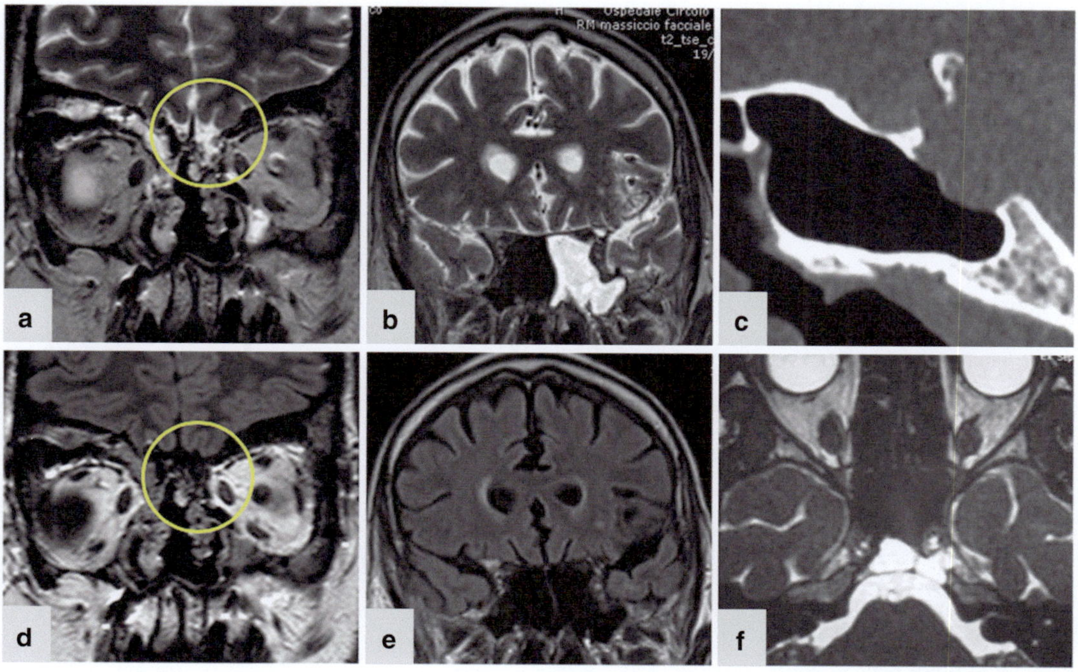

Fig. 13.3 Indications for skull base reconstruction. Olfactory cleft CSF leak: MRI T2 signal of the fluid component (**a**) and suppression of CSF signal in T2-FLAIR sequence (**d**), both highlighted by a yellow ring. Sphenoid sinus lateral recess CSF leak: MRI T2 signal of the fluid component (**b**) and suppression of CSF signal in T2-FLAIR sequence (**e**). Transclival ecchordosis physaliphora in a 40-year-old female: the bony skull base defect is visible at the upper clivus in preoperative CT scan (**c**) and it is confirmed by MRI T2 where a signal of the fluid component is present (**f**)

that impaired the application of the technique in narrow sinonasal spaces [48].

Another open issue is represented by the working area and surgical volumes related to endoscopic endonasal surgery. At present, because of the straightness and rigidness of the instruments, the surgeon has to remove important structures such as nasal septum, turbinates, and others in order to obtain an adequate visualization of the surgical field. A forthcoming technological development of endoscopic skull base surgery will be the introduction of flexible endoscopes and instruments to perform more minimally invasive procedures, allowing fewer traumas to the nose and paranasal sinuses, minimizing such postoperative sinonasal problems. In 2015, Schuler et al. described a preclinical pioneering cadaveric evaluation of the Flex© System, a computer-assisted flexible endoscope that covers a three-dimensional working space and has a flexibility of 180°, thus improving visualization of the surgical field [49].

A future technology that might be applied to endoscopic skull base surgery will be the use of virtual augmented reality (AR) combined with image guidance systems, which may have many interesting implications, such as to locate, through a virtual-reality environment, the lesion and its adjacent structures.

Robot-assisted surgery is continuing to advance in multiple specialties and the instrumentations are improving day after day. The reported benefits of robotic surgery are excellent three-dimensional visualization and the ability to accomplish two-handed surgery through small incisions or openings. In 2007, O'Malley et al. performed preclinical experiments using the Da Vinci Surgical System, developing a new cervical-transoral robotic surgery (c-TORS) approach which proved to ensure access the

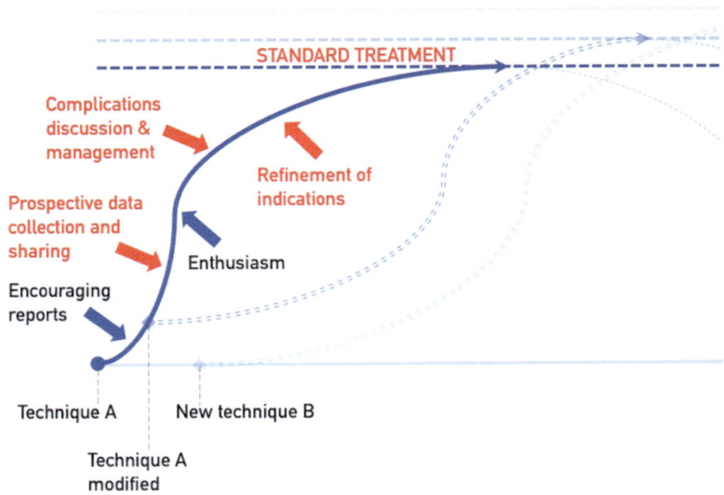

Fig. 13.4 The modified Scott's parabola shows how refinements of current techniques and newly developed techniques create a new standard of treatment

nasopharynx, clivus, sphenoid, pituitary sella, and suprasellar anterior fossa [50]. Such advances may be applied also to skull base reconstruction in the next future.

The dynamic role of a given surgical technique has been theorized in an elegant way by Scott et al. who developed a parabola that describes the rise and fall of a new surgical technique [51]. Figure 13.4 depicts a modified Scott's parabola, showing how refinements of current techniques and newly developed techniques are gradually acknowledged and create a new standard of treatment. When applying the concept of Scott's parabola to endoscopic skull base reconstruction techniques, we can expect promising evolutions within the foreseeable future, given that limits of endoscopic skull base surgery have not yet been set.

Acknowledgments MTZ is a PhD student of the "Biotechnologies and Life Sciences" course at Università degli Studi of Insubria, Varese, Italy.

Conflict of Interest All the authors declare no conflict of interest and no financial relationship to disclose.

Copyright and Permissions We declare that the manuscript text and all related figures are originals and no further permissions are needed.

References

1. Onerci TM, Ferguson BJ. Nasal polyposis. In: Pathogenesis, medical and surgical treatment. New York: Springer; 2010.
2. Stammberger H. Functional endoscopic sinus surgery. Philadelphia: BC Decker; 1991. p. 1–15.
3. Mosher HP. The symposium on the ethmoid: the surgical anatomy of the ethmoidal labyrinth. Trans Am Acad Ophthalmol Otolaryngol. 1929;34: 376–410.
4. Dandy W. Pneumocephalus (intracranial pneumatocele or aerocele). Arch Surg. 1926;12(5):949–82.
5. Dohlman G. Spontaneous cerebrospinal rhinorrhoea: case operated by rhinologic methods. Acta Otolaryngol Suppl. 1948;67:20–3.
6. Hirsch O. Successful closure of cerebrospinal fluid rhinorrhea by endonasal surgery. Arch Otolaryngol. 1952;56(1):1–12.
7. Wigand WE. Transnasal ethmoidectomy under endoscopic control. Rhinology. 1981;19:7–15.
8. Mattox DE, Kennedy DW. Endoscopic management of cerebro-spinal fluid leaks and cephaloceles. Laryngoscope. 1990;100:857–62.
9. Lanza DC, O'Brien DA, Kennedy DW. Endoscopic repair of cerebrospinal fluid fistulae and encephaloceles. Laryngoscope. 1996;106:1119–25.
10. Waitz G, Wigand ME. Results of endoscopic sinus surgery for the treatment of inverted papillomas. Laryngoscope. 1992;102:917–22.
11. Samaha M, Metson R. Image-guided resection of fibro- osseous lesions of the skull base. Am J Rhinol. 2003;17:115–8.

12. De Divitis E, Cappabianca P, Cavallo LM. Endoscopic trans-sphenoidal approach: adaptability of the procedure to different sellar lesions. Neurosurgery. 2002;51:699–707.
13. Thomas RF, Monacci WT, Mair EA. Endoscopic image-guided transethmoid pituitary surgery. Otolaryngol Head Neck Surg. 2002;127:409–16.
14. Yuen AP, Fung CF, Hung KN. Endoscopic cranionasal resection of anterior skull base tumor. Am J Otolaryngol. 1997;18:431–3.
15. Thaler ER, Kotapka M, Lanza DC, Kennedy DW. Endoscopically assisted anterior cranial skull base resection of sinonasal tumors. Am J Rhinol. 1999;13:303–10.
16. Stammberger H, Anderhuber W, Walch C, Papaefthymiou G. Possibilities and limitations of endoscopic management of nasal and paranasal sinus malignancies. Acta Otorhinolaryngol. 1999;53:199–205.
17. May M, Hoffmann DF, Sobol SM. Video endoscopic sinus surgery: a two-handed technique. Laryngoscope. 1990;100(4):430–2.
18. Hegazy HM, Carrau RL, Snyderman CH, Kassam A, Zweig J. Transnasal endoscopic repair of cerebrospinal fluid rhinorrhea: a meta-analysis. Laryngoscope. 2000;110(7):1166–72.
19. Mattavelli D, Schreiber A, Ferrari M, Accorona R, Bolzoni Villaret A, Battaglia P, Castelnuovo P, Nicolai P. Three-layer reconstruction with iliotibial tract after endoscopic resection of sinonasal tumors. World Neurosurg. 2017;101:486–92.
20. Wormald PJ, McDonogh M. 'Bath-plug' technique for the endoscopic management of cerebrospinal fluid leaks. J Laryngol Otol. 1997;111(11):1042–6.
21. Hadad G, Bassagasteguy L, Carrau R, et al. A novel reconstructive technique after endoscopic expanded endonasal approaches: vascular pedicle nasoseptal flap. Laryngoscope. 2006;116(10):1882–6.
22. Leng LZ, Brown S, Anand VK, Schwartz TH. Gasket-seal watertight closure in minimal-access endoscopic cranial base surgery. Neurosurgery. 2008;62(5):342–3.
23. Raza SM, Schwartz TH. Multi-layer reconstruction during endoscopic endonasal surgery: how much is necessary? World Neurosurg. 2015;83(2):138–9.
24. Schick B, Wolf G, Romeike BF, Mestres P, Praetorious M, Plinkert PK. Dural cell culture. A new approach to study duraplasty. Cells Tissues Organs. 2003;173(3):129–37.
25. Cappabianca P, Esposito F, Cavallo LM, et al. Use of equine collagen foil as dura mater substitute in endoscopic endonasal transsphenoidal surgery. Surg Neurol. 2006;65(2):144–9.
26. Kassam A, Carrau RL, Snyderman CH, Gardner P, Mintz A. Evolution of reconstructive techniques following endoscopic expanded endonasal approaches. Neurosurg Focus. 2005;19(1):E8.
27. Illing E, Chaaban MR, Riley KO, Woodworth BA. Porcine small intestine submucosal graft for endoscopic skull base reconstruction. Int Forum Allergy Rhinol. 2013;3(11):928–32.
28. Draf W, Schick B. How I do it: endoscopic-microscopic anterior skull base reconstruction. Skull Base. 2007;17(1):53–8.
29. Kassam AB, Thomas A, Carrau RL, et al. Endoscopic reconstruction of the cranial base using a pedicled nasoseptal flap. Neurosurgery. 2008;63(1):44–53.
30. Nyquist GG, Anand VK, Singh A, Schwartz TH. Janus flap: bilateral nasoseptal flaps for anterior skull base reconstruction. Otolaryngol Head Neck Surg. 2010;142(3):327–31.
31. Fortes FSG, Carrau RL, Snyderman CH, et al. The posterior pedicle inferior turbinate flap: a new vascularized flap for skull base reconstruction. Laryngoscope. 2007;117(8):1329–32.
32. Prevedello DM, Barges-Coll J, Fernandez-Miranda JC, et al. Middle turbinate flap for skull base reconstruction: cadaveric feasibility study. Laryngoscope. 2009;119(11):2094–8.
33. Simal Julián JA, Miranda Lloret P, Cárdenas Ruiz-Valdepeñas E, Barges Coll J, Beltrán Giner A, Botella AC. Middle turbinate vascularized flap for skull base reconstruction after an expanded endonasal approach. Acta Neurochir. 2011;153(9):1827–32.
34. Perez-Pinas I, Sabate J, Carmona A, Catalina-Herrera CJ, Jimenez-Castellanos J. Anatomical variations in the human paranasal sinus region studied by CT. J Anat. 2000;197:221–7.
35. Battaglia P, Turri-Zanoni M, De Bernardi F, Dehgani Mobaraki P, Karligkiotis A, Leone F, Castelnuovo P. Septal flip flap for anterior skull base reconstruction after endoscopic resection of sinonasal cancers: preliminary outcomes. Acta Otorhinolaryngol Ital. 2016;36(3):194–8.
36. Bozkurt G, Leone F, Arosio AD, Dehgani Mobaraki P, Elhassan HA, Seyhun N, Turri-Zanoni M, Castelnuovo P, Battaglia P. Septal flip flap for anterior skull base reconstruction after endoscopic transnasal craniectomy: long-term outcomes. World Neurosurg. 2019;128:409–16.
37. Fortes FS, Carrau RL, Snyderman CH, et al. Transpterygoid transposition of a temporoparietal fascia flap: a new method for skull base reconstruction after endoscopic expanded endonasal approaches. Laryngoscope. 2007;117(6):970–6.
38. Bolzoni Villaret A, Nicolai P, Schreiber A, Bizzoni A, Farina D, Tschabitscher M. The temporo-parietal fascial flap in extended transnasal endoscopic procedures: cadaver dissection and personal clinical experience. Eur Arch Otorhinolaryngol. 2013;270(4):1473–9.
39. Ketcham A, Wilkins R, Vanburen J, Smith R. A combined intracranial facial approach to the paranasal sinuses. Am J Surg. 1963;106:698–703.
40. Cantù G, Solero CL, Pizzi N, Nardo L, Mattavelli F. Skull base reconstruction after anterior craniofacial resection. J Craniomaxillofac Surg. 1999;27(4):228–34.
41. Yoshioka N, Rhoton AL. Vascular anatomy of the anteriorly based pericranial flap. Neurosurgery. 2005;57(1):11–6.

42. Castelnuovo PG, Belli E, Bignami M, Battaglia P, Sberze F, Tomei G. Endoscopic nasal and anterior craniotomy resection for malignant nasoethmoid tumors involving the anterior skull base. Skull Base. 2006;16(1):15–8.
43. Zanation AM, Snyderman CH, Carrau RL, Kassam AB, Gardner PA, Prevedello DM. Minimally invasive endoscopic pericranial flap: a new method for endonasal skull base reconstruction. Laryngoscope. 2009;119(1):13–8.
44. Oliver CL, Hackman TG, Carrau RL, et al. Palatal flap modifications allow pedicled reconstruction of the skull base. Laryngoscope. 2008;118(12):2102–6.
45. Herr MW, Lin DT. Microvascular free flaps in skull base reconstruction. Adv Otorhinolaryngol. 2013;74:81–91.
46. Cherubino M, Turri-Zanoni M, Battaglia P, Giudice M, Pellegatta I, Tamborini F, Maggiulli F, Guzzetti L, Di Giovanna D, Bignami M, Calati C, Castelnuovo P, Valdatta L. Chimeric anterolateral thigh free flap for reconstruction of complex cranio-orbito-facial defects after skull base cancers resection. J Craniomaxillofac Surg. 2017;45(1):87–92.
47. Turri-Zanoni M, Zocchi J, Lambertoni A, Giovannardi M, Karligkiotis A, Battaglia P, Locatelli D, Castelnuovo P. Endoscopic endonasal reconstruction of anterior skull base defects: what factors really affect the outcomes? World Neurosurg. 2018;116:436–43.
48. Castelnuovo P, Battaglia P, Turri-Zanoni M, Volpi L, Bignami M, Dallan I. Transnasal skull base reconstruction using a 3-d endoscope: our first impressions. J Neurol Surg B Skull Base. 2012;73(2):85–9.
49. Schuler PJ, Scheithauer M, Rotter N, Veit J, Duvvuri U, Hoffmann TK. A single-port operator-controlled flexible endoscope system for endoscopic skull base surgery. HNO. 2015;63(3):189–94.
50. O'Malley BW Jr, Weinstein GS. Robotic anterior and midline skull base surgery: preclinical investigations. Int J Radiat Oncol Biol Phys. 2007;69(2):125–8.
51. Scott JW. Scott's parabola: the rise and fall of a surgical technique. Br Med J. 2001;323:1477.

14 Operative Room Set-Up and Instrumentation

Revadi Govindaraju, Bing Zhou, and Narayanan Prepageran

14.1 Introduction

The surgical repair procedure of cerebrospinal fluid (CSF) leaks varies according to the site or sites of leak, size of defect, presence of meningoencephalocele, and other factors such as previous repair done and the type of reconstruction of skull base defect required. In cases where the site of leak is not identified preoperatively and to improve localization intraoperatively, intrathecal injection of fluorescein may be performed in the operative room prior to repair [1–3]. In addition to this, co-morbidity or predisposing factor such as Idiopathic intracranial hypertension (IIH) may necessitate lumbar puncture/drain for diagnostic or therapeutic purposes performed in the operative room [4]. This procedure is not limited to patients with IIH since there are surgeons who routinely place lumbar drain in all cases and others who use it only on select cases of high flow leaks, large skull base defects, or revision cases [3, 5]. Image guidance surgery appears to be useful in particular for complicated cases to locate the defect confidently and as a teaching tool for trainees [6, 7].

In order to accommodate the various requirements, the operative room should be equipped sufficiently and set up for an efficient workflow.

14.2 Operative Room Set-Up and Manpower

The operative room set-up should be tailored according to the operating preference of the surgeon. In our institution, the usual set-up is for the anesthetic working console and personnel to be at the foot end of the table. The camera system and the monitor are at the head end of table, slightly off-centered to the left of patient (Fig. 14.1a). In a standard two-handed single surgeon endoscopic procedure as seen in Fig. 14.1b, the surgeon stands on the patient's right and the nursing staff and instrument table on the same or opposite side. If the case is more complex and is performed utilizing a four-handed technique, it is performed in a brain suite (Fig. 14.1c). The main surgeon stands on the right of patient and second surgeon on the opposite side. The brain suite is fully equipped with image guidance system, wall mounted imaging viewer, and connected to an magnetic resonance imaging (MRI) facility in the adjoining room to facilitate intraoperative MRI if required (Fig. 14.1d).

For a simple repair procedure, the single surgeon may require an assistant surgeon/trainee who

R. Govindaraju · N. Prepageran (✉)
Department of Otorhinolaryngology-Head and Neck Surgery, Faculty of Medicine, Universiti Malaya, Jln Profesor Diraja Ungku Aziz, Kuala Lumpur, Malaysia

B. Zhou
Department of Otorhinolaryngology-Head and Neck Surgery, Beijing Tongren Hospital, Capital Medical University, Beijing, China
e-mail: entzhou@263.net

A. A. AlQahtani et al. (eds.), *CSF Rhinorrhea*, https://doi.org/10.1007/978-3-030-94781-1_14

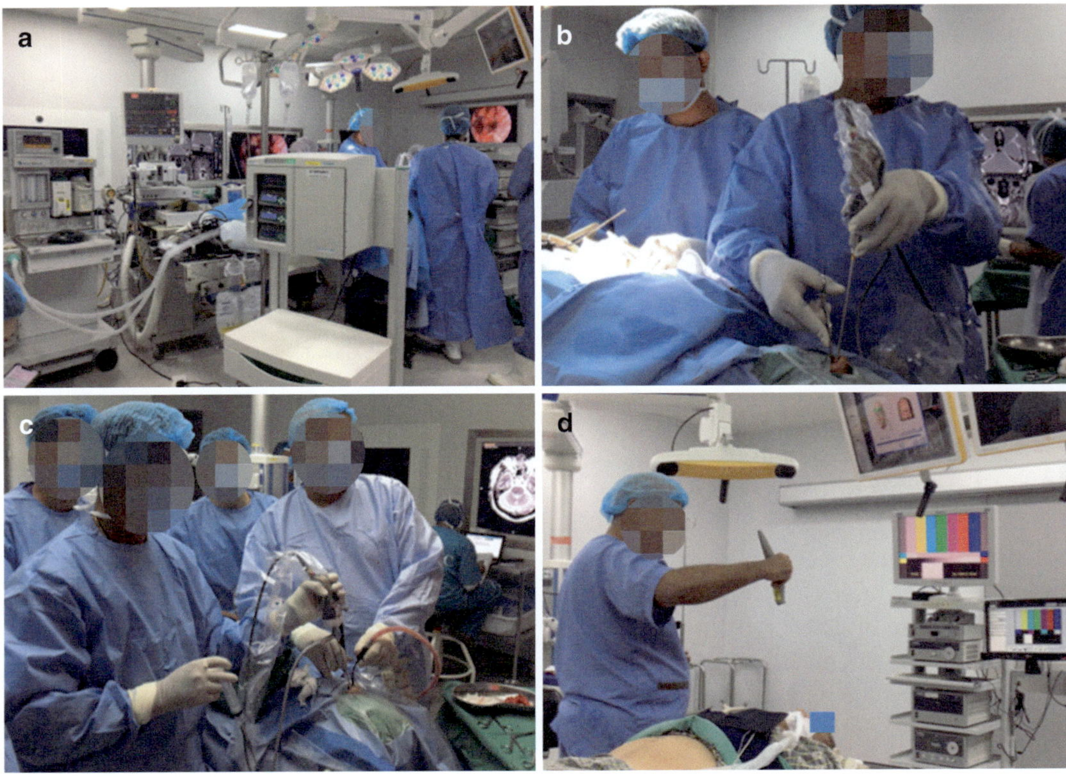

Fig. 14.1 Operative room set-up overview. (**a**) Anesthetic working console and personnel at the foot end of table; monitor and camera system console placed in front of the surgeons, (**b**) surgeon position in a two-handed technique, and (**c**) the positioning of surgeons in 4-handed technique. (**d**) Image guidance system; both monitor and camera array are suspended from the ceiling allowing ease and flexibility for adjustments

performs suctioning intraoperatively when cautery is used, for graft harvesting and to assist in setting up the image guidance system. A scrub nurse, a runner, and a general attendant may be sufficient to assist the surgery. In a more complex repair procedure, the requirement for nursing staff increases as the injection of intrathecal injection or lumbar puncture/drain procedure may run concurrently as the preparation for the actual surgery is going on.

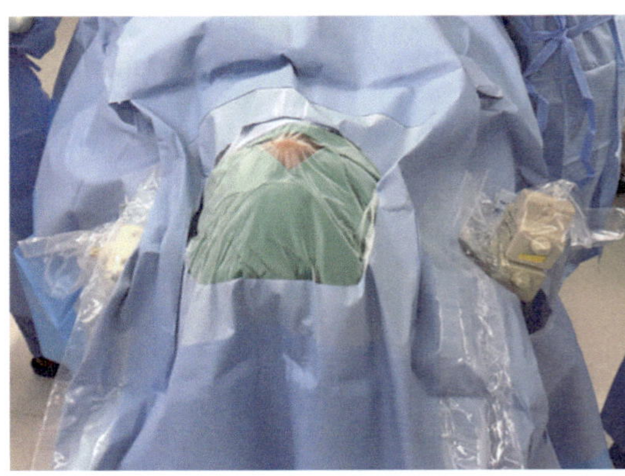

Fig. 14.2 Face draping done leaving the nose exposed and reference frame of image guidance system in transparent sterile draping

14.3 Patient Position

The standard head position used in our institution is a neutral position with a slight extension secured with either a 3-point fixation or using soft gel pillow; the head may be turned slightly towards the surgeon (Fig. 14.2). The head position however, may vary based on the surgeon preference. Some surgeons alter the degree of flexion or extension depending on the site of the defect; a neutral position when approaching sphenoid sinus but a more hyperextended position may be assumed for anterior locations [8].

Reverse Trendelenburg position (RTP) in 20° tilt allows for surgery to be carried out with good visualisation of the anterior skull base [8]. This position has also been shown to reduced blood loss in functional endoscopic sinus surgery (FESS) without compromising surgical technique [9].

The use of angled endoscopes may offer additional benefit for leak sites in a more anterior location, e.g., adjacent to the frontal recess or when an angled view is necessary [8]. The operating table should also be able to provide adequate tilt in other directions, especially in a case when head-down position (Trendelenburg position) is required to ensure intrathecal injection has received distribution to the site of leak [1, 7].

14.4 Image Guidance System (IGS)

The use of neuronavigational system have become indispensable in any skull base surgery. The system incorporates a computer workstation, tracking system, surgical instruments, data transfer hardware and software [10]. The set-up and available space of the operative room should take into account the requirements of the specific system, its advantages, and disadvantages/limitations.

Some of the earlier systems are big and will need a separate tower to place them next to the endoscopic/video equipment stack. Monitors suspended from ceiling or wall mounted monitors are other options for space constraints. More recently, the physical attributes of the system have become smaller with monitors incorporating both endoscopic images and preoperative imaging that it can even fit into an office-setting (e.g., Fusion Compact by Medtronic, Jacksonville, FL) [11].

The type of tracking system used is also vital in designing the operative room set-up. The optical tracking systems require that the line-of-sight be maintained between the instrument tracker and the camera array. Conversely, the electromagnetic navigation system avoids the need for that but uses instruments with copper coils attached to it to detect the changes of electromagnetic (EM) field from an EM emitter attached to the operating table. Each system affects the way a surgeon stands and holds the instruments to avoid disruption of the tracking. To avoid this, newer products have been introduced that uses flat EM field generators that can be placed under the patient's head (TruDi and StealthStation IGS platforms). Other technological advancements include the development of microsensors incorporated into navigation suction instruments that is not affected by bending of the instruments. These malleable instruments have been recently offered by Fiagon ENT Navigation (Fiagon AG Medical Technologies), Stryker TGS Navigation System (Stryker), and TruDi Navigation [10].

Apart from the physical consideration and physics of the system, the computer workstation should be able to run the operating system used (e.g., Microsoft/LINUX) [11]. Triplanar imaging in neuronavigational surgery using hybrid or fused images of both computed tomography (CT) and MRI are technological features to be sought for in the newer IGS systems for better characterization of any skull base defect with herniated intracranial content [11]. The CT would give details of the bony defect and the MRI allows delineation of the herniation content to avoid undue complications such as injury to the vessel and brain.

14.5 Prepping and Draping

Once registration for image guidance is completed and lumbar drain or intrathecal injection have been performed as required, the patient is returned to supine position for skin prepping and draping. The choice of face prepping is variable, but in our institution normal saline alone has been the practice, with no adverse effect of surgical site infection observed. The donor site for graft is usually the abdomen or thigh: both need separate prepping with povidone-iodine and surgery is conducted with instruments separate from the nasal cavity to avoid surgical site infection. Surgeons who prefer fat/cartilage graft from the ear alternatively will need similar prepping with povidone-iodine and surgical site draped separately. Chlorhexidine is best avoided for ear as there have been reports of ototoxicity and also ocular toxicity [12]. Practices vary and there are surgeons who use chlorhexidine for abdomen and thigh and povidone-iodine solution for face and nostrils [13]. Finally, sterile draping for the face is performed leaving the nose exposed and the reference frame of IGS covered by a transparent sterile drape to allow the camera to detect the light-emitting diodes (Fig. 14.2).

14.6 Surgical Instruments, Devices, and Biomaterials

Surgery for spontaneous CSF leaks would generally involve standard endoscopic sinus surgery (ESS) steps for access. The extent of surgery is dictated by the site of leak. A leak from the cribriform plate or lateral lamella would require a complete ethmoidectomy, with or without middle turbinectomy. Sphenoid sinus leaks are trickier in particular if it occurs at the sphenoid sinus lateral recess; in such cases approaches vary from trans-pterygoid, transnasal transsphenoidal and trans-ethmoidal approaches to access the site of the leak. Intraoperative iatrogenic cause of CSF leaks would require less exploration of the nasal cavity and the paranasal sinus.

A general ESS set is therefore essential to assist in the repair with the addition of bone rongeurs, drills/burs for bony removal in trans-pterygoid and transsphenoidal approaches.

Hopkins rigid endoscope in various angles should be available, though the most valuable would be the 0°endoscope. Technological advancement has seen further improvements in sinus visualization with the availability of endoscopes with mobile prisms allowing the surgeon to choose variable angles between 15 and 90°. This is also coupled with recent advancement in high definition cameras such as Olympus Viscera system [14]. Availability of such resources would enhance a surgical experience.

14.6.1 Special Dissectors (Intracranial Intradural)

Special dissectors or probes are useful to gently elevate mucosa around the defect in the cribriform plate or lateral lamella which can be easily fractured. In case of a meningoencephalocele, special dissectors, e.g., Rhoton microdissector set (Codman, Johnson & Johnson company, Raynham, MA) can also be used to palpate and delineate the bony defect (Fig. 14.3a–c). Once the dural herniation is reduced, angled probes can be used to palpate beneath the defect to elevate the dura if extradural graft placement is required (Fig. 14.3d). When the underlying bone is more solid or in the instance of thick scarred tissue superficial to site of defect as seen in Fig. 14.4a, b, a microcurette would also do the trick to expose the bare bone around the defect.

14.6.2 Electrocautery Devices

The conventional electrocautery used is the bipolar as the skull base defect is at the interface between the brain and nose. A straight bipolar cautery is useful to reduce the herniation of a meningoencephalocele if the lesion is in the medial or paramedian position but if the pathology is more laterally placed such as in the sphenoid sinus lateral recess, the use of a more angled cautery will be less frustrating. Insulated monopolar cautery with or without suction or with tips straight or bent are tools best reserved for hemostasis when creating access or for elevation of local flaps. It should not be directly used at the site of skull base defect (Fig. 14.5).

14.6.3 Other Instruments Used for Removal of Encephalocele

Encephaloceles have also been successfully removed using other instruments such as Coblator, which uses radiofrequency coblation technology [2, 7]. Herniated dura or encephalocele may also be resected carefully with thru-cut forceps [3]. This is preferably done after ensuring dural or encephalocele vessels have been cauterized to avoid intracranial hemorrhage [7]. Most surgeons suggest the use of the bipolar cautery to remove the last portion or the base of the encephalocele in combination with other devices [2, 3].

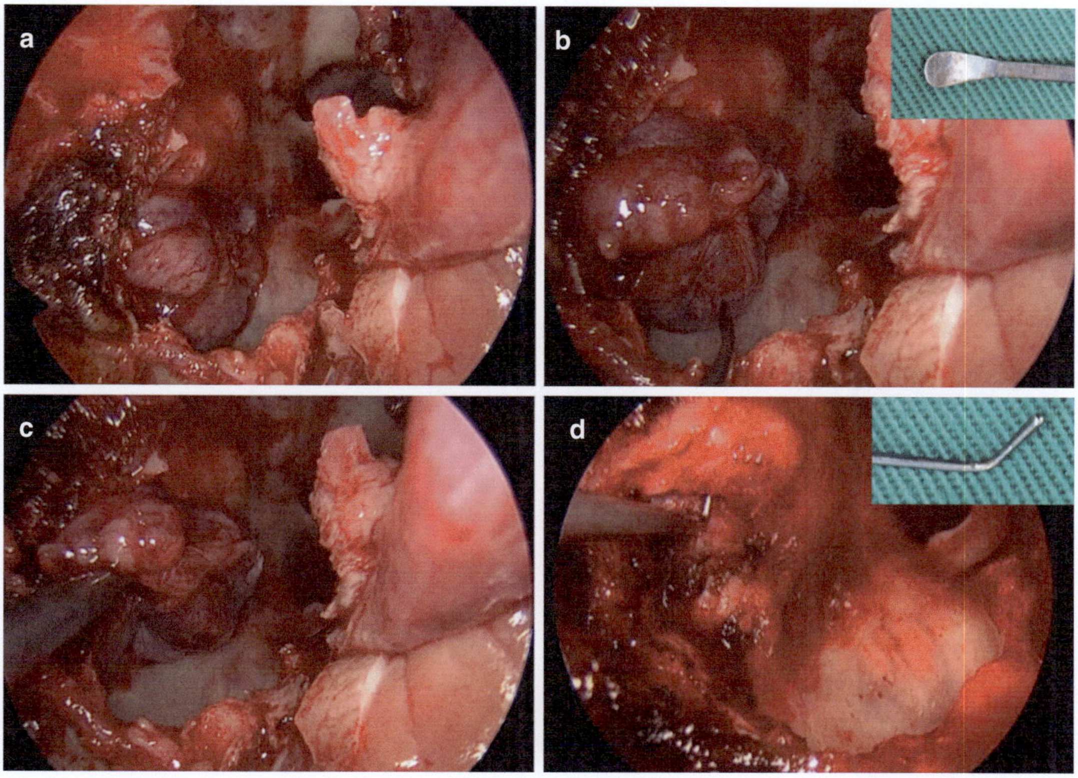

Fig. 14.3 In a repair of (**a**) sphenoid sinus lateral recess meningoencephalocele, (**b**, **c**) an elevator from the microdissector set (inset shows a close-up image) is used to palpate and delineate the bony defect in the recess and (**d**) subsequently after reduction of the herniation, 40° angled probe (inset shows a close-up image) is used to palpate around the defect

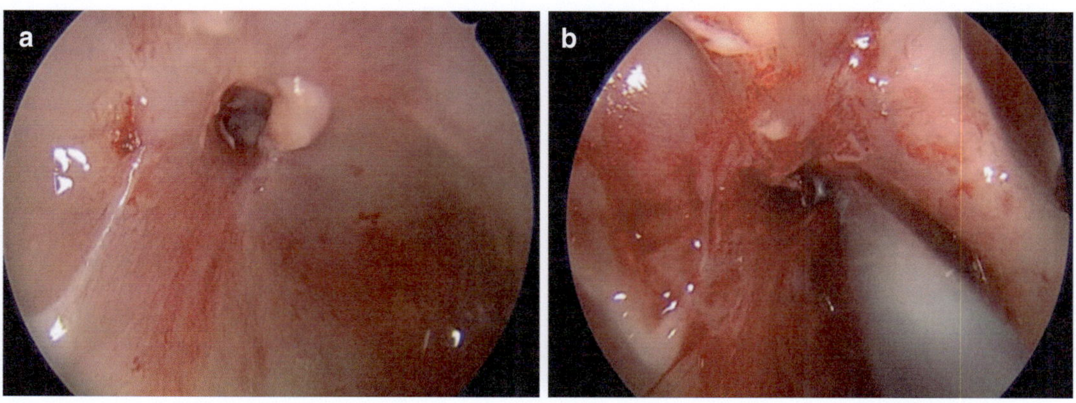

Fig. 14.4 (**a**) In the case of a CSF leak with surrounding scarred tissue, (**b**) a microcurette is used to dissect the scarred tissue and expose the bare bone surrounding it

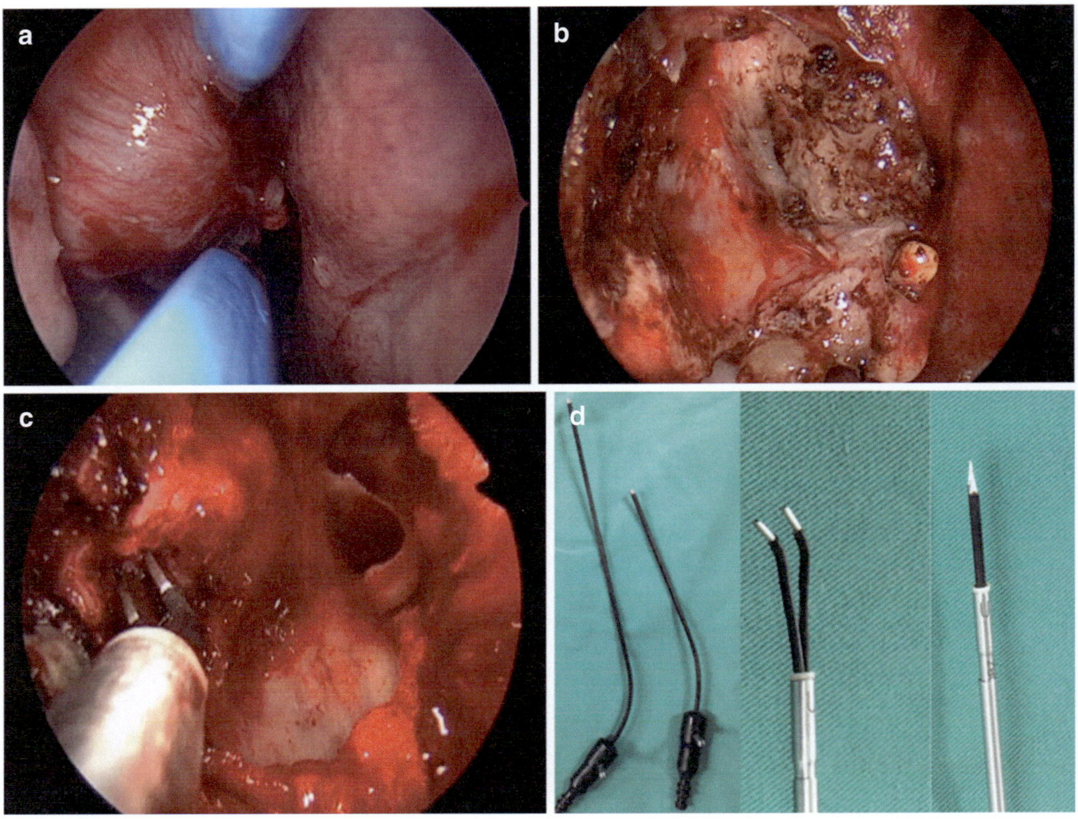

Fig. 14.5 Electrocautery used for reduction of the herniated meningoencephalocele. (**a**) A standard straight bipolar cautery instrument is used when the meningoencephalocele is easily accessible and allows a complete reduction of the herniated content (**b**). (**c**) An angled bipolar cautery is used to cauterize a small bleeding vessel in a sphenoid sinus lateral recess meningoencephalocele post-reduction. (**d**) Images (from left to right) of suction monopolar cautery's of different lengths, angled bipolar cautery, and a straight bipolar cautery

14.6.4 Special Graft Positioning Instruments/Seekers

Graft placement into the defect can be performed using sinus ostium seekers or double ended ball probes (Fig. 14.6a, b). These probes allow small amount of fat to be pushed in each time into the defect. Similarly, the special dissectors would also serve the same function for graft positioning (Fig. 14.6c, d). For larger defects, some surgeon prefers olive-tipped antral suction probe (without suction attached) or straight curette [15].

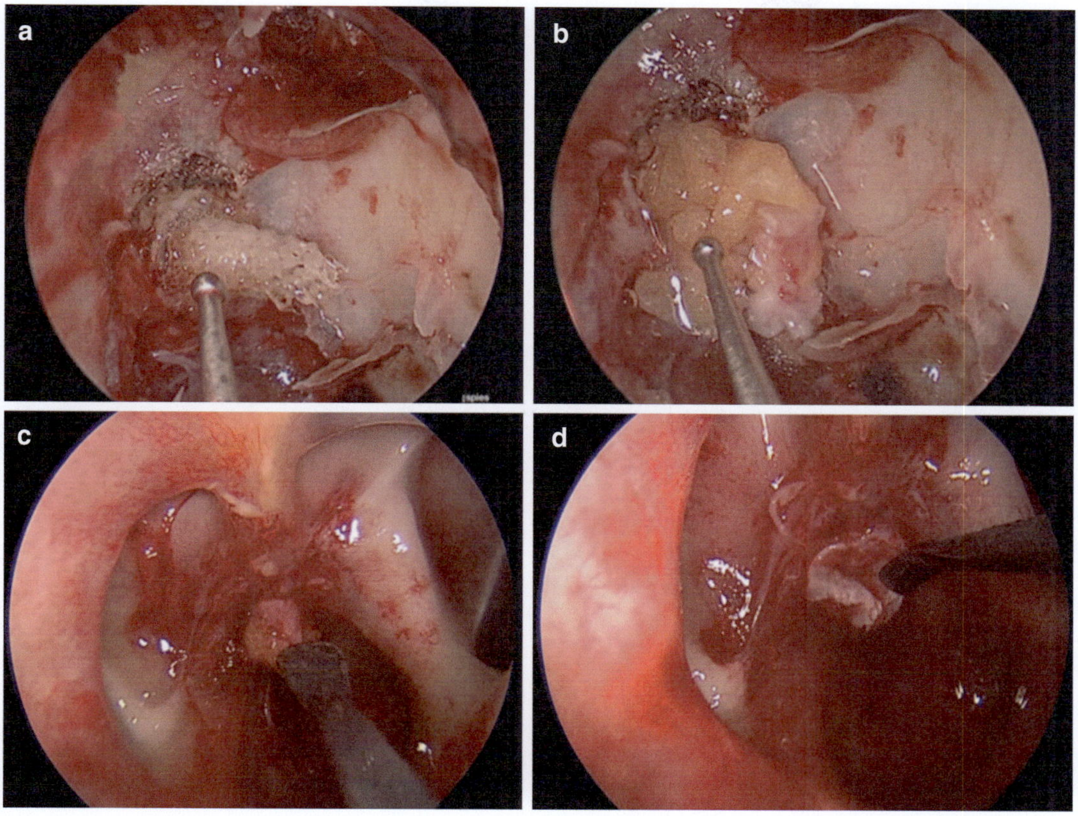

Fig. 14.6 Sinus ostium seeker used to position (**a**) hemostats, e.g., Surgicel and (**b**) fat graft into the skull base defect causing the CSF leak. Special microdissector used in neurosurgery is used similar to a sinus ostium seeker for positioning of (**c**) fat graft and (**d**) fascia lata

14.6.5 Set-up of the Suction During or After Positioning of the Reconstructive Material

Post-graft placement, the assessment of a watertight seal requires suctioning to clear the fluid around the grafts. In our institution, small square neuro patties (1/2″ × 1/2″, Codman, Johnson & Johnson Company, Raynham, MA) are placed as a protective layer when suctioning is used during and after graft placements (Fig. 14.7a, b) without having to set the suction pressure to a lower level. Neuro-patties are also useful as adjunct to gauge the defect size of an encephalocele by using it to reduce the herniation intracranially (Fig. 14.7c, d).

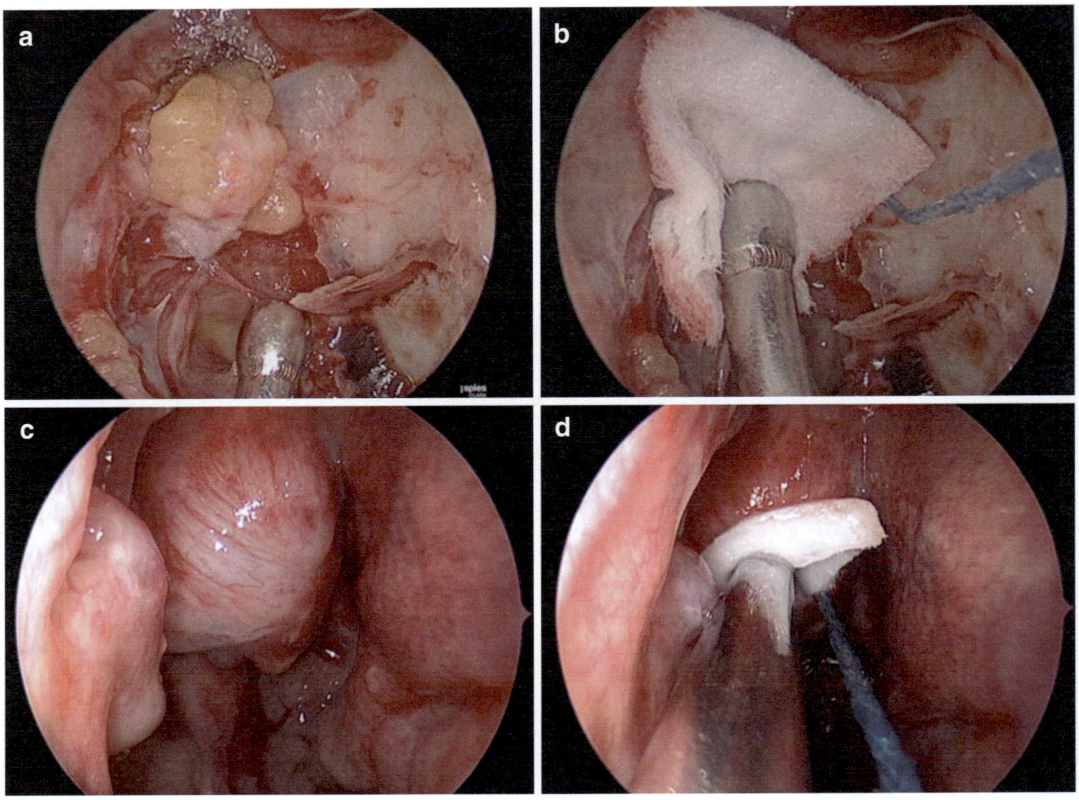

Fig. 14.7 Neuro patty may serve various functions. (**a**, **b**) Neuro patty is used to protect the graft from being suctioned out as the area is cleared of fluid before Valsalva is performed to check for a watertight seal. (**c**, **d**) Suction catheter over a neuro patty gently pushing the herniation; this will allow the surgeon to check the reducibility of the herniation without traumatizing the mucosa and at the same time delineate the bony defect

14.6.6 Sealants, Hemostatic Agents, and Nasal Packing

Fibrin sealants activate coagulation cascades and are useful to improve the graft adhesion to the defect edges. The commercially available sealant comes in various forms, preparation, and delivery system, e.g., DuraSeal (COVIDIEN, Bedford, MA), TISSEEL (Baxter Int Inc.), and Evicel (Johnson & Johnson Corporation) (Fig. 14.8a) The grafts can also be further supported by other absorbable and non-absorbable materials.

Commonly used absorbable hemostatic agents include oxidized cellulose polymer (e.g., Surgicel) (Fig. 14.8b), gelatin foams (e.g., Gelfoam) (Fig. 14.8c), and synthetic biodegradable foams (NasoPore, Stryker) [16].

In some cases, the grafts are further reinforced with non-absorbable nasal packing such as polyvinyl acetate foams (Merocel, MEDTRONIC, XOMED, Jacksonville, FL), carboxymethylcellulose-coated fabric tampons (RAPID-RHINO, Smith & Nephew), or simple materials consisting of Vaseline-soaked gauze or even Foley's catheter (Fig. 14.8d). In selected cases of frontal recess CSF leak repairs, glove fingers with Merocel within or silicone stents would help maintain patency of the outflow tract [7, 17].

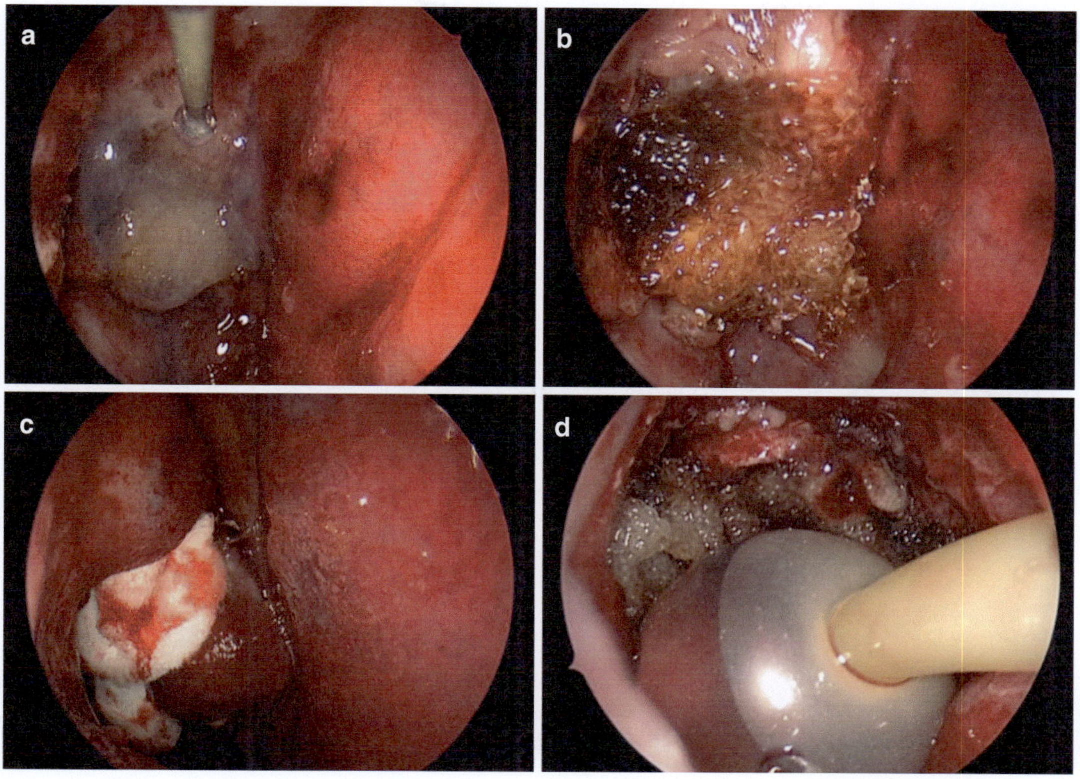

Fig. 14.8 Final stages of repair of CSF leak. (**a**) Tissue sealant such as TISSEEL is applied over the graft. Subsequent layers may involve more hemostats such as (**b**) surgicel and (**c**) gelfoam. (**d**) Foleys catheter balloon is inflated adjacent to the repair site in some cases of large defect with CSF leak

14.7 Conclusion

The basis of a surgical repair of CSF leak is common across the techniques described and utilized. However, along with technical variations present, there are myriads of instruments, devices, and biomaterials available at the surgeons' disposal to choose from to perform the procedure.

References

1. Wormald PJ, McDonogh M. The bath-plug closure of anterior skull base cerebrospinal fluid leaks. Am J Rhinol. 2003;17(5):299–305.
2. Smith N, Riley KO, Woodworth BA. Endoscopic coblator-assisted management of encephaloceles. Laryngoscope. 2010;120(12):2535–9.
3. Nyquist GG, Schwartz TH. Endoscopic management of cerebrospinal fluid rhinorrhea. Head Neck Surg. 2011;22(3):229–31.
4. Martin TJ, Loehrl TA. Endoscopic CSF leak repair. Curr Opin Otolaryngol Head Neck Surg. 2007;15:35–9.
5. Bedrosian JC, Anand VK, Schwartz TH. The endoscopic endonasal approach to repair of iatrogenic and noniatrogenic cerebrospinal fluid leaks and encephaloceles of the anterior cranial fossa. World Neurosurg. 2014;82(6):86–94.
6. Paludetti G, Sergi B, Rigante M, Campioni P, Galli J. New techniques and technology to repair cerebrospinal fluid rhinorrhea. Acta Otorhinolaryngol Ital. 2004;24(3):130–6.
7. Illing EA, Woodworth BA. Management of frontal sinus cerebrospinal fluid leaks and encephaloceles. Otolaryngol Clin N Am. 2016;49(4):1035–50.
8. Gonen L, Monteiro E, Klironomos G, Alghonaim Y, Vescan A, Zadeh G, Gentili F. Endoscopic endonasal repair of spontaneous and traumatic cerebrospinal fluid rhinorrhea: a review and local experience. Neurosurg Clin N Am. 2015;26(3):333–48.
9. Gan EC, Habib AR, Rajwani A, Javer AR. Five-degree, 10-degree, and 20-degree reverse Trendelenburg position during functionalendoscopic sinus surgery: a double-blind randomized controlled trial. Int Forum Allergy Rhinol. 2014;4(1):61–8.

10. Schmale IL, Vandelaar LJ, Luong AU, Citardi MJ, Yao WC. Image-guided surgery and intraoperative imaging in rhinology: clinical update and current state of the art. Ear Nose Throat J. 2020;100(10):475–86. https://doi.org/10.1177/0145561320928202.
11. Citardi MJ, Yao W, Luong A. Next-generation surgical navigation systems in sinus and skull base surgery. Otolaryngol Clin N Am. 2017;50(3):617–63.
12. Corby M, Meller C, Park S. Does perioperative skin preparation reduce surgical site infection? Laryngoscope. 2018;128(9):1987–9.
13. Ditzel Filho LFS, Prevedello DM, Patel MR, Otto BA, Carrau RL. Perioperative considerations: planning, intraoperative and postoperative management. Curr Otorhinolaryngol Rep. 2013;1(4):183–90.
14. Khanna A, Sama A. New instrumentations in the operating room for sinus surgery. Curr Opin Otolaryngol Head Neck Surg. 2018;26(1):13–20.
15. Chin D, Harvey RJ. Endoscopic reconstruction of frontal, cribiform and ethmoid skull base defects. Adv Otorhinolaryngol. 2013;74:104–18.
16. Massey CJ, Singh A. Advances in absorbable biomaterials and nasal packing. Otolaryngol Clin N Am. 2017;50(3):545–63.
17. Patron V, Roger V, Moreau S, Babin E, Hitier M. State of the art of endoscopic frontal sinus cerebrospinal fluid leak repair. Eur Ann Otorhinolaryngol Head Neck Dis. 2015;132(6):347–52.

Role of the Anesthesiologist

15

Alexandre B. Todeschini, Marco Echeverria-Villalobos, and Sergio D. Bergese

15.1 Introduction

There is evidence of primitive anesthetic procedures from pre-Colombian South America suggesting that coca leaves were chewed and placed in the wounds for numbing the area. This is one of the earliest evidence of anesthesia recorded. Its real advances, however, were developed in the late nineteenth and twentieth century [1]. Neurosurgery was born even earlier before any evidence of anesthetic procedures was produced by mankind. Anthropological specimens with successful trephinations date back to the Neolithic period. It was born to treat the damage sustained in fights, disputes, and wars when men realized that a blow to the head could quickly bring down an opponent or to alleviate spiritual ailments [2, 3].

Despite its ancient roots, modern neurosurgery would only develop after two important advances: infection control and anesthesiology. Anesthesia meant that surgeons no longer required heavy restraints on the patient during surgery and could perform the procedure slower and more carefully, and it allowed patients to undergo surgery without pain [1]. Both specialties grew and changed considerably, with new anesthetic agents and new surgical techniques. The contribution of proper anesthesia to the development of neurosurgery cannot be overstated. The pain and discomfort that were once considered necessary and noble in a patient's convalescence are now treated and prevented in patient-centered care, which led to improvements in patient outcome and satisfaction [1, 2].

15.2 The Need for Neuro-anesthesiologists

The collaboration between anesthesia and neurosurgery benefited both specialties and, slowly, the field of neuro-anesthesia emerged, as the specific requirements of neurosurgery were not fully met by the anesthesia used during general surgical procedures [4]. Despite the specific requirements and expertise involved, the Society of Neuroscience Anesthesia and Critical Care would only be founded in 1972 and still today there is opposition to the idea of every neurosurgical case, such as a CSF leak, requiring a neuro-anesthesiologist [5, 6]. The idea that specialized training is needed for anesthesia in neurosurgical cases is not new.

A. B. Todeschini · M. Echeverria-Villalobos
Department of Anesthesiology, Wexner Medical Center, The Ohio State University College of Medicine, Columbus, OH, USA
e-mail: Marco.EcheverriaVillalobos@osumc.edu

S. D. Bergese (✉)
Department of Anesthesiology, School of Medicine, Stony Brook University Health Sciences Center, Stony Brook, NY, USA

Department of Neurological Surgery, School of Medicine, Stony Brook University Health Sciences Center, Stony Brook, NY, USA
e-mail: sergio.bergese@stonybrookmedicine.edu

A. A. AlQahtani et al. (eds.), *CSF Rhinorrhea*, https://doi.org/10.1007/978-3-030-94781-1_15

Harvey William Cushing (April 8, 1869–October 7, 1939), oftentimes referred to as the Father of American Neurosurgery, also had remarkable contributions to anesthesia such as introducing the concept of anesthesia induction (using ethyl chloride), the introduction of the first anesthesia records (which he called "ether charts"), the monitoring of blood pressure and precordial auscultation (heart monitoring). Lastly, he was also the first to have a neuro-anesthesiologist working with him [2, 7].

"The Chief," recognizing the need for careful and expert management of the patient under anesthesia, was the first to have the same etherizer working with him constantly. His colleague, Dr. Samuel Griffith Davis, can be called the first neuro-anesthesiologist [7]. Dr. Cushing himself explained thoroughly the need for an expert in 1909: "*In cranial operations in particular, not only because of the cramped field and the need of a covering for the anesthetist, but also because the cardio-respiratory centers in the medulla are often already embarrassed through pressure, anesthetization by an expert is absolutely essential.*" He goes further to praise Dr. Griffith Davis: "*It is due entirely to his skill that in over three hundred cranial operations there has been a complete absence of the calamities usually assigned to anesthesia*" [8]. These considerations by Dr. Cushing still apply today. There may be situations when a neuro-anesthesiologist will not be available and a general anesthesiologist can be in charge of these cases, but it is preferable to always perform this complex type of surgery under the experienced and expert gaze of a neuro-anesthesiologist.

15.3 Antibiotics Administration

The risk of postoperative meningitis after endonasal skull base surgery varies between 0.3% and 7%. Antibiotics are often used to decrease this already small risk because of the serious sequelae this infection may cause, therefore avoiding a single case brings significant benefit, despite the risk of selecting more resistant strains [9, 10].

The ideal prophylactic antibiotic regimen is still debated, regarding both the drugs to be used and the optimal duration. Antibiotics should have no or few and only mild side-effects, low cost, and broad-spectrum. The duration of use is also debated [10]. In 1991, Carrau et al. analyzing skull base surgeries concluded that infection rates were lowest when antibiotics were used for 24–48 h after surgery when compared to shorter than 24 h duration or longer than 48 h [11]. Other studies, analyzing more aggressive antibiotic regimens, suggested that patients should receive IV prophylactic antibiotics until discharge and oral antibiotics until nasal packing is removed. The guidelines vary among institutions [10].

At our institution, we routinely conduct screening cultures of a nasal swab preoperatively. If the nasal screening is negative or positive only for methicillin-susceptible *Staphylococcus aureus* (MSSA) Cefepime 2 g IV before incision and a new dose every 4 h (2 g) is used. If the nasal screening is pending or positive for methicillin-resistant *Staphylococcus aureus* (MRSA), Vancomycin 1.5 g IV before incision and a new dose every 12 h (1 g) are also given. After surgery, Cefepime IV 2 g every 8 h is administered at least during the initial 24 h after the end of surgery. Patients then are advanced to PO cefuroxime *or* sulfamethoxazole-trimethoprim until nasal packing is removed, usually as an outpatient procedure.

The use of PO antibiotics, while the nasal packing is in place, is necessary to avoid the proliferation of *Staphylococcus aureus* and the possible occurrence of toxic shock syndrome (TSS), described by Todd et al. in 1978 [12]. This syndrome is characterized by elevated hyperthermia, headache, confusion, conjunctival hyperemia, cutaneous rash, vomiting and diarrhea, and oliguria, eventually leading to refractory shock. Laboratory findings include acute renal failure, elevated liver enzymes and failure, and disseminated intravascular coagulation [13]. The high morbidity and mortality associated with this syndrome warrants prevention while nasal packing is in place, a significant risk factor first described by Thomas et al. and corroborated by other studies [13–15].

Despite the variation in drugs and durations, taking into account the serious sequelae meningitis and TSS may cause, it is reasonable to use antibiotics for every skull base case. Our institutional protocol, outlined above, has been met with success and a low infection rate (according to in-house analysis, unpublished data).

15.4 Intracranial Hypertension

Understanding the origin of a skull base defect is paramount for successful correction. In spontaneous (i.e., non-traumatic or postoperative) defects, there is strong evidence suggesting that it is associated with idiopathic intracranial hypertension (IIH) [9, 16–18]. IIH is frequently associated with female sex and obesity (body mass index >30 kg/m^2). Patients frequently have either direct evidence of IIH (opening pressure higher than 15 cmH_2O measured through a lumbar tap) or indirect imaging signs (encephalocele, empty sella, enlarged Meckel's cave, and increased CSF in the optic nerve sheaths) [18].

CSF rhinorrhea may be a "physiological" way for the body to control the elevated pressure by creating an opening in an area where the cranial vault is thinner. Once this "escape valve" is closed during surgery, pressure can build progressively. Controlling elevated ICP should be a part of the management in these cases. Options to be considered include acetazolamide (a diuretic which inhibits carbonic anhydrase and reduces CSF production), shunt diversion procedures (ventriculo- or lumbar-peritoneal shunts), and weight loss. There is no consensus regarding the management of ICP in the treatment of CSF rhinorrhea. However, different studies have shown that controlling ICP significantly increases success rates of CSF leak correction when compared to cases with no postoperative control of ICP [9, 18].

At our institution, 24–36 h after repair surgery to correct the leak, a spinal tap is performed to measure opening pressure. If it is elevated, a CSF diversion procedure is scheduled (usually, a lumbar-peritoneal shunt).

15.5 Obesity and OSA

The association of CSF leaks and obesity may create further challenges for the anesthesiologist. Obesity is associated with an increased incidence of hypertension, diabetes, cardiovascular disease, obstructive sleep apnea (OSA), and obesity hypoventilation syndrome (OHS). Different issues may interfere with the management of the obese patient, from mask ventilation to postoperative care [19]. Excess body fat is usually associated with a reduction in chest wall and total lung compliance, creating a restrictive defect [20]. Airway management can be treacherous in obese patients. Detailed reviews of such management have been published [21–23]. To summarize, the obese patient, particularly if morbidly obese (body mass index >40 k/m^2), should be pre-oxygenated in a sitting position to increase tolerance to apnea during muscle paralysis [24]. Induction of anesthesia should be performed in the head elevated laryngoscopy position (HELP) to facilitate ventilation and intubation. The "ramped" position, which is similar to the HELP, can also improve the view during laryngoscopy when compared to the standard position [25]. Both these steps may be challenging and should be done by an experienced anesthesia care provider, assisted by a second person (preferably an anesthesiologist) accustomed with difficult airway management and with the necessary tools for the management of any complications readily available [19].

The presence of OSA, which is frequently associated with obesity, further complicates management. OSA patients have an increased incidence of systemic hypertension (from sympathetic activation), pulmonary hypertension, and right and left ventricle hypertrophy. These comorbidities lead to more complications, particularly involving respiration and intubation (difficult intubation and ventilation, unexpected reintubation, ICU admissions) [19, 26]. In endoscopic endonasal approaches, particularly those with dural opening such as a CSF rhinorrhea repair, the use of continuous postoperative airway pressure (CPAP) is not recommended for at least 7 days. Special attention to these patients is required after surgery to allow early intervention in the case of respiratory depression and need for assisted ventilation [27].

15.6 Blood Pressure Management During Surgery

Providing adequate cerebral perfusion pressure (CPP) and cerebral blood flow (CBF) is the most important objective of neuro-anesthesia, which are intimately related to blood pressure. It is important to understand the regulation of CPP and CBF in a healthy brain and how pathological states, anesthetic agents and the opening of the cranial vault can influence this relationship [28].

Permissive (alternatively called controlled or induced) hypotension is a decrease of 20–30% from the baseline mean arterial pressure. It has been used in neurosurgery to help reduce intra-operative blood loss and improve visualization during surgery. However, these benefits have not been proven, particularly in endoscopic endonasal approaches (EEA), where significant bleeding is not common. The potential risks related to this practice include cerebral ischemia and greater retraction injury from impaired blood flow, inadequate hemostasis and rebleeding after the surgery, cardiovascular complications, and renal dysfunction [29]. Considering these factors, anesthesiologists advocate a normotensive state or only a mild hypotension (15% reduction from baseline) should be used during EEAs, avoiding mean arterial pressure (MAP) below 60–65 mmHg [30]. Maintaining MAP during EEA above 70 mmHg during the entire procedure should be the objective during an EEA, and bleeding is usually controlled locally with minimal difficulty [29, 30].

15.7 Valsalva Maneuver

This maneuver was described by the Italian anatomist Antonio Maria Valsalva (1666–1723) to force out from the middle ear foreign bodies or pus [31]. In an awake patient, it is achieved by asking him while sitting to exhale against a resistance (closed mouth, glottis, or hand) to increase intrathoracic pressure to 40 mmHg for 15–20 s followed by sudden release and return to normal breathing. Under general anesthesia and endotracheal intubation, it can be performed by transferring ventilation to manual mode, closing the adjustable pressure-limiting valve, and compressing the breathing circuit bag for 15–20 s to elevate the intrathoracic pressure to the desired levels (40–45 mmHg). Before this procedure, the anesthesia care provider must ensure adequate depth of anesthesia or neuromuscular blockade to prevent patient effort against the forced ventilation. It decreases venous return to the heart leading to engorgement of cerebral veins, reducing CPP and CBF, and increased intracranial pressure (ICP) [32–34].

The Valsalva maneuver is used to identify the CSF leaks during the early stages of the procedure and to locate possible bleeding points that could become active with patient activity after emergence from anesthesia [33]. It can lead to complications that both the anesthesiologist and the surgeon must be attentive to before, during, and after the maneuver (after intrathoracic pressure has returned to normal). Some of these complications are: decrease in the MAP and possible ischemic complications, rupture of intracranial aneurysms, increment in intraocular pressure, macular or retinal hemorrhages, recurrence of a CSF leak from displacement of the skull base reconstruction, and a possible vacuum-effect at the end of the maneuver, from the egress of CSF during and normalization of ICP, leading to trapped pneumocephalus [32].

The Valsalva maneuver is useful to identify the exact location (or locations) of the skull base defect during surgery before reconstruction is completed. Its use after can displace the reconstruction and cause the defect to open again before the end of the procedure or if it is not noticed by the surgical team, it can lead to a persistent postoperative CSF leak [32, 33].

15.8 Emergence from Anesthesia

Early postoperative complications during the emergence period can have serious effects and may require re-intervention and can cause permanent sequelae or death. The role of the anesthesiologist is key to prevent these complications [35]. During the emergence period after the end of surgery, the anesthesiologist should minimize coughing, hypertension, hypoxia, and hypercapnia, which can lead to hemorrhage, cerebral edema, and elevated ICP [36]. A fresh reconstruction of the skull base to correct a CSF leak is put under stress in these conditions and can fail.

Hypertension, a consequence of sympathetic stimulation with an increase in circulating catecholamine and oxygen consumption, is a risk factor for hemorrhage, causing a recrudescence of bleeding from loosely coagulated vessels at lower pressures. Control of hemodynamic changes is always required at the end of a neurosurgical procedure. A prophylactic infusion of esmolol can be considered if the likelihood of a hypertensive episode is high. During the emergence, the anesthesia care provider should always have an antihypertensive agent (labetalol, urapidil, nicardipine, clevidipine) available at this stage, should it be needed [36–39].

Intracranial hypertension peaks can also be minimized by careful emergence procedures. Tracheal stimulation is a well-documented cause of increases in ICP, coughing, and cerebral hyperemia. The use of lidocaine in the laryngotracheal mucosa (instilled in the endotracheal tube) minimizes the physiological responses to this stimulus and its complications [36].

The anesthesiologist also has to be attentive to other important factors for a smooth emergence. Hypothermia should be avoided with air warming blankets to prevent shivering, which increases oxygen consumption and ICP. Pain prevention should begin in the operating room and extend into the postoperative care [36].

15.9 Postoperative Care

After the procedure, the patient is extubated in the operating room and transferred to the post-anesthesia care unit (PACU) where close neurological and hemodynamic monitoring is maintained usually in a 2:1 patient-to-nurse ratio. Once fully awake, usually after 2–3 h the patient can be transferred to a postoperative unit [40]. Headache is the main complaint after surgery and should be managed with narcotics or non-steroidal anti-inflammatory medications. Postoperative nausea and vomiting (PONV) can affect up to 40% of patients, mainly women and non-smokers, leading to a peak in ICP from the retching effort that could undo the recent reconstruction. No specific guideline for PONV prophylaxis or treatment in EEA or rhinorrhea repair is available but we recommend its routine use, particularly in non-smokers and women who are more susceptible to it [36, 41]. Retching and vomiting lead to peaks of ICP and blood pressure and a decrease in cerebral perfusion. A triple therapy prophylaxis is recommended to avoid this common complication. Some of the drugs that may be used are dexamethasone, promethazine, ondansetron, and aprepitant [42].

If any signs of complications arise in the PACU, the patient should be reassessed by the neurosurgical and anesthesia team to decide the proper course, which may include imaging exams, return to the operating room or intensive care unit (ICU) monitoring [40].

Not every patient needs to be monitored in ICU after surgery. ICU should be planned for those patients with a serious previous illness and an American Society of Anesthesiologists (ASA) score of >3, who would require ICU monitoring regardless of the procedure. Patients who suffered intraoperative complications such as excessive blood loss and transfusions should also be considered for ICU observation after surgery [40]. Other variables that have been identified in multivariate analysis as risk factor for postoperative complications and may warrant ICU observation are diabetes and older age [43, 44]. In otherwise healthy patients and uncomplicated procedures, patients can be transferred from PACU when fully awake to the ward for continued care and observation by the surgical team, concluding the role of the anesthesiologist in CSF rhinorrhea correction [40].

15.10 Enhanced Recovery After Surgery (ERAS) in Neurosurgery

The Enhanced Recovery After Surgery (ERAS) was first described in cardiac surgery in 1994, called the fast-track recovery, to reduce extubation time, ICU, and hospital stay with comparable rates of morbidity and mortality [45]. This concept expanded to other specialties improving outcomes when properly adopted [46, 47]. Eventually, in 2001, a European group of surgeons started the Enhanced Recovery After Surgery (ERAS) Study group and developed a model of interventions for the entire perioperative period seeking to reduce the physiologic response to the surgical insult [48].

Twenty-four core elements are distributed along the patients' pathway administered by different departments and professionals, working in synergy between one element and the next. The protocols should be under continuous audit, implementing changes as new evidence comes to light [49], resulting in different levels of effectiveness with reduced length of stay, complications, and readmissions [50, 51].

Despite the acceptance and success that ERAS protocols have with other specialties, the ERAS Society still does not have a neurosurgical protocol for craniotomies or EEA [52]. Few randomized control trials and narrative reviews on ERAS for craniotomies have been published, but the initial results suggest that adopting ERAS guidelines may, in the future, improve surgical outcomes. Table 15.1 reviews some of the guidelines that have been extrapolated from other specialties into the incipient ERAS protocol for elective craniotomies adopted in early studies [53–55]. It is important to remember that a CSF rhinorrhea correction, despite not having external incisions, is, nonetheless, a craniotomy, in which the craniotomy is hidden within the sinonasal cavity.

Table 15.1 Suggestions for an ERAS protocol in craniotomies

Preoperative counseling to patients and family on the objectives and expectations of surgery
Abstinence from alcohol and smoking for 1 month before surgery
Perioperative carbohydrate loading should be encouraged with clear, carbohydrate-rich liquids
Mechanical antithrombotic prophylaxis (graduated compression stockings, intermittent pneumatic compression)
Routine prophylactic antibiotic use
Minimize scalp shaving (if any needed)
Local anesthetic infiltration and scalp blocks
No recommendation on the anesthetic protocol at the moment (short versus longer acting anesthetics or TIVA versus pure inhalational anesthetics)
Non-opioid analgesia using IV acetaminophen, gabapentinoids, and non-steroidal anti-inflammatory medications. Opioids should be considered a rescue medication
Routine postoperative nausea and vomiting prophylaxis with serotonin receptor antagonists and dexamethasone
Minimally invasive craniotomies and endoscopic skull base approaches are possibly superior to other approaches
Avoiding hypothermia
Fluid balance through non-invasive cardiac output monitoring to determine volume status
Early removal of bladder catheters and surgical drains
Encourage early mobilization
Frequent audits to assess impact and encourage compliance

15.11 Conclusion

The anesthesiologist plays a pivotal role in any surgical procedure, being responsible for the well-being and homeostasis of the patient while the surgical team is concerned with the technical aspects of the surgery. The anesthesiologist should be integrated into the surgical team for the best outcomes possible.

As discussed above, many variables influence the outcome and the anesthesiologist needs to be aware of them to help ensure the best possible outcome. A well-trained and experienced professional should be in charge of the anesthesia procedures and the immediate postoperative care until the patient is fully awake and ready to be discharged to the floor, under the sole care of the surgical team.

Disclosures Funding Source: No funding was obtained for this study.

Financial Disclosure: The authors have no significant financial relationships to disclose.

Submission Statement: The contents of this manuscript have not been copyrighted or published previously.

IRB Review Statement/Ethics Guidelines: This manuscript did not seek IRB review or approval. This is a narrative review based on previously published articles and author experience. As such it did not involve any study on patients, chart reviews or data collection, therefore, not requiring IRB review.

References

1. Chivukula S, Grandhi R, Friedlander RM. A brief history of early neuroanesthesia. Neurosurg Focus. 2014;36(4):E2.
2. Goodrich J, Flamm E. Historical overview of neurosurgery. Youmans Neurol Surg. 2011;1:3–38.
3. Liu CY, Apuzzo MLJ. The genesis of neurosurgery and the evolution of the neurosurgical operative environment: part I - prehistory to 2003. Neurosurgery. 2003;52(1):3–19.
4. Frost EA. A history of neuroanesthesia. The wondrous story of anesthesia. New York: Springer; 2014. p. 871–85.
5. Ghaly RF. Do neurosurgeons need neuroanesthesiologists? Should every neurosurgical case be done by a neuroanesthesiologist? Surg Neurol Int. 2014;5:76.
6. Mashour GA, Lauer K, Greenfield MLVH, Vavilala M, Avitsian R, Kofke A, et al. Accreditation and standardization of neuroanesthesia fellowship programs: results of a specialty-wide survey. J Neurosurg Anesthesiol. 2010;22(3):252–5.
7. Molnar C, Nemes C, Szabo S, Fulesdi B. Harvey cushing, a pioneer of neuroanesthesia. J Anesth. 2008;22(4):483–6.
8. Cushing H. Some principles of cerebral surgery. J Am Med Assoc. 1909;52(3):184–95.
9. Oakley GM, Orlandi RR, Woodworth BA, Batra PS, Alt JA. Management of cerebrospinal fluid rhinorrhea: an evidence-based review with recommendations. Int Forum Allergy Rhinol. 2016;6(1):17–24.
10. Johans SJ, Burkett DJ, Swong KN, Patel CR, Germanwala AV. Antibiotic prophylaxis and infection prevention for endoscopic endonasal skull base surgery: our protocol, results, and review of the literature. J Clin Neurosci. 2018;47:249–53.
11. Carrau RL, Snyderman C, Janecka IP, Sekhar L, Sen C, Damico F. Antibiotic-prophylaxis in cranial base surgery. Head Neck J Sci Spec. 1991;13(4):311–7.
12. Todd J, Kapral F, Fishaut M, Welch T. Toxic shock syndrome associated with phage group-I staphylococci. Pediatr Res. 1978;12(4):500.
13. Kojaoghlanian T. Toxic shock syndrome. Introduction to clinical infectious diseases. New York: Springer; 2019. p. 301–7.
14. Thomas SW, Baird IM, Frazier RD. Toxic shock syndrome following submucous resection and rhinoplasty. J Am Med Assoc. 1982;247(17):2402–3.
15. Hull HF, Mann JM, Sands CJ, Gregg SH, Kaufman PW. Toxic shock syndrome related to nasal packing. Arch Otolaryngol. 1983;109(9):624–6.
16. Schlosser RJ, Wilensky EM, Grady MS, Bolger WE. Elevated intracranial pressures in spontaneous cerebrospinal fluid leaks. Am J Rhinol. 2003;17(4):191–5.
17. Schlosser RJ, Woodworth BA, Wilensky EM, Grady MS, Bolger WE. Spontaneous cerebrospinal fluid leaks: a variant of benign intracranial hypertension. Ann Otol Rhinol Laryngol. 2006;115(7):495–500.
18. Teachey W, Grayson J, Cho DY, Riley KO, Woodworth BA. Intervention for elevated intracranial pressure improves success rate after repair of spontaneous cerebrospinal fluid leaks. Laryngoscope. 2017;127(9):2011–6.
19. Brodsky JB. Thoracic anesthesia for morbidly obese patients and obese patients with obstructive sleep apnea. In: Principles and practice of anesthesia for thoracic surgery. New York: Springer; 2011. p. 377–88.
20. Pelosi P, Croci M, Ravagnan I, Tredici S, Pedoto A, Lissoni A, et al. The effects of body mass on lung volumes, respiratory mechanics, and gas exchange during general anesthesia. Anesth Analg. 1998;87(3):654–60.
21. Cattano D, Corso RM. Airway management of the patient with morbid obesity. Cases Emerg Airway Manage. 2015;2015:63–70.
22. Kristensen MS. Airway management and morbid obesity. Eur J Anaesthesiol. 2010;27(11):923–7.
23. Langeron O, Birenbaum A, Le Sache F, Raux M. Airway management in obese patient. Minerva Anestesiol. 2014;80(3):382–92.
24. Altermatt FR, Munoz HR, Delfino AE, Cortinez LI. Pre-oxygenation in the obese patient: effects of position on tolerance to apnoea. Br J Anaesth. 2005;95(5):706–9.
25. Collins JS, Lemmens HJM, Brodsky JB, Brock-Utne JG, Levitan RM. Laryngoscopy and morbid obesity: a comparison of the "sniff" and "ramped" positions. Obes Surg. 2004;14(9):1171–5.
26. Vasu TS, Doghramji K, Cavallazzi R, Grewal R, Hirani A, Leiby B, et al. Obstructive sleep apnea syndrome and postoperative complications clinical use of the STOP-BANG questionnaire. Arch Otolaryngol. 2010;136(10):1020–4.

27. Choi DL, Reddy K, Weitzel EK, Rotenberg BW, Vescan A, Algird A, et al. Postoperative continuous positive airway pressure use and nasal saline rinses after endonasal endoscopic skull base surgery in patients with obstructive sleep apnea: a practice pattern survey. Am J Rhinol Allergy. 2019;33(1):51–5.
28. Randell T, Niskanen M. Management of physiological variables in neuroanaesthesia: maintaining homeostasis during intracranial surgery. Curr Opin Anesthesiol. 2006;19(5):492–7.
29. Soghomonyan S, Stoicea N, Sandhu GS, Pasternak JJ, Bergese SD. The role of permissive and induced hypotension in current neuroanesthesia practice. Front Surg. 2017;4:1.
30. Amorocho MC, Fat I. Anesthetic techniques in endoscopic sinus and skull base surgery. Otolaryngol Clin N Am. 2016;49(3):531.
31. Yale SH. Antonio maria valsalva (1666-1723). Clin Med Res. 2005;3(1):35–8.
32. Kumar CM, Van Zundert AAJ. Intraoperative valsalva maneuver: a narrative review. Can J Anaesth. 2018;65(5):578–85.
33. Haldar R, Khandelwal A, Gupta D, Srivastava S, Rastogi A, Singh PK. Valsalva maneuver: its implications in clinical neurosurgery. Neurology. 2016;64(6):1276–80.
34. Porth CJM, Bamrah VS, Tristani FE, Smith JJ. The valsalva maneuver - mechanisms and clinical implications. Heart Lung. 1984;13(5):507–18.
35. Bruder N, Ravussin P. Recovery from anesthesia and postoperative extubation of neurosurgical patients: a review. J Neurosurg Anesthesiol. 1999;11(4):282–93.
36. Bruder NJ. Awakening management after neurosurgery for intracranial tumours. Curr Opin Anaesthesiol. 2002;15(5):477–82.
37. Lim SH, Chin NM, Tai HY, Wong M, Lin TK. Prophylactic esmolol infusion for the control of cardiovascular responses to extubation after intracranial surgery. Ann Acad Med. 2000;29(4):447–51.
38. Bergese SD, Puente EG. Clevidipine butyrate: a promising new drug for the management of acute hypertension. Exp Opin Pharmacol. 2010;11(2):281–95.
39. Brower KI, Murphy C, Arias-Morales CE, Rankin D, Palettas M, Bergese SD. Safety and efficacy of intravenous clevidipine for the perioperative control of acute hypertension in neurosurgical patients: a dose update. Clin Med Insights. 2017;9:2517.
40. Bui JQ, Mendis RL, van Gelder JM, Sheridan MM, Wright KM, Jaeger M. Is postoperative intensive care unit admission a prerequisite for elective craniotomy? J Neurosurg. 2011;115(6):1236–41.
41. Dumont AS, Nemergut EC 2nd, Jane JA Jr, Laws ER Jr. Postoperative care following pituitary surgery. J Intensive Care Med. 2005;20(3):127–40.
42. Bergese SD, Puente EG, Antor MA, Viloria AL, Yildiz V, Kumar NA, et al. A prospective, randomized, double-blinded, double-dummy pilot study to assess the preemptive effect of triple therapy with aprepitant, dexamethasone, and promethazine versus ondansetron, dexamethasone and promethazine on reducing the incidence of postoperative nausea and vomiting experienced by patients undergoing craniotomy under general anesthesia. Front Med. 2016;3:29.
43. Hanak BW, Walcott BP, Nahed BV, Muzikansky A, Mian MK, Kimberly WT, et al. Postoperative intensive care unit requirements after elective craniotomy. World Neurosurg. 2014;81(1):165–72.
44. Hecht N, Spies C, Vajkoczy P. Routine intensive care unit-level care after elective craniotomy: time to rethink. World Neurosurg. 2014;81(1):66–8.
45. Engelman RM, Rousou JA, Flack JE, Deaton DW, Humphrey CB, Ellison LH, et al. Fast-track recovery of the coronary bypass patient. Ann Thorac Surg. 1994;58(6):1742–6.
46. Bardram L, Funch-Jensen P, Jensen P, Crawford ME, Kehlet H. Recovery after laparoscopic colonic surgery with epidural analgesia, and early oral nutrition and mobilisation. Lancet. 1995;345(8952):763–4.
47. Kehlet H, Mogensen T. Hospital stay of 2 days after open sigmoidectomy with a multimodal rehabilitation programme. Br J Surg. 1999;86(2):227–30.
48. Kehlet H, Wilmore DW. Evidence-based surgical care and the evolution of fast-track surgery. Ann Surg. 2008;248(2):189–98.
49. Ljungqvist O, Scott M, Fearon KC. Enhanced recovery after surgery: a review. JAMA Surg. 2017;152(3):292–8.
50. Gustafsson UO, Hausel J, Thorell A, Ljungqvist O, Soop M, Nygren J, et al. Adherence to the enhanced recovery after surgery protocol and outcomes after colorectal cancer surgery. Arch Surg. 2011;146(5):571–7.
51. Group EC. The impact of enhanced recovery protocol compliance on elective colorectal cancer resection: results from an international registry. Ann Surg. 2015;261(6):1153–9.
52. ERAS Society. ERAS/guidelines/list of guidelines. 2019. Available from http://erassociety.org/guidelines/list-of-guidelines.
53. Hagan KB, Bhavsar S, Raza SM, Arnold B, Arunkumar R, Dang A, et al. Enhanced recovery after surgery for oncological craniotomies. J Clin Neurosci. 2016;24:10–6.
54. Mishra RK, Kapoor I, Mahajan C, Prabhakar H. Enhanced recovery after surgery: neuroanaesthetic perspective. J Neuroanaesthesiol Crit Care. 2017;4(1):17–22.
55. Wang Y, Liu B, Zhao T, Zhao B, Yu D, Jiang X, et al. Safety and efficacy of a novel neurosurgical enhanced recovery after surgery protocol for elective craniotomy: a prospective randomized controlled trial. J Neurosurg. 2018;1:1–12.

Synthetic Materials for Skull Base Reconstruction

16

Ghassan Alokby and Jarrett Walsh

16.1 Introduction

Significant advances in endoscopic sinus and skull base surgery can be attributed to the development of angled telescopes, navigation systems, and high definition cameras coupled with a better understanding of the endoscopic anatomy of the nasal cavity and ventral skull base [1, 2]. As a consequence of these advancements, skull base defects are now able to be managed through transnasal approaches using autografts [3]. The first endoscopic cerebrospinal fluid (CSF) leak repair was described by Wigand in 1981 [4] with the same principles for CSF leak repair applied subsequently for the repair of the defects resulting from endoscopic resection of skull base and intracranial tumors [5]. The use of vascularized flaps laid the ground for further advancements in endoscopic skull base approaches as the repair of complex and large defects that resulted from tumor resections were repaired with a success rate similar to the open approaches [5, 6].

Various grafts can be used for skull base repair, and given the multitude of options, we can match graft material to the size and type of defect to provide an optimal repair. Autografts such as nasal mucosa, abdominal fat, and fascia lata make an ideal graft from the point that they are derived from the same hosts, making them well tolerated, without the risks of immunological reaction or infection transmission. However, autografts have their limitations. A separate donor site may be required to obtain the grafts, with the risks related to the additional procedure such as infection, hematoma or seroma formation, cosmetic concerns, and longer operation time. Another limitation is the availability of enough tissue to reconstruct larger defects commonly resulting from oncological resection [7–9].

Using synthetic dural substitutes may address many of the limitations of autografts. However, there are certain criteria in the dural substitute that are essential to proper wound healing. Any external material implanted to a patient must be well tolerated by the host, limiting any foreign body reactions to integrate well with the surrounding tissue [7]. The implant needs to have good handling so that it can be well positioned at the defect site allowing good approximation to the surrounding tissues. Finally, it needs to have the sufficient strength to form a water-tight barrier [1, 7, 10]. Although the use of synthetic dural substitutes will result in additional expense, the cost may be offset by shorter operative time [8].

Many materials have been used in dural repair or as a substitute with varied outcomes. In the mid-1900s, polymer derived materials, such as

G. Alokby
Department of Otolaryngology, Head and Neck Surgery, King Faisal Specialist Hospital and Research Center, Riyadh, Saudi Arabia

College of medicine, Alfaisal University, Riyadh, Saudi Arabia

J. Walsh (✉)
Department of Otolaryngology – Head and Neck Surgery, University of Iowa, Carver College of Medicine, Iowa City, IA, USA
e-mail: jarrett-walsh@uiowa.edu

A. A. AlQahtani et al. (eds.), *CSF Rhinorrhea*, https://doi.org/10.1007/978-3-030-94781-1_16

Dacron and Orlon, were popular. However, high infection rates, the inability of the material to integrate with the surrounding dura, and foreign body encapsulation were commonly encountered and lead to discontinuation of their use [7]. Newer materials introduced have shown to be well tolerated and effective in repair skull base defects [3, 9]. The main principles for skull base repair remain constant regardless of the material being used: visualization, clearance of obstructive tissue, and close approximation. Clear visualization of any defect is imperative for complete closure. Any tissue adjacent or herniating through the defect should be cauterized and removed so that all edges of the defect are clearly seen. The bony edges of the defect should be well identified and smoothed, which may make the defect larger. However, having a well-defined defect with smooth edges helps in the final principle, close approximation. Having the graft material approximated closely to bare bone and avoiding significant overlay of graft material on mucosa will lead to quicker closure and avoid the formation of a mucocele [11, 12]. A water-tight closure should be achieved using a meticulous surgical technique and optimal choice of reconstructive material that can withstand the nasal environment and may need to be supplemented with the vascularized flaps in cases with high risk of postoperative CSF leak [6, 10, 13].

When applying these principles, many dural substitutes have been shown to have an outcome similar to autograft [8, 9, 14, 15]. In this chapter, we will present a collection of reconstruction materials classified by source material: xenografts, allografts, alloplastic, and other synthetic materials.

16.2 Xenograft

A variety of bovine-derived collagen matrices are available as dural substitutes and are typically used as part of multilayer repair [9, 16–18]. The primary differences in available bovine collagen matrices are donor site and post-harvest processing. DuraGen (Integra LifeSciences, Plainsboro, NJ), Dura-guard (Synovis, St. Paul, MN), and Durepair (TEI Biosciences, Boston, MA; distributed by Medtronic Neurosurgery, Goleta, CA) are examples of commonly used bovine-derived collagen matrix. All have proven to be well tolerated by the host without causing foreign body reactions [7].

Evaluation of the three collagen matrix derived grafts using a canine duraplasty model has previously been performed to compare their in vivo properties. Although all three materials are derived from bovine collagen, the difference in their physical properties, porosity, and cross-linking influenced operative tissue handling and postoperative resorption, vascularization, and tissue integration. Ultimately this comparative study concluded that all three materials are safe and effective in healing dura efficiently. However, the delicate nature of DuraGen makes it more suitable as in inlay layer for low flow leak, whereas Durepair and Duraform were found to be effective in both low- and high-flow leaks [7].

Oakley et al. published their experience with 120 cases repaired using DuraGen. It was used as the first inlay layer for reconstruction and followed by a free mucosal graft for defects less than 1 cm. Larger defects included DuraGen with a vascularized flap or a combination of both graft and flap. In their series, postoperative CSF leaks were reported in 3.3% of the patients. Other reported complications were meningitis (3.3%), other intracranial infections (2.5%), intracranial bleeding (1.7%), and epistaxis (1.7%) [9].

Dura-Guard (Synovis, St. Paul, MN) is produced by processing sheets of bovine pericardium. It is reported to be more durable than DuraGen and can effectively be used as part of multilayer repair of the skull base [7]. Nyquist et al. published a series of 32 patients where Dura-Guard was used interchangeably with fascia lata as an inlay layer for skull base defects. It was supported by a rigid buttress with or without vascularized flap depending on the size of the defect. In this series there was no postoperative CSF leak in 93.5% of the cases [19].

Unlike the previously mentioned collagen-based materials, a newer xenograft that has application in skull base reconstruction is porcine intestinal submucosa extracellular matrix (Biodesign, Cook Medical Bloomington, IN) [20, 21]. Biodesign is acellular, resorbable, and was initially used as a tissue substitute in various surgical procedures, such as repair of abdominal hernias and for gynecologic and urologic procedures [21]. Ultimately, this material was identified as having potential for dural repair.

Illing et al. published their experience with 155 cases of CSF leak repaired using Biodesign. The etiologies of CSF leaks included traumatic, spontaneous, congenital and related to tumor resections. The graft material was used as a part of a multilayer repair. The success rate in closing the defect was 94%. They concluded that porcine small intestinal submucosa is a safe material that can be used for skull base reconstruction [21].

16.3 Allograft

Allogenic dermis, pericardium, and fascia lata have all been used for skull base reconstruction [14, 22–24]. AlloDerm (LifeCell Corp, Woodlands, TX) is an allogenic, acellular dermal graft that is formed from cadaveric skin. It is processed using a high ionic strength solution to separate the epidermis from the dermis followed by processing with sodium deoxycholate to remove cellular components from the dermal matrix. This processing reduces major histocompatibility class I and II molecules to decrease risk for immunologic rejection of the material [25]. The remaining dermal framework is freeze-dried and rehydrated before use [8, 25].

Early vascularization and tissue integration is an important criterion for any material used in dural repairs, to reduce the risk of infection and extrusion of the graft [25]. Taufique et al. studied explanted AlloDerm from two patients after 11 and 17 months of the initial skull base reconstruction. Upon histological evaluation, there was evidence that AlloDerm undergoes revascularization when used for skull base reconstruction [25].

Several authors have published their experience with AlloDerm as a multilayer or as a stand-alone reinstruction material. Schimdt et al. described using a thin layer of AlloDerm as an inlay graft followed by an onlay graft of thick AlloDerm in defects in the lateral recess of the sphenoid with vascularized flaps preserved for large defects. They have reported four cases that were successfully treated with this approach with no postoperative CSF leak [24].

Lorenz et al. reported 8 cases of skull base repair using septal bone or cartilage layered between sheets AlloDerm, placed intracranially and overlayed with a mucosal free graft sealed with fibrin glue. The reconstruction was supported by both absorbable and non-absorbable nasal packing. Failure rates were reported at 4% [26]. Leong et al. presented a series of 16 patients, who had skull base repair in a multilayer fashion using acellular dermal allograft following resection of anterior skull base neoplasms [27]. Eloy et al. reported 10 cases that underwent purely endoscopic trans-cribriform resection of anterior skull base tumors. The repair of the skull base consisted of an inlay fascia lata graft, inlay/onlay acellular dermis graft, and vascularized flap. No postoperative CSF leak was reported in this series [23].

Germani et al. presented a series of 55 patients with anterior skull base defects. 55% of the cases were repaired using AlloDerm as part of a multilayer repair or as a stand-alone reconstruction layer. The remaining 45% of the cases had their defect repaired using bone and mucosal graft; bone, cartilage, and mucosal graft; bone paste, lyophilized dura, and mucosal graft; or mucosal graft alone. There was no postoperative CSF leak in 97% of the cases in the AlloDerm group and in 92% of the cases in the non-AlloDerm group. There were no statistical differences in closure or complication rates between groups with respect to the type of repair or defect size [8].

Gaynor et al. presented a retrospective cohort study comparing AlloDerm to fat in repair of sellar defects. Out of 429 patients who underwent the procedure, Intraoperative CSF leak occurred in 160 cases (35.5%). 95 of those patients underwent repair with AlloDerm and 46 underwent repair with fat autograft, with postoperative CSF leak rates of 8.4% and 15.2%, respectively. 19 patients underwent repair with other techniques or no repair at all, with postoperative leak rate of 0% [15].

Another allogenic material that can be used for skull base reconstruction is derived from cadaveric pericardium. Tutoplast® Pericardium (Tutogen Medical GmbH) is an allogeneic natural collagen matrix that is processed via a proprietary tissue sterilization process. Multiple washes are performed to remove cellular components of the pericardium. Oxidative and solvent treatments reduce immunogenicity of the final product. Finally, the tissue is terminally sterilized with low-dose irradiation. Cavallo et al. published a series of 21 patients with suprasellar lesions where skull base reconstruction was carried out using a multilayer repair consisting of Tutoplast pericardium in combination with another layer of solid support at the bone layer (Lactosorb, Walter Lorenz Surgical). CSF leak rate was 9.5%. No patients in the series developed meningitis [28].

Divitiis et al. published a series of 11 patients diagnosed with meningioma who underwent transnasal endoscopic resection. The anterior cranial floor was reconstructed in a multilayered fashion with collagen sponge matrix, Tutoplast, and resorbable solid material (Lactosorb). Three patients developed postoperative CSF leak that was successfully repaired by revision surgery [29]. In another series, Cavallo et al. used the same technique in the repair of the skull base following the resection of 21 cases of craniopharyngioma. The postoperative CSF leak rate was 16.7% [30].

16.4 Alloplastic

Inorganic and synthetic materials have been used for skull base repair from the 1890s, including inert metal foils and rubber as the earliest reported repair materials [31]. By the middle of the twentieth century, a variety of synthetic polymers were available and used for dural closure. Dacron, a non-absorbable polymer made from polyethylene terephthalate (PETE), was widely used through the 1980s. Dacron was initially used independently, but was subsequently incorporated in a silicone coating for dural implantation [31, 32]. By the end of the century, silicone grafts with or without Dacron were being abandoned due to concerns for associated bleeding, infection, and delayed cortical adhesion [33, 34]. Significant attention in the past several decades has focused on absorbable materials, able to integrate or guide surrounding tissue regrowth, while avoiding the risks for cortical adhesion, hemorrhage, and infection realized with non-absorbable materials. While many of these materials are used in duraplasty and subsequent cranioplasty, there are studies that have followed the potential use of alloplastic materials into the realm of skull base dural repair and closure.

Absorbable polymers of polygalactin 910 (Vicryl) and poly-p-dioxanone (PDS) are often known as common suture materials, however, their combination in the form of a woven patch has been marketed as Ethisorb (Codman, Raynham, MA) and has shown utility in dural closure. Arndt et al. demonstrated the utility of this patch in 8 patients with transnasal repair using layers of Ethisorb to form a "sandwich" around the skull base defect with an overlying mucosal graft for final closure. The success rate of this series was 100%, without significant complications [35].

Another synthetic material considered for dural closure is polyurethane (Neuro-Patch, Aesculap, Tuttlingen, Germany). Initially described as a material with potential use in the 1990s, the largest reported series of dural repairs with this material was published in 2003. Postoperative leak was noted in 9 of the 70 patients [36, 37].

One of the most recent advances in alloplastic dural repair is the FDA approval of a microspun poly(lactic-co-glycolic acid) (PGLA) and poly(dioxanone) matrix (Cerafix Dura Substitute, Acera Surgical, St. Louis, MO) [38]. Currently the material is only indicated for dural defects of less than 31.7 cm^2 [39]. The initial case report of its use in four patients shows excellent closure and no graft-related complications at 6 month follow-up [40].

While not technically an alloplastic material, fibrin sealants can be used as an adjuvant for closure of dural defects, especially in a multilayer closure. While prospective and retrospective series regarding the use of fibrin sealants abound, only three randomized control trials were noted in a large systematic literature review published by Esposito et al. [41]. This report demonstrated that water-tight closure was significantly improved in the fibrin sealant group. However, postoperative CSF leak rates were noted to be higher in the sealant group over the control group. The overall postoperative leak rates were noted to be 4.5% in the fibrin sealant group as compared to 2% in the control group [42]. In a recent evidence-based review with recommendations focusing on management of cerebrospinal fluid rhinorrhea repair, Oakley et al. address the use of fibrin sealants. Similar to the systematic review, a paucity of high-level data results in an overall recommendation as "option" with a value judgment of "surgeon preference," citing its increased cost without clear supporting evidence [3]. Additional studies by Eloy et al. further question the need of fibrin sealants for skull base defect repairs. In their series of 74 patients, a 0% postoperative leak rate was reported in closures without use of fibrin sealants versus 2.4% in the group repaired with the use of fibrin sealant [43].

In addition to dural repair, alloplastic materials are commonly used as a rigid support for bony skull base defects. Similar to dural repair, rigid materials are available in absorbable and non-absorbable forms. Commonly used bioabsorbable polymers introduced in the last two decades include poly-P-dioxanone (PDS, Ethicon, Somerville, NJ), poly(D,L)lactic acid (Resorb-X sellar plate; KLS Martin, Jacksonville, FL), and co-polymers of poly(D,L)lactic acid with glycolic acid (Lactosorb, Zimmer Biomet, Jacksonville, FL). These materials are available as plates or mesh with balanced malleability, to easily shape the material to the defect size and allow for placement, and rigidity, to oppose intracranial pressures on the repair site.

Potter et al. describe a series of 28 patients with closure of anterior skull base defects with Resorb-X sellar plates, noting only 1 (3.2%) postoperative CSF leak, only after a second surgical intervention for persistent pituitary tumor [44]. Al-Asousi et al. report a case series including 7 skull base repairs using PDS sheets as the rigid component of a multilayer repair. There were no reported postoperative leaks with no significant postoperative complications noted in the limited series [45]. Finally, a collection of techniques including Lactosorb as a component of a multilayer closure has been presented by Cavallo et al. [28].

Non-absorbable materials used in the repair of skull base defects are also often used as part of a multilayer closure. Current options in non-absorbable materials include titanium mesh, cements, and porous polyethylene (Medpor; Stryker, Kalamazoo, MI). Titanium implants are a consideration due to their excellent biocompatibility. Titanium mesh has the added benefit of intraoperative shaping to meet the specific contours of defects. For application in known defect sizes, the option for pre-manufactured titanium plates is available, but at the cost of limited intraoperative manipulation of the graft. A potential downside to rigid titanium grafting is migration or exposure of the plate over time, which may lead to complications such as infection, crusting, or bleeding. The need for MRI evaluation of the skull base defect postoperatively should be considered before placing titanium, as some attenuation of signal is possible in tissues adjacent to the implant site.

Cements have been used as part of bone reconstruction in various anatomic sites. Common cement base materials include hydroxyapatite and poly-methyl methacrylate (PMMA). Hydroxyapatite has the capacity to be molded in situ before hardening and may promote induction of osteoneogenesis, properties that have contributed to its use in skull base repair [46, 47]. One potential concern with hydroxyapatite cement is crack formation on curing, which requires removal of fragmented cement and addition of layered cement to obtain a complete adequate seal [47]. PMMA cements have been reported for skull base closure, specifically the use of the high-viscosity variety [48]. Cited benefits of the high-viscosity variety include improved working consistency over low-viscosity variants, which allows for use in endoscopic repairs and reduces risk of local extravasation and migration. Unfortunately, there is limited long-term follow-up data for the endoscopic application of PMMA cements.

Finally, Medpor implants have the biocompatibility of non-absorbable implants with the capacity of integration of surrounding tissues like absorbable implants [49]. Medpor is available in plate form, allowing for ease of application for endoscopic repairs, and can be cut to size. Liebelt et al. present a series of 200 consecutive patients with sellar defects, of which 136 were repaired with Medpor plates. Other patients closed with nasal bone grafting did not require rigid closure. Two patients (1.5%) in the Medpor group had postoperative CSF leak, compared to one patient (1.6%) in the nasal bone group. Other complications were not significantly different between groups [50].

16.5 Surgical Technique

In this section, we will describe the skull base reconstruction using AlloDerm. The skull base defect is prepared for closure, initially, by optimizing exposure. All edges of the defect must be clearly seen. Mucosa adjacent to the bony edges of the defect must be reflected away or removed to expose the surrounding bone. Likewise, the dural defect must be properly visualized. The dural edge to be repaired is elevated from the surrounding cranial bone by applying a saline soaked neurosurgical pledget and elevating the dura gently. An intermediate thickness Alloderm graft, approximately 1mm thick, is optimal for anterior skull base closure given the balance of compliance and strength. The Alloderm should be prepared by rehydrating in sterile saline prior to repair of the defect. The defect is measured carefully to calculate the size of Alloderm needed. A neurosurgical pledget of known size may be used to estimate the defect size, alternatively a small ruler can be placed for measurement of larger defects. An additional 2 cm should be added to each side of the calculated defect size to estimate the size of the graft material required. If a 2 × 3-cm defect is being repaired, the Alloderm should be 6 × 7-cm in size. The graft is gently centered over the defect. Using a curved probe or other instrument, the edges are gently tucked intracranially, ensuring that the free edge is visible during placement and remains extracranial. The Alloderm is effectively doubled back on itself on the cranial side of the bony edges, creating a pocket circumferentially (Fig. 16.1a, b). Oxidized regenerated cellulose, Surgicel (Ethicon, Somerville, NJ), is wrapped around a plug of dry Gelfoam (Pfizer, New York, NY) and is used as a wedge into the circumferential pocket, each piece cut to the approximate length of the defect edge. Alternating opposite sides are supported with plugs to keep the graft in place and maintain a circumferential water-tight seal around the bony defect during plug placement. The intranasal ends of the graft are allowed to fold back and contact surrounding bone circumferentially (Fig. 16.2). Any reflected mucosa is then draped back over the edges of the repair. The end result is a hammock-like structure that supports the dural defect and is anchored circumferentially on the bony edges of the defect, essentially forming a water-tight gasket by the wedges of oxidized regenerated cellulose and gel foam (Figs. 16.3 and 16.4). Gelfoam or other absorbable material is placed over the graft surface to protect the graft from adhesion to any nasal packing. A merocel pack is applied to the edge of the graft and hydrated to apply reinforcement from below. The merocel pack generally remains in place for 1 week.

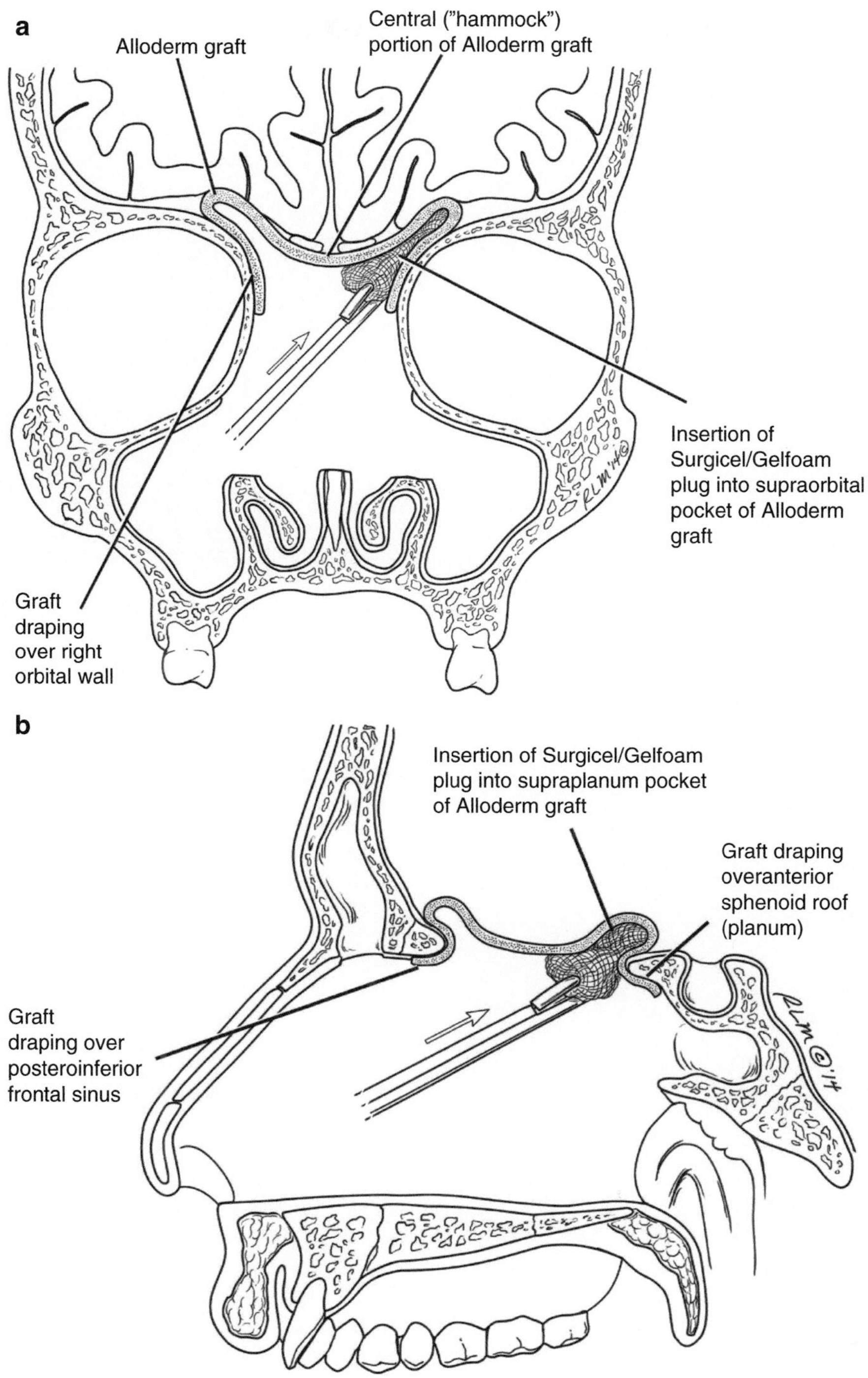

Fig. 16.1 Inlay/onlay technique for placement of allograft closures in the anterior skull base. Resorbable gelfoam and oxidized regenerated cellulose are used to form plugs that secure the graft circumferentially along the superior edge of the defect. Excess graft is draped over exposed bone to promote the formation of a tight seal (**a**, **b**)

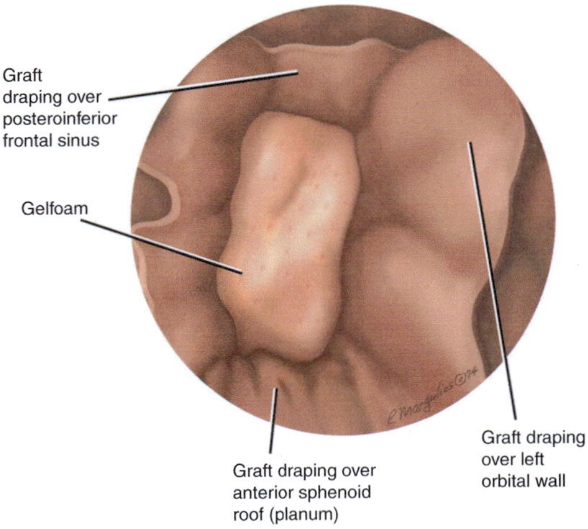

Fig. 16.2 Final repair of skull base defect with care to support the central "hammock" portion and ensure that draping edges are well seated without folds to prevent CSF leakage

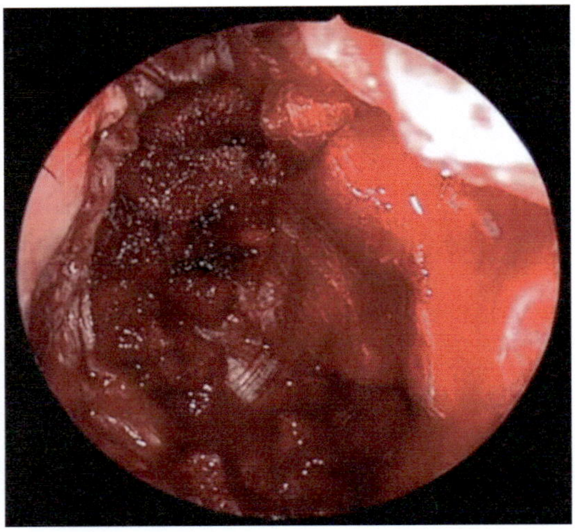

Fig. 16.3 Endoscopic view using a 70° nasal endoscope of the skull base repair following anterior skull base resection using Tutoplast® Fascia Lata

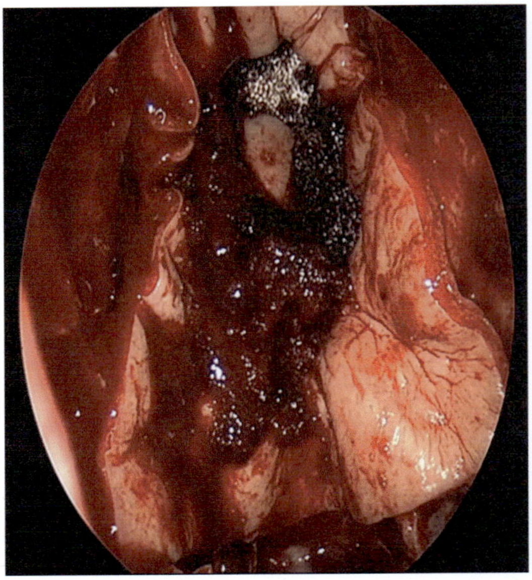

Fig. 16.4 Endoscopic view using a 70° nasal endoscope of the skull base repair following anterior skull base resection using AlloDerm

References

1. Snyderman CH, et al. Technologic innovations in neuroendoscopic surgery. Otolaryngol Clin N Am. 2009;42(5):883–90.
2. Snyderman CH, et al. What are the limits of endoscopic sinus surgery? The expanded endonasal approach to the skull base. Keio J Med. 2009;58(3):152–60.
3. Oakley GM, et al. Management of cerebrospinal fluid rhinorrhea: an evidence-based review with recommendations. Int Forum Allergy Rhinol. 2016;6(1):17–24.
4. Wigand ME. Transnasal ethmoidectomy under endoscopical control. Rhinology. 1981;19(1):7–15.
5. Zanation AM, et al. Reconstructive options for endoscopic skull base surgery. Otolaryngol Clin N Am. 2011;44(5):1201–22.

6. Patel MR, et al. How to choose? Endoscopic skull base reconstructive options and limitations. Skull Base. 2010;20(6):397–404.
7. Zerris VA, et al. Repair of the dura mater with processed collagen devices. J Biomed Mater Res B Appl Biomater. 2007;83(2):580–8.
8. Germani RM, et al. Endoscopic reconstruction of large anterior skull base defects using acellular dermal allograft. Am J Rhinol. 2007;21(5):615–8.
9. Oakley GM, et al. Collagen matrix as an inlay in endoscopic skull base reconstruction. J Laryngol Otol. 2018;132(3):214–23.
10. Snyderman CH, et al. Endoscopic reconstruction of cranial base defects following endonasal skull base surgery. Skull Base. 2007;17(1):73–8.
11. Bedrosian JC, Anand VK, Schwartz TH. The endoscopic endonasal approach to repair of iatrogenic and noniatrogenic cerebrospinal fluid leaks and encephaloceles of the anterior cranial fossa. World Neurosurg. 2014;82(6 Suppl):86–94.
12. Alokby G, Casiano RR. Endoscopic resection of sinonasal and ventral skull base malignancies. Otolaryngol Clin N Am. 2017;50(2):273–85.
13. Roxbury CR, et al. Layered sellar reconstruction with avascular free grafts: Acceptable alternative to the nasoseptal flap for repair of low-volume intraoperative cerebrospinal fluid leak. Am J Rhinol Allergy. 2016;30(5):367–71.
14. Karnezis TT, et al. Factors impacting cerebrospinal fluid leak rates in endoscopic sellar surgery. Int Forum Allergy Rhinol. 2016;6(11):1117–25.
15. Gaynor BG, et al. Acellular dermal allograft for sellar repair after transsphenoidal approach to pituitary adenomas. J Neurol Surg B Skull Base. 2013;74(3): 155–9.
16. Learned KO, et al. MR imaging evaluation of endoscopic cranial base reconstruction with pedicled nasoseptal flap following endoscopic endonasal skull base surgery. Eur J Radiol. 2013;82(3):544–51.
17. Kassam AB, et al. Endoscopic endonasal pituitary transposition for a transdorsum sellae approach to the interpeduncular cistern. Neurosurgery. 2008; 62(3):57–72.
18. Zanation AM, et al. Nasoseptal flap reconstruction of high flow intraoperative cerebral spinal fluid leaks during endoscopic skull base surgery. Am J Rhinol Allergy. 2009;23(5):518–21.
19. Nyquist GG, et al. Endoscopic endonasal repair of anterior skull base non-traumatic cerebrospinal fluid leaks, meningoceles, and encephaloceles. J Neurosurg. 2010;113(5):961–6.
20. Marchioni D, et al. Endoscopic transnasal surgery of clival lesions: our experience. Eur Arch Otorhinolaryngol. 2018;275(5):1149–56.
21. Illing E, et al. Porcine small intestine submucosal graft for endoscopic skull base reconstruction. Int Forum Allergy Rhinol. 2013;3(11):928–32.
22. Fiorindi A, et al. Banked fascia lata in sellar dura reconstruction after endoscopic transsphenoidal skull base surgery. J Neurol Surg B Skull Base. 2015; 76(4):303–9.
23. Eloy JA, et al. Triple-layer reconstruction technique for large cribriform defects after endoscopic endonasal resection of anterior skull base tumors. Int Forum Allergy Rhinol. 2013;3(3):204–11.
24. Schmidt RF, et al. Surgical nuances for the endoscopic endonasal transpterygoid approach to lateral sphenoid sinus encephaloceles. Neurosurg Focus. 2012;32(6):5.
25. Taufique ZM, et al. Revascularization of alloderm used during endoscopic skull base surgery. J Neurol Surg B Skull Base. 2019;80(1):46–50.
26. Lorenz RR, et al. Endoscopic reconstruction of anterior and middle cranial fossa defects using acellular dermal allograft. Laryngoscope. 2003;113(3): 496–501.
27. Leong JL, Citardi MJ, Batra PS. Reconstruction of skull base defects after minimally invasive endoscopic resection of anterior skull base neoplasms. Am J Rhinol. 2006;20(5):476–82.
28. Cavallo LM, et al. Skull base reconstruction in the extended endoscopic transsphenoidal approach for suprasellar lesions. J Neurosurg. 2007;107(4): 713–20.
29. de Divitiis E, et al. Endoscopic transnasal resection of anterior cranial fossa meningiomas. Neurosurg Focus. 2008;25(6):E8.
30. Cavallo LM, et al. The endoscopic endonasal approach for the management of craniopharyngiomas involving the third ventricle. Neurosurg Rev. 2013;36(1):27–37.
31. Maher CO, et al. Evaluation of a novel propylene oxide—treated collagen material as a dural substitute. J Neurosurg. 2003;99(6):1070–6. https://doi.org/10.3171/jns.2003.99.6.1070.
32. Maier W. Biomaterials in skull base surgery. GMS Curr Top Otorhinolaryngol. 2009;8:7. https://doi.org/10.3205/cto000059.
33. Simpson D, Robson A. Recurrent subarachnoid bleeding in association with dural substitute. J Neurosurg. 1984;60(2):408–9. https://doi.org/10.3171/jns.1984.60.2.0408.
34. Robertson SC, Menezes AH. Hemorrhagic complications in association with silastic dural substitute: pediatric and adult case reports with a review of the literature. Neurosurgery. 1997;40(1):201–5. https://doi.org/10.1097/00006123-199701000-00046.
35. Arndt S, et al. Ethisorb/ethisorb durapatch for the transnasal duraplasty procedure? Laryngo-Rhino-Otologie. 2006;85(4):260–4. https://doi.org/10.1055/s-2005-921055.
36. Sakas DE, et al. Biologically inert synthetic dural substitutes. J Neurosurg. 1990;73(6):936–41. https://doi.org/10.3171/jns.1990.73.6.0936.
37. Raul JS, et al. Use of polyester urethane (neuro-patch) as a dural substitute. Prospective study of 70 cases. Neuro-Chirurgie. 2003;49(2-3):83–9.
38. MacEwan MR, et al. Novel nanofabricated dura substitute effectively repairs dural defects independent of

defect size in a canine duraplasty model. Interdiscip Neurosurg. 2018;14:150–5. https://doi.org/10.1016/j.inat.2018.08.006.
39. Cerafix product insert. Cerafix product insert. Acera Surgical, Inc. https://secureservercdn.net/198.71.233.197/fcb.4f8.myftpupload.com/wp-content/uploads/2018/12/MKG-20004-Cerafix-IFU.pdf. Accessed 3 Oct 2019.
40. Schmalz P, et al. Use of an absorbable synthetic polymer dural substitute for repair of dural defects: a technical note. Cureus. 2018;10:e2127. https://doi.org/10.7759/cureus.2127.
41. Esposito F, et al. Fibrin sealants in dura sealing: a systematic literature review. PLoS ONE. 2016;11(4):e0151533. https://doi.org/10.1371/journal.pone.0151533.
42. Green A, Alexander L, et al. A multicentre, prospective, randomized, controlled study to evaluate the use of a fibrin sealant as an adjunct to sutured dural repair. Br J Neurosurg. 2015;29(1):11–7. https://doi.org/10.3109/02688697.2014.948808.
43. Eloy A, Anderson J, Choudhry OJ, et al. Endoscopic nasoseptal flap repair of skull base defects: is addition of a dural sealant necessary? Otolaryngology. 2012;147(1):161–6. https://doi.org/10.1177/0194599812437530.
44. Potter A, Nicholas J, et al. Bioabsorbable plate cranial base reconstruction: cranial base reconstruction. Laryngoscope. 2015;125(6):1313–5. https://doi.org/10.1002/lary.24991.
45. Al-Asousi A, Fahad, et al. The use of polydioxanone plates for endoscopic skull base repair. Am J Rhinol Allergy. 2017;31(2):122–6. https://doi.org/10.2500/ajra.2017.31.4411.
46. Marchac D, Greensmith A. Long-term experience with methylmethacrylate cranioplasty in craniofacial surgery. J Plast Reconstr Aesthet Surg. 2008;61(7):744–52. https://doi.org/10.1016/j.bjps.2007.10.055.
47. Kitano A, Masahiko A, Taneda M. Icing and multilayering technique of injectable hydroxyapatite cement paste for cranial base reconstruction after transsphenoidal surgery: technical note. Operat Neurosurg. 2007;61:53–4. https://doi.org/10.1227/01.neu.0000289713.80178.ce.
48. Moliterno A, Jennifer A, et al. High-viscosity polymethylmethacrylate cement for endoscopic anterior cranial base reconstruction. J Neurosurg. 2010;113(5):1100–5. https://doi.org/10.3171/2010.3.JNS09453.
49. Park J, Guthikonda M. The Medpor™ sheet as a sellar buttress after endonasal transsphenoidal surgery: technical note. Surg Neurol. 2004;61(5):488–92. https://doi.org/10.1016/S0090-3019(03)00581-0.
50. Liebelt BD, et al. Sellar floor reconstruction with the medpor implant versus autologous bone after transnasal transsphenoidal surgery: outcome in 200 consecutive patients. World Neurosurg. 2015;84(2):240–5. https://doi.org/10.1016/j.wneu.2015.02.025.

Free Autologous Grafts

17

Yazeed Abdulilah Alsuliman, Marc A. Tewfik,
and Peter-John Wormald

17.1 Free Autologous Grafts

Since Dandy first described the successful repair of the skull base in 1926 and then with the era of endoscopic skull base surgery, many operative techniques have been adopted to reach a successful watertight closure of skull base defects. Those techniques have employed a wide range of closure materials, including simple autografts, allografts, xenografts, synthetic materials, local flaps, or even free flaps.

This chapter will explore the different free autografts used in skull base reconstruction, their indications, limitations, and technical considerations.

Y. A. Alsuliman
Division of Otolaryngology, Head and Neck Surgery, Department of Surgery, King Fahad Medical City, Riyadh, Saudi Arabia

M. A. Tewfik (✉)
Department of Otolaryngology - Head and Neck Surgery, McGill University Health Center, Montreal, QC, Canada
e-mail: marc.tewfik@mcgill.ca

P.-J. Wormald
Department of Surgery, Otolaryngology - Head and Neck Surgery, The University of Adelaide, Adelaide, SA, Australia
e-mail: peterj.wormald@adelaide.edu.au

17.2 Types of Autologous Grafting Materials

Before intranasal vascularized tissue flaps were described, skull base reconstruction was limited to free autografts. Many autologous graft materials have been described in the literature concerning skull base reconstruction. Those include fascia, fat, mucosa, bone, and cartilage [1]. They can be used as a single layer, but more often are used in conjunction with other grafts and/or flaps (Table 17.1).

Table 17.1 Types of autologous free grafts

Type of autologous graft	Donor site	Common uses
Mucosa	• Nasal septum • Middle/inferior turbinate • Nasal floor	• Overlay single or supporting layer
Fat	• Thigh • Abdomen • Ear lobe	• Fill up dead space • Bath plug technique
Fascia	• Fascia lata • Rectus fascia • Temporalis fascia	• Overlay or underlay single or supporting layer
Bone	• Nasal septum • Mastoid • Calvarium • Iliac crest	• Prevent herniation of intracranial contents in large defects • Gasket seal technique
Cartilage	• Nasal septum • Conchal	

A. A. AlQahtani et al. (eds.), *CSF Rhinorrhea*, https://doi.org/10.1007/978-3-030-94781-1_17

17.3 Free Mucosal Grafts

As for all free grafts, mucosal grafts depend on the recipient site's blood supply to heal and therefore need to be placed on a well-vascularized bed. Mucosal grafts have the advantage of being harvested locally from the nasal cavity without adding wound related morbidity. Typically, they are harvested from septum, middle turbinate, inferior turbinate, or nasal floor. Because these different nasal subsites typically have different mucosal thicknesses, those with naturally thick mucosa such as the inferior turbinate mucosa and superior septum should be harvested in split-thickness. This way, they will remain thinner and require less nourishment by the underlying vascularized bed in order to survive.

Donor site-related morbidity should be considered when choosing to harvest nasal mucosa. Harvesting mucosa from an intact middle turbinate is technically challenging and can risk a skull base injury [2]. If middle turbinectomy has been performed for exposure purposes, its mucosa can be harvested on the instrument table with no additional risks. Taking septal mucosal graft can adversely affect the future use of a pedicled septal flap and often results in an exposed cartilage that takes time to remucosalize leading to prolonged crusting, cartilage necrosis, or septal perforation. Nasal floor mucosa is another safe alternative option which has been reported to remucosalize relatively fast despite its theoretical risk of nasal vestibule stenosis if performed too far anteriorly [3]. Mucosa can only be used as an overlay graft (over the intranasal surface of the bone), and care should be taken to apply the mucosal side outwardly to avoid the risk of mucocele formation.

Mucosal grafts have a relative rapid healing process. It takes around 6 days for the mucosa to be fixed to the skull base and there is a microscopic evidence of re-epithelization by postoperative day 12. However, complete remucosalization can take up to 90 days [4]. Hoseman et al. have found that mucosal grafts contract by 20% during healing process, and for this reason, the surgeon should take this in consideration to harvest a proper sized graft [5].

17.4 Fat Grafts

Using fat graft can play an effective role in reaching watertight closure of skull base defects as well as filling up dead space in advanced skull base approaches such as trans-clival ones. Fat grafts are typically harvested from the thigh, abdomen, or ear lobe. Although most studies show no difference in the viability of fat grafts harvested from different donor sites, one study shows that more adipose-derived stem cells are found within the fat grafts harvested from the lower abdomen or inner thigh [6]. Those stem cells have a unique wound healing potential. In animal models, adipose stem cells are found to be able to promote epithelization and vascularization [7]. That was the basis of Fonmarty et al. study that reported a successful anterior skull base reconstruction after resecting malignant tumors using en bloc fat graft as a single layer in overlay fashion [8]. After non-vascularized fat grafting, a very dynamic remodeling of adipose tissue was observed [9]. Many adipocytes die within the 2 weeks of transplantation, but the adipose-derived stem cells remain alive and partially regenerate the adipose tissue by week 3, whereas the remaining dead cells get replaced with fibrotic tissue [10].

Despite the safety and effectiveness of the use of fat in skull base surgery, some authors have described complications. Taha et al. reported 1% complication rate of autologous fat grafting including fat necrosis with subsequent CSF leak and lipoid meningitis as a result of dissemination of fat into the subarachnoid space [11].

Fat can safely be placed intradurally, but care must be taken not to let small globules of fat dissociate from the main graft that can then translocate within the CSF space. An adequately sized graft has the advantage of acting as a buttress upon which subsequent layers can rest, applying pressure to these from the intracranial side, and protecting delicate intracranial structures. Care must be taken not to place excessive fat intradurally as this can compress major anatomical structures and can also impact the accuracy of postoperative images [12, 13].

The bath-plug closure is one the techniques that utilizes fat graft for reconstructing the skull base. This technique was described to provide dural seal by placing the fat plug intracranially and use a stitch to expand the fat plug which then allows the natural pressure from the CSF to maintain this seal [14].

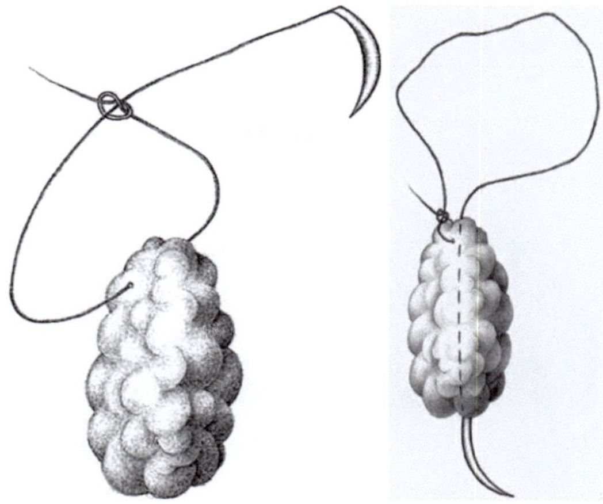

Fig. 17.1 Making a knot with a 4-0 vicryl suture at one end of the fat plug and passed down its length

17.5 The Fat Bath-Plug Surgical Technique

Once the site of the leak has been identified, the dural defect is enlarged until the bony edges of the defect is delineated. Prolapsed meningocele or meningoencephalocele is resected after carefully checking that the prolapsed tissue does not contain intracranial blood vessels. The residual tissue is cauterized with bipolar diathermy to ensure hemostasis. The nasal mucosa surrounding the defect is stripped away for at least 5 mm. A fat graft is then harvested from the ear lobe that is about the same diameter as the defect and 1.5–2 cm long. If the size of the defect is larger than 12 mm, the fat can be taken from the abdomen but defects larger than 1.5 cm are not suitable for this technique. The ear lobe fat is preferable as the fat globules are tightly knitted and easy to work with. Next, a 4-0 vicryl suture is passed through one end of the fat plug and knotted, then the suture is passed down the length of the fat plug (Fig. 17.1). The fat graft is introduced gently and gradually through the defect knot first using malleable frontal sinus probe. Once fully introduced, the suture is pulled while an instrument supports the fat plug as it protrudes through the defect as the suture is pulled (Fig. 17.2a, b). This will expand the fat on the intracranial surface of the defect and as the fat plug is now larger than the defect and the fat prolapses through the defect, a tight seal is achieved. A free mucosal graft is slid up the suture and placed in overlay fashion and supported with fibrin glue and Gelfoam. The vicryl suture is cut just below the graft and supporting material (Fig. 17.3).

17.6 Fascia Grafts

Fascia grafts such as fascia lata and temporalis fascia are another great option that is utilized by many skull base surgeons for reconstruction purposes. Fascia lata in particular is a very popular grafting material due to its strength, availability, and pliability. Although many surgeons prefer adding a pedicled flap for reconstructing large skull base defects, fascia lata alone has been used successfully in the past as a double layer (underlay and overlay) in repairing such defects (Fig. 17.4) [15]. Nicolai et al. have also utilized fascia in a "three layer technique" covering skull base defects after resecting large sinonasal malignant tumors, by using fascia intradurally, then intracranial extradurally (underlay), and covering it with an extracranial (overlay) mucosal graft [16]. Tachibana et al. investigated the healing process of fascia lata graft in an animal study and

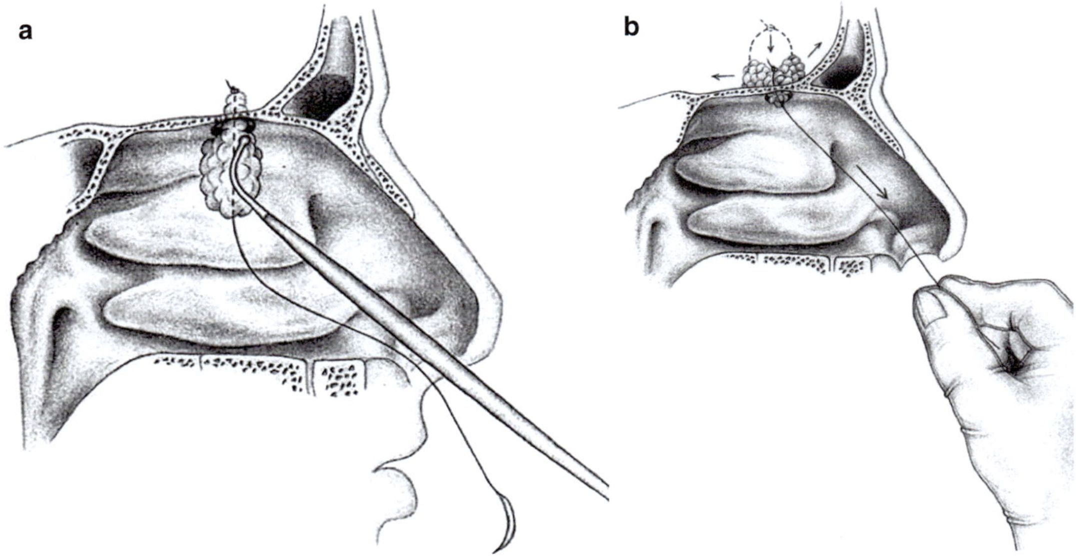

Fig. 17.2 (**a**) The fat graft is gently introduced into the skull base defect using a curved frontal sinus probe. (**b**) Then the suture is pulled while the plug is supported to allow the plug to expand and seal the defect

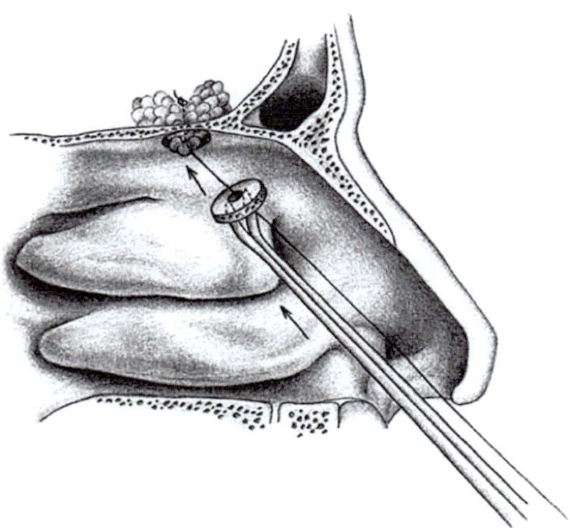

Fig. 17.3 The mucosal graft is slid up the length of the suture and placed to cover the fat plug in overlay fashion

found that fascial graft was already tightly connected to adjacent dura at 1 week and tolerated high intracranial pressure even without a supporting vascular flap [17].

17.7 Surgical Technique of Harvesting Fascia Lata

The leg is positioned so that it is slightly flexed at the knee and internally rotated, and a soft roll is applied under the knee. A longitudinal linear incision is made along the center of the lateral thigh with a length that is suitable to harvest a proper sized graft. Usually, a 3–5 cm incision is adequate (Fig. 17.5). Next, a blunt dissection of the overlying fat is made, and the fascia lata is exposed. A proximal and distal transverse incisions are made on the fascia (this defines the length of the graft). An anterior and posterior fasciotomy incisions are also made (defines the width of the graft). The fascia is bluntly dissected off the underlying muscle, and fascia graft is delivered and kept in wet dressing until used. Hemostasis is then to be completed with electrocautery and drain can be placed if necessary, and the wound is closed in two layers. The fascia

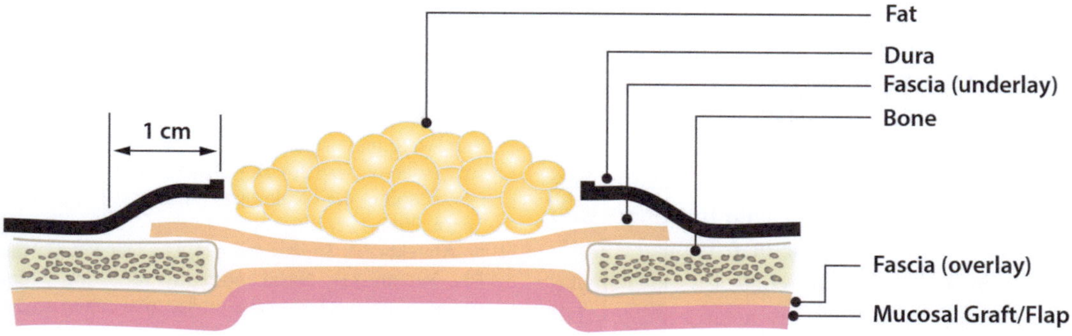

Fig. 17.4 Demonstration of an example of multilayer closure technique of skull base defect in which fat is used intradurally to seal the CSF leak, then fascia lata is used in underlay and overlay layers, and finally an overlay mucosal graft/flap is used

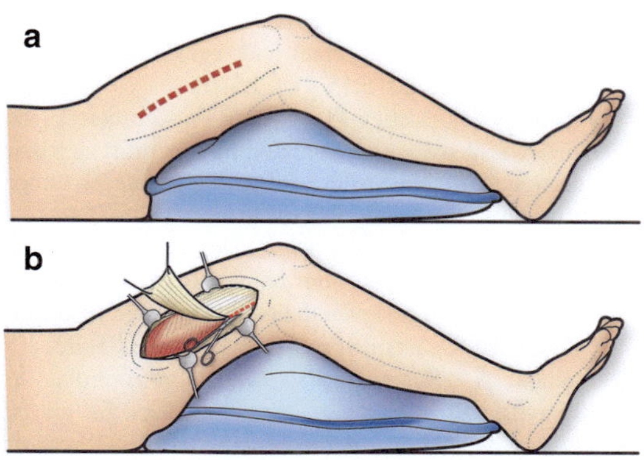

Fig. 17.5 (**a**) Shows the proper positioning of the leg before harvesting fascia lata graft. (**b**) Shows the incision site and a fascia lata cut from underlying muscle

lata defect is usually closed either primarily or if the graft taken is large, a vicryl mesh is sutured into the defect. This prevents the complication of muscle prolapse through the fascia lata defect in the postoperative period.

17.8 Bone/Cartilage Grafts

The need for bone or cartilage grafts in skull base reconstruction is controversial. Rigid reconstruction may be needed to prevent herniation of intracranial contents. In at risk patients (chronic cough, overweight), some surgeons believe that it is beneficial in large defects to support the reconstruction with either a bone graft or titanium plate as an underlay between the underlay and onlay reconstruction layers [18]. Gasket-seal watertight closure is one of the reconstruction techniques that can use a bone graft as part of multilayer reconstruction [19].

In this technique, often an underlay is placed intracranially, then an onlay graft (commonly fascia lata) is placed over the defect and must exceed the bony defect by around 1 cm circumferentially. To ensure that the edges of this graft remain in contact with the edges of the defect, a bone or cartilage graft that is roughly the same size of the defect is gently pushed into the defect and wedged on the edges of the defect forming a watertight seal. A popular donor site for bone and cartilage grafts is the nasal septum which is faster and easier in endoscopic approaches, and it also avoids adding remote donor site morbidity.

17.9 Outcomes of Various Autologous Graft Materials

The current literature uses the absence of recurrent cerebrospinal fluid (CSF) leak as a definition of successful skull base repair [20]. A meta-analysis study that evaluated the outcomes of endoscopic skull base repair with different types grafts and techniques has shown a success rate of 90–97% regardless of the type of graft [21].

This applies for small defects, but for large ones, a vascularized flap has significantly better outcome in comparison with free grafts with CSF leak rates post repair of 6.7% and 15.6%, respectively. There is no consensus as to what size defines a small versus a large defect, but many authors use a 1–2 cm limit to define a small defect [22–24].

Evidence for clear cut comparison of success rates between different types of grafts is currently unavailable. Most studies are retrospective and do not control for the many variables such as what supporting reconstructive material was used, the particular repair technique, type of packing, use of a lumbar drain usage, etc. [25].

17.10 Single Layer Versus Multilayer Grafts in Skull Base Repair

Regardless of the type of reconstruction material, the multilayer closure approach is believed to have the advantage resisting positive pressure (high intracranial pressure or high flow CSF leak) and negative pressure (pneumocephalus) gradients [26]. However, some studies have showed that a single-layer closure technique has similar outcomes to multilayer approach in experienced hands with a meticulous technique [23, 27]. The single layer reconstruction has also been shown to be effective after resecting sellar tumors with no intraoperative CSF leak [28]. In general, we believe that a multi-layer reconstruction technique is superior to a single-layer closure and should be the reconstruction technique of choice.

References

1. Zanation AM, Thorp BD, Parmar P, Harvey RJ. Reconstructive options for endoscopic skull base surgery. Otolaryngol Clin N Am. 2011;44(5): 1201–22.
2. Prevedello DM, Barges-Coll J, Fernandez-Miranda JC, Morera V, Jacobson D, Madhok R, et al. Middle turbinate flap for skull base reconstruction: cadaveric feasibility study. Laryngoscope. 2009;119(11): 2094–8.
3. Suh JD, Ramakrishnan VR, DeConde AS. Nasal floor free mucosal graft for skull base reconstruction and cerebrospinal fluid leak repair. Ann Otol Rhinol Laryngol. 2012;121(2):91–5.
4. de Almeida JR, Snyderman CH, Gardner PA, Carrau RL, Vescan AD. Nasal morbidity following endoscopic skull base surgery: a prospective cohort study. Head Neck. 2011;33(4):547–51.
5. Hosemann W, Goede U, Sauer M. Wound healing of mucosal autografts for frontal cerebrospinal fluid leaks--clinical and experimental investigations. Rhinology. 1999;37(3):108–12.
6. Pu LL. Towards more rationalized approach to autologous fat grafting. JPRAS. 2012;65(4):413–9.
7. Shingyochi Y, Orbay H, Mizuno H. Adipose-derived stem cells for wound repair and regeneration. Expert Opin Biol Ther. 2015;15(9):1285–92.
8. Fonmarty D, Bastier PL, Lechot A, Gimbert E, de Gabory L. Assessment of abdominal fat graft to repair anterior skull base after malignant sinonasal tumor extirpation. Otolaryngology. 2016;154(3):540–6.
9. Eto H, Kato H, Suga H, Aoi N, Doi K, Kuno S, et al. The fate of adipocytes after nonvascularized fat grafting: evidence of early death and replacement of adipocytes. Plast Reconstr Surg. 2012;129(5):1081–92.
10. Sunaga A, Sugawara Y, Katsuragi-Tomioka Y, Kobayashi E. The fate of nonvascularized fat grafts: histological and bioluminescent study. Plast Reconstr Surg Glob Open. 2013;1(6):e40.
11. Taha AN, Almefty R, Pravdenkova S, Al-Mefty O. Sequelae of autologous fat graft used for reconstruction in skull base surgery. World Neurosurg. 2011;75(5-6):692–5.
12. Kremer P, Forsting M, Ranaei G, Wuster C, Hamer J, Sartor K, et al. Magnetic resonance imaging after transsphenoidal surgery of clinically non-functional pituitary macroadenomas and its impact on detecting residual adenoma. Acta Neurochir. 2002;144(5): 433–43.
13. Slavin ML, Lam BL, Decker RE, Schatz NJ, Glaser JS, Reynolds MG. Chiasmal compression from fat packing after transsphenoidal resection of intrasellar tumor in two patients. Am J Ophthalmol. 1993;115(3):368–71.
14. Wormald PJ, McDonogh M. 'Bath-plug' technique for the endoscopic management of cerebrospinal fluid leaks. J Laryngol Otol. 1997;111(11):1042–6.
15. Gil Z, Abergel A, Leider-Trejo L, Khafif A, Margalit N, Amir A, et al. A comprehensive algorithm for anterior skull base reconstruction after oncological resections. Skull Base. 2007;17(1):25–37.
16. Nicolai P, Battaglia P, Bignami M, Bolzoni Villaret A, Delu G, Khrais T, et al. Endoscopic surgery for malignant tumors of the sinonasal tract and adja-

cent skull base: a 10-year experience. Am J Rhinol. 2008;22(3):308–16.
17. Tachibana E, Saito K, Fukuta K, Yoshida J. Evaluation of the healing process after dural reconstruction achieved using a free fascial graft. J Neurosurg. 2002;96(2):280–6.
18. Wang EW, Vandergrift WA, Schlosser RJ. Spontaneous CSF leaks. Otolaryngol Clin N Am. 2011;44(4):845–56.
19. Leng LZ, Brown S, Anand VK, Schwartz TH. "Gasket-seal" watertight closure in minimal-access endoscopic cranial base surgery. Neurosurgery. 2008;62(5):342–3.
20. Prickett KK, Wise SK, Delgaudio JM. Choice of graft material and postoperative healing in endoscopic repair of cerebrospinal fluid leak. Arch Otolaryngol. 2011;137(5):457–61.
21. Hegazy HM, Carrau RL, Snyderman CH, Kassam A, Zweig J. Transnasal endoscopic repair of cerebrospinal fluid rhinorrhea: a meta-analysis. Laryngoscope. 2000;110(7):1166–72.
22. Bernal-Sprekelsen M, Rioja E, Ensenat J, Enriquez K, Viscovich L, Agredo-Lemos FE, et al. Management of anterior skull base defect depending on its size and location. Biomed Res Int. 2014;2014:346873.
23. Germani RM, Vivero R, Herzallah IR, Casiano RR. Endoscopic reconstruction of large anterior skull base defects using acellular dermal allograft. Am J Rhinol. 2007;21(5):615–8.
24. Nyquist GG, Anand VK, Mehra S, Kacker A, Schwartz TH. Endoscopic endonasal repair of anterior skull base non-traumatic cerebrospinal fluid leaks, meningoceles, and encephaloceles. J Neurosurg. 2010;113(5):961–6.
25. Prickett KK, Wise SK. Grafting materials in skull base reconstruction. Adv Otorhinolaryngol. 2013;74:24–32.
26. DeConde AS, Suh JD, Ramakrishnan VR. Treatment of cerebrospinal fluid rhinorrhea. Curr Opin Otolaryngol. 2015;23(1):59–64.
27. Banks CA, Palmer JN, Chiu AG, O'Malley BW Jr, Woodworth BA, Kennedy DW. Endoscopic closure of CSF rhinorrhea: 193 cases over 21 years. Otolaryngology. 2009;140(6):826–33.
28. Tabaee A, Anand VK, Brown SM, Lin JW, Schwartz TH. Algorithm for reconstruction after endoscopic pituitary and skull base surgery. Laryngoscope. 2007;117(7):1133–7.

Local Pedicled Flaps

18

Paolo Castelnuovo, Federico Russo,
and Paolo Battaglia

18.1 Introduction

The overall goals of skull base reconstruction include separation of the cranial cavity from the sinonasal tract, preventing cerebrospinal fluid leaks (CSF-L), pneumocephalus and intracranial infections, such as ascending bacterial meningitis and abscesses, and protection of cranial nerves and major vessels against desiccation and infection.

Early endoscopic reconstructive techniques were based on experience with the repair of defects following spontaneous CSF leaks and accidental or iatrogenic trauma. Multiple reports have validated that small skull base defects can be reconstructed with a wide variety of free grafting techniques, achieving success in more than 95% of the patients [1, 2].

However, when applied to the larger and more complex skull base defects, these techniques might be inadequate. In these cases, reconstruction is challenging not only because of the size of the defects but also because of the site and effects of gravity (high flow of cerebrospinal fluid at the middle and posterior skull base) and the proximity of delicate neurovascular structures, not surrounded by bony borders (such as optic chiasm, internal carotid artery, VI cranial nerve, olfactory threads).

Subsequent refinements of the free grafting techniques, such as multilayer repair, reduced the CSF leak rate of the anterior skull base [3], but it remained high for large defects located at the middle and posterior skull base [4]. Therefore, many pedicled vascularised flaps have been developed over the years (i.e. the Hadad-Bassagasteguy flap) for reconstruction of complex and high-flow skull base defects, with a decrease in CSF leak incidence to <5% [5, 6].

The vascularised flap techniques employ tissues that maintain a connection with the donor site (pedicle) and are transferred to the receiver site, which has to be adjacent, through sliding and rotation movements. They have their own vascularisation. An ideal flap should be simple to design, resist trauma, produce little to no morbidity, provide an adequate surface area and have an arc of rotation that permits its transposition without the tendency to return to its original position.

Pedicle vascularised flaps, when applied directly to close a defect or placed over traditional fascia grafts, should provide very strong support and rapid re-epithelialisation, especially in critical areas. Different vascularised flaps for skull base reconstruction are described in literature.

Supplementary Information The online version contains supplementary material available at [https://doi.org/10.1007/978-3-030-94781-1_18].

P. Castelnuovo (✉) · F. Russo · P. Battaglia
Division of Otorhinolaryngology, Department of Surgical Specialties, Head and Neck Surgery and Forensic Dissection Research Center, University of Insubria, Varese, Italy

A. A. AlQahtani et al. (eds.), *CSF Rhinorrhea*, https://doi.org/10.1007/978-3-030-94781-1_18

18.2 Hadad-Bassagasteguy Flap

The Hadad-Bassagasteguy flap (HBF) [7] is a vascular pedicled flap supplied by the posterior nasoseptal arteries. These arteries arise from the posterior nasal artery, one of the terminal branches of the maxillary artery. The posterior nasoseptal arteries supply the entire length of the nasal septum and anastomose with the ethmoidal arteries, the greater palatine artery and the anterior facial artery. The flap is designed according to the size and shape of the defect, although it is best to overestimate the size and then trim the flap if needed. Harvesting of the HBF includes the use of two horizontal parallel incisions along the nasal septum. An inferior incision is made over the maxillary crest and a superior incision is made 1–2 cm below the most superior aspect of the septum to preserve the olfactory epithelium [8] following an ideal line that passes through the axilla of superior and middle turbinate. A vertical incision at the muco-cutaneous junction joins these two horizontal incisions, anteriorly. Posteriorly, the superior incision extends laterally over the rostrum of the sphenoid sinus at the inferior aspect of the sphenoid ostium, till the tail of superior turbinate, while the inferior incision extends along the posterior free border of the nasal septum and then laterally along the arch of the posterior choana, till the tail of middle turbinate (Video 18.1). A strip of the mucosa between the sphenoid rostrum incisions contains the posterior septal arteries and forms a relatively long and narrow pedicle that facilitates a long reach and wide arc of rotation. It is also important to raise the pedicle to a level that is as close as possible to the sphenopalatine foramen to gain maximum length (Fig. 18.1). Maximal length of the flap is obtained by placing the anterior vertical incision at the muco-cutaneous junction. A wider flap can be harvested by placing the inferior incision at the lateral nasal floor in the inferior meatus, taking care to preserve the Hasner valve (Video 18.2). All incisions can be modified according to reconstructive requirements.

The elevation of the flap starts anteriorly with a Cottle dissector or similar instrument. The septal incisions may be completed with scissors

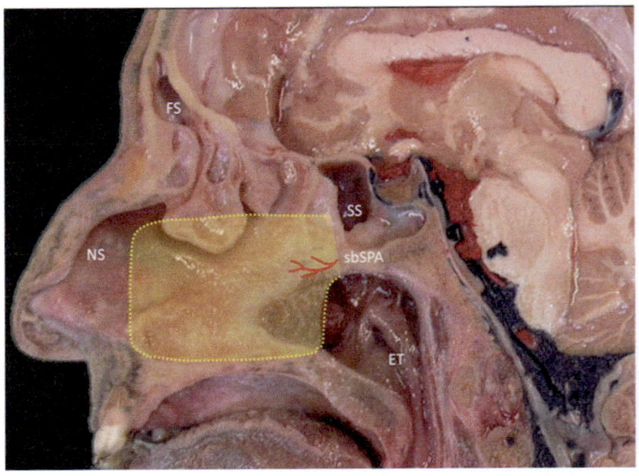

Fig. 18.1 Hadad-Bassagasteguy (HBF). Sagittal view (cadaver specimen). The yellow dotted line shows the incisions to harvest HBF. *NS* nasal septum, *FS* frontal sinus, *SS* sphenoidal sinus, *ET* Eustachian tube, *sbSPA* septal branches of the sphenopalatine artery

or other sharp instruments, as necessary. Elevation of the flap from the anterior surface of the sphenoid sinus is completed with the preservation of the posterolateral vascular pedicle. Once harvested, the flap can be stored into the nasopharynx or inside the antrum until the extirpative phase of the surgery is concluded [9]. In some cases, extensive sphenoidotomy is required to repair clival or Sternberg's canal CSF-L, risking to damage HBF pedicle. In this situation, a rescue flap approach can be used, which consists of partially harvesting the most superior and posterior aspects of the flap to protect its pedicle and provide access to the sphenoid. In particular, a horizontal incision is performed over the surface of the sphenoid, at the level of the sphenoid ostium. This incision is continued medially over the sphenoid rostrum and then anteriorly into the nasal septum (for approximately one-third to one-half of the septum following the sagittal plane, parallel to a line that passes through the axillas of ethmoidal turbinates). Using an elevator, a mucosal flap is created by raising the mucosa immediately below the incision in a submucopericondrial/subperiosteal fashion, until it is freed at the level of the floor of the sphenoid or choanae. A wide sphenoidotomy can be performed above and below the rescue flap pedicle, preserving the previously raised (rescue) flap [10].

The endoscopic transpterygoid approach classically involves the coagulation and transection of the sphenopalatine artery (SPA) at the level of its foramen, adopting the contralateral HBF for skull base reconstruction. However, using some surgical tricks, the pedicle of the ipsilateral nasoseptal flap can be preserved during the endoscopic transpterygoid approach. In particular, it is necessary to extend the inferior mucosal incision laterally to the medial pterygoid plate and inferiorly to the sphenopalatine foramen to achieve maximal mobility of the vascular pedicle. Identification, coagulation and transection of the SPA branches are mandatory to lateralise the pterygopalatine fossa content and the nasoseptal flap pedicle. Once the vidian nerve is sacrificed, the base of the pterygoid bone can be drilled without injury to the vascular pedicle. In this way, the ipsilateral HBF is available for skull base reconstruction after endoscopic transpterygoid approach [11].

A double elevation of HBF from both the sides of the nasal septum is described, too [12].

Usually, silicone splints are used in the postoperative period to protect the denuded septum and facilitate the re-epithelialisation and left in site for 15–21 days.

The HBF has become a mainstay reconstructive option for CSF-L due to its versatility, wide arc of rotation, generous size and relative ease to harvest. Factors that may predict difficulty in raising HBF include a deviated septum, septal spurs, an existing perforation, and prior septal surgery. Furthermore, the HBF may not be available in revision surgeries in which it has already been used, in previous extended sphenoidotomy or pterygopalatine fossa surgery. Potential morbidity exists with the use of the NSF. If the superior incision to harvest the flap is made too high along the skull base, olfactory fibres can be injured, resulting in hypo/anosmia. However, if the flap is elevated on one side, patients should have functioning olfactory fibres on the contralateral side, but potential for complete anosmia exists, and several patients have complained decreased olfaction after surgery. Moreover, nasal crusting at the donor site might be present for several weeks after surgery [5]. The likelihood of this complication is considerably reduced if a silicone splint is left in place for 3 weeks. The HBF flap, though not the only option, is the preferred one for the reconstruction of anterior, middle and posterior skull base defects, from the posterior wall of frontal sinus back to the clivus and from orbit to orbit [7]. However, the HBF may not be adequate for the repair of anterior defects, such as the CSF-L of the posterior wall of the frontal sinus. The posterior location of its pedicle can lead to tension and retraction of the flap with incomplete closure of the defect's anterior border. In fact, in case of CSF-L of the posterior wall of frontal sinus, other flaps have been described, such as the one pedicled at the level of the septal branches of the anterior ethmoidal arteries.

18.3 Anterior and Posterior Ethmoidal Artery Septal Flap

The anterior ethmoidal artery septal flap (AEA flap or Castelnuovo's flap) [13] is a mucosal flap based on the septal branches of the anterior ethmoidal artery, first described by Castelnuovo et al. for the repair of septal perforations. Its harvesting includes a gentle lateralisation of the middle turbinate, paying attention not to fracture the lateral lamella, to expose the upper part of the nasal septum and to gain a wider operation space. A posterior vertical incision along the nasal septum, following an ideal line passing through the septal projection of the superior turbinate's axilla, is performed. The incision is started 1–2 cm below the most superior aspect of the septum, preserving the olfactory epithelium, and it is continued along the nasal floor, reaching the lateral wall of the inferior meatus. An anterior vertical incision, parallel to the previous one, is carried out along the nasal septum at the level of the septal projection of the middle turbinate's axilla, starting 1–2 cm below the cribriform plate, continuing along the nasal floor and reaching the inferior meatus. A horizontal incision on the sagittal plane, along the inferior meatus, is made to join the most lateral aspect of the previous vertical incisions (Fig. 18.2). All incisions can be modified and tailored to obtain a longer and a wider flap, according to reconstructive requirements. The subperiosteal/subperichondral eleva-

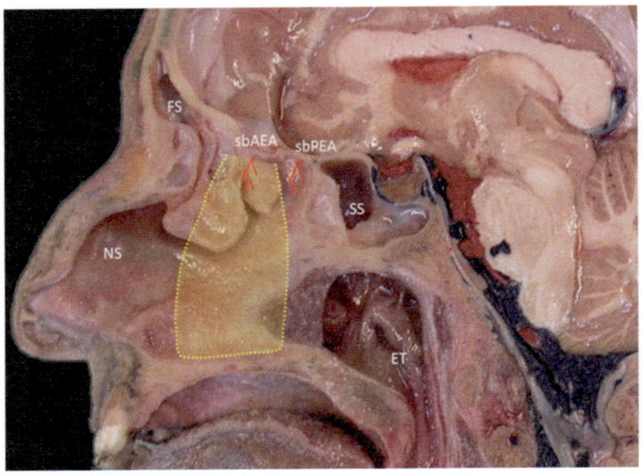

Fig. 18.2 Anterior ethmoidal artery flap (AEA flap). Sagittal view (cadaver specimen). The yellow dotted line shows the incisions to harvest AEA flap. *NS* nasal septum, *FS* frontal sinus, *SS* sphenoidal sinus, *ET* Eustachian tube, *sbAEA* septal branch of the anterior ethmoidal artery, *sbPEA* septal branch of the posterior ethmoidal artery

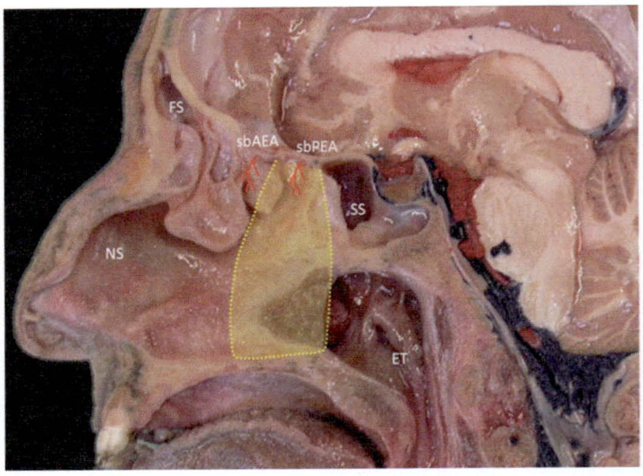

Fig. 18.3 Posterior ethmoidal artery flap (PEA flap). Sagittal view (cadaver specimen). The yellow dotted line shows the incisions to harvest PEA flap. *NS* nasal septum, *FS* frontal sinus, *SS* sphenoidal sinus, *ET* Eustachian tube, *sbAEA* septal branch of the anterior ethmoidal artery, *sbPEA* septal branch of the posterior ethmoidal artery

tion of the flap is performed starting from the anterior incision.

Thanks to the anterior location of its pedicle and its geometry, the AEA flap can be rotated to repair ipsilateral CSF-L of the posterior wall of the frontal sinus and the frontal infundibulum [14], preserving the frontal sinus drainage pathway (Video 18.3) [15]. Furthermore, this flap can be used to cover the exposed bone at the level of the posterior wall of frontal sinus after frontal sinusotomies that require drilling of the frontal sinus floor (according to Draf type IIb and III), reducing post-operative restenosis rate [16]. In literature, a mucosal septal flap supplied by septal branches of posterior ethmoidal artery (PEA flap) has also been described. Its harvesting includes two parallel vertical incisions along the nasal septum, extended along the floor of the nasal cavity, reaching the inferior meatus. The anterior one is made along an ideal line passing through the septal projection of the superior turbinate's; the posterior one is carried out anteriorly to the anterior sphenoidal wall. A sagittal incision along the inferior meatus is made to connect the most lateral aspect of the previous vertical incisions (Fig. 18.3). Once harvested, the PEA flap can be rotated to cover ipsilateral defects of the lateral recess of the sphenoid sinus, due to the posterior location of its pedicle and its flexibility [14]. Ethmoidal arteries-based flaps (AEA and PEA flaps) are easy, quick and convenient to harvest, provide a large coverage area with a robust blood supply and have been proved to be reliable pedicle flaps that can be used to repair CSF-L in certain cases. In particular, the AEA flap's main indication is the management of defects of the posterior wall of frontal sinus, where it represents the first choice. In fact, as previously demonstrated, the posterior location of HBF pedicle can lead to tension and retraction of the flap with incomplete closure of the anterior border of the defect. As described also for the HBF, various factors, such as a deviated septum, septal spur, existing perforations and prior septal surgeries, may make the harvesting of ethmoidal arteries-based flaps difficult. Similarly, nasal crusting at the donor site is prolonged for several weeks after surgery. To note, the harvesting of AEA and PEA flaps involves sacrifice of the septal branches of the sphenopalatine artery; therefore, once it is set up, it will not be possible to use ipsilateral HBF for any revision surgery.

18.4 Septal Flip-Flap

The septal flip-flap (SFF) [17] consists of mucoperichondrium and mucoperiosteum from the nasal septum, and its pedicle is based on the septal branches of ethmoidal arteries. Its harvesting includes the removal of nasal septum mucoperichondrium–mucoperiosteum ipsilateral to the defect. The septal cartilage and perpendicular plate of the ethmoid are removed. An anterior vertical incision in the contralateral septal mucosa is performed, starting superiorly at the level of the posterior wall of the frontal sinus and carried out anteriorly, reaching the frontal beak, and downward reaching the nasal floor. A posterior vertical incision is carried out from the sphenoidal planum to the nasal floor. In this step, the septal branches of the SPA passing over the nasal choana are cauterised and cut. Finally, the two vertical incisions are connected through a horizontal incision back to front at the level of the contralateral nasal floor, including the inferior meatus if necessary (Fig. 18.4).

In this way, SFF is superiorly hinged and freely rotated to cover the anterior skull base defects (Video 18.4).

Similarly, a contralateral superiorly based mucoperiosteal nasal septal flap, with a creation of window at the highest aspect of the nasal septum to allow transfer of the flap to the affected side, has been described in literature [18]. SFF is simple and quick to harvest, and it is able to repair huge defects of the anterior skull base thanks to its vascular pedicle, which is both anatomically consistent and capable of supporting a large mucosal surface area. The origin of the pedicle and its geometry ensure an arc of rotation that is ideal for the reconstruction of the ethmoid roof and very anterior skull base defects, and it can also cover the medial orbital wall. In fact, SPA-based flaps, such as Hadad flap, middle and inferior turbinate flap, can be pulled down by the pedicle itself for gravitational and geometrical reasons, especially in the posterior ethmoidal roof, where the creation of a dead space between the flap and the skull base could compromise the reconstruction [19].

The restricted indication for the reconstruction of the sella and the clivus due to the width of the pedicle that constrains the arc of rotation should be mentioned as a limitation of the flap. From a technical viewpoint, previous septoplasty and cauterisation of ethmoidal arteries for epistaxis or other reasons should be considered as restrictions precluding the use of the SFF.

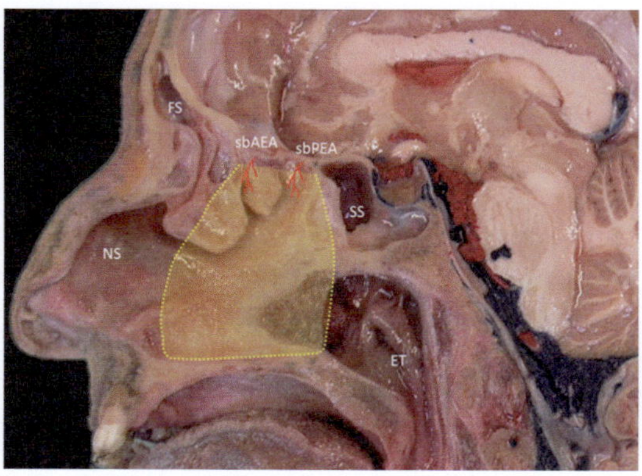

Fig. 18.4 Septal flip flap (SFF). Sagittal view (cadaver specimen). The yellow dotted line shows the incisions to harvest SFF. *NS* nasal septum, *FS* frontal sinus, *SS* sphenoidal sinus, *ET* Eustachian tube, *sbAEA* septal branch of the anterior ethmoidal artery, *sbPEA* septal branch of the posterior ethmoidal artery

18.5 Bipedicled Anterior Septal Flap

The bipedicled anterior septal flap (BASF) [20] is supplied by septal branches of the superior labial artery and nasopalatine artery (anastomosis between the sphenopalatine and greater palatine arteries that is transmitted through the incisive canal). To harvest BASF, a posterior vertical incision is made on the septal mucosa, medial to the natural sphenoid ostium, from the choanal arch to 1 cm below the skull base. A second anterior vertical incision immediately posterior to the incisive canal from the nasal floor to a line parallel to the top of the choanal arch is performed. After that, an inferior horizontal incision joins the inferior aspect of the posterior vertical incision and the superior aspect of the anterior vertical incision. A superior horizontal incision is carried out from the superior aspect of the posterior vertical incision to the superior aspect of the dorsal septum, 1 cm below the skull base. Finally, the anterior-most incision is made from the anterior aspect of the superior horizontal incision to the caudal margin of the septum at the level of the middle septal angle (Fig. 18.5). A mucoperichondrial flap is elevated starting from

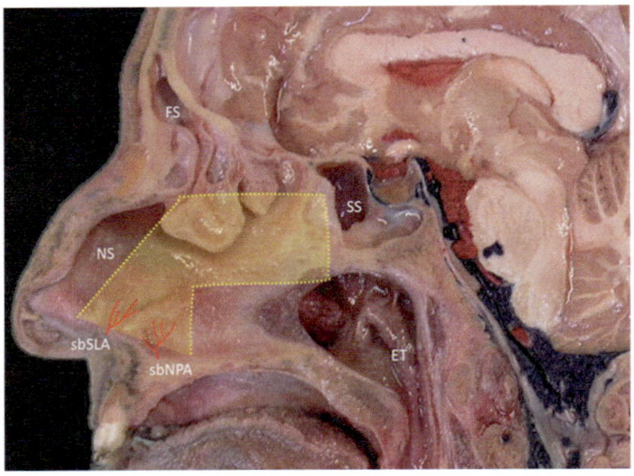

Fig. 18.5 Bepedicled anterior septal flap (BASF). Sagittal view (cadaver specimen). The yellow dotted line shows the incisions to harvest BASF. *NS* nasal septum, *FS* frontal sinus, *SS* sphenoidal sinus, *ET* Eustachian tube, *sbSLA* septal branch of the superior labial artery, *sbNPA* septal branch of the nasopalatine artery

the anterior incision. According to its anatomic characteristics and its surface area of 916 mm^2, the BASF's main indication is the anterior skull base repair at the level of the posterior wall of the frontal sinus. Furthermore, this flap is used to cover the exposed bone at the level of frontal beak or anterior wall of the frontal sinus after Draf type IIB/III, reducing the post-operative restenosis rate. The BASF has a lower morbidity than other septal flaps. In fact, the harvesting of HBF, for example, requires an incision anteriorly to the caudal septal margin resulting in prolonged, symptomatic crusting and obstruction at the level of the internal valve. Contrarily, the mucosa of the BAS flap is harvested from the postero-superior septum resulting in a donor site that may be less symptomatic. The restricted indication for the reconstruction of the most anterior aspect of the skull base due to its anterior pedicle should be mentioned as a limitation of the flap. Previous septoplasty should be considered a contraindication to harvest the BASF.

18.6 Posterior Pedicle Inferior Turbinate Flap

The posterior pedicle inferior turbinate flap (PPITF) [21] is based on the inferior turbinate artery, a terminal branch from the postero-lateral nasal artery, which is a terminal branch from the sphenopalatine artery. The inferior turbinate is gently medialised to better expose the entire medial surface of the inferior turbinate and allow visualisation of the mucosa from the inferior meatus. The flap may be designed according to the size of the defect, but it is best to harvest the entire turbinate to assure adequate coverage. A wider flap may be harvested by extending the lower incision to include the lateral mucoperiosteum of the turbinate and even the inferior meatus. It is best to identify first the sphenopalatine artery as it exits the sphenopalatine foramen and to follow it distally to identify the postero-lateral nasal artery. Two parallel incisions are performed following the sagittal plane of the inferior turbinate, the superior one just above the inferior turbinate, at fontanelle level, and the inferior one following the caudal margin of the turbinate. A vertical cut made along the anterior head of the turbinate connects the two previous incisions (Fig. 18.6). The mucoperiosteum is elevated starting from the anterior aspect of the inferior turbinate, providing about 4.97 cm^2 of surface area [22]. Care must be taken to avoid injuring the vascular pedicle as it enters at the superior aspect of its lateral attachment, approximately 1.0 and 1.5 cm from its posterior tip. One disadvantage of using the PPITF is the formation of crusting over the inferior tur-

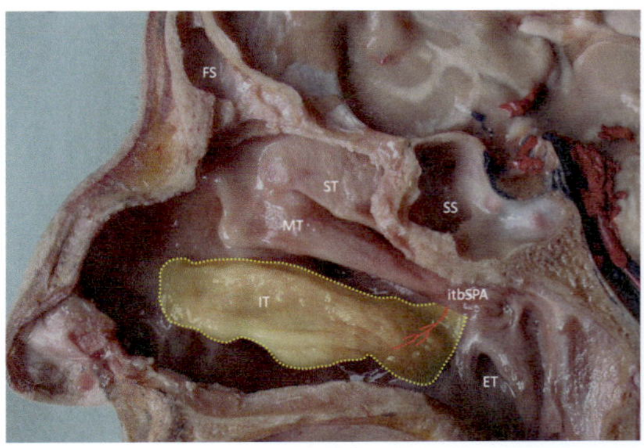

Fig. 18.6 Posterior pedicle inferior turbinate flap (PPITF). Sagittal view of the lateral nasal wall (cadaver specimen). The yellow dotted line shows the incisions to harvest PPITF. *ST* superior turbinate, *MT* middle turbinate, *IT* inferior turbinate, *FS* frontal sinus, *SS* sphenoidal sinus, *ET* Eustachian tube, *itbSPA* inferior turbinate branch of the sphenopalatine artery

binate in the post-operative period. The re-mucosalisation of the donor site was observed after a period of 3–4 weeks. In addition, in patients with prior inferior turbinectomy or turbinate atrophy, the mucosal surface may have inadequate size; therefore, these are relative contraindications to the PPITF. The use of an inferior turbinate pedicled flap is limited by its size and configuration and is a better option for the reconstruction of more posterior and inferior defects such as in the clivus; to increase its coverage, it is possible to raise bilateral PPITFs (when feasible), or an inferior turbinate flap in conjunction with another pedicled flap to address larger defects.

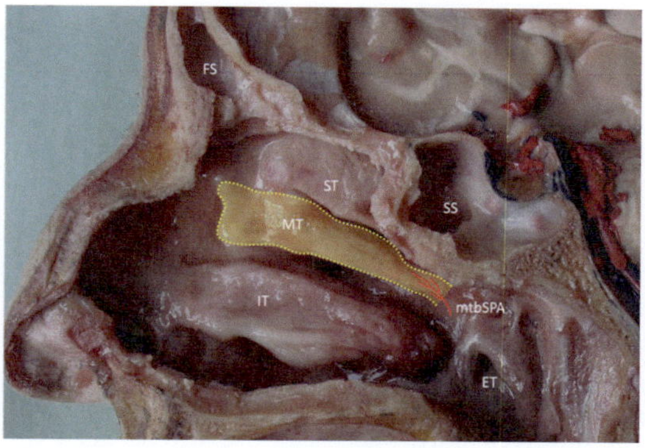

Fig. 18.7 Posterior pedicle middle turbinate flap (PPMTF). Sagittal view of the lateral nasal wall (cadaver specimen). The yellow dotted line shows the incisions to harvest PPMTF. *ST* superior turbinate, *MT* middle turbinate, *IT* inferior turbinate, *FS* frontal sinus, *SS* sphenoidal sinus, *ET* Eustachian tube, *mtbSPA* middle turbinate branch of the sphenopalatine artery

18.7 Posterior Pedicle Middle Turbinate Flap

The posterior pedicle middle turbinate flap (PPMTF) [23] is supplied by the middle turbinate branch of the sphenopalatine artery that runs through the posterior attachment and constitutes its pedicle.

Its harvesting entails a vertical incision at the head of the turbinate and a horizontal incision at the medial aspect of the middle turbinate (MT) mucosa, respecting the attachment to the cribriform plate. Subperiosteal elevation of the mucoperiosteum from the bony component is carried out, while the turbinate bone and attachments are still intact. After the bone is removed, a cut is made through the MT's axilla, detaching it from the lateral wall of the nasal cavity and skull base. The incision is extended dorso-caudally along the sagittal plane until the mucosa is completely divided and unfolded in the same way as opening a book (Fig. 18.7). Elevation of the flap is completed preserving its posterior pedicle, which contains the MT branch of the sphenopalatine artery. The pedicle, however, may be dissected back to the sphenopalatine foramen to increase its length and mobility and, henceforth, its reach and arc of rotation.

A significant limitation of the PPMTF is the technical difficulty involved with its harvesting due to the anatomical variability that occurs in 25% of subjects [24]. The most common anomalies include concha bullosa, paradoxical MT and unilateral hypoplasia. Potential complications exist during PPMTF harvesting. If the incisions on the medial and lateral aspect of the turbinate are made too high along the skull base, the cribriform plate and lateral lamella can be injured, which can result in CSF-L. The surface area of the PPMTF is somewhat limited at 5.6 cm^2 [23].

The superior position of the middle turbinate pedicle flap allows it to reach defects of the cribriform plate, planum sphenoidale, sella and fovea ethmoidalis area.

18.8 Turbinal Flap

The turbinal flap (TF) [25] consists of middle and superior turbinate mucosa, and it is supplied by the ethmoidal arteries system. Harvesting of the TF includes vertical incision at the middle turbinate's anterior edge, from the axilla down to its inferior border. Subperiosteal elevation of the mucoperiosteal layers on both medial and lateral sides of the middle and superior turbinates, and their common lamina is performed. Sectioning of the lateral mucoperiosteal layer close to the skull base from the anterior edge of the middle turbinate to the posterior insertion of the superior turbinate is carried out, before removing middle and superior concha's bony framework. Whereupon, the turbinal branches of the SPA at the tail of the MT are cauterised and cut, and the posterior insertion of middle and superior turbinates to the skull base is sectioned. Finally, the lateral mucoperiosteal layer is rotated inferiorly (Fig. 18.8). According to its anatomic characteristic and its surface area of 8.6 cm^2, the TF's main indication is the anterior skull base repair at the level of the ethmoid roof, preserving the entire olfactory mucosa (Video 18.5). Conversely, the posterior wall of the frontal sinus and the planum sphenoidalis may be only partially covered by such flap. When the medial mucoperiosteal layer is sufficient for the reconstruction, harvesting of the TF is easier and faster. In fact, similarly to what described for the PPMTF, TF harvesting is demanding and time-consuming, and the most technically difficult step is the dissection of the lateral mucoperiosteal layer. Further limitation of the TF regards its thickness, as the middle and superior turbinates' mucosa is very thin compared to the nasal septum and inferior turbinate. Moreover, the dissection of the pedicle upward to the common lamina of the turbinates could result in a minimal CSF leak, otherwise easily repairable by the flap itself.

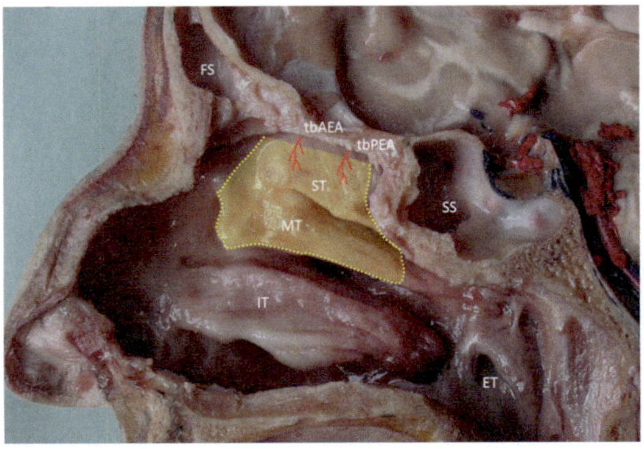

Fig. 18.8 Turbinal flap (TF). Sagittal view of the lateral nasal wall (cadaver specimen). The yellow dotted line shows the incisions to harvest TF. *ST* superior turbinate, *MT* middle turbinate, *IT* inferior turbinate, *FS* frontal sinus, *SS* sphenoidal sinus, *ET* Eustachian tube, *tbAEA* turbinal branch of the anterior ethmoidal artery, *tbPEA* turbinal branch of the posterior ethmoidal artery

18.9 Anterior Pedicle Lateral Nasal Wall Flap

The anterior pedicle lateral nasal wall flap (APLWF) [20] is based on branches of the facial (angular and lateral nasal) and anterior ethmoidal artery. The APLWF harvesting begins with a pedicle's posterior incision, following the lacrimal bone, anterior to the uncinated process, extending posteriorly on a sagittal plane over the superior aspect of the inferior turbinate. A maxillary antrostomy can be performed to facilitate the priory described incision, and resection of the middle turbinate can facilitate the incision and harvesting process. At the most posterior aspect of this incision, the SPA and its branches must be cauterised and cut. At the level of inferior turbinate's tail, this incision joins a perpendicular incision that runs medially to cross the floor of the nose and reach the septum. The pedicle's anterior incision is carried out from the most caudal aspect of the nasal bone to the upper aspect of the inferior turbinate, following the pyriform aperture. It continues anterior to the head of the inferior turbinate and then intersects another perpendicular incision that also crosses the floor of the nose to reach the septum. The two horizontal incisions on the floor of the nose are joined by another sagittal incision that follows the maxillary crest at the junction of the floor of the nose and nasal septum. The APLWF can be tailored according to the size of the defect, either decreasing the surface area of the nasal floor (with a more lateral incision) or including the most inferior aspect of the nasal septum mucoperiosteum (placing the incision higher on the nasal septum). A separate vertical incision over the head of the inferior turbinate is extended laterally to intersect the pedicle's anterior incision to allow the elevation of the mucoperiosteal lining of the nasal and meatal sides of the inferior turbinate. The flap is elevated subperiosteally, and the dissection is continued along the medial aspect of the inferior turbinate. The opening of the lacrimal duct is spared by curving the anterior horizontal incision around it or performing an elliptical incision around the opening. Once the incisions around the nasolacrimal duct are completed, the mucosa is

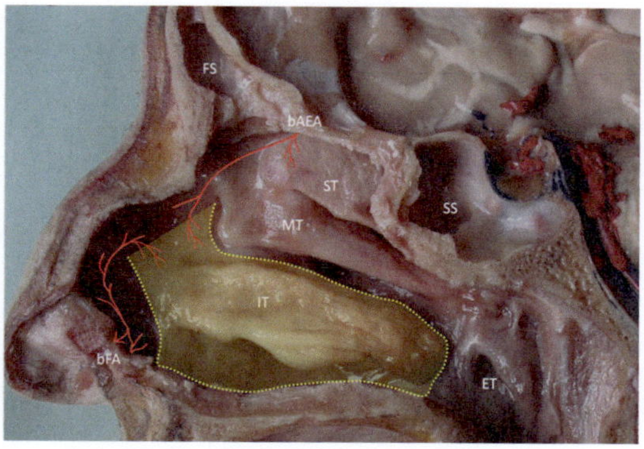

Fig. 18.9 Anterior pedicle lateral nasal wall flap (APLWF). Sagittal view of the lateral nasal wall (cadaver specimen). The yellow dotted line shows the incisions to harvest APLWF. *ST* superior turbinate, *MT* middle turbinate, *IT* inferior turbinate, *FS* frontal sinus, *SS* sphenoidal sinus, *ET* Eustachian tube, *bAEA* branch of the anterior ethmoidal artery, *bFA* branches of the facial artery

elevated medially. The residual bone is removed (Fig. 18.9). Surgical experience and endoscopic skills are required to harvest APLWFs. A potential complication during APLWF harvesting is the opening of nasolacrimal duct. Donor site morbidity includes transitory nasal crusting, which continues until a complete re-mucosalisation occurs. The flap dimensions are sufficient to reconstruct the area from the posterior wall of frontal sinus to the sella turcica (antero-posterior) and from orbit to orbit (latero-lateral).

18.10 Surgical Technique: General Aspects

The criterion that guides the CSF-leak repair procedure is 'integration of the borders'. No matter what type of technique or flaps is used, the preparatory stage of duraplasty must include appropriate exposure of the defect, undermining of the dural margins (when possible), and smoothing of the defect's edges to get a tensioactive effect for the flap. As a general rule, meticulous management of the tissues is required for obtaining the best integration, and a dedicated surgical team is recommended to perform the reconstruction.

The flap, which is usually either mucoperichondrial or mucoperiosteal and harvested from the ipsilateral or contralateral nasal cavity, is put in place with the mucosa side facing the nasal cavity, and it is firmly secured by applying pressure from the centre outwards, to prevent air from remaining trapped between the graft and the defect surface. Furthermore, as for any overlay technique, the receptor site must be stripped of its mucosal layer in the area that needs to be covered by the flap, to avoid the formation of mucoceles [26].

The flap has to cover all the defect area without overlapping the frontal and/or sphenoidal sinusotomy(ies). Particular care has to be given to the vascular pedicle, which must not be rotated with acute angles or stretched out. For this reason, it is important to remove bony edges surrounding its origin, in order to allow free movements of the flap, thus increasing its range of motion and length. At last, the flap is properly fixed with OxiCell® and fibrin glue along the borders but, preferably, not under it; this avoids a gap between graft and receiving site.

The introduction of vascularised flaps reduced the rate of post-operative CSF-L from 20% to nearly 5% so that they have become a common method of closure in many skull base procedures. Available data refers mainly to HBF due to the fact that it is the most used [27]. High-flow CSF leaks typically benefited from the use of a vascularised pedicled flap rather than a free tissue grafts, with post-operative success rates of 94% versus 82%, respectively. These results were partially dependent on anatomic location of the repair site, with superior results noted with the use of vascularised pedicled flaps for transclival approaches, whereas no clear differences were noted between the use of vascularised and non-vascularised closures in other subsites [28].

In spite of the fact that the widespread use of pedicled flaps has improved the outcome of duraplasty procedures, a reconstruction technique must be chosen according to some anatomical-mechanical factors and oncological factors. The anatomical-mechanical factors are linked to the site of the defect and its borders, since collimation of the borders is very important. The three cranial fossae differ because of their adjacent structures:

- In the anterior cranial fossa, the epidural detachment is not very difficult, over the roof of the orbit, and is necessary for receiving the extradural intracranial layer of the plasty, which should normally be spread out within the epidural space to guarantee sealing of the duraplasty. The olfactory fissure is an exception in this case because it is impossible to detach the epidural plane (olfactory foramina) without tearing the dura itself. In the light of these considerations, the reconstruction of olfactory fissure CSF-L is based on overlay technique, using graft or flap in the case of larger defects [29].
- In the middle fossa, the main issues are the optic nerve, the chiasm that is vascularised by the small arterial branches of the superior hypophyseal artery structure (in fact, the visual field can be harmed by even the slightest damage or only compression), the pituitary stalk (functional damage can result from minor trauma or manoeuvres) and the internal carotid artery. In this area, epidural detachment must be handled very gently or even avoided, using the Gasket-seal closure technique, eventually covered by vascularised flap to provide stronger stability and promote rapid re-epithelialisation.
- In the posterior cranial fossa, the critical points encountered are where the VI cranial nerve passes through the dura and crosses the Dorello canal, and the high cerebrospinal fluid flow. If these aspects are considered, it is evident that the best reconstruction option is the multilayer technique with free grafts or gasket seal covered by vascularised flap, to cope with a greater force of gravity.

Intracranial content has to be covered with protective material. Two options frequently used are: heterologous (such as Integra DuraGen®, a collagen matrix) and autologous materials, such as fascia lata, that can be inserted intracranially (intradurally and extradurally).

References

1. Hegazy HM, Carrau RL, Snyderman CH, Kassam A, Zweig J. Transnasal endoscopic repair of cerebrospinal fluid rhinorrhea: a meta-analysis. Laryngoscope. 2000;110(7):1166–72.
2. Locatelli D, Rampa F, Acchiardi I, Bignami M, De Bernardi F, Casteltselnuovo P. Endoscopic endonasal approaches for repair of cerebrospinal fluid leaks: nine year experience. Neurosurgery. 2006;58:246–57.
3. Castelnuovo PG, Delú G, Locatelli D, Padoan G, Bernardi FD, Pistochini A, Bignami M. Endonasal endoscopic duraplasty: our experience. Skull Base. 2006;16(1):19–24.
4. Kassam A, Carrau RL, Snyderman CH, Gardner P, Mintz A. Evolution of reconstructive techniques following endoscopic expanded endonasal approaches. Neurosurg Focus. 2005;19(1):E8.
5. El Sayed IH, Roediger FC, Goldberg AN, Parsa AT, McDermott MW. Endoscopic reconstruction of skull base defects with the nasal septal flap. Skull Base. 2008;18(6):385–94.
6. Kassam A, Carrau RL, Horowitz M, Snyderman C, Hirsch BE. The role of fibrin sealants in cranial base surgery. New York: Medscape Neurology & Neurosurgery; 2002.
7. Hadad G, Bassagasteguy L, Carrau RL, Mataza JC, Kassam A, Snyderman CH, Mintz A. A novel reconstructive technique after endoscopic expanded endonasal approaches: vascular pedicle nasoseptal flap. Laryngoscope. 2006;116(10):1882–6.
8. Baban MIA, Battaglia P, Mohammed MH, Locatelli D, Shawkat A, Turri-Zanoni M, Castelnuovo P. How to preserve the olfaction in harvesting the nasoseptal flap in endoscopic skull base surgery. Oper Tech Otolaryngol. 2020;31:7–12. https://doi.org/10.1016/j.otot.2020.03.001.
9. Kassam AB, Thomas A, Carrau RL, Snyderman CH, Vescan A, Prevedello D, Mintz A, Gardner P. Endoscopic reconstruction of the cranial base using a pedicled nasoseptal flap. Neurosurgery. 2008;63(1):44–52.
10. Rivera-Serrano CM, Snyderman CH, Gardner P, Prevedello D, Wheless S, Kassam AB, Carrau RL, Germanwala A, Zanation A. Nasoseptal "rescue" flap: a novel modification of the nasoseptal flap technique for pituitary surgery. Laryngoscope. 2011;121(5):990–3.
11. Pinheiro-Neto CD, Paluzzi A, Fernandez-Miranda JC, Scopel TF, Wang EW, Gardner PA, Snyderman CH. Extended dissection of the septal flap pedicle for ipsilateral endoscopic transpterygoid approaches. Laryngoscope. 2014;124(2):391–6.
12. Nyquist GG, Anand VK, Singh A, Schwartz TH. Janus flap: bilateral nasoseptal flaps for anterior

skull base reconstruction. Otolaryngol Head Neck Surg. 2010;142(3):327–31.
13. Castelnuovo P, Ferreli F, Khodaei I, Palma P. Anterior ethmoidal artery septal flap for the management of septal perforation. Arch Facial Plast Surg. 2011;13(6):411–4.
14. Mao S, Li M, Li D, Lin H, Ye H, Tang R, Su K, Zhang W. Septal floor rotational flap pedicled on ethmoidal arteries for endoscopic skull base reconstruction. Laryngoscope. 2019;129(12):2696–701.
15. Bozkurt G, Zocchi J, Russo F, Pietrobon G, Karligkiotis A, Elhassan HA, Seyhun N, Bignami M, Castelnuovo P. Frontal sinus preservation during cerebrospinal fluid leak repair. J Craniofac Surg. 2019;30(8):763–8.
16. Seyedhadi S, Mojtaba MA, Shahin B, Hoseinali K. The Draf III septal flap technique: a preliminary report. Am J Otolaryngol. 2013;34(5):399–402.
17. Battaglia P, Turri-Zanoni M, De Bernardi F, Dehgani Mobaraki P, Karligkiotis A, Leone F, Castelnuovo P. Septal flip flap for anterior skull base reconstruction after endoscopic resection of sinonasal cancers: preliminary outcomes. Acta Otorhinolaryngol Ital. 2016;36(3):194–8.
18. Eviatar E, Gavriel H. Endoscopic contralateral superiorly based mucoperiosteal nasal septal flap for closure of cerebrospinal fluid leak. J Neurol Surg B Skull Base. 2013;74:126–9.
19. Bozkurt G, Leone F, Arosio AD, Dehgani Mobaraki P, Elhassan HA, Seyhun N, Turri-Zanoni M, Castelnuovo P, Battaglia P. Septal flip flap for anterior skull base reconstruction after endoscopic transnasal craniectomy: long-term outcomes. World Neurosurg. 2019;128:409–16.
20. Hadad G, Rivera-Serrano CM, Bassagaisteguy LH, Carrau RL, Fernandez-Miranda J, Prevedello DM, Kassam AB. Anterior pedicle lateral nasal wall flap: a novel technique for the reconstruction of anterior skull base defects. Laryngoscope. 2011;121(8):1606–10.
21. Murakami CS, Kriet D, Ierokomos A. Nasal reconstruction using the inferior turbinate mucosal flap. Arch Facial Plast Surg. 1999;1:97–100.
22. Fortes FS, Carrau RL, Snyderman CH, Prevedello D, Vescan A, Mintz A, Gardner P, Kassam AB. The posterior pedicle inferior turbinate flap: a new vascularized flap for skull base reconstruction. Laryngoscope. 2007;117(8):1329–32.
23. Prevedello DM, Barges-Coll J, Fernandez-Miranda JC, Morera V, Jacobson D, Madhok R, dos Santos MC, Zanation A, Snyderman CH, Gardner P, Kassam AB, Carrau R. Middle turbinate flap for skull base reconstruction: cadaveric feasibility study. Laryngoscope. 2009;119(11):2094–8.
24. Perez-Pinas I, Sabate J, Carmona A, Catalina-Herrera CJ, Jimenez-Castellanos J. Anatomical variations in the human paranasal sinus region studied by CT. J Anat. 2000;197:221–7.
25. Schreiber A, Mattavelli D, Ferrari M, Rampinelli V, Lancini D, Belotti F, Rodella LF, Nicolai P. The turbinal flap: an additional option for anterior skull base reconstruction. Cadaveric feasibility study and case report. Int Forum Allergy Rhinol. 2017;7(2):199–204.
26. Karligkiotis A, Meloni F, Herman P, Castelnuovo P. How to avoid mucocele formation under pedicled nasoseptal flap. Am J Otolaryngol. 2014;35(4):546–7.
27. Harvey RJ, Parmar P, Sacks R, Zanation AM. Endoscopic skull base reconstruction of large dural defects: a systematic review of published evidence. Laryngoscope. 2012;122:452–9.
28. Clavenna MJ, Turner JH, Chandra RK. Pedicled flaps in endoscopic skull base reconstruction: review of current techniques. Curr Opin Otolaryngol Head Neck Surg. 2015;23(1):71–7.
29. Turri-Zanoni M, Zocchi J, Lambertoni A, Giovannardi M, Karligkiotis A, Battaglia P, Locatelli D, Castelnuovo P. Endoscopic endonasal reconstruction of anterior skull base defects: what factors really affect the outcomes? World Neurosurg. 2018;116:436–43.

Regional Pedicled Flaps for Skull Base Reconstruction

19

Nyall R. London Jr, Ricardo L. Carrau, and Adam Zanation

19.1 Introduction

Among other structural functions, the skull base serves to separate the anterior, middle, and posterior cranial fossae from the sinonasal cavity. Restoring this separation is a key element of any reconstructive technique. Advances in endoscopic endonasal surgery have led to the creation of large dural and skull base defects, requiring the development of appropriate skull base reconstructive methods to prevent postoperative cerebrospinal fluid (CSF) leak and meningitis [1]. While free grafting may be adequate for small low CSF flow defects, vascularized reconstruction with local, regional, or free flap techniques has become a mainstay in reconstruction of larger high CSF flow settings [2–4]. The most commonly utilized vascularized tissue transfer is the nasoseptal flap (NSF) [5–7]. However, in the setting of a malignancy requiring oncologic resection of the nasal septum or loss of its integrity or blood supply from previous surgery, an NSF or alternative intranasal flap may not be available, necessitating the use of alternative reconstructive techniques [8]. A regional pedicled flap may be a viable reconstruction option for a sizable skull base defect if a NSF is unavailable. The most commonly utilized regional pedicled flaps include the pericranial and temporoparietal fascia flaps (TPFF). Additional regional flaps include the occipital, palatal, facial buccinator, pedicled buccal fat pad, and salpingopharyngeus flap [9]. In this chapter, we will describe the anatomy, technique, and reported outcomes with each of these regional pedicled flap options.

N. R. London Jr
Department of Otolaryngology - Head and Neck Surgery, The Ohio State University, Columbus, OH, USA

Department of Otolaryngology - Head and Neck Surgery, Johns Hopkins School of Medicine, Baltimore, MD, USA

National Institute on Deafness and Other Communication Disorders, NIH, Bethesda, MD, USA
e-mail: nlondon2@jhmi.edu

R. L. Carrau
Department of Otolaryngology - Head and Neck Surgery, The Ohio State University, Columbus, OH, USA

Department Neurological Surgery, The Ohio State University, Columbus, OH, USA

A. Zanation (✉)
Department of Otolaryngology - Head and Neck Surgery, University of North Carolina at Chapel Hill, Chapel Hill, NC, USA

Department Neurosurgery, University of North Carolina at Chapel Hill, Chapel Hill, NC, USA
e-mail: adam_zanation@med.unc.edu

19.2 Trans-frontal Pericranial Flap

The pericranial flap has been utilized to reconstruct skull base defects long prior to the advent of endoscopic techniques [10]. This flap, supplied by the ipsilateral supratrochlear and supraorbital

A. A. AlQahtani et al. (eds.), *CSF Rhinorrhea*, https://doi.org/10.1007/978-3-030-94781-1_19

arteries, can readily cover defects of the anterior skull base, anteroposteriorly from the frontal sinus to the sella turcica, and laterally from orbit to orbit [11]. Length of the flap necessary has been estimated at 11–12.5 cm to cover the defects of the anterior skull base, 14–15.5 cm for parasellar defects, and 18–20.5 cm for clival defects [12]. While it may be feasible to reach a purely posterior skull base defect, one should consider its potential impact on olfaction rather than when using an alternative reconstructive option [11]. During open craniofacial resections, the pericranial flap is easily delivered through inferior aspect of the supraorbital bar or craniotomy (i.e., below the bone grafts). Multiple techniques have been described for delivering the pericranial flap through the frontal sinus into the anterior skull base when the tumor resection is performed via an endoscopic technique (i.e., trans-frontal pericranial flap). These variations include the "mailbox slot," "money box approach," or nasion window [9, 13, 14]. Although traditionally harvested through a coronal incision, harvesting the pericranial flap through an endoscopic assisted technique has been reported [12, 15, 16].

To harvest a pericranial flap through a coronal incision, the patient is placed in a supine position, and the head is positioned on a horseshoe or fixated with a three-pin Mayfield clamp. The hair is shaved or parted at the intended coronal incision site. If parted, the hair is displaced anterior and posterior to the incision with lubricating jelly, and it is fixed in position with staples. The head and face are then prepped with iodoform solution and draped in standard fashion.

An incision through the dermis, galea, and pericranium from temporal line to temporal line is carried with a 10 blade extending laterally over the superficial layer of the deep temporal fascia down to the level of the auricle. A scalpel, rather than electrocautery, is used for the incisions and dissection to reduce the risk of alopecia. We prefer to raise the flap in a subperiosteal plane and harvest the pericranial flap off the galea after the resection is completed. This helps to keep the pericranial flap from desiccating during the remainder of the operation and yields a thicker flap. However, we recognize that others prefer raising the scalp in a subgaleal plane leaving the pericranium over the cranium and then elevating it off the bone before the craniotomy [17]. To increase the pericranial flap length, the scalp posterior to a coronal incision carried through the galea may be elevated posteriorly in a subgaleal plane prior to incising the pericranium.

As the subperiosteal dissection is brought anteriorly, the supraorbital and supratrochlear neurovascular bundles are identified and are released from the respective notches. However, in the presence of a complete foramen, its inferior aspect is opened in an inverted V fashion using a 2–4 mm osteotome. This allows the inferior mobilization of the neurovascular bundles. After dural reconstruction has been performed, the pericranial flap is mobilized through the median frontal sinus respecting the drainage pathways of the frontal sinus (for endoscopic resection and reconstruction) or beneath the orbital or cranial bone grafts (for a subcranial resection). The pericranial flap reconstruction may also be reinforced with additional grafts such as a fascia lata graft or bolstered with packing inserted through the nasal cavity.

The pericranial flap is generally regarded as a robust regional flap with good outcomes. One study including 16 patients undergoing skull base reconstruction with a pericranial flap noted no flap failures [16]. Another study including 10 patients undergoing pericranial flap reconstruction noted no evidence of postoperative cerebrospinal fluid (CSF) leak and; furthermore, 8/10 patients underwent radiation therapy without subsequent flap complications [10]. A third study of 26 patients undergoing anterior skull base reconstruction noted partial or total flap necrosis in three patients and one case of minor CSF accumulation under the scalp [18]. Lastly, another report described a patient with delayed radionecrosis of the pericranial flap after proton therapy, corticosteroids, hyperbaric oxygen, and bevacizumab resulting in a CSF leak, meningitis, and frontal lobe herniation through the original skull base defect [19].

To minimize postoperative pericranial flap complications (trans-frontal technique), it has been suggested that the medial border of the flap should not extend past the midline. Furthermore, a Draf III sinusotomy is important to avoid mucocele formation [16].

19.3 Temporoparietal Fascia Flap

The temporoparietal fascia flap (TPFF), based on the superficial temporal artery and vein and delivered through a transpterygoid approach, is another regional flap option ideal for middle or posterior cranial fossa defects [20, 21]. An alternative corridor to the anterior skull base through a supraorbital epidural approach has also recently been reported [22]. A length of 15 cm is generally regarded as the minimum required length to reconstruct most defects; however, a longer flap length may be necessary to reach the defects of the craniocervical junction [21].

An ipsilateral endoscopic transpterygoid approach is often performed prior to harvesting a TPFF. An incision is made through the dermis with a 10 blade and ultimately extended laterally down to the auricle (Fig. 19.1a). A scalpel is utilized to perform this incision as well as the subsequent dissection in lieu of electrocautery to reduce the risk of alopecia. The galea (medially) or temporoparietal fascia (laterally) are identified with sharp dissection. The dissection then continues superficial to this plane, and deep to the hair follicles and subcutaneous fat, with sharp dissection (Fig. 19.1b). Sharp dissection is performed both in an anterior as well as a posterior direction so as to harvest adequate tissue for reconstruction. Anteriorly, one must consider the location of the frontal branch of the facial nerve; thus, the flap is usually elevated posterior to the hairline. After this has been completed, an incision is made medially through the galea and pericranium down to the frontal bone. We prefer harvesting and incorporating both the layers in order to increase the robustness of the flap. The flap is then raised off the bone with a periosteal elevator from a medial to lateral direction (Fig. 19.1c). As the dissection proceeds laterally, the superficial layer of the deep temporal fascia is identified, and raising the flap continues superficial to this layer. The superficial temporal artery and vein are identified and preserved, and dissection continues until the pedicle has been appropriately optimized for rotation through the infratemporal fossa. An incision is then made through the superficial layer of the deep temporal fascia, which is then dissected from the muscle following a plane posterior to the zygomatic arch and into the infratemporal fossa (Fig. 19.1d). Occasionally, a lateral canthotomy may be necessary to release the temporalis muscle from the lateral orbital wall to allow for optimal transfer of the flap into the nasal cavity. A guide wire is introduced into the sinonasal cavity and a percutaneous tracheostomy dilators utilized to distend the corridor through the infratemporal fossa (Fig. 19.1e). After this has been achieved, the flap is tied to the guide wire, which is pulled through the infratemporal fossa and into the sinonasal cavity as the flap is guided externally (Fig. 19.1f). The flap can then be accommodated to reconstruct the skull base defect (Fig. 19.1g).

There are few studies analyzing the outcomes of the TPFF for skull base reconstruction. One study including seven patients (presenting four chordomas and three nasopharyngeal cancers) noted no TPFF failures [16]. The TPFF is commonly used for a wide range of other reconstructive purposes as a pedicled or free flap including auricular, orbital, laryngeal, and cutaneous oncologic defect repair [23–25]. A retrospective study of 82 cases of TPFF in 71 patients for a range of reconstructive purposes reported no significant complications and a partial necrosis in only 2 of 82 flaps [26]. It is important to note that for skull base reconstruction, kinking or damage to the superficial artery or vein during rotation through the infratemporal fossa will lead to flap death. Additionally, a prior temporal artery biopsy or injury to the superficial artery or vein may compromise its vascular flow. Additional risks of the TPFF harvest include alopecia, given the plane of dissection near the hair follicles. Injury to the frontal branch of the facial nerve or the internal maxillary artery can also occur with this approach [16]. Use of an endoscopic harvest of a temporoparietal fascia flap has also been reported in an effort to improve donor site morbidity [27].

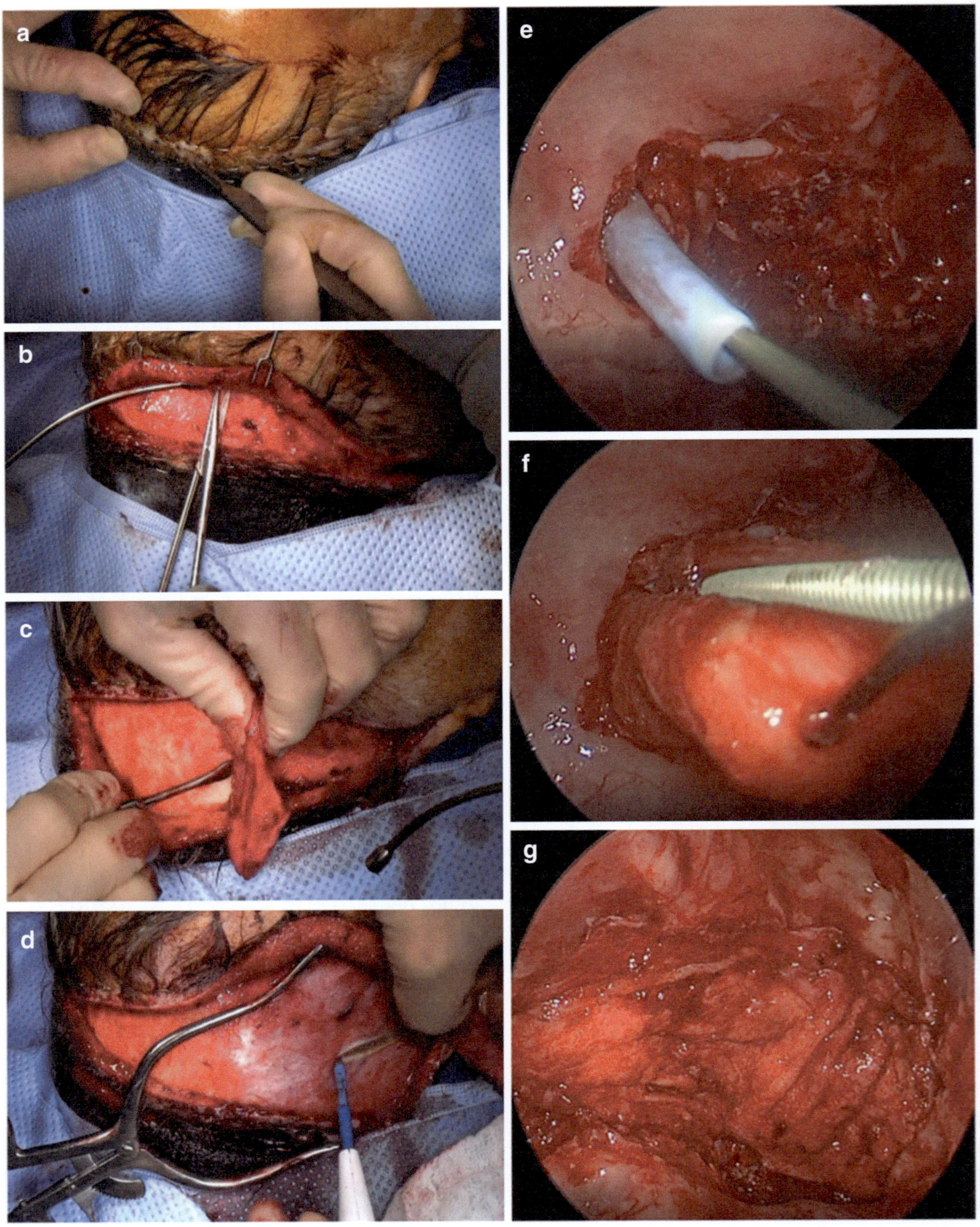

Fig. 19.1 (**a**) The hair is parted and reinforced with staples. Incision is made with a 10 blade. (**b**) The flap is raised in an anterior and posterior direction using sharp dissection. (**c**) After the pericranium is raised from the frontal bone, the flap is transitioned to superficial to the superficial layer of the deep temporal fascia. (**d**) Incision is made in the superficial layer of the deep temporal fascia to allow for transposition of the flap into the infratemporal fossa. (**e**) A percutaneous tracheal dilator is utilized to enlarge the corridor through the infratemporal fossa. (**f**) The TPFF is secured to a guide wire and introduced into the sinonasal cavity. (**g**) The TPFF is then optimally placed to reconstruct the defect

19.4 Occipital Flap

The occipital flap has been described for multiple head and neck reconstructive purposes including the pharynx, lateral temporal bone, and scalp [28–30]. This flap, based on the occipital artery and with an average pedicle length of 8 cm, may be advantageous in regard to not be compromised by previous skull base surgery or radiation due to its distant location from the skull base [31]. The occipital flap may be ideal for the reconstruction of clival or middle cranial fossa defects [16, 31].

A transverse incision is made along the mastoid process, and the vascular pedicle is exposed after transecting the sternocleidomastoid, splenius capiti, and longus capiti muscles [31]. One must be vigilant for a large tributary vein at the mastoid tip joining the transverse segment which if present must be carefully ligated so as not to injure the pedicle [16, 31]. The pedicle is traced and the galea-pericranium is incised. Some have suggested that in order to minimize the risk of damaging the pedicle, the dissection should proceed to a level that allows adequate rotation without kinking of the pedicle and that tracing the pedicle all the way to the external carotid artery is unnecessary and places the vein at risk [16, 31]. Once the flap is harvested, it may then be introduced into the sinonasal cavity through a transpharyngeal, transpterygoid, or prevertebral corridor [16, 31, 32]. In a large series of 330 skull base reconstructions, the occipital flap was used only once [16].

19.5 Oliver Palatal Flap

The palatal flap, based on the descending palatine artery, has been classically used for cleft palate reconstruction; however, the palatal flap can also be used for the reconstruction of defects of the planum, sella, and clivus [16, 33]. The Oliver flap is raised in a subperiosteal plane, and the greater palatine foramen is enlarged with a high-speed drill [33, 34]. A wide maxillary antrostomy is created and the posterior maxillary wall removed. The descending palatine artery is mobilized from the pterygopalatine canal and the palatal flap is then passed through the enlarged greater palatine foramen into the sinonasal cavity [33]. The flap is considered a last option in skull base reconstruction due to its complexity and the potential for oronasal fistula [16, 34]. However, one study reported the use of the flap in two patients with successful results [16].

19.6 Facial Buccinator Flap

The facial buccinator flap is based on a modification of the facial artery musculomyomucosal (FAMM) and buccinator flaps and can be used for reconstruction of defects of the anterior skull base [35]. First, the parotid duct is identified and not incorporated into the flap [36]. The anterior margin of the flap is approximately 1cm from the oral commissure and the posterior margin near the retromolar trigone [36]. The flap incorporates the mucosa, submucosal tissue, and a portion of the buccinator muscle [36]. To allow mobilization into the sinonasal cavity, the proximal facial artery is ligated, and blood supply for the flap is derived from reverse flow from the angular artery [16]. The flap may then be pivoted at the superior gingivobuccal sulcus and delivered into the sinonasal cavity through a maxillary window [35, 36]. Utilization of this flap has been reported for a patient with osteoradionecrosis and resultant anterior cranial fossa CSF leak [16, 36].

19.7 Pedicled Buccal Fat Pad Flap

The buccal fat pad flap, pedicled on the internal maxillary artery (IMA), may be harvested endoscopic endonasal after removing the posterior wall of the maxillary sinus. Alternatively, it may be harvested via a skin incision or a buccal mucosal incision (pedicle based on the TFA and FA). It can be used to reconstruct moderate size defects such as sellar and clival defects and the middle cranial fossa [37].

19.8 Salpingopharyngeus Flap (Dicle Flap)

The Dicle flap (named after Dicle University in Turkey) is a pedicled myomucosal flap supplied by branches of the ascending pharyngeal artery. The salpingopharyngeus muscle originates from the lateral lamina of the Eustachian tube (torus tubarius) and descends at the anterior margin of the fossa of Rosenmüller to form the salpingopharyngeal fold. Its inferior aspect inserts into the palatopharyngeal muscle and the superior edge of the thyroid cartilage. It can be used to reconstruct the defects of the inferior clivus and craniovertebral junction, and for the protection of the petrous and paraclival segments of internal carotid artery. Caveats of this flap include the need for secondary healing of the donor site, potential Eustachian tube dysfunction, and dysphagia [38].

19.9 Conclusions

The most commonly used vascularized tissue flap for reconstruction of skull base defects is the NSF. However, in the setting of malignancy or previous surgery, an alternative regional flap reconstruction may be necessary. While the pericranial and TPFF are the most commonly utilized extranasal regional flaps, additional options including the occipital, palatal, facial buccinator, pedicled buccal fat, and salpingopharyngeus flap have been utilized. The pericranial and facial buccinator flaps are classically described for anterior skull base defects while the TPFF, occipital, and salpingopharyngeus flaps are ideally situated for reconstruction of posterior or clival defects. The palatal flap may also be used for clival defects as well as for reconstruction of the sella turcica and planum. Many of these flaps are technically challenging, and the morbidity compared to alternative options should be weighed when selecting these techniques.

Conflict of Interest The authors have no relevant conflicts of interest to disclose.

References

1. de Lara D, Ditzel Filho LF, Prevedello DM, Carrau RL, Kasemsiri P, Otto BA, et al. Endonasal endoscopic approaches to the paramendian skull base. World Neurosurg. 2014;82(6):121–9. https://doi.org/10.1016/j.wneu.2014.07.036.
2. Clavenna MJ, Turner JH, Chandra RK. Pedicled flaps in endoscopic skull base reconstruction: review of current techniques. Curr Opin Otolaryngol Head Neck Surg. 2015;23(1):71–7. https://doi.org/10.1097/MOO.0000000000000115.
3. Hachem RA, Elkhatib A, Beer-Furlan A, Prevedello D, Carrau R. Reconstructive techniques in skull base surgery after resection of malignant lesions: a wide array of choices. Curr Opin Otolaryngol Head Neck Surg. 2016;24(2):91–7. https://doi.org/10.1097/MOO.0000000000000233.
4. Kang SY, Eskander A, Hachem RA, Ozer E, Teknos TN, Old MO, et al. Salvage skull base reconstruction in the endoscopic era: vastus lateralis free tissue transfer. Head Neck. 2018;40(4):E45–52. https://doi.org/10.1002/hed.25094.
5. Hadad G, Bassagasteguy L, Carrau RL, Mataza JC, Kassam A, Snyderman CH, et al. A novel reconstructive technique after endoscopic expanded endonasal approaches: vascular pedicle nasoseptal flap. Laryngoscope. 2006;116(10):1882–6.
6. Reuter G, Bouchain O, Demanez L, Scholtes F, Martin D. Skull base reconstruction with pedicled nasoseptal flap: technique, indications, and limitations. J Craniomaxillofac Surg. 2019;47(1):29–32. https://doi.org/10.1016/j.jcms.2018.11.012.
7. Shastri KS, Leonel LCPC, Patel V, Charles-Pereira M, Kenning TJ, Peris-Celda M, et al. Lengthening the nasoseptal flap pedicle with extended dissection into the pterygopalatine fossa. Laryngoscope. 2019;130:18–24. https://doi.org/10.1002/lary.27984.
8. London NR, Ishii M, Gallia G, Boahene KDO. Technique for reconstruction of large clival defects through an endoscopic-assisted tunneled retropharyngeal approach. Int Forum Allergy Rhinol. 2018;8(12):1454–8. https://doi.org/10.1002/alr.22187.
9. Kim GG, Hang AX, Mitchell C, Zanation AM. Pedicled extranasal flaps in skull base reconstruction. Adv Otorhinolaryngol. 2013;74:71–80. https://doi.org/10.1159/000342282.
10. Patel MR, Shah RN, Snyderman CH, Carrau RL, Germanwala AV, Kassam AB, et al. Pericranial flap for endoscopic anterior skull-base reconstruction: clinical outcomes and radioanatomic analysis of preoperative planning. Neurosurgery. 2010;66(3):506–12. https://doi.org/10.1227/01.NEU.0000365620.59677.FF.
11. Tang IP, Carrau RL, Otto BA, Prevedello DM, Kasemsiri P, Ditzel L, et al. Technical nuances of commonly used vascularised flaps for skull base reconstruction. J Laryngol Otol. 2015;129(8):752–61. https://doi.org/10.1017/S002221511500167X.

12. Klatt-Cromwell CN, Thorp BD, Del Signore AG, Ebert CS, Ewend MG, Zanation AM. Reconstruction of skull base defects. Otolaryngol Clin N Am. 2016;49:107–17.
13. Majer J, Herman P, Verillaud B. "Mailbox slot" pericranial flap for endoscopic skull base reconstruction. Laryngoscope. 2016;126(8):1736–8. https://doi.org/10.1002/lary.25686.
14. Santamaria A, Langdon C, López-Chacon M, Cordero A, Enseñat J, Carrau R, et al. Radio-anatomical analysis of the pericranial flap "money box approach" for ventral skull base reconstruction. Laryngoscope. 2017;127(11): 2482–9. https://doi.org/10.1002/lary.26574.
15. Zanation AM, Snyderman CH, Carrau RL, Kassam AB, Gardner PA, Prevedello DM. Minimally invasive endoscopic pericranial flap: a new method for endonasal skull base reconstruction. Laryngoscope. 2009;119(1):13–8. https://doi.org/10.1002/lary.20022.
16. Patel MR, Taylor RJ, Hackman TG, Germanwala AV, Sasaki-Adams D, Ewend MG, et al. Beyond the nasoseptal flap: outcomes and pearls with secondary flaps in endoscopic endonasal skull base reconstruction. Laryngoscope. 2014;124:846–52. https://doi.org/10.1002/lary.24319.
17. Chakravarthi S, Gonen L, Monroy-Sosa A, Khalili S, Kassam A. Endoscopic endonasal reconstructive methods to the anterior skull base. Semin Plast Surg. 2017;31:203–13. https://doi.org/10.1055/s--0037-1607274.
18. Yano T, Tanaka K, Kishimoto S, Lida H, Okazaki M. Reliability of and indications for pericranial flaps in anterior skull base reconstruction. J Craniofac Surg. 2011;22(2):482–5. https://doi.org/10.1097/SCS.0b013e318207b714.
19. Battaglia P, Turri-Zanoni M, Castelnuovo P, Prevedello DM, Carrau RL. Brian herniation after endoscopic transnasal resection of anterior skull base malignancies. Neurosurgery. 2015;11:457–62. https://doi.org/10.1227/NEU.0000000000000859.
20. Fortes FS, Carrau RL, Snyderman CH, Kassam A, Prevedello D, Vescan A, et al. Transpterygoid transposition of a temporoparietal fascia flap: a new method for skull base reconstruction after endoscopic expanded endonasal approaches. Laryngoscope. 2007;117(6):970–6.
21. Veyrat M, Verillaud B, Herman P, Bresson D. How I do it. The pedicled temporoparietal fascia flap for skull base reconstruction after endonasal endoscopic approaches. Acta Neurochir. 2016;158(12):2291–4.
22. Ferrari M, Vural A, Schreiber A, Mattavelli D, Gualtieri T, Taboni S, et al. Side-door temporoparietal fascia flap: a novel strategy for anterior skull base reconstruction. World Neurosurg. 2019;126:e360–70. https://doi.org/10.1016/j.wneu.2019.02.056.
23. Collar RM, Zopf D, Brown D, Fung K, Kim J. The versatility of the temporoparietal fascia flap in head and neck reconstruction. J Plast Reconstr Aesthet Surg. 2012;65(2):141–8. https://doi.org/10.1016/j.bjps.2011.05.003.
24. Mavropoulos JC, Bordeaux JS. The temporoparietal fascia flap: a versatile tool for the dermatologic surgeon. Dermatol Surg. 2014;40:113–9. https://doi.org/10.1097/dss.0000000000000114.
25. Baujat B, Struk S, Lesnik M, de Crouy CO, Barbut J, Lefevre M, et al. Fascia temporalis free flap for cricotracheal reconstruction: a novel approach. Ann Thorac Surg. 2017;104(3):1040–6. https://doi.org/10.1016/j.athoracsur.2017.02.078.
26. Mokal NJ, Ghalme AN, Kothari DS, Desai M. The use of the temporoparietal fascia flap in various clinical scenarios: a review of 71 cases. Indian J Plast Surg. 2013;46(3):493–501. https://doi.org/10.4103/0970-0358.121988.
27. Yano H, Fukui M, Yamada K, Nishimura G. Endoscopic harvest of free temporoparietal fascial flap to improve donor-site morbidity. Plast Reconstr Surg. 2001;107(4):1003–9.
28. de Magalhães RP, Brandão LG, Magalhães MG, Ferraz AR. Galeal pedicle flap of the occipital region for pharynx reconstruction: anatomic and clinical considerations. Plast Reconstr Surg. 1998;102(6): 2124–8.
29. Kwon H, Kim HJ, Yim YM, Jung SN. Reconstruction of scalp defect after Moyamoya disease surgery using an occipital pedicle V-Y advancement flap. J Craniofac Surg. 2008;19:1075–9.
30. Moore MG, Lin DT, Mikulec AA, McKenna MJ, Varvares MA. The occipital flap for reconstruction after lateral temporal bone resection. Arch Otolaryngol Head Neck Surg. 2008;134(6):587–91. https://doi.org/10.1001/archotol.134.6.587.
31. Rivera-Serrano CM, Snyderman CH, Carrau RL, Durmaz A, Gardner PA. Transpharyngeal and transpterygoid transposition of a pedicled occipital galeopericranial flap: a new flap for skull base reconstruction. Laryngoscope. 2011;121(5):914–22. https://doi.org/10.1002/lary.21376.
32. Durmaz A, Fernandez-Miranda J, Snyderman CH, Rivera-Serrano C, Tosun F. Prevertebral corridor: posterior pathway for reconstruction of the ventral skull base. J Craniofac Surg. 2011;22(3):848–53. https://doi.org/10.1097/SCS.0b013e31820f7d86.
33. Oliver CL, Hackman TG, Carrau RL, Snyderman CH, Kassam AB, Prevedello DM, et al. Palatal flap modifications allow pedicled reconstruction of the skull base. Laryngoscope. 2008;118(12):2102–6. https://doi.org/10.1097/MLG.0b013e318184e719.
34. Zanation AM, Thorp BD, Parmar P, Harvey RJ. Reconstructive options for endoscopic skull base surgery. Otolaryngol Clin N Am. 2011;44(5):1201–22. https://doi.org/10.1016/j.otc.2011.06.016.
35. Rivera-Serrano CM, Oliver CL, Sok J, Prevedello DM, Gardner P, Snyderman CH, et al. Pedicled facial buccinator (FAB) flap: a new flap for reconstruction of skull base defects. Laryngoscope.

2010;120(10):1922–30. https://doi.org/10.1002/lary.21049.

36. Farzal Z, Lemos-Rodriguez AM, Rawal RB, Overton LJ, Sreenath SB, Patel MR, et al. The reverse-flow facial artery buccinator flap for skull base reconstruction: key anatomical and technical considerations. J Neurol Surg B Skull Base. 2015;76(6):432–9. https://doi.org/10.1055/s-0035-1551669.

37. Markey J, Benet A, El-Sayed IH. The endonasal endoscopic harvest and anatomy of the buccal fat pad flap for closure of skull base defects. Laryngoscope. 2015;125(10):2247–52.

38. Gun R, Oyama K, Kapucu B, Wang L, Al Qahtani AA, Otto BA, et al. Salpingopharyngeus myomucosal flap. J Craniofac Surg. 2014;25(6):1967–70.

Free Tissue Transfer for Orbital and Skull Base Reconstruction

20

Nyall R. London Jr, Stephen Y. Kang, and Sidharth V. Puram

20.1 Introduction

Microvascular free tissue transfer allows for the recruitment of new donor tissue from an area distant to the defect. This versatile technique is particularly useful for large tissue defects, to bring non-irradiated tissue into the field, revision surgery, or when alternative reconstructive options have been exhausted [1, 2]. The goal of skull base reconstruction is to recreate the separation between the intracranial space, sinonasal cavity, and external environment, thus reducing leakage of cerebrospinal fluid (CSF), pneumocephalus, and risk of meningitis [3]. Good results have been reported in open skull base free flap reconstruction with a 94% flap success rate and CSF leak and meningitis rates from 5% to 11.8% and 2% to 5.9%, respectively [4, 5]. The most commonly utilized tissue donor sites for skull base repair include rectus abdominis, vastus lateralis, anterolateral thigh, radial forearm, latissimus dorsi, and osteocutaneous free flaps [2–7]. As with any free flap, risks include flap failure, wound breakdown, and donor site morbidity. In this chapter, we describe advances in endoscopic-assisted and open approaches for free tissue transfer reconstruction of the orbit and skull base.

N. R. London Jr
Department of Otolaryngology-Head and Neck Surgery, The Ohio State University, Columbus, OH, USA

Department of Otolaryngology-Head and Neck Surgery, Johns Hopkins School of Medicine, Baltimore, MD, USA
e-mail: nlondon2@jhmi.edu

S. Y. Kang
Department of Otolaryngology-Head and Neck Surgery, The Ohio State University, Columbus, OH, USA
e-mail: Stephen.Kang@osumc.edu

S. V. Puram (✉)
Department of Otolaryngology-Head and Neck Surgery, The Ohio State University, Columbus, OH, USA

Department of Otolaryngology-Head and Neck Surgery, Washington University School of Medicine, St. Louis, MO, USA

Department of Genetics, Washington University School of Medicine, St. Louis, MO, USA
e-mail: sidpuram@wustl.edu

20.2 Endoscopic-Assisted Skull Base Free Tissue Transfer Reconstruction

Advancements in endoscopic skull base surgery have led to the creation of large skull base defects of the anterior, middle, and posterior cranial fossa. Typically, these defects can be reconstructed with a pedicled local flap such as the nasoseptal flap or a regional flap such as a pericranial or temporoparietal fascia flap [8, 9]. However, these reconstructive options may not be available due

A. A. AlQahtani et al. (eds.), *CSF Rhinorrhea*, https://doi.org/10.1007/978-3-030-94781-1_20

to disease involvement or as a result of previous surgery. Furthermore, these reconstructive techniques may fail as a result of radiation-induced osteoradionecrosis of the skull base. Given the increasing movement from open to endoscopic approaches for treating malignancies and diseases of the sinonasal cavity and skull base, there is a need for refinement of endoscopic-assisted free flap techniques.

Endoscopic-assisted skull base free flap reconstruction is challenging. These patients are often high-risk and self-selected, having undergone multiple prior failed locoregional resections [7]. Frequently, these patients may have a history of proton beam, radiation therapy, or infected operative fields [7]. Recipient vessels for microvascular anastomosis are often far from the defect site. Furthermore, these techniques have only been recently described, and published reports are typically single cases with the largest case series including four patients [7].

The corridor utilized for delivery of the free flap pedicle from the sinonasal cavity to the recipient vessel depends on the location of the defect at the anterior or posterior skull base. For anterior skull base defects, variations of an anterior maxillotomy (Caldwell-Luc) and medial maxillectomy have been reported to allow for pedicle anastomosis in the neck [7, 10, 11]. Use of an anterior maxillotomy for pedicle delivery has also been reported for the reconstruction of a posterior clival defect [12]. However, a transcervical approach for free flap reconstruction of the clivus and craniocervical junction with pedicle delivery through a prevertebral/retropharyngeal plane may provide a more direct route for pedicle anastomosis [2, 13]. A prevertebral/retropharyngeal route for free flap delivery may, on the other hand, compromise the airway or swallowing function [2].

Our technique for free flap reconstruction of an anterior skull base defect first begins with meticulous debridement of the sinonasal cavity and anterior skull base (Fig. 20.1a, b). After the defect has been prepared, we then prepare the corridor for the free flap pedicle. This first begins with an endoscopic medial maxillectomy and removal of adjacent sinonasal mucosa to allow for flap adherence (Fig. 20.1c) [7]. An incision is then made in the gingivobuccal sulcus, and the anterior maxillary wall and infraorbital nerve are identified. A wide anterior maxillotomy is then performed, and the infraorbital nerve is preserved. We have noted that it is important to have a wide anterior maxillotomy and medial maxillectomy to allow an unhindered passage of the pedicle to prevent constriction [7]. A transcervical incision is then made, and the marginal mandibular nerve preserved. A vastus lateralis flap is then raised. We do not utilize a skin paddle to allow for the mucosalization of the flap within the sinonasal cavity. The thinned vastus lateralis flap is passed into the sinonasal cavity, and the pedicle is tunneled and passed below the marginal mandibular nerve (Fig. 20.1d, e). Microvascular anastomosis is performed in standard fashion to recipient vessels within the neck (Fig. 20.1f). When situating the flap for skull base defect reconstruction, it is important to completely obliterate any dead space between the flap and the skull base [7]. The flap is then supported with non-absorbable packing and nasal trumpets to aid in flap adherence to the skull base and optimal healing (Fig. 20.1g). The nasal cavity is debrided on a routine basis in the outpatient setting ,and the flap typically mucosalizes in the first several months (Fig. 20.1h). With this approach, we have experienced a high success rate in endoscopic reconstruction, with only a single instance of delayed flap failure (Fig. 20.2).

20.3 Orbital Reconstruction

Orbital exenteration is a common indication for cranial base microvascular reconstruction [3]. Frequently, adjuvant radiation is indicated in these scenarios, and optimal volume reconstruction of the orbital cavity with free tissue transfer is commonly performed. Our institution prefers a closed orbital reconstructive approach with optimal volume reconstruction of the orbital defect as described by Chepeha et al. [14]. These authors defined closed orbital reconstruction as an approach that uses free tissue to restore the volume to the orbit and maintain the placement

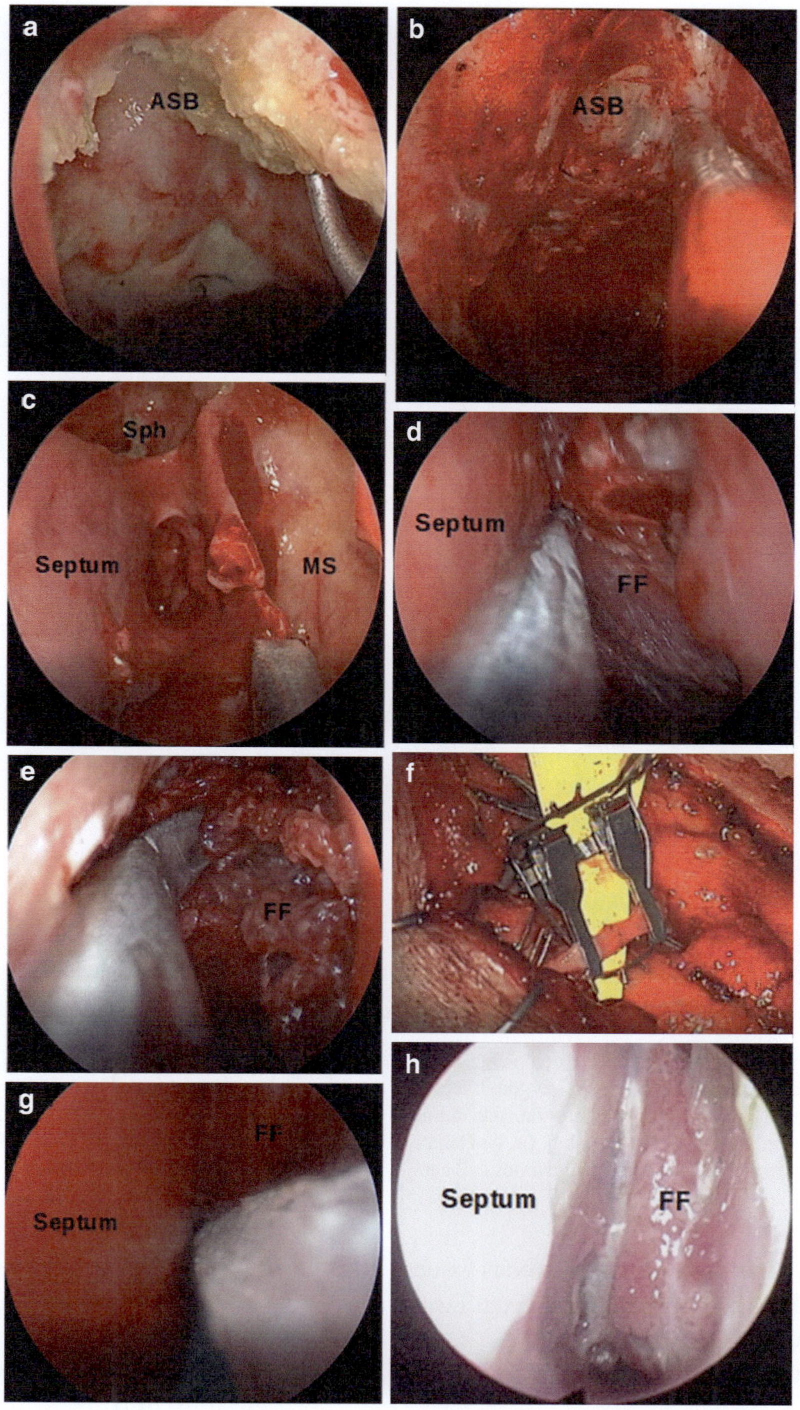

Fig. 20.1 Microvascular free tissue reconstruction of the anterior skull base. (**a**, **b**) The anterior skull base was debrided and osteoradionecrotic bone removed in preparation for free flap reconstruction. (**c**) A left endoscopic medial maxillectomy was performed. (**d**) The vastus lateralis flap was pulled through the left medial maxillectomy. (**e**) The free flap is positioned against the anterior skull base defect through the right nasal cavity. (**f**) Microvascular anastomosis is performed. (**g**) The free flap is supported with non-absorbable packing (white) and nasal trumpets (green). (**h**) Outpatient endoscopic three months post-op demonstrates a mucosalized flap. *ASB* anterior skull base, *FF* free flap, *MS* maxillary sinus, *Sph* sphenoid sinus

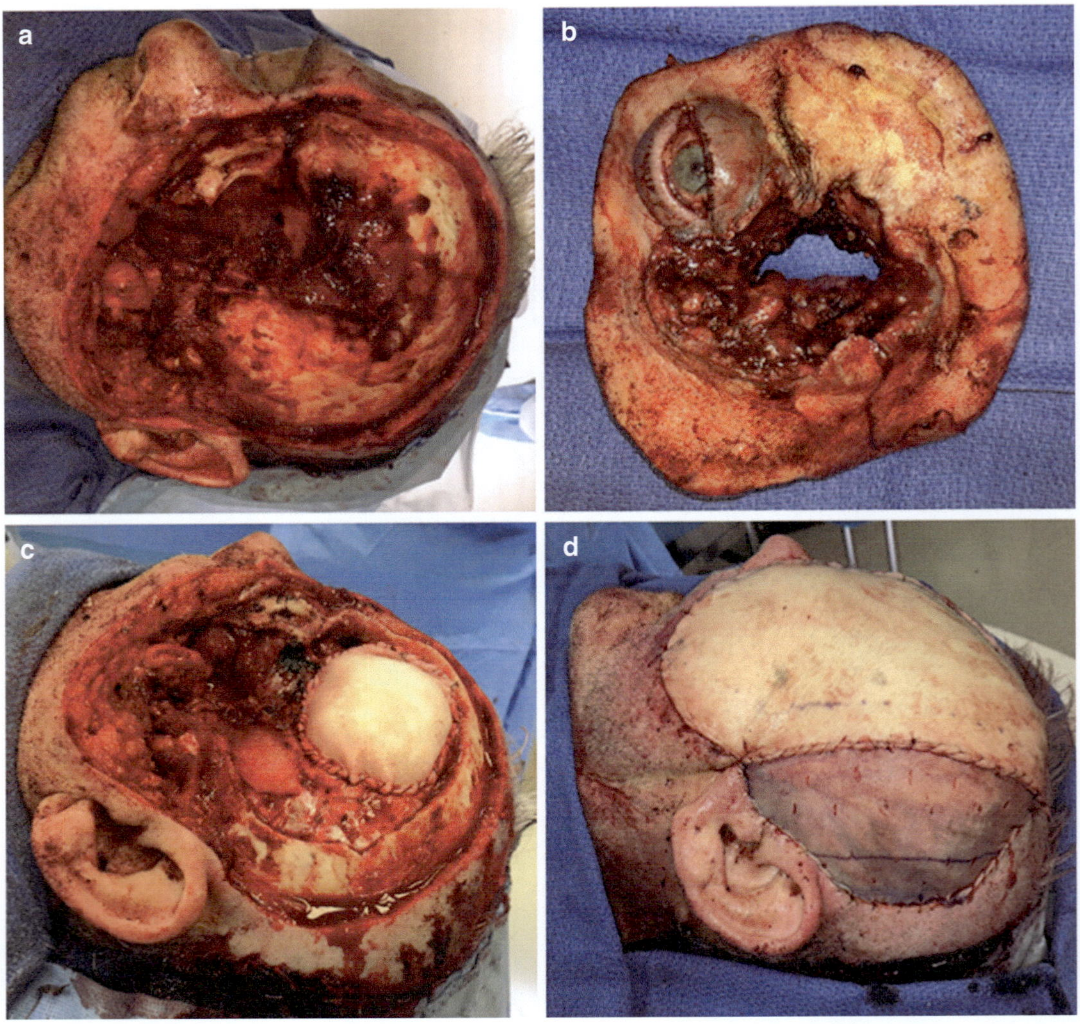

Fig. 20.2 Free tissue reconstruction of a composite, open skull base defect (fronto-temporal-orbital-zygomatic craniectomy, maxillectomy, orbital exenteration, and dural resection) using an anterolateral thigh flap. (**a**, **b**) Defect and soft tissue resection of an invasive squamous cell carcinoma extending through skull base to dura. (**c**) Defect after dural reconstruction. (**d**) Reconstruction with anterolateral thigh free flap with split thickness skin graft over the vastus muscle of the flap

and structure of the surrounding cutaneous tissue such as the brow and eyelids, if preserved [14]. Critical factors to consider when considering microvascular reconstruction include:

- Is the orbital rim intact?
- Is there an intracranial defect, i.e., dura exposed?
- Will the patient receive adjuvant radiation treatment?
- Is the orbital cavity a closed space?
- Will the pedicle reach the recipient vessels?

20.3.1 Reconstructive Approaches to Common Orbital Defects

20.3.1.1 Orbital Defect with Intact Orbital Rim

Our approach to this defect is to fill the volume of the orbital cavity with soft tissue. The keys to successful reconstruction of this defect are: (a) increased volume reconstruction of the defect in anticipation of flap atrophy after adjuvant radiation and (b) use of adipofascial soft tissue, without muscle, which avoids flap contracture. Since the orbit is a closed, contained space, avoidance of flap atrophy in this space is critical [15]. As such, one of the most commonly utilized donor sites is the radial forearm, which can be harvested with a beavertail of fat that can be rolled and tucked into the orbital defect with the distal portion of the radial forearm utilized as the skin paddle. Importantly, a radial forearm free flap also offers the advantage of a long pedicle, which is necessary to reach recipient vessels in the neck. Another excellent option is a perforator-based rectus abdominis flap, which can be harvested as an adipofascial flap without muscle, which avoids postoperative contracture within the orbit. The perforator-based rectus abdominis flap also provides a pedicle length that is often >13 cm [15]. The anterolateral thigh can also be used although it has a shorter pedicle than the rectus donor site.

20.3.1.2 Orbital Defect Without Orbital Rim

Orbital exenteration defects that include the partial or total resection of the orbital rim represents a common reconstructive challenge. The osteocutaneous forearm is an ideal donor site for this defect as it permits soft tissue reconstruction of the orbital defect and bone that can be customized to restore the structure of the orbital rim [14]. This technique is well described in the literature. When greater than 30–40% of the orbital rim is missing, this defect may require a different donor site that provides greater bone length [16]. In these cases, the scapula/parascapular donor site can provide adequate bone length that can be cut as well as a soft tissue adipofascial skin paddle that can reconstruct the volume of the orbital cavity [16].

20.3.1.3 Total Maxillectomy Defect with Orbital Exenteration

These defects present the challenge of a large volume defect with the need to provide bone reconstruction of the orbital rim and malar eminence. These can be approached with two general approaches: (a) two microvascular free flaps or (b) use of the subscapular system. With the first approach, the total maxillectomy defect can be reconstructed with the fibula donor site utilizing the osteotomy technique described by Fritz et al. [17]. Often, a second soft tissue free flap, such as the radial forearm with beavertail, rectus, or anterolateral thigh flap, will be utilized to separately reconstruct the volume of the orbital cavity once the orbital rim and malar eminence is reconstructed with bone. Alternatively, the subscapular system can be utilized, harvesting the lateral border of the scapula with parascapular/scapular skin paddles and also offers the additional advantage of including the latissimus dorsi paddle and avoiding the need for using two separate flaps. When using the scapula donor site for skull base reconstruction, we often prefer a scapular tip flap based on the angular artery to the scapular tip off of the thoracodorsal system [18]. Advantages of this technique include freedom and mobility between the latissimus skin paddle and the scapular tip, avoidance of two flaps, and a long pedicle that obviates the need for vein grafting [18].

20.4 Open Skull Base Free Flap Reconstruction

Reconstruction of open skull base defects using free tissue transfer represents a relatively recent advent in reconstructive surgery. Although a variety of pedicled-based flaps had been used in the past, including temporoparietal fascia or trapezius flaps [19, 20], these reconstructive options were limited by their ability to reach cranial defects as well as the intrinsically limited versatility of the donor tissue. The widespread adoption of free tissue reconstruction has enabled a dramatically altered approach to skull base defects.

On the most fundamental level, reconstruction of open skull base defects requires a multidisciplinary effort that combines the expertise of a skull base neurosurgeon with a head and neck microvascular free flap surgeon. In an ideal situation, these two individuals work together on both extirpative surgery and the reconstruction. In our institutional experience, before inset of free tissue, the native wound should first be reconstructed with similar material to what has been resected. Thus, if dura has been resected, we typically advocate for the application of collagen matrix or a similar allograft to reconstruct this layer [21]. In addition to providing an additional layer of protection against CSF leak, this approach also adds an additional barrier against infection and exposure to the surrounding environment [21]. Typically, a metal plate/mesh is then placed to further buttress this coverage and provide a layer of strength that recapitulates the resected bone. However, this additional coverage may not always be possible depending on the location and nature of the defect. With these layers in place, the microvascular team can then assess what free tissue may provide the best form of reconstruction.

20.4.1 Preparation of Recipient Vessels

In determining which free tissue may offer the best option, there are several major considerations including pedicle length, consideration related to the defect, and tissue characteristics of the donor tissue, which will be the focus of the remainder of this chapter. In all skull base reconstructive cases, we recommend routinely prepping and draping the leg and foot for possible saphenous vein grafts. Prior to any free tissue transfer harvest, it is imperative to evaluate what vessels may be present and to completely dissect out these supplying vessels. In many skull base reconstructive cases, patients have undergone prior treatment, often including radiation, which adds a further layer of complexity and challenge to identification of vessels with adequate caliber and flow [22]. The superficial temporal artery and vein are the most common sites to be initially explored and dissected—typically through a superficial, preauricular approach—due to their relative proximity to most open skull base defects. However, the caliber of these vessels is highly variable which makes their use and reliability unpredictable. In cases where these vessels are not tenable, saphenous vein grafts may be used to connect a flap utilized at the skull base to the facial artery and vein at the level of the mandible or even the distal angular branches of the facial. Additional recipient vessels in the neck can certainly be used, but risk of anastomotic failure rises with an increased length in the vein graft: A recent retrospective review of interposition vein grafts in 309 head and neck free flaps (among 6025 total flaps) revealed flap compromise and failure rates of 8.2% and 3.2%, with prior radiation and length of graft significantly influencing outcomes in multivariate analyses [23].

20.4.2 Pedicle Length

The required length and caliber of the recipient vessels will also necessarily be defined by the pedicle length and caliber of the flap itself. For example, a radial forearm free flap (RFFF) for an anterior cranial defect is likely to reach the ipsilateral facial artery and vein, owing to its 10–14 cm pedicle length. Similarly, the latissimus dorsi affords a relatively long 6–8 cm pedicle based on the thoracodorsal artery and vein, which can be afforded even greater length by tracing these into the subscapular system up to the axillary artery and vein. In contrast, an anterolateral thigh (ALT) flap or rectus abdominis flap is unlikely to provide a pedicle length longer than 5–6 cm; thus, requiring vein grafts if the superficial temporal vessels are not a viable option. Careful planning with regard to the recipient vessels is of utmost importance when selecting free tissue for skull base reconstruction.

20.4.3 Defect Considerations

Although pedicle length is critical when choosing a flap, the nature of the defect is often the overriding consideration. Skull base defects can range from simple skin and soft tissue deficits over a plate/mesh with underlying dura/reconstructed dura to composite defects after fronto-temporal-orbital-zygomatic craniotomy with soft tissue resection. In our experience, we rarely utilize osteocutaneous flaps for open skull base reconstruction as the residual cranial bone is often adequate to provide structural support, with the notable exception of orbital defects (see Sect. 20.3). Instead, we have found that the risk of CSF leak along with the size and depth of the defect remains primary considerations. In cases where CSF leak is a concern due to resection of the dura, we strongly advocate overlying the defect with muscle [24]. Typically, an anterolateral thigh free flap can be harvested to provide for adequate muscle coverage from the vastus lateralis with an overlying fasciocutaneous paddle. If residual skin remains that allow adequate closure, then a muscle only vastus lateralis free flap may be utilized (see 'Sect. 20.2). The rectus and latissimus dorsi flaps serve as an alternative to the ALT when muscle is needed, but generally the bulk of these flaps precludes routine use in small to medium sized skull base defects. In contrast, if a defect merely requires coverage (e.g., over alloplastic plate or mesh), then the RFFF offers versatile fasciocutaneous tissue that may be contoured to most defects, while maintaining full coverage of hardware and a generous pedicle length [25]. In cases where patients may be receiving postoperative adjuvant radiation therapy, this vascularized tissue coverage is critical to preventing plate exposure and hardware extrusion.

20.4.4 Flap Donor Tissue Qualities

The final major consideration in free tissue reconstruction of open skull base defects relates to the intrinsic tissue qualities of the donor flap. As mentioned, osteocutaneous flaps are rarely used in this context because bone is not usually needed and because the soft tissue component of osteocutaneous flaps has limited size and mobility (with the exception of a scapula system-based flap). Thus, fasciocutaneous (e.g., RFFF) and myofasciocutaneous (e.g., ALT, rectus) flaps tend to be major workhorses for skull base defects. Because RFFF can provide thin, pliable fascia and skin that has adequate diameter, these tissue qualities favor its use in cranioplasties when covering hardware [25]. In contrast, an ALT can be harvested to 25 × 8 cm with primary closure in most individuals and offers an even larger skin paddle, if required, with the additional benefit of associated vastus lateralis muscle. The tissue quality of the ALT is highly variable in an individual based on their BMI and age [26, 27], with some patients having ALT flaps that mimic a RFFF while in others a significant component of subcutaneous fat is present and leads to significant thickness of the ALT. For large scalp defects that may about the skull base, the latissimus dorsi offers a broad swath of muscle with excellent coverage that will eventually thin over time after denervation. This flap can be covered with a skin graft to accelerate healing, acellular regenerative materials such as Integra, or left to granulate and heal by secondary intention. In contrast, for deep defects, the rectus abdominis flap has intrinsic qualities of tissue bulk owing to the thick dermis, substantial subcutaneous tissue, and associated rectus muscle. Cranial defects that extend to the supra-orbital region may benefit from a bulky flap such as the rectus, which can provide coverage as well as replenish the lost orbital volume. Clearly, the intrinsic tissue qualities of each reconstructive option are important considerations when choosing a flap.

It should be clear that choice of free tissue for open skull base reconstruction cannot be approached in an algorithmic fashion. We recommend thoughtful consideration of the above factors—pedicle length, defect size and quality, and donor flap tissue features—as the main drivers of this decision. We have found that careful discussion with other head and neck reconstructive surgeons is particularly helpful, given the complexities and nuances associated with these cases. Importantly, in the vast majority of cases, free flap elevation can proceed in parallel with the primary ablation once the defect is defined. However, it is imperative to confirm adequate vessels are available prior to harvesting the flap and the initiation of ischemia. One of the major challenges within this field remains the small and rare nature of these cases, which severely precludes meaningfully powered prospective and even retrospective review of outcomes. As centers of excellence increasingly develop and foster expertise in skull base surgery, it will be imperative to conduct multi-institutional studies to further add objectivity to this important area.

20.5 Conclusions

Free tissue transfer reconstruction of the skull base and orbit through endoscopic-assisted open approaches is particularly useful for large defects, to bring non-irradiated tissue into the field, revision surgery, or when alternative reconstructive options have been exhausted. In the setting of a maxillectomy, orbital exenteration, skin involvement, or large tissue defect, an open approach for reconstruction may be indicated, and these techniques were addressed here. When defects are localized to the skull base, endoscopic-assisted approaches may be useful to attain the benefits of free tissue transfer and avoid some of the morbidity of an open approach. Endoscopic-assisted approaches are continuing to be refined and with time, larger outcome studies with these techniques can be performed.

Conflict of Interest The authors have no relevant conflicts of interest to disclose.

References

1. Hachem RA, Elkhatib A, Beer-Furlan A, Prevedello D, Carrau R. Reconstructive techniques in skull base surgery after resection of malignant lesions: a wide array of choices. Curr Opin Otolaryngol Head Neck Surg. 2016;24(2):91–7. https://doi.org/10.1097/MOO.0000000000000233.
2. London NR, Ishii M, Gallia G, Boahene KDO. Technique for reconstruction of large clival defects through an endoscopic-assisted tunneled retropharyngeal approach. Int Forum Allergy Rhinol. 2018;8(12):1454–8. https://doi.org/10.1002/alr.22187.
3. Wang W, Vincent A, Sokoya M, Kohlert S, Kadakia S, Ducic Y. Free-flap reconstruction of skull base and orbital defects. Semin Plast Surg. 2019;33(1):72–7. https://doi.org/10.1055/s-0039-1677881.
4. Llorente JL, Lopez F, Camporro D, Fueyo A, Rial JC, de Leon RF, et al. Outcomes following microvascular free tissue transfer in reconstructing skull base defects. J Neurol Surg B Skull Base. 2013;74(5):324–30. https://doi.org/10.1055/s-0033-1353364.
5. Macía G, Picón M, Nunez J, Almeida F, Alvarez I, Acero J. The use of free flaps in skull base reconstruction. Int J Oral Maxillofac Surg. 2016;45(2):158–62. https://doi.org/10.1016/j.ijom.2015.09.001.
6. Rowe D, Emmett J. Reconstruction of the base of skull defect – lessons learned over 25 combined years. J Neurol B Skull Base. 2016;77(2):161–8. https://doi.org/10.1055/s-0036-1579779.
7. Kang SY, Eskander A, Hachem RA, Ozer E, Teknos TN, Old MO, et al. Salvage skull base reconstruction in the endoscopic era: vastus lateralis free tissue transfer. Head Neck. 2018;40(4):45–52. https://doi.org/10.1002/hed.25094.
8. Hadad G, Bassagasteguy L, Carrau RL, Mataza JC, Kassam A, Snyderman CH, et al. A novel reconstructive technique after endoscopic expanded endonasal approaches: vascular pedicle nasoseptal flap. Laryngoscope. 2006;116(10):1882–6.
9. Reuter G, Bouchain O, Demanez L, Scholtes F, Martin D. Skull base reconstruction with pedicled nasoseptal flap: technique, indications, and limitations. J Craniomaxillofac Surg. 2019;47(1):29–32. https://doi.org/10.1016/j.jcms.2018.11.012.
10. Kato H, Mizuta K, Yamada N, Ueda N, Ito Y. A new route for passing a free flap vascular pedicle using contralateral facial vessels as recipient vessels in skull base reconstruction. Plast Reconstr Surg. 2012;130(1):212–4. https://doi.org/10.1097/PRS.0b013e3182550121.
11. Patel MR, Taylor RJ, Hackman TG, Germanwala AV, Sasaki-Adams D, Ewend MG, et al. Beyond the nasoseptal flap: outcomes and pearls with secondary flaps in endoscopic endonasal skull base reconstruction. Laryngoscope. 2014;124:846–52. https://doi.org/10.1002/lary.24319.
12. Hackman TG. Endoscopic adipofascial radial forearm flap reconstruction of a clival defect. Plast Reconstr Surg Glob Open. 2016;4(11):21109.
13. Kakarala K, Richmon JD, Durand ML, Borges LF, Deschler DG. Reconstruction of a nasopharyngeal defect from cervical spine osteoradionecrosis. Skull Base. 2010;20(4):289–92. https://doi.org/10.1055/s-0030-1249244.
14. Chepeha DB, Wang SJ, Marentette LJ, Bradford CR, Boyd CM, Prince ME, Teknos TN. Restoration of the orbital aesthetic subunit in complex midface defects. Laryngoscope. 2004;114(10):1706–13. https://doi.org/10.1097/00005537-200410000-00006.
15. Kang SY, Spector ME, Chepeha DB. Perforator based rectus free tissue transfer for head and neck reconstruction: new reconstructive advantages from an old friend. Oral Oncol. 2017;74:163–70. https://doi.org/10.1016/j.oraloncology.2017.06.029.
16. Moyer JS, Chepeha DB, Prince ME, Teknos TN. Microvascular reconstruction of the orbital complex. Facial Plast Surg Clin North Am. 2009;17(2):225–37. https://doi.org/10.1016/j.fsc.2009.01.011.
17. Shipchandler TZ, Waters HH, Knott PD, Fritz MA. Orbitomaxillary reconstruction using the layered fibula osteocutaneous flap. Arch Facial Plast Surg. 2012;14(2):110–5. https://doi.org/10.1001/archfacial.2011.1329.
18. Chepeha DB, Khariwala SS, Chanowski EJ, Zumsteg JW, Malloy KM, Moyer JS, Prince ME, Sacco AG, Lee JS. Thoracodorsal artery scapular tip autogenous

transplant: vascularized bone with a long pedicle and flexible soft tissue. Arch Otolaryngol Head Neck Surg. 2010;137(10):958–64. https://doi.org/10.1001/archoto.2010.166.
19. Rosen HM. The extended trapezius musculocutaneous flap for cranio-orbital facial reconstruction. Plast Reconstr Surg. 1985;75(3):318–27.
20. Collar RM, Zopf D, Brown D, Fung K, Kim J. The versatility of the temporoparietal fascia flap in head and neck reconstruction. J Plast Reconstr Aesthet Surg. 2012;65(2):141–8. https://doi.org/10.1016/j.bjps.2011.05.003.
21. Roxbury CR, Saavedra T, Ramanathan M Jr, Lim M, Ishii M, Gallia GL, Reh DD. Layered sellar reconstruction with avascular free grafts: Acceptable alternative to the nasoseptal flap for repair of low-volume intraoperative cerebrospinal fluid leak. Am J Rhinol Allergy. 2016;30(5):367–71. https://doi.org/10.2500/ajra.2016.30.4356.
22. Krag C, De Rose G, Lyczakowski T, Freeman CR, Shapiro SH. Free flaps and irradiated recipient vessels: an experimental study in rabbits. Br J Plast Surg. 1982;35(3):328–36.
23. Di Taranto G, Chen SH, Elia R, Sitpahul N, Chan JCY, Losco L, Cigna E, Ribuffo D, Chen HC. Outcomes following head neck free flap reconstruction requiring interposition vein graft or vascular bridge flap. Head Neck. 2019;41(9):2914–20. https://doi.org/10.1002/hed.25767.
24. Djalilian HR, Gapany M, Levine SC. Reconstruction of complicated skull base defects utilizing free tissue transfer. Skull Base. 2002;12(4):209–13.
25. Herr MW, Lin DT. Microvascular free flaps in skull base reconstruction. Adv Otorhinolaryngol. 2013;74:81–91. https://doi.org/10.1159/000342283.
26. Akdeniz Doğan ZD, Çavuş Özkan M, Tuncer FB, Saçak B, Çelebiler Ö. A comparative clinical study of flap thickness: medial sural artery perforator flap versus anterolateral thigh flap. Ann Plast Surg. 2018;81(4):472–4. https://doi.org/10.1097/SAP.0000000000001488.
27. De Virgilio A, Iocca O, Di Maio P, Malvezzi L, Pellini R, Mercante G, Spriano G. Head and neck soft tissue reconstruction with anterolateral thigh flaps with various components: Development of an algorithm for flap selection in different clinical scenarios. Microsurgery. 2019;39(7):590–7. https://doi.org/10.1002/micr.30495.

21 Repair of Cerebrospinal Fluid Leaks of the Anterior Cranial Fossa

Alhanouf Alqabbani, Abdulaziz A. AlQahtani, and Paolo Castelnuovo

21.1 Surgical Approaches and Exposure

21.1.1 Frontal Sinus Wall Defect

The frontal sinus wall defect is one of the most difficult areas to repair endoscopically. The two main goals of frontal sinus wall defect repair are reliable repair of the skull base defect and maintain patency of the frontal sinus [1]. It was suggested by Woodworth et al. to divide frontal sinus CSF leaks into three types based on the anatomic site of the defect: (1) those immediately adjacent to the frontal recess, (2) those with direct involvement of the frontal recess, and (3) those located within the frontal sinus proper [1]. This anatomic classification can determine the surgical approach required which includes exclusive endoscopic, endoscopic-assist, and external approaches.

A. Alqabbani
Department of Otorhinolaryngology/Head and Neck Surgery, King Abdullah bin Abdulaziz University Hospital, Riyadh, Saudi Arabia

A. A. AlQahtani (✉)
Department of Otorhinolaryngology/Head and Neck Surgery, King Fahad Medical City, Riyadh, Saudi Arabia

P. Castelnuovo
Division of Otorhinolaryngology, Department of Biotechnology and Life Sciences, University of Insubria, Varese, Italy

Endoscopic access to the site of CSF leak in frontal sinus is improved with the usage of angled scope and properly designed instruments. To get access to the defect, all air cells of the frontal sinus outflow tract, such as agger nasi cells antero-laterally or suprabullar cells posteriorly, must be removed to increase the chance of long-term frontal sinus patency. Preserving the mucosa surrounding the outflow tract, but not surrounding the defect, will also increase long-term patency as stripping the mucosa will ultimately lead to scar tissue formation. Anterior ethmoidectomy and skull base skeletonization will provide adequate exposure to the posterior aspect of frontal recess. The extent of frontal sinosotomy is determined based on the location of the defect. It should be individualized for each case using escalating approach. A Draf 2A/2B frontal sinusotomy is usually used when the reconstruction involves areas anterior to the anterior ethmoidal artery and medial to an imaginary line along the lamina papyracia (Fig. 21.1). Endoscopic Modified Lothrop Procedure (Draf 3) is indicated when the defect is within a higher and lateral position in the frontal sinus proper. This wide exposure is needed to allow proper instrumentations, facilitates the flap/graft placement, and ensures a functioning frontal cavity [2]. Far lateral frontal sinus defect is mostly difficult to access endoscopically. Therefore, an osteoplastic flap or endoscopic-assist frontal trephination is required.

A. A. AlQahtani et al. (eds.), *CSF Rhinorrhea*, https://doi.org/10.1007/978-3-030-94781-1_21

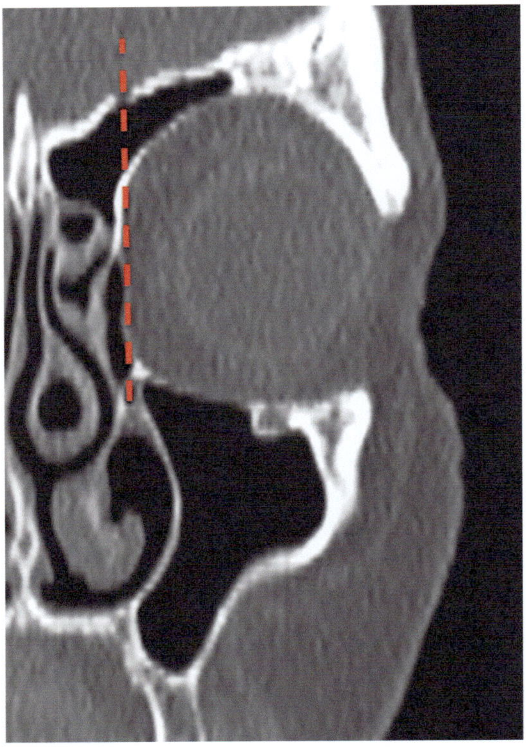

Fig. 21.1 Computed tomography, coronal view of frontal sinus with dotted red line that split frontal sinus proper into medial and lateral compartment

21.1.2 Ethmoid Roof and Olfactory Cleft Defect

Ethmoid roof defect can be approached with standard trans-ethmoid endoscopic approach. For adequate exposure, complete anterior and posterior ethmoidectomy is usually indicated [3].

Olfactory cleft CSF leak is one of the challenging sites to repair because of narrow working space and poor visualization. It is accessed through direct paraseptal approach. Tow techniques are usually used to access and reconstruct the olfactory cleft defect: (a) middle turbinate resection technique (Fig. 21.2) and (b) middle turbinate preserving technique (Fig. 21.3) [4, 5]. For both techniques, anterior and posterior ethmoidectomy with or without sphenoidotomy is usually needed. It allows adequate lateralization of middle turbinate if the surgeon decided to use the preserving technique. Middle turbinate resection is the technique of choice for the authors, especially when the defect extend lateral to the middle turbinate attachment or for narrow olfactory cleft. The middle turbinate is removed with the entire lamella of the ethmoturbinals to obtain

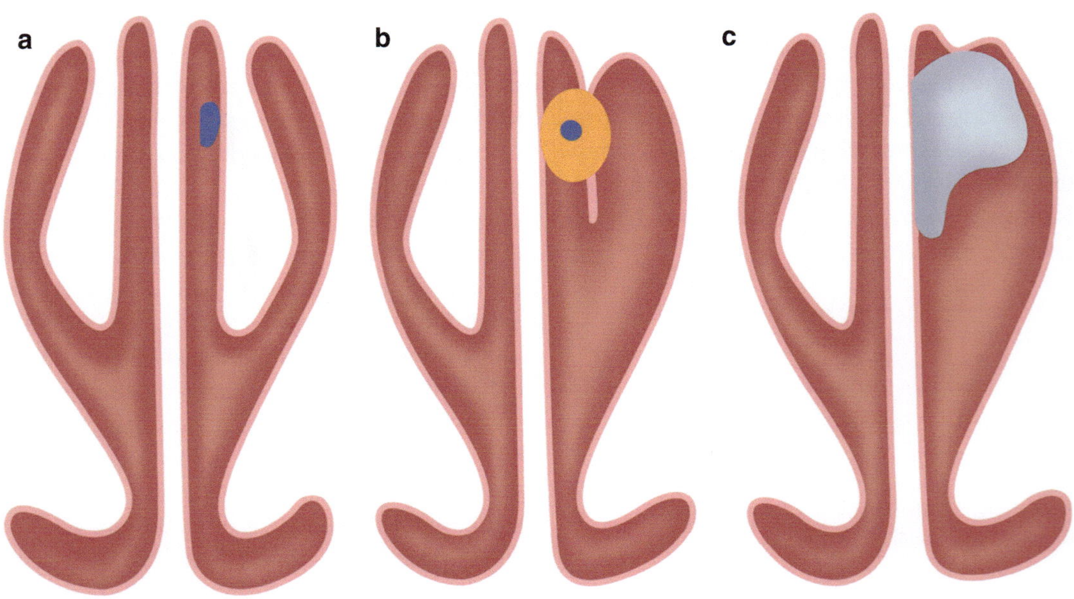

Fig. 21.2 Schematic drawing showing repair of olfactory cleft CSF leak. Small meningocele is shown in (**a**). Middle turbinate is resected up to the cribriform plate and the mucosa around the defect is stripped (**b**). The graft is applied over the defect and extended over the septum and ethmoid roof (**c**)

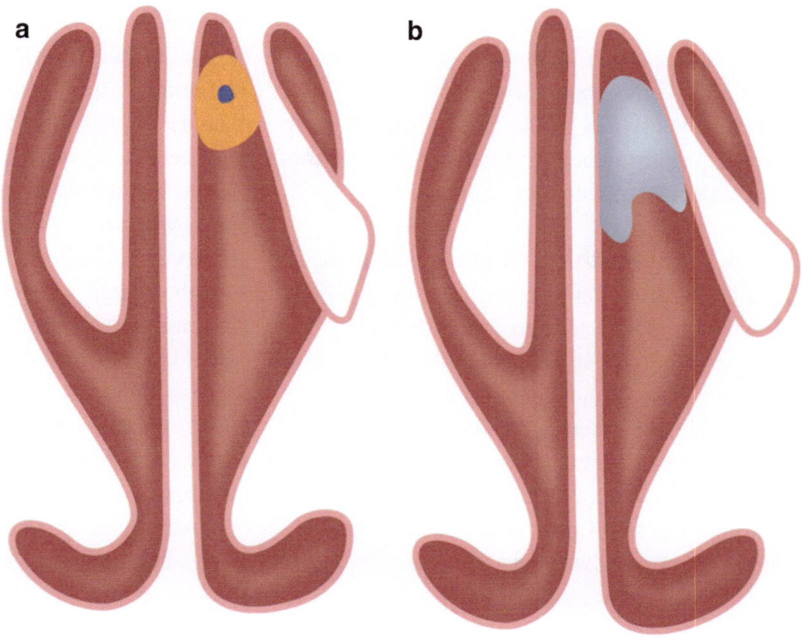

Fig. 21.3 Schematic drawing showing repair of olfactory cleft CSF leak with middle turbinate preservation. After ethmoidectomy, middle turbinate is lateralized for better exposure of the defect (**a**). The graft is applied in an inverted U-shape fashion (**b**)

a smooth surface for the proper implantation of the graft. Here, the muco-periosteal layer of middle turbinate can be used for grafting by furnishing it over the upper nasal septum, cribriform, and fovea ethmoidalis [4].

21.2 Reconstruction Technique

21.2.1 Preparation of the Defect Site

21.2.1.1 Resection of Meningocele/Meningoencephalocele

It is important to amputate the herniated meninges and encephalocele to reach the bony defect of skull base. It cannot be pushed back to the intra-cranium, as it has a risk to increase the intracranial pressure, induce CNS infection, and/or herniate again [6]. The prolapsed brain tissue is non-functioning brain parenchyma that is safe to be resected [7]. Radiological images including CTA and MRA are of paramount importance to investigate the presence of vascular structures looping within the herniated part. Medial Orbito-Frontal Artery (MOFA) is a branch of A2 segment of the anterior cerebral artery that runs around the gyrus rectus of the inferio-medial surface of frontal lobe and can be present within the encephalocele. Presence of vascular structure may necessitate an open craniotomy for proper hemostatic control. Meningocele/meningoencephalocele is usually resected by using bipolar electro-cautery and sharp dissection or by using tissue ablation devices. Powered instrument like microdebrider must not be used to evacuate the encephalocele. It is important to resect the herniated portion till the bony edges are delineated, and the meninges are retracted above the defect.

21.2.1.2 Demucosalization

The one most important step in reconstruction is to avoid mucosal entrapment between graft/flap and the defect. The surgeon should remove the mucosa surrounding the defect for at least 3–5 mm [8]. Mucosal entrapment between the graft/flap and the defect can affect the graft stability and healing. Also, it may lead to mucocele formation as a late complication [9]. Bleier et al. reported a 3.6% mucocele rate after CSF leak repair using the vascularized flap. Verilaud et al.

and Di Rocco et al. have reported an incidence of mucocele formation after skull base reconstruction in pediatric population at 50% and 14%, respectively [10, 11]. The higher incidence in younger age group is mostly related to the growing and developing sinuses with age.

21.2.1.3 Smoothing of Bony Margins

During the formation of encephalocele, the bony edges of the defect tend to evert over time. It is necessary to remove and smoothen the edges and any bony projections around the defect. This maneuver often worsened the CSF leak and increases the size of defect, but it is critical to obtain an eventual delineated ground for the graft/flap. Diamond burr drill is usually used to achieve this step. Care must be taken not to over widen the defect or create another one.

21.2.1.4 Dura Undermining

In large size defects and in case of a multi-layer reconstruction in ethmoidal and frontal sinus defects, the dura should be undermined carefully to create a subdural space. This step is important for applying the intracranial extradural layer. About 3–5 mm space all around the edges is considered enough. Angled elevator is usually used to execute this step. Area like cribriform plate cannot be undermined because of thin bone, adherent dura, and presence of olfactory filaments penetrating the plate. In other areas like fovea ethmoidalis, around the anterior ethmoid artery, undermining the dura necessitates electrocautery and incising the artery.

Finally, when local flap is used for reconstruction, involved sinus walls should be marsupialized, and any sharp bony edges along the way have to be removed. This will allow the flap to contour the walls of the cavity from the origin of the pedicle to the reconstruction site [8].

21.2.2 Single Layer vs. Multilayer Technique

The goal of defect repair is to create stable scaffold for rapid ingrowth of granulation and re-epithelialization by sinonasal mucosa [12]. Repair with single layer such as free mucosal graft can be successfully utilized in simple, small defect <10 mm [8]. It is typically applied for cribriform plate defect with a reported success rate of 94.9% [5]. Acellular dermal allograft, AlloDerm, has been used as a single-layer graft to repair large defects (2 cm) with little or no additional morbidity. A single piece of AlloDerm is positioned intracranially, with the margins of the graft material extending extracranially, to overlay the bony margins of the defect [12]. However, multilayer repair decreases the risk of recurrence of CSF leak, and potentially minimizes pneumocephalus with reported success rate of >90% [13, 14]. Multilayer repair includes combination of different planes of graft/flap placement, i.e., underlay/overlay and different combination of graft materials: autologous, non-autologous, and vascularized flap.

21.2.3 Underlay Vs. Overlay Technique

21.2.3.1 Underlay Technique

The graft is placed in the subdural and/or epidural spaces. Different options of graft materials can be used as an underlay layer. Bone or cartilage cannot be utilized as a first layer and should not be in direct contact with the brain. It is recommended to make the underlay graft one third larger in diameter than the defect proper as this works to compensate for shrinking of the graft during healing [15].

21.2.3.2 Overlay Technique

The graft/flap is placed extracranially over the bone. One should be vigilant not to leave sinonasal mucosa between the graft/flap and the bone [15]. It is recommended that the layer must cover leak margins by at least 5 mm [16].

Underlay and overlay techniques are frequently combined, especially when large dural defect exist. It can be done with two-grafts technique or three-grafts technique as described by Castelnuovo et al. [4]. In two-grafts technique, one graft is inserted under the skull base defect between the bone and the dura and the other placed as an overlay. In the three-graft technique, the first graft is inserted deep to the dura (intracranial and intradural), the second one inserted between bone and dura (intracranial and extradural), and the third placed as an overlay (extracranial).

Other techniques for leak repair include suturing the dura mater under endoscopic visualization as described by Cukurova et al. [3]. Tension-free closure is required for this technique, and it is limited to large bony defects with small dural defects.

21.3 Use of Supporting Materials

Supporting materials is commonly used to increase stability of the graft/flap. There are no standardized recommendations about the material option or the duration. Options may vary, and it includes absorbable, non-absorbable inflatable packs or balloon of a Foley's catheter. In case of Foley's catheter, the balloon has to be inflated under endoscopic visualization (usually about 20 ml required). Over inflation should be avoided as this can cause displacement of the reconstruction and/or compression of the vascular pedicle. The balloon may be deflated after a few days and subsequently removed at about 1 week post surgery [8]. Rigid silicon sheet is another option that can be used as an inverted "U" and held in place by nasal packing [16].

Tissue sealants such as fibrin matrix and synthetic compounds are available and can be applied around the graft to secure it [17]. Use of sealants is thought to increase the adhesion of the graft and prevent the need for nasal packing [18]. However, there is an argument that it is not required and merely contributes to unnecessary surgical costs. Eloy et al. reported no statistically significant difference in recurrence CSF leakage between two groups of patients with high-flow CSF leaks where in one group dural sealant was used and the other group was not [19]. Finally, absorbable gelatin sponge or oxidized regenerated cellulose is frequently used to separate the graft from the packing material. It helps to prevent avulsion of the graft or flap during pack removal [18].

21.4 Repair of Defects Following Skull Base Resection

Repair of defects following skull base resection is challenging not only because of the size of the defects but also because of the lack of supporting structures, the effects of gravity, and high-flow CSF leak [20]. When dealing with tumors encroaching the anterior skull base, the ethmoidal roof and cribriform plate are completely removed unilaterally or bilaterally, based on the extension and histology of the tumor [21]. Endoscopic endonasal transcribriform resection of anterior skull base tumors results in large skull base defects that often extend from the posterior wall of the frontal sinus to the tuberculum sellae in the sagittal plane, and from one medial orbital wall to the other in the coronal plane [22, 23]. Repair of such large defect necessitates multilayer reconstruction and vascularized flap, which have better result compared to other reconstructive options. Multilayer reconstructions with vascularized flaps have reduced postoperative CSF leak rates of between 5% and 10% [14]. Hundred percent success rate has been reported in some case series with multilayer reconstruction after endoscopic skull base resection [24]. Multilayer reconstruction with grafts is only another successful method as mentioned earlier (Fig. 21.4) [4].

In cases of unilateral ethmoid roof resection without removal of the crista galli, there is no horizontal bony edge medially to support and hold the graft. Therefore, the medial graft edge should run superiorly against the falx cerebri. If bilateral olfactory fossa resection with the removal of crista galli is indicated, then it allows the subdural graft to be supported on the contralateral ethmoid roof [8]. As mentioned earlier, the intradural graft should be 30% larger than the dural defect to secure all edges during manipulation of the subsequent layer and to overcome delayed graft shrinkage [25].

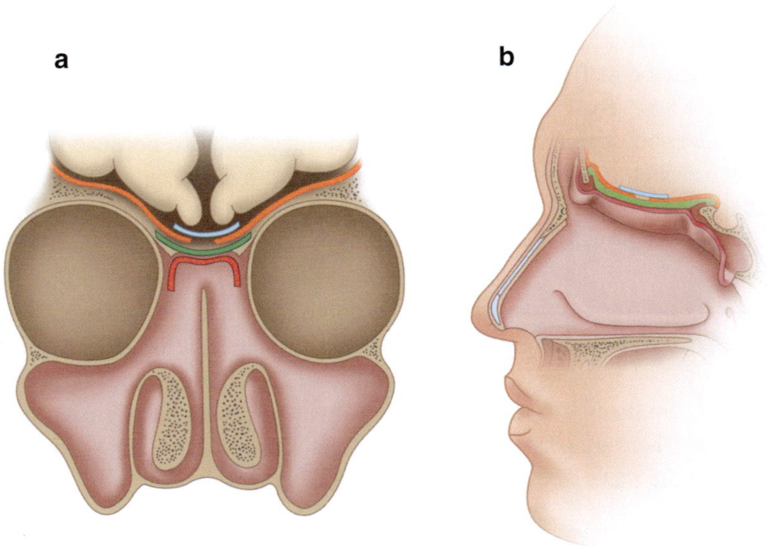

Fig. 21.4 Multilayer reconstruction after endoscopic skull base resection is shown in this schematic drawing. Two to three layers are applied to seal the leak as demonstrated in the coronal and sagittal view (**a**, **b**)

References

1. Woodworth B, Schlosser R, Palmer J. Endoscopic repair of frontal sinus cerebrospinal fluid leaks. J Laryngol Otol. 2005;119(9):709–13. https://doi.org/10.1258/0022215054797961.
2. Chin D, Snidvongs K, Kalish L, Sacks R, Harvey RJ. The outside-in approach to the modified endoscopic Lothrop procedure. Laryngoscope. 2012;122:1661–9.
3. Cukurova I, Cetinkaya EA, Aslan IB, Ozkul D. Endonasal endoscopic repair of ethmoid roof cerebrospinal fluid fistula by suturing the dura. Acta Neurochir. 2008;150(9):897–900.
4. Castelnuovo PG, Delú G, Locatelli D, et al. Endonasal endoscopic duraplasty: our experience. Skull Base. 2006;16(1):19–24. https://doi.org/10.1055/s--2005-922096.
5. Luk LJ, Ikeda A, Wise SK, DelGaudio JM. Middle turbinate friendly technique for cribriform cerebrospinal fluid leak repair. Otolaryngology. 2019;161(3):522–8. https://doi.org/10.1177/0194599819847944.
6. Nyquist GG, Anand VK, Mehra S, Kacker A, Schwartz TH. Endoscopic endonasal repair of anterior skull base non-traumatic cerebrospinal fluid leaks, meningoceles, and encephaloceles. J Neurosurg. 2010;113(5):961–6. https://doi.org/10.3171/2009.10.JNS08986.
7. Celin S. Contemporary diagnosis and management of anterior skull base encephalocele and cerebrospinal fluid leaks. In: Arriaga MA, Day JD, editors. Neurosurgical issues in otolaryngology: principles and practice of collaboration. Philadelphia: Lippincott Williams & Wilkins; 1999. p. 199–204.
8. Chin D, Harvey R. Endoscopic reconstruction of frontal, cribiform and ethmoid skull base defects. Adv Otorhinolaryngol. 2013;74:104–18.
9. Bleier BS, Wang EW, Vandergrift WA, Schlosser RJ. Mucocele rate after endoscopic skull base reconstruction using vascularized pedicled flaps. Am J Rhinol Allergy. 2011;25(3):186–7. https://doi.org/10.2500/ajra.2011.25.3587.
10. Verillaud B, Genty E, Leboulanger N, Zerah M, Garabédian EN, Roger G. Mucocele after transnasal endoscopic repair of traumatic anterior skull base fistula in children. Int J Pediatr Otorhinolaryngol. 2011;75(9):1137–42. https://doi.org/10.1016/j.ijporl.2011.06.005.
11. Di Rocco F, Couloigner V, Dastoli P, Sainte-Rose C, Zerah M, Roger G. Treatment of anterior skull base defects by a transnasal endoscopic approach in children. J Neurosurg Pediatr. 2010;6(5):459–63. https://doi.org/10.3171/2010.8.PEDS09325.
12. Germani RM, Vivero R, Herzallah IR, Casiano RR. Endoscopic reconstruction of large anterior skull base defects using acellular dermal allograft. Am J Rhinol. 2007;21(5):615–8.
13. DeConde AS, Suh JD, Ramakrishnan VR. Treatment of cerebrospinal fluid rhinorrhea. Curr Opin Otolaryngol Head Neck Surg. 2015;23(1):59–64. https://doi.org/10.1097/MOO.0000000000000124.
14. Harvey RJ, Parmar P, Sacks R, Zanation AM. Endoscopic skull base reconstruction of large dural defects: a systematic review of published evidence. Laryngo-

scope. 2012;122(2):452–9. https://doi.org/10.1002/lary.22475.
15. Lund VJ, Stammberger H, Nicolai P, et al. European position paper on endoscopic management of tumours of the nose, paranasal sinuses and skull base. Rhinol Suppl. 2010;22:1–143.
16. Castelnuovo P, Mauri S, Locatelli D, Emanuelli E, Delù G, Giulio GD. Endoscopic repair of cerebrospinal fluid rhinorrhea: learning from our failures. Am J Rhinol. 2001;15(5):333–42.
17. Mathias T, Levy J, Fatakia A, McCoul ED. Contemporary approach to the diagnosis and management of cerebrospinal fluid rhinorrhea. Ochsner J. 2016;16(2):136–42.
18. Hegazy HM, Carrau RL, Snyderman CH, Kassam A, Zweig J. Transnasal endoscopic repair of cerebrospinal fluid rhinorrhea: a meta-analysis. Laryngoscope. 2000;110:1166–72.
19. Eloy JA, Choudhry OJ, Friedel ME, Kuperan AB, Liu JK. Endoscopic nasoseptal flap repair of skull base defects: is addition of a dural sealant necessary? Otolaryngology. 2012;147(1):161–6. https://doi.org/10.1177/0194599812437530.
20. Snyderman CH, Kassam AB, Carrau R, Mintz A. Endoscopic reconstruction of cranial base defects following endonasal skull base surgery. Skull Base. 2007;17(1):73–8. https://doi.org/10.1055/s--2006-959337.
21. Castelnuovo P, Turri-Zanoni M, Battaglia P, Antognoni P, Bossi P, Locatelli D. Sinonasal malignancies of anterior skull base: histology-driven treatment strategies. Otolaryngol Clin N Am. 2016;49(1):183–200.
22. Casiano RR, Numa WA, Falquez AM. Endoscopic resection of esthesioneuroblastoma. Am J Rhinol. 2001;15:271–9.
23. Liu JK, Christiano LD, Patel SK, Tubbs RS, Eloy JA. Surgical nuances for removal of olfactory groove meningiomas using the endoscopic endonasal transcribriform approach. Neurosurg Focus. 2011;30:E3.
24. Eloy JA, Patel SK, Shukla PA, Smith ML, Choudhry OJ, Liu JK. Triple-layer reconstruction technique for large cribriform defects after endoscopic endonasal resection of anterior skull base tumors. Int Forum Allergy Rhinol. 2013;3(3):204–11. https://doi.org/10.1002/alr.21089.
25. Turri-Zanoni M, Zocchi J, Lambertoni A, Giovannardi M, Karligkiotis A, Battaglia P, Locatelli D, Castelnuovo P. Endoscopic endonasal reconstruction of anterior skull base defects: what factors really affect the outcomes? World Neurosurg. 2018;116:436–43.

Repair of Cerebrospinal Fluid Leaks of the Middle Cranial Fossa

22

Joao Paulo Almeida, Vijay K. Anand,
and Theodore H. Schwartz

22.1 Introduction

The management of skull base pathology has been significantly impacted with the development of endoscopic skull base surgery [1–5]. When performed by experienced teams, this technique has been associated with improved tumor resection rates and an overall lower rate of complications if compared to classic transcranial approaches in selected cases [6–14]. Endoscopic endonasal approaches (EEA), however, also have their limitations, such as difficult maneuverability in certain areas, 2D visualization, and difficulties in skull base reconstruction. Further understanding of skull base anatomy and the development of new surgical techniques, instruments, and high-definition/3D endoscopes have contributed to overcome some of those challenges. However, cerebrospinal fluid (CSF) leakage still is reported after EEA [15–19].

In the early phase of EEA, CSF leaks were considered one of the most important limitations of extended approaches. At that time, reconstruction after extended approaches relied on non-vascularized flaps (mucosal grafts, fat grafts, fascia lata, dura substitutes), and high CSF leak rates (20–50%) were not uncommon [16–20]. The rise of the vascularized nasoseptal flap (Hadad-Bassagasteguy) significantly changed the outcomes associated with skull base reconstruction and is considered a landmark in the modern age of EEA (after 2006) [21]. In the last 10 years, additional techniques have been reported, such as the gasket seal [22–24] and button [25, 26] techniques, as well as the use of fluorescein for identification of CSF leaks [17, 27–30] and protocols for the use of lumbar drains for management of CSF leaks in endoscopic cases [15, 18, 31]. Those have further improved the rates of postoperative CSF leak and, therefore, outcomes of endoscopic surgery.

Management of CSF leaks may be performed with the use of different techniques and materials [32, 33]. Adequate selection should take into consideration the location and severity of the leak as well as patient characteristics (body

Supplementary Information The online version contains supplementary material available at [https://doi.org/10.1007/978-3-030-94781-1_22].

J. P. Almeida
Department of Neurosurgery, Mayo Clinic Florida, Jacksonville, FL, USA
e-mail: almeida.joao@mayo.edu

V. K. Anand
Department of Otolaryngology, Weill Cornell Medical College, New York Presbyterian Hospital, New York, NY, USA

T. H. Schwartz (✉)
Department of Neurological Surgery, Weill Cornell Medical College, New York Presbyterian Hospital, New York, NY, USA
e-mail: schwarh@med.cornell.edu

A. A. AlQahtani et al. (eds.), *CSF Rhinorrhea*, https://doi.org/10.1007/978-3-030-94781-1_22

mass index—BMI, sleep apnea, previous surgeries) [16]. As a general rule, treatment selection aims to minimize morbidity while achieving maximum efficacy in the reconstruction of the skull base. In the current chapter, we discuss different techniques for management of CSF leaks after EEA in the sella, suprasellar, and lateral sphenoid sinus regions. A management protocol is presented, and surgical videos are included to illustrate some of the techniques here described.

22.2 Repair of Skull Base After Trans-sellar Approach for Pituitary Adenomas

22.2.1 Surgical Exposure (Fig. 22.1)

The technique used in our center has been previously described and has undergone some minor modifications since those earlier papers [34, 35]. Our philosophy has been to adopt different approaches according to the extent of the tumor and chance of CSF leak [16]. If the tumor is a large macroadenoma with >2 cm of suprasellar extension, then a lumbar drain is placed, and 0.2 ml of 10% fluorescein (AK-Fluor, AKORN) is injected in 10 ml of CSF to help visualize CSF leaks. Likewise, for these large tumors with high chance of a large leak, a vascularized nasoseptal (NS) flap based on the posterior septal artery is raised. If a flap is likely to be used, then the mucosa of the sphenoid must be removed to prevent a mucocele. Direct contact of the flap to the sphenoid bone is necessary for optimal skull base reconstruction. If mucosa is left between the flap and the bone, there is a chance of suboptimal closure and postoperative leak, as well as a chance of development of postoperative sphenoidal mucoceles [36]. The flap, besides useful for skull base reconstruction, is also important as a substitute for the sphenoidal mucosa. It facilitates re-epithelization of the sphenoidal sinus and minimizes chances of crusting and infections [37].

If a flap is not being used, then maximal preservation of the mucosa is the goal. The nasociliary beat frequency and the properties of the mucus layer are important in the defense against upper airways infections [38, 39]. Therefore, disturbance of the integrity of the nasal mucosa may impair the physiology of the nasal cavity and lead to olfactory changes, delayed surgical heal-

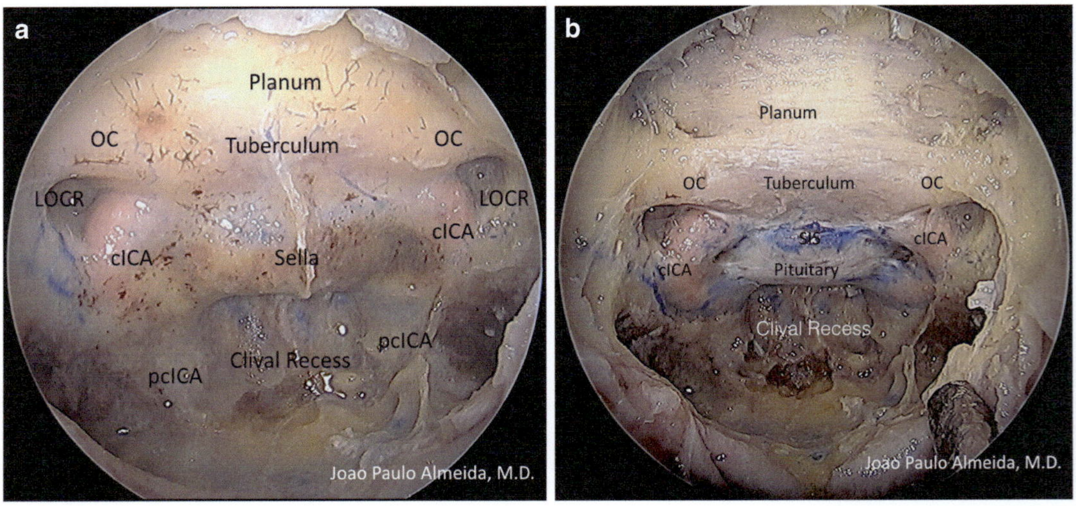

Fig. 22.1 Surgical exposure for sellar and suprasellar lesions. (**a**) Skull base exposure after a wide sphenoidotomy allows identification of the planum, tuberculum, sella, and clival recess in the midline; paramedian structures include the optic canals (OC), lateral optic carotid recesses (LOCR), clinoid segment of the internal carotid artery (cICA), and paraclival segment of the internal carotid artery (pICA). Copyrights: Joao Paulo Almeida, MD. (**b**) Dura exposure of the sella and suprasellar lesion after an extended transtuberculum transplanum approach. Copyrights: Joao Paulo Almeida, MD

ing, crusting, and sinusitis. Maximum preservation of the mucosa is recommended, and surgical techniques have been developed with the goal of minimizing mucosa disruption and/or substituting the resected mucosa with autografts.

22.2.2 Graded Reconstruction Based on the Severity of the Leak

Techniques for skull base reconstruction are selected according to the characteristics of the lesion, location, and severity of the leak [16, 40].

22.2.2.1 No Leak: Nothing Vs Surgicel Vs Gelfoam

This group of patients has a very low risk rate of postoperative CSF leak and therefore requires a less complex reconstruction. In theory, if no intraoperative leak were observed, there would be no need for reconstruction. However, intraoperative CSF leak is not always clearly identifiable, and CSF leaks may still develop after surgery, secondary to a new tear in the thinned diaphragm/suprasellar arachnoid layers. Our group has analyzed and demonstrated the benefits of intrathecal fluorescein for the identification of intraoperative CSF leaks and reconstruction of skull base defects. Fluorescein has been injected routinely in a large series of cases, via lumbar puncture or lumbar drain, for the identification of CSF leaks, with sensitivity and specificity of 92.9% and 100%, respectively [17]. This has contributed to our management of CSF leaks and to the development of our institutional protocol for skull base reconstruction. The most common techniques for closure in cases of pituitary adenomas with no CSF leak include the use of Surgicel, Gelfoam, and/or free mucosal grafts. The results of simple closure of the sellar defect with Surgicel have been reported in microscopic and endoscopic series. Seda et al. describe the effectiveness of a layer of hemostatic agents in the sella, in cases that did not have a CSF leak (no postoperative leak observed in those cases in that study) [41]. Recently, Varma et al. [42] reported the results of Surgicel for reconstruction in 150 patients who underwent EEA and had no intraoperative CSF. No additional material (Gelfoam, fascia lata, dura substitute, or sealant) was used. Two patients (1.3%) had a postoperative CSF in this cohort. The authors concluded that this technique is effective in patients undergoing endoscopic resection of sellar masses. Another material used in those cases is free mucosa grafts [32, 43, 44]. As reported by Kuan et al. in 2018, this technique has been safe and effective in most of those patients (postoperative leak rate: 0.9%) [44]. The current Weill Cornell protocol for skull base reconstruction [16] considers pathological characteristics, locations, and expected CSF leak flow for technique and material section. For sellar tumors (pituitary adenomas/Rathke's cleft cyst/intrasellar craniopharyngiomas) <2.5 cm in diameter or with <1 cm suprasellar extension, lumbar drain and vascularized flaps are generally not used. Cases with no CSF leak are closed with Gelfoam (Pfizer) for hemostasis. While we used to use a MEDPOR (Porex Corp.) buttress placed as an inlay, covered with DuraSeal (Covidien) or Adherus (Surgical one), we no longer feel that a buttress is required in this situation. The sealant is used in cases where there is a small, unappreciated CSF leak that may lead to a postoperative leak. Following this protocol, no postoperative CSF leaks have been observed in a cohort of 126 patients [16]. Other groups have used a similar technique, with good results. The protocol reported by Conger et al [45] favored the use of collagen sponge over the gland and arachnoid followed by repositioning of the sphenoid mucosa and then a final layer of collagen sponge over the sella, for skull base reconstruction in cases of sellar tumors with no intraoperative CSF leak. Fat graft was recommended in cases with large sellar dead space, and a rigid buttress (MEDPOR or vomer) was used in selected cases, such as those with BMI > 30 kg/m^2. No postoperative leak was observed in those patients in this study. Ruggeri et al. in 2019 reported the use of collagen matrix and fibrin glue for those cases with no postoperative CSF leak reported in this subgroup [46].

22.2.2.2 Small Weeping Leak: Gelfoam Vs Fat Graft with or Without Buttress with or Without Nasoseptal Flap

In our experience, cases with low-flow leaks (i.e., small "weeping" leak, confirmed by Valsalva maneuver, without obvious or with only small diaphragmatic defect) [40] are closed with Gelfoam, Alloderm, or a fat graft and a MEDPOR buttress followed by sealant covering the reconstruction. Patients are kept in bed for 24 h with the head of the bed at 30°. No postoperative CSF leaks have been observed with the use of this technique [16]. Lumbar drains and/or vascularized flaps are not used for those cases, and this has not affected the outcomes in our institution. A nasoseptal flap can be used in these cases, but it is probably not necessary. It is our preference to avoid the use of vascularized NS flaps in those cases to minimize nasal morbidity (olfactory dysfunction, crusting, delayed healing). A similar management strategy has been applied by other groups [45], with a similar rate of success. The systematic review published by Soudry et al. [32] reported an overall 93% success reconstruction rate for sellar tumors. Studies that performed reconstruction based on free graft/biomaterials had a successful reconstruction in 87–100% of cases, while those who used a vascularized NS flap had success rates of 94–100%. A systematic review published by our group demonstrated similar results, with an overall postoperative CSF leak of 5.6% in patients who underwent EEA for pituitary adenomas [16].

22.2.2.3 Large Arachnoid Tear: Fat Graft or Duraform with or Without Floor Reconstruction with or Without Nasoseptal Flap

Patients with large macroadenomas (>2.5 cm; >1 cm suprasellar extension) may present with high-flow CSF leaks after tumor resection, secondary to opening of suprasellar cisterns. Differently from the other patient groups reported above, this group of patients is usually managed with use of a vascularized nasoseptal flap. Our current technique relies on a multi-layer reconstruction that includes a fat graft or Alloderm covered with a nasoseptal flap, and then a sealant to keep the flap in place [16, 23]. While we used to use a MEDPORE buttress, we have moved away from the use of MEDPORE since it can be extruded, and the flap is usually adequate to hold the fat or Alloderm in place. Additionally, a lumbar drain is placed at the beginning of surgery and kept for 24 h, draining at a rate of 5 mL/h. The drain is removed in the evening on the first postoperative day, and patients are mobilized on the second postoperative day. This provides 12 h for the small lumbar dural puncture hole to close prior to ambulation and allows early mobilization of the patients. In circumstances in which a high-flow leak is expected but none is observed, we place only Gelfoam or Alloderm in the sella rather than fat, and although the nasoseptal flap is still used because it was harvested at the beginning of the procedure, the lumbar drain is removed immediately after the operation. The vascularized nasoseptal flap may not be available in cases of reoperations. In those cases, a non-vascularized graft (fascia lata) may be used although results may be slightly inferior (87–100% of success vs 94–100% success) [32]. As previously reported [47], the use of a vascularized nasoseptal flap has been associated with a significantly lower rate of CSF leak (2.4% vs 0% for pituitary adenoma surgery). Although the impact of the combined use of rigid reconstruction, vascularized flap, and lumbar drain is not clear, our experience has demonstrated that this technique has been associated with excellent outcomes and no additional complications. In fact, the application of our reconstruction protocol at Weill Cornell has virtually eliminated postoperative CSF leaks after pituitary adenoma surgery [15, 16, 24, 27, 28, 47]. Other groups have reported different techniques [3, 25, 38, 40, 45, 48]. A multi-layer reconstruction with the use of vascularized flap but no rigid reconstruction has been commonly reported for the management of pituitary adenomas with high-flow leak. Paluzzi et al. [48] observed that the use of the flap has significantly reduced the CSF leak rate after pituitary adenoma resection (11.5% vs 2.9%). On the contrary, other groups have also reported good results with the use of a multi-layer technique that does not routinely include a vascularized flap [45]. A multi-layer reconstruction based on fat graft, rigid reconstruction, and collagen matrix has been associated with good postoperative CSF leak rates even if no vascularized flap was used routinely (CSF leak 1.4%) [45].

22.2.3 When to Consider Using a Lumbar Drain: Evidences for or Against

The use of lumbar drain (LD) has been a matter of debate in endoscopic skull base surgery [1, 15, 18, 31]. Although its use has been recommended by some centers, including the senior authors, it is not universally accepted as effective. The concept behind the use of lumbar drains is to facilitate healing of the dural reconstruction by lowering intracranial pressure and providing an alternative drainage route of CSF from the subarachnoid space [15, 16, 23, 47]. However, LDs are not free of complications and may be associated with post-puncture headaches, infections, tension pneumocephalus, and uncal herniation, which raises issues regarding the risk/benefit ratio, particularly in light of the questionable utility [15, 16, 23, 47]. In our experience, LDs are considered for all cases in which an intraoperative high-flow CSF leak is expected. Therefore, LDs are usually used for the resection of pituitary adenomas larger than 2.5 cm with >2 cm of suprasellar extension. The adoption of an LD arose from experience with patients who had small postoperative CSF leaks that stopped with lumbar drainage [23]. The hypothesis is that if the LD had been used immediately after surgery, the leak would not have occurred in the first place. This has been a safe technique in our center and has become a standard approach in our current protocol. In fact, the routine use of NS flaps has been associated with a more frequent use of LDs in our center (55.1% before routine NS flap vs 82.4% after NS flap introduction) [47]. The flap ensures complete coverage of the dural defect and allows for safer use of LD, minimizing chances of tension pneumocephalus. Evidence for use of LD is limited, and the benefit of routine use of lumbar drains after pituitary adenoma surgery is questioned in the literature. Systematic reviews have not demonstrated benefit of routine use of lumbar drains [1, 31]; however, most included studies were retrospective case series with heterogeneous inclusion criteria [31]. Recently, a randomized trial demonstrated a significant positive impact of LD in cases of intradural pathology (8.2% vs 21.2%, $p = 0.017$). However, no benefits were reported for pituitary adenomas with suprasellar extension [18]. The experience at Weill Cornell, however, demonstrates the safety and efficacy of LD in cases of pituitary adenomas with high-flow CSF leaks [16, 23, 24, 28, 34, 35, 47].

22.2.4 Intrathecal Fluorescein

Intrathecal fluorescein has been routinely applied in our EEA procedures. It is safe and allows identification of CSF leaks that could otherwise not be identified [17, 27–30, 49]. It is important to mention this is an off-label use of fluorescein; all patients are informed about the off-label use and potential complications prior to surgery. Our protocol consists of intravenous premedication with dexamethasone (10 mg) and diphenhydramine (50 mg), followed by intrathecal injection of 0.25 ml of 10% of intrathecal fluorescein (ITF) (AK-Fluor, Akorn). Fluorescein is diluted in 10 mL of withdraw CSF and administered over several minutes, either through a lumbar puncture (adenomas <2.5 cm and no suprasellar extensions) or lumbar drain (large adenomas with suprasellar extension) [27, 29]. The sensitivity and specificity of low-dose ITF for detecting intraoperative CSF leaks is 92.9% and 100%, respectively. The negative predictive value and positive predictive value are 88.8% and 100%, respectively [17]. Most observed side effects were nonspecific, transient, and likely not caused by fluorescein, including malaise (57.4%), headaches (51.9%), dizziness (31.5%), and nausea/vomiting (24.1%); there were no seizures. In a larger study of 203 pituitary patients, we did not find any evidence of side effects related to the ITF [17, 49].

22.3 Repair of Skull Base Defect After Transtuberculum Transplanum Approach

22.3.1 Surgical Exposure (Fig. 22.1, Video 22.1)

Most steps of this approach are similar to those described above for the trans-sellar approach. However, some significant differences should be noticed, including all cases will undergo insertion of LD at the start of the case, and ITF will be injected via the LD; and an NS flap will be raised in all cases, in order to improve the reconstruction at the end of the procedure.

To maximize exposure of the tuberculum and planum region, posterior ethmoidectomy is completed as well as a wide sphenoidotomy. That allows visualization of the sella, tuberculum, planum, medial and lateral optico-carotid recess (OCR), carotid parasellar carotid, and optic canal [5, 15, 20]. Infrachiasmatic lesions will include tuberculum sella meningiomas and craniopharyngiomas. In those cases, bone removal is tailored to allow exposure of the suprasellar cisterns below the chiasm (i.e., tuberculum region). The tuberculum (or suprasellar notch) and medial OCR are routinely drilled out [5]. The sella bone is removed in selected cases of suprasellar meningiomas to maximize dura exposure and maneuverability. A transplanum extension is necessary in cases of meningiomas (or other suprasellar tumors) located anterior and/or superior to the optic chiasm. In those cases, bone removal, at the midline, can extend from planum to the sella, and from medial wall of orbit to medial wall of orbit [20]. Once again, the approach should be tailored to the size and extension of the tumor, to avoid excessively large openings and unnecessary herniation of the frontal lobe during the procedure. Intraoperative surgical neuronavigation can help to achieve this goal and is routinely used for EEA in our center.

22.3.2 Dealing with Mucosa and Bone Around Defect

The sphenoid sinus mucosa is extensively removed, since an NS flap is routinely used for reconstruction in those cases. The bone adjacent to the skull base defect should be free of mucosa, to facilitate attachment of the flap to the skull base. The NS flap, covering the posterior wall of the sphenoid sinus, will facilitate reepithelization of the sinus and minimize chances of sphenoidal crusting and infection.

22.3.3 Reconstruction Technique

As reported for sellar tumors/pituitary adenomas, multiple techniques are reported for skull base reconstruction after resection of suprasellar tumors. Different materials including fascia lata, fat graft, dura substitutes, and sealants are used. Techniques such as the gasket seal closure and button closure have also been routinely applied. Patient and tumor characteristics must be considered when planning the reconstruction. Unlike pituitary adenomas, all cases that require EEA to the suprasellar space may be considered associated with high-flow leaks and will benefit of multilayer reconstruction and vascularized reconstruction [5, 15, 16, 20].

22.3.3.1 Inlay, Onlay Multilayer Closure with NS Flap

A well-known technique for reconstruction is based on multilayer repair of the skull base defect, with vascularized and non-vascularized materials, to replace tissues transgressed during the approach [3, 4, 19, 50]. This reconstruction is based on an inlay layer of dural substitute (Duragen, Integra Life Sciences, Boston, MA), as to "replace" the arachnoid layer, covered with a vascularized mucosal flap. The flap is held in place with a layer of dural sealant and supported by fat autograft or Gelfoam. A Foley catheter balloon or Merocel is used, as a buttress for the reconstruction. The addition of the NS flap significantly improved the results of this multilayer technique. As reported by Koutourousiou et al. [51], before the introduction of the flap, CSF leak rate of suprasellar meningiomas was 69.2%; after the introduction of the flap, this rate went down to 16.1% and the same group reports a recent CSF leak rate of 11.7% in the last years. The importance of vascularized reconstruction is even more noticeable when results of craniopharyngioma surgery are assessed. CSF leak rate of 58–60% have been reported prior to the adoption of the NS flap; however, with the use of the vascularized flap, the overall CSF leak rate has been significantly lowered (21–23.4%) [50, 52]. An important difference between craniopharyngiomas and meningiomas is the occurrence of intraventricular extensions in the former. This increases the CSF leak flow over the skull base repair and is at least partially responsible for higher leak rates observed in such cases. Recently, cases of postoperative encephalocele have been reported after resection of anterior and posterior fossa tumors that did not undergo reconstruction with a rigid buttress [53, 54]. Although evidence still is limited and long-term follow-up is needed, this may represent a significant limitation of reconstructions such as this, without rigid bone repair.

22.3.3.2 Button Closure with NS Flap

The button technique was described by the Thomas Jefferson University group in 2010 [25, 26], in order to improve CSF leaks after resection of intradural tumors. This technique consists of a two-layer fascia lata "button" graft to seal the dural defect. The "button" is constructed of two pieces of fascia lata attached to one another by suture. One layer is inserted inside the defect as an inlay while the other layer lies over the dura. An NS flap is then placed against the skull base over the button graft. This technique has been associated with an overall low CSF leak rate (11.2%) after resection of craniopharyngiomas [55] and may be an interesting option in cases that will not accommodate a gasket seal closure. Our institution has begun employing the button closure with increasing frequency, particularly if there are no bony edges to use the gasket (see below) and has used two layers of Alloderm, rather than fascia lata, to avoid making an incision in the patient's thigh.

22.3.3.3 Gasket Seal Closure with NS Flap

The gasket seal technique was initially described by the senior authors of this chapter in 2008 [24]. It is a routine part of our protocol for the reconstruction of intradural cases associated with high-flow CSF leaks, such as suprasellar meningiomas and craniopharyngiomas. For those cases, a combination of techniques and materials are used, including perioperative lumbar drains, ITF, gasket seal, and NS flap. For the gasket seal to be effective, the defect in the skull base must be surrounded by a rim of bone. The diameters of this defect are measured either with a ruler or with a cottonoid. For many years, the soft tissue graft we used was derived from fascia lata grafts harvested from the thigh. We tend to use the left thigh so that harvesting does not disrupt the endonasal procedure. The fascia lata graft is fashioned in the same dimensions of the cranial base defect but with an additional 1 cm of diameter so as to extend beyond the edge of the cranial base defect. The fascia lata graft is placed over the defect as an overlap. A piece of MEDPOR is cut to be the same size as the defect and placed over the fascia lata graft and countersunk into the defect so that the edges of the buttress are wedged just beyond the bony edges of the defect, holding it in place. The center of the fascia lata graft is intracranial, whereas the edges remain in the sinus cavity, similar to a cauliflower leaf. The fascia lata, which is circumferentially wedged between the bony edge of the cranial defect and the graft, creates a watertight gasket seal. More recently, we have begun using Alloderm to avoid a thigh incision and have had good success. Care is necessary when inserting the rigid reconstruction to avoid neurovascular injuries, due to the proximity to the internal carotid artery and optic nerve. Previous reports have demonstrated the safety and efficacy of this strategy, with an overall postoperative CSF leak <10% [15, 16, 23, 24, 28, 47, 56]. The Weill Cornell experience with EEA for suprasellar meningiomas and craniopharyngiomas was recently described, demonstrating CSF leak rates of 8% and 3.7%, respectively [5, 15]. Regarding the suprasellar meningioma study, it is important to mention that leaks were only observed in two cases that did not have an LD inserted due to their high BMI and inability to access the thecal space. Therefore, no leak was observed in cases that completely followed the recommended protocol.

22.3.3.4 Use of Fat

In our experience, fat may be used in selected cases, to obliterate the intracranial cavity left after resection of large suprasellar meningiomas. It is not routinely used, however, if the third ventricle is widely open, such as in some cases of craniopharyngiomas, a fat graft is not used to avoid the graft falling into the floor of the third ventricle and causing obstructive hydrocephalus. In our center, the use of fat for reconstruction in the suprasellar space has decreased in the last years. In some cases, we have used Alloderm rather than fat to avoid an abdominal incision. Other groups, however, have reported successful strategies based on the use of fat. The Naples group recently published the results of a new reconstruction technique, named "Triple F" technique [57]. The first "F" stands for autologous fat, to be used as a cork stopper across the intra-extradural space and to eliminate dead space, the second "F" refers to the use of an NS flap, to cover the skull base defect, and the third "F" stands for "flash," or early patient mobilization out of bed. The authors reported their experience with 25 cases that underwent transtuberculum transplanum approaches for resection of multiple tumors, including craniopharyngiomas, meningiomas, and giant pituitary adenomas. CSF leak was noted in only one case (1/25, 4%), which was adequately treated with additional application of fibrin glue. Those results are similar to those obtained with the gasket seal closure and represent a significant achievement.

22.3.4 Evidence for and Against Use of LD

As described, LDs are routinely used at Weill Cornell for cases that will require extended approaches to the tuberculum and planum region. Although not universally accepted, this approach is an important component of our management protocol and has been associated with excellent results [5, 15, 16]. The main criticisms regarding the use of LDs include its questionable efficacy and its potential risks of complications (tension pneumocephalus, tonsil herniation, meningitis, headaches). Although some authors have advocated against the use of LD [31], recent studies demonstrated some evidence in favor of use of LD. Cohen et al. [15] demonstrated that LD may be useful to prevent postoperative CSF leak, particularly in patients with elevated BMI. In that study, only two leaks were observed, and those two patients had not received an LD due to impossibility of insertion of the drain. The best evidence to date is originated from the results of a trial recently published, which demonstrated an overall lower CSF leak rate in patients that received an LD for 72 h after surgery (8.2% vs 21.2% (odds ratio 3.0, 95% confidence interval 1.2–7.6, $p = 0.017$)) [18]. Post hoc analysis of location of the defect and its effect on CSF leak rates demonstrated a statistically significant positive impact of LD in anterior and posterior fossa cases. A positive effect was also observed in suprasellar tumors; however, no statistical significance was observed (LD group: 4.7% vs control group 9.5%, $p = 0.43$). Regarding complications secondary to LD, that study confirmed our previous findings and demonstrated the safety of LDs since only three complications (3.5%) were observed: two patients had spinal headaches that were managed with blood patches and one patient had a retained catheter that was observed without consequence.

22.3.5 Use of Fluorescein

All patients that undergo extended endoscopic surgery by the senior authors will receive ITF via a lumbar drain, according to the protocol previously described [16]. This has been a safe adjunct for identification and repair of CSF leaks, without significant associated morbidity. As leak will inevitably occur during resection of intradural tumors, ITF main role in those cases is to maximize the dura repair at the end of surgery. It improves the visualization of minimal CSF leak flow around a suboptimal reconstruction and then allows correction of the repair, in cases that otherwise could have presented with a postoperative CSF leak.

22.4 Endoscopic Repair of Sternberg's Canal and Other Defects of the Lateral Recess of the Sphenoid Sinus

22.4.1 Debate About Whether It Is Really a "Sternberg Canal" Leak

CSF leaks arising from the sphenoid sinus account for 10% of spontaneous and secondary fistulas. Most sphenoid sinus leaks occur spontaneously, and almost half of spontaneous leaks are believed to originate in the sphenoid. The relatively high rate of spontaneous CSF leaks in the sphenoid sinus might indicate a structural predisposition to dehiscence inherent to the sphenoid bone anatomy and/or development [58, 59].

In 1888, Maximilian Sternberg described the course of the canal as originating between the lesser sphenoid wing and sphenoid body posteriorly, running along the lateral wall of the sphenoid sinus, medial to foramen rotundum (FR), medial to the Vidian canal (VC), and ending at the vaginal process of the nasopharynx anteriorly. This delineates the fusion plane between alisphenoid, basisphenoid, and presphenoid. He noted that a persistent canal is almost ubiquitously present in the skulls of 3- to 4-year-old children and in approximately 4% of adult skulls [60]. There is, however, a fair amount of debate in the literature surrounding the potential contribution of Sternberg's canal to the occurrence of spontaneous CSF leaks. Many authors have pointed to Sternberg's canal as a potential site of sphenoid sinus encephaloceles, while others contend that this is not likely based on the location of sphenoid CSF leaks relative to the expected site of Sternberg's canal [58, 60, 61]. In 2009, Tomazic and Stammberger published a five-patient series and described Sternberg's canal as "located in the posterior part of the lateral sphenoid sinus wall inferior and lateral to the maxillary nerve" [62]. They argue that the canal is a source of spontaneous CSF leak when there is an extensive lateral pneumatization of the sphenoid sinus wall. Once this communicates with the patent canal, a leak may ensue. In contrast to this view, Baranano [61] and Illing et al. [63] contend that, by definition, Sternberg's canal must exist medial to the superior orbital fissure, and thus, medial to foramen rotundum (FR) and V2. They argue that Sternberg's canal is not likely to give rise to lateral sphenoid sinus CSF leaks since most occur lateral to V2. A recent study by the Weill Cornell group (unpublished data) supports the findings of Baranano and Illing. In our series, of 103 repaired CSF leaks, 17 arose from the lateral sphenoid. Only three of those cases could possibly be consistent with a Sternberg's canal leak, and even these cases were questionable, since the defects did not follow the course of the classic Sternberg's canal. The cases we report of "possible" Sternberg's canal defects were very similar clinically to the defects that occurred lateral to FR and which were certainly not related to Sternberg's canal. No significant differences between the two groups in terms of the degree of extensive pneumatization of the sphenoid sinus, BMI, average age at time of surgery, sex, presence of arachnoid pits, meningitis, evidence of increased ICP, encephalocele, and postoperative leak were observed. Moreover, most patients in this series were obese middle-aged women, a common feature of spontaneous CSF leaks. Our findings suggest that these characteristics predispose the middle fossa to spontaneous sphenoid leaks irrespective of their precise location and that the etiology of both Sternberg's canal and non-Sternberg's canal sphenoid defects does not differ in this regard. Therefore, the minority of leaks that arise medial to FR may be related to dehiscence of the sphenoid wall in the region of Sternberg's canal but definitive causative proof is lacking.

22.4.2 Surgical Exposure: Transpterygoid Approach (Fig. 22.2, Video 22.2)

The transmaxillary transpterygoid approach provides access to the lateral recess of the sphenoid sinus and, therefore, is the endoscopic endonasal approach used for repair of middle fossa/lat-

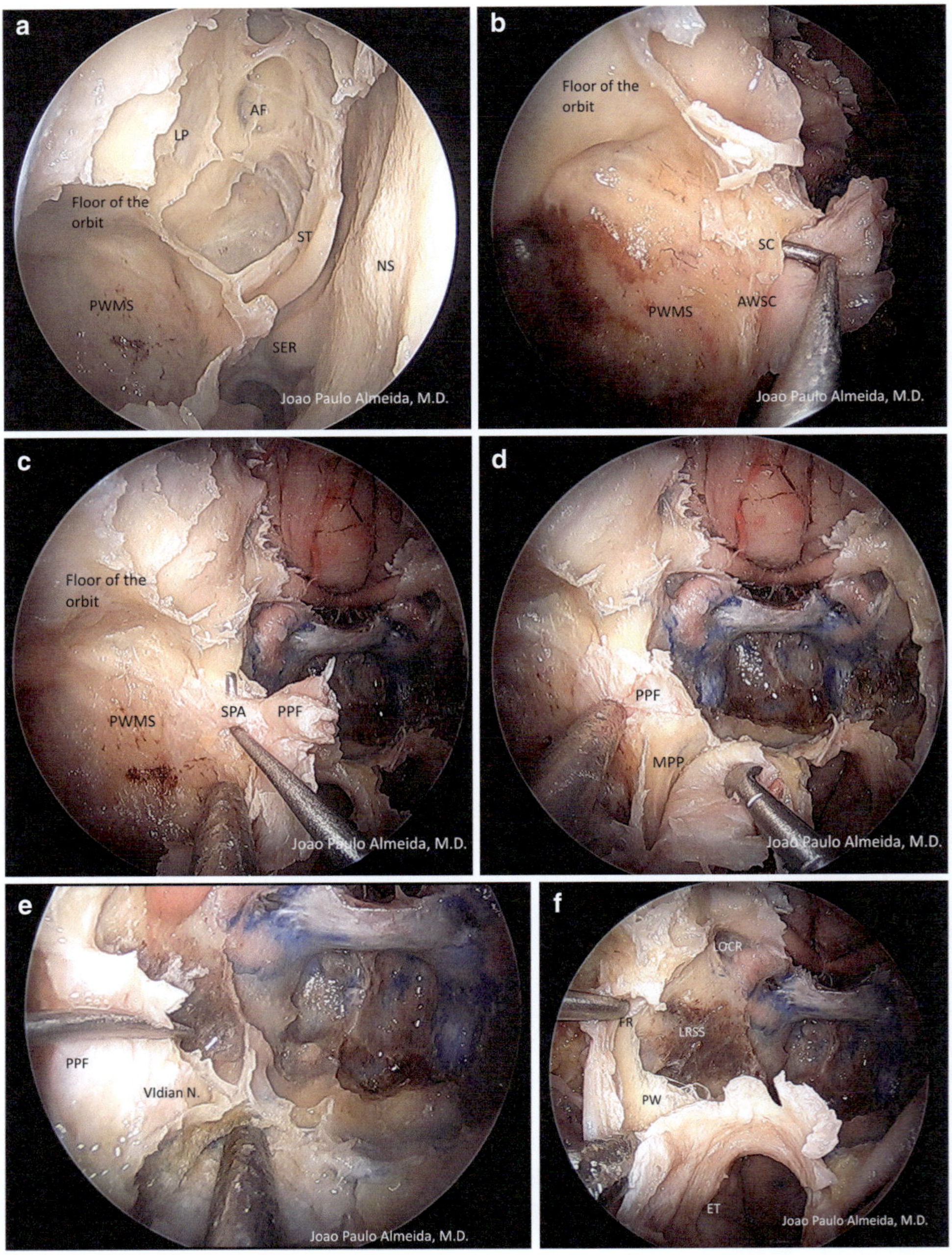

Fig. 22.2 Transpterygoid approach—right side. (**a**) Exposure after right middle turbinectomy, uncinectomy, ethmoidectomy, and maxillary antrostomy. *LP* lamina papyracea, *PWMS* posterior wall of the maxillary sinus, *ST* superior turbinate, *AF* anterior fossa, *SER* sphenoethmoidal recess, *NS* nasal septum. Copyrights: Joao Paulo Almeida, MD. (**b**) Exposure of the sphenopalatine canal. *PWMS* posterior wall of the maxillary sinus, *AWSC* anterior wall of the sphenopalatine canal (composed by the orbital process of the vertical part of the palatine bone), *SC* sphenopalatine canal. Copyrights: Joao Paulo Almeida, MD. (**c**) Exposure of the sphenopalatine artery. *PWMS* posterior wall of the maxillary sinus, *SPA* sphenopalatine artery, *PPF* pterygopalatine fossa contents. Copyrights: Joao Paulo Almeida, MD. (**d**) Exposure of the pterygoid process after transection of the SPA. *MPP* medial pterygoid process, *PPF* pterygopalatine fossa contents. Copyrights: Joao Paulo Almeida, MD. (**e**) Exposure of the Vidian nerve and canal after displacement of the contents of the PPF and partial drilling of the MPP. *PPF* pterygopalatine fossa contents. Copyrights: Joao Paulo Almeida, MD. (**f**) Exposure of the lateral recess of the sphenoid sinus, after transection of the Vidian nerve and disconnection of its attachment to the pterygopalatine ganglion. *LRSS* lateral recess of the sphenoid sinus, *FR* foramen rotundum, *PW* pterygoid wedge, *LOCR* lateral optic carotid recess, *ET* Eustachian tube. Copyrights: Joao Paulo Almeida, MD

eral recess of the sphenoid sinus leaks [64]. All patients will have an LD inserted at the beginning of surgery, and fluorescein is used for the identification of the leak. The procedure itself is initiated with a rigid 0-degree endoscope; 1% lidocaine with 1:100,000 epinephrine is used to vasoconstrict the sphenopalatine artery at the sphenopalatine foramen, in addition to infiltrating the uncinate process and vertical lamella of the middle turbinate, in the side of the defect. A middle turbinectomy, uncinectomy, and ethmoidectomy are completed, and the medial wall of the maxillary ostium is opened. A contralateral vascularized NS flap is then harvested for skull base repair at the end of surgery. That is followed by resection of the posterior third of the septum, which allows for a binostril, four-handed surgical technique. After a wide maxillary antrostomy is done, the mucosa and bone of the posterior wall of the maxillary sinus are removed, and the anterior and posterior walls of the sphenopalatine canal are resected. That leads to exposure of the sphenopalatine artery, which is then coagulated and transected. The contents of the pterygopalatine fossa are pushed laterally to reveal the Vidian nerve, the medial pterygoid plate, and the pterygoid “wedge.” The foramen rotundum and the maxillary nerve (V2) are observed at the superior margin of the fossa, traveling laterally and superiorly toward the inferior orbital fissure. The maxillary nerve can be traced posteriorly to identify the foramen rotundum. The attachment of the Vidian nerve to the pterygopalatine ganglion can be cut and disconnected, which maximizes the mobilization of the contents of the pterygopalatine fossa and exposure to the lateral recess of the sphenoid sinus.

22.4.3 Dealing with Mucosa and Bone Around Defect

The mucosa of the sphenoid sinus and lateral recess are stripped away to fully expose the bone anatomy of the sinus, facilitate the adhesion of the vascularized flap, and minimize chances of postoperative mucocele. Intrasphenoidal septations should be extensively drilled out to facilitate the positioning of the flap at the end of the procedure. Venous bleeding originated from the mucosa is easily controlled with the use of warm irrigation and hemostatic powder/Gelfoam.

22.4.4 Reconstruction Technique

According to our current protocol, spontaneous CSF leaks undergo multi-layer reconstruction. In this situation, we use an inlay of Duraguard covered with an onlay of fat and an NS flap, kept in place with dural sealant. Lumbar drainage is used for 3 days at 5 ml/h because these patients often have benign intracranial hypertension. Patients are placed on acetazolamide for 2 weeks after discharge to keep the CSF pressure down. In case of CSF leak recurrence, a ventriculoperitoneal shunt may be offered to address the intracranial hypertension and maximize chances of success of the reconstruction.

22.4.5 Correction of CSF Leaks in the Lateral Recess of the Sphenoid Sinus: Current Results

At Weill Cornell, the multi-layer reconstruction with the use of a vascularized NS flap led to effective repair of the CSF leak in all cases [16]. As for other skull base defects, the introduction of the NS flap improved the results of lateral recess of sphenoid sinus reconstruction. A previous multi-institutional study that assessed endoscopic reconstruction without an NS flap observed a rate of successful CSF leak repair of 85% [64], a good outcome but still inferior to the excellent results achieved with the vascularized reconstruction. Other centers have reported similar good outcomes after endoscopic repair of such leaks, with successful results of 85–100% [65–70].

22.5 Limitations and Surgical Challenges of Sellar, Suprasellar, and Lateral Sphenoid CSF Leak Repair

Although significant technical improvements have occurred in the last 10 years, skull base repair still requires attention and may be associated with significant complications after EEA. Important questions, such as what is the best reconstruction technique, are now being answered. The accumulation of data since the advent of EEA has led to the development of modern protocols for skull base reconstruction associated with low rates of postoperative CSF leak [16, 47]. However, further studies are necessary to elucidate important questions, such as the role of lumbar drains in sellar and suprasellar surgery and the impact on the quality of life and nasal function after different reconstruction techniques.

Our current protocol [16] favors the use of lumbar drains and NS flap in cases with suprasellar extension. Although our experience is positive, the use of LD may lead to severe complications if inappropriately used. The combination of the gasket seal technique and NS flap significantly reduces the chances of leaks and minimizes chances of LD-associated epidural collections and tension pneumocephalus. If the surgeon is not confident on the reconstruction, an LD likely should not be inserted.

Multi-layer reconstruction based on vascularized NS flap has become the workhorse for skull base reconstruction in cases associated with high-flow CSF leak. However, that tissue is not always available, such as in some reoperation cases. Additional vascularized techniques, such as variations of the NS flap and middle and inferior turbinate flap techniques [71, 72], have been developed as an attempt to aid in reconstruction in such cases, but are more technically demanding and may not lead to similar rates of success.

Finally, there is a need for additional trial assessing different techniques for skull base reconstruction, regarding its effectiveness and preservation of quality of life.

22.6 Conclusions

EEA for the management of sellar and parasellar lesions has significantly improved in the last 15 years. Extended approaches, once associated with high rates of postoperative CSF leaks, now have leak rates of <5%, similar to those of open approaches. The development of new techniques and materials for skull base reconstruction and the design of protocols for tailored reconstruction have significantly changed the results of endoscopic approaches. Cases that present with low-flow CSF leak do not require routine vascularized reconstruction; simpler techniques such as reconstruction with fat graft or collagen matrix are usually enough for those cases. Extended approaches to the suprasellar or parasellar space (lateral recess of the sphenoid sinus leaks) will benefit of multi-layer reconstruction with vascularized nasoseptal flap. LD is safe and associated with excellent results in those cases.

Anatomical knowledge, adequate case selection, and surgical experience remain the fundamental aspects of skull base surgery and should be considered for the reconstruction of the skull base, a major aspect of all endoscopic procedures.

References

1. Wang EW, Gardner PA, Zanation AM. International consensus statement on endoscopic skull-base surgery: executive summary. Int Forum Allergy Rhinol. 2019;9:127–44.
2. Snyderman CH, Carrau RL, Kassam AB, Zanation A, Prevedello D, Gardner P, et al. Endoscopic skull base surgery: principles of endonasal oncological surgery. J Surg Oncol. 2008;97(8):658–64.
3. Kassam AB, Gardner PA, Snyderman CH, Carrau RL, Mintz AH, Prevedello DM. Expanded endonasal approach, a fully endoscopic transnasal approach for the resection of midline suprasellar craniopharyngiomas: a new classification based on the infundibulum. J Neurosurg. 2008;108(4):715–28.
4. Kassam AB, Prevedello DM, Carrau RL, Snyderman CH, Thomas A, Gardner P, et al. Endoscopic endonasal skull base surgery: analysis of complications in the authors' initial 800 patients. J Neurosurg. 2011;114(6):1544–68.

5. Ordonez-Rubiano EG, Forbes JA, Morgenstern PF, Arko L, Dobri GA, Greenfield JP, et al. Preserve or sacrifice the stalk? Endocrinological outcomes, extent of resection, and recurrence rates following endoscopic endonasal resection of craniopharyngiomas. J Neurosurg. 2018;2018:1–9.
6. Shetty SR, Ruiz-Trevino AS, Omay SB, Almeida JP, Liang B, Chen YN, et al. Limitations of the endonasal endoscopic approach in treating olfactory groove meningiomas. A systematic review. Acta Neurochir. 2017;159(10):1875–85.
7. Dhandapani S, Singh H, Negm HM, Cohen S, Anand VK, Schwartz TH. Cavernous sinus invasion in pituitary adenomas: systematic review and pooled data meta-analysis of radiologic criteria and comparison of endoscopic and microscopic surgery. World Neurosurg. 2016;96:36–46.
8. Komotar RJ, Starke RM, Raper DM, Anand VK, Schwartz TH. Endoscopic endonasal versus open repair of anterior skull base CSF leak, meningocele, and encephalocele: a systematic review of outcomes. J Neurol Surg Part A. 2013;74(4):239–50.
9. Tabaee A, Anand VK, Barron Y, Hiltzik DH, Brown SM, Kacker A, et al. Endoscopic pituitary surgery: a systematic review and meta-analysis. J Neurosurg. 2009;111(3):545–54.
10. Komotar RJ, Starke RM, Raper DM, Anand VK, Schwartz TH. Endoscopic endonasal compared with anterior craniofacial and combined cranionasal resection of esthesioneuroblastomas. World Neurosurg. 2013;80(1-2):148–59.
11. Komotar RJ, Starke RM, Raper DM, Anand VK, Schwartz TH. Endoscopic endonasal compared with microscopic transsphenoidal and open transcranial resection of craniopharyngiomas. World Neurosurg. 2012;77(2):329–41.
12. Komotar RJ, Starke RM, Raper DM, Anand VK, Schwartz TH. Endoscopic skull base surgery: a comprehensive comparison with open transcranial approaches. Br J Neurosurg. 2012;26(5):637–48.
13. Komotar RJ, Starke RM, Raper DM, Anand VK, Schwartz TH. Endoscopic endonasal versus open transcranial resection of anterior midline skull base meningiomas. World Neurosurg. 2012;77(5-6): 713–24.
14. Komotar RJ, Starke RM, Raper DM, Anand VK, Schwartz TH. Endoscopic endonasal compared with microscopic transsphenoidal and open transcranial resection of giant pituitary adenomas. Pituitary. 2012;15(2):150–9.
15. Cohen S, Jones SH, Dhandapani S, Negm HM, Anand VK, Schwartz TH. Lumbar drains decrease the risk of postoperative cerebrospinal fluid leak following endonasal endoscopic surgery for suprasellar meningiomas in patients with high body mass index. Operat Neurosurg. 2018;14(1):66–71.
16. Patel KS, Komotar RJ, Szentirmai O, Moussazadeh N, Raper DM, Starke RM, et al. Case-specific protocol to reduce cerebrospinal fluid leakage after endonasal endoscopic surgery. J Neurosurg. 2013;119(3):661–8.
17. Raza SM, Banu MA, Donaldson A, Patel KS, Anand VK, Schwartz TH. Sensitivity and specificity of intrathecal fluorescein and white light excitation for detecting intraoperative cerebrospinal fluid leak in endoscopic skull base surgery: a prospective study. J Neurosurg. 2016;124(3):621–6.
18. Zwagerman NT, Wang EW, Shin SS, Chang YF, Fernandez-Miranda JC, Snyderman CH, et al. Does lumbar drainage reduce postoperative cerebrospinal fluid leak after endoscopic endonasal skull base surgery? A prospective, randomized controlled trial. J Neurosurg. 2018;2018:1–7.
19. Fraser S, Gardner PA, Koutourousiou M, Kubik M, Fernandez-Miranda JC, Snyderman CH, et al. Risk factors associated with postoperative cerebrospinal fluid leak after endoscopic endonasal skull base surgery. J Neurosurg. 2018;128(4):1066–71.
20. Mascarenhas L, Moshel YA, Bayad F, Szentirmai O, Salek AA, Leng LZ, et al. The transplanum transtuberculum approaches for suprasellar and sellar-suprasellar lesions: avoidance of cerebrospinal fluid leak and lessons learned. World Neurosurg. 2014;82(1-2):186–95.
21. Hadad G, Bassagasteguy L, Carrau RL, Mataza JC, Kassam A, Snyderman CH, et al. A novel reconstructive technique after endoscopic expanded endonasal approaches: vascular pedicle nasoseptal flap. Laryngoscope. 2006;116(10):1882–6.
22. Shin J, Forbes J, Lehner K, Tomasiewicz H, Schwartz TH, Phillips CD. Skull base 3D modeling of rigid buttress for gasket-seal closure using operative endoscopic imaging: cadaveric feasibility. J Neurol Surg Part B Skull Base. 2019;80(1):67–71.
23. Garcia-Navarro V, Anand VK, Schwartz TH. Gasket seal closure for extended endonasal endoscopic skull base surgery: efficacy in a large case series. World Neurosurg. 2013;80(5):563–8.
24. Leng LZ, Brown S, Anand VK, Schwartz TH. "Gasket-seal" watertight closure in minimal-access endoscopic cranial base surgery. Neurosurgery. 2008;62(5):342–3.
25. Luginbuhl AJ, Campbell PG, Evans J, Rosen M. Endoscopic repair of high-flow cranial base defects using a bilayer button. Laryngoscope. 2010;120(5): 876–80.
26. Campbell PG, McGettigan B, Luginbuhl A, Yadla S, Rosen M, Evans JJ. Endocrinological and ophthalmological consequences of an initial endonasal endoscopic approach for resection of craniopharyngiomas. Neurosurg Focus. 2010;28(4):8.
27. Banu MA, Kim JH, Shin BJ, Woodworth GF, Anand VK, Schwartz TH. Low-dose intrathecal fluorescein and etiology-based graft choice in endoscopic endonasal closure of CSF leaks. Clin Neurol Neurosurg. 2014;116:28–34.
28. Jakimovski D, Bonci G, Attia M, Shao H, Hofstetter C, Tsiouris AJ, et al. Incidence and significance of intraoperative cerebrospinal fluid leak in endoscopic pituitary surgery using intrathecal fluorescein. World Neurosurg. 2014;82(3):513–23.

29. Placantonakis DG, Tabaee A, Anand VK, Hiltzik D, Schwartz TH. Safety of low-dose intrathecal fluorescein in endoscopic cranial base surgery. Neurosurgery. 2007;61(3):161–5.
30. Tabaee A, Placantonakis DG, Schwartz TH, Anand VK. Intrathecal fluorescein in endoscopic skull base surgery. Otolaryngol Head Neck Surg. 2007;137(2):316–20.
31. Bakhsheshian J, Hwang MS, Friedman M. What is the evidence for postoperative lumbar drains in endoscopic repair of CSF leaks? Laryngoscope. 2015;125(10):2245–6.
32. Soudry E, Turner JH, Nayak JV, Hwang PH. Endoscopic reconstruction of surgically created skull base defects: a systematic review. Otolaryngol Head Neck Surg. 2014;150(5):730–8.
33. Sigler AC, D'Anza B, Lobo BC, Woodard TD, Recinos PF, Sindwani R. Endoscopic skull base reconstruction: an evolution of materials and methods. Otolaryngol Clin N Am. 2017;50(3):643–53.
34. Hofstetter CP, Shin BJ, Mubita L, Huang C, Anand VK, Boockvar JA, et al. Endoscopic endonasal transsphenoidal surgery for functional pituitary adenomas. Neurosurg Focus. 2011;30(4):10.
35. Hofstetter CP, Mannaa RH, Mubita L, Anand VK, Kennedy JW, Dehdashti AR, et al. Endoscopic endonasal transsphenoidal surgery for growth hormone-secreting pituitary adenomas. Neurosurg Focus. 2010;29(4):6.
36. Kim BY, Shin JH, Kim SW, Hong YK, Jeun SS, Kim SW, et al. Risk factors predicting nasoseptal flap failure in the endoscopic endonasal transsphenoidal approach. J Craniofac Surg. 2017;28(2):468–71.
37. Nyquist GG, Anand VK, Singh A, Schwartz TH. Janus flap: bilateral nasoseptal flaps for anterior skull base reconstruction. Otolaryngol Head Neck Surg. 2010;142(3):327–31.
38. Alobid I, Ensenat J, Marino-Sanchez F, Rioja E, de Notaris M, Mullol J, et al. Expanded endonasal approach using vascularized septal flap reconstruction for skull base tumors has a negative impact on sinonasal symptoms and quality of life. Am J Rhinol Allergy. 2013;27(5):426–31.
39. Alobid I, Ensenat J, Marino-Sanchez F, de Notaris M, Centellas S, Mullol J, et al. Impairment of olfaction and mucociliary clearance after expanded endonasal approach using vascularized septal flap reconstruction for skull base tumors. Neurosurgery. 2013;72(4): 540–6.
40. Esposito F, Dusick JR, Fatemi N, Kelly DF. Graded repair of cranial base defects and cerebrospinal fluid leaks in transsphenoidal surgery. Neurosurgery. 2007;60(4):295–303.
41. Seda L, Camara RB, Cukiert A, Burattini JA, Mariani PP. Sellar floor reconstruction after transsphenoidal surgery using fibrin glue without grafting or implants: technical note. Surg Neurol. 2006;66(1):46–9.
42. Chaskes MB, Fastenberg JH, Vimawala S, Nyquist GF, Rabinowitz MR, Chitguppi C, et al. A simple onlay sellar reconstruction does not increase the risk of postoperative cerebrospinal fluid leak in well-selected patients. J Neurol Surg. 2021;82(3):231–5.
43. Scagnelli RJ, Patel V, Peris-Celda M, Kenning TJ, Pinheiro-Neto CD. Implementation of free mucosal graft technique for sellar reconstruction after pituitary surgery: outcomes of 158 consecutive patients. World Neurosurg. 2019;122:506–11.
44. Kuan EC, Yoo F, Patel PB, Su BM, Bergsneider M, Wang MB. An algorithm for sellar reconstruction following the endoscopic endonasal approach: a review of 300 consecutive cases. J Neurol Surg. 2018;79(2):177–83.
45. Conger A, Zhao F, Wang X, Eisenberg A, Griffiths C, Esposito F, et al. Evolution of the graded repair of CSF leaks and skull base defects in endonasal endoscopic tumor surgery: trends in repair failure and meningitis rates in 509 patients. J Neurosurg. 2018;130(3): 861–75.
46. Ruggeri AG, Cappelletti M, Giovannetti F, Priore P, Pichierri A, Delfini R. Proposal of standardization of closure techniques after endoscopic pituitary and skull base surgery based on postoperative cerebrospinal fluid leak risk classification. J Craniofac Surg. 2019;30(4):1027–32.
47. McCoul ED, Anand VK, Singh A, Nyquist GG, Schaberg MR, Schwartz TH. Long-term effectiveness of a reconstructive protocol using the nasoseptal flap after endoscopic skull base surgery. World Neurosurg. 2014;81(1):136–43.
48. Paluzzi A, Fernandez-Miranda JC, Tonya Stefko S, Challinor S, Snyderman CH, Gardner PA. Endoscopic endonasal approach for pituitary adenomas: a series of 555 patients. Pituitary. 2014;17(4):307–19.
49. Zhang M, Azad TD, Singh H, Salam S, Jain S, Anand VK, et al. Lumbar puncture for the injection of intrathecal fluorescein: should it be avoided in a subset of patients undergoing endoscopic endonasal resection of sellar and parasellar lesions? J Neurol Surg. 2018;79(6):554–8.
50. Radovanovic I, Dehdashti AR, Turel MK, Almeida JP, Godoy BL, Doglietto F, et al. Expanded endonasal endoscopic surgery in suprasellar craniopharyngiomas: a retrospective analysis of 43 surgeries including recurrent cases. Operat Neurosurg. 2019;17:132–42.
51. Koutourousiou M, Fernandez-Miranda JC, Stefko ST, Wang EW, Snyderman CH, Gardner PA. Endoscopic endonasal surgery for suprasellar meningiomas: experience with 75 patients. J Neurosurg. 2014;120(6):1326–39.
52. Koutourousiou M, Gardner PA, Fernandez-Miranda JC, Tyler-Kabara EC, Wang EW, Snyderman CH. Endoscopic endonasal surgery for craniopharyngiomas: surgical outcome in 64 patients. J Neurosurg. 2013;119(5):1194–207.
53. Battaglia P, Turri-Zanoni M, Castelnuovo P, Prevedello DM, Carrau RL. Brain herniation after endoscopic transnasal resection of anterior skull base malignancies. Neurosurgery. 2015;11:457–62.
54. Jalessi M, Sharifi G, Jahanbakhshi A, Parsa K, Yazdanifard P. Third ventricle herniation into the

sphenoid sinus following endoscopic transnasal transsphenoidal fenestration of Rathkes cleft cyst. Turk Neurosurg. 2014;24(1):63–6.
55. Park HR, Kshettry VR, Farrell CJ, Lee JM, Kim YH, Won TB, et al. Clinical outcome after extended endoscopic endonasal resection of craniopharyngiomas: two-institution experience. World Neurosurg. 2017;103:465–74.
56. Leng LZ, Greenfield JP, Souweidane MM, Anand VK, Schwartz TH. Endoscopic, endonasal resection of craniopharyngiomas: analysis of outcome including extent of resection, cerebrospinal fluid leak, return to preoperative productivity, and body mass index. Neurosurgery. 2012;70(1):110–23.
57. Cavallo LM, Solari D, Somma T, Cappabianca P. The 3f (fat, flap & flash) technique for skull base reconstruction after endoscopic endonasal suprasellar approach. World Neurosurg. 2019;126: 439–46.
58. Shetty PG, Shroff MM, Fatterpekar GM, Sahani DV, Kirtane MV. A retrospective analysis of spontaneous sphenoid sinus fistula: MR and CT findings. AJNR Am J Neuroradiol. 2000;21(2):337–42.
59. Schuknecht B, Simmen D, Briner HR, Holzmann D. Nontraumatic skull base defects with spontaneous CSF rhinorrhea and arachnoid herniation: imaging findings and correlation with endoscopic sinus surgery in 27 patients. AJNR Am J Neuroradiol. 2008;29(3):542–9.
60. Thakur JD, Manzi B, Savardekar AR, Singh MP, Menger R, Nanda A. Commentary: Maximilian Sternberg (1863-1934): the man behind Sternberg's canal and his contribution to the modern-day skull base anatomy and neuroscience-historical vignette. Neurosurgery. 2018;83(3):120–4.
61. Baranano CF, Cure J, Palmer JN, Woodworth BA. Sternberg's canal: fact or fiction? Am J Rhinol Allergy. 2009;23(2):167–71.
62. Tomazic PV, Stammberger H. Spontaneous CSF-leaks and meningoencephaloceles in sphenoid sinus by persisting Sternberg's canal. Rhinology. 2009;47(4):369–74.
63. Illing E, Schlosser RJ, Palmer JN, Cure J, Fox N, Woodworth BA. Spontaneous sphenoid lateral recess cerebrospinal fluid leaks arise from intracranial hypertension, not Sternberg's canal. Int Forum Allergy Rhinol. 2014;4(3):246–50.
64. Tabaee A, Anand VK, Cappabianca P, Stamm A, Esposito F, Schwartz TH. Endoscopic management of spontaneous meningoencephalocele of the lateral sphenoid sinus. J Neurosurg. 2010;112(5):1070–7.
65. Zoli M, Farneti P, Ghirelli M, Giulioni M, Frank G, Mazzatenta D, et al. Meningocele and meningoencephalocele of the lateral wall of sphenoidal sinus: the role of the endoscopic endonasal surgery. World Neurosurg. 2016;87:91–7.
66. Janakiram TN, Subramaniam V, Parekh P. Endoscopic endonasal repair of sphenoid sinus cerebrospinal fluid leaks: our experience. Indian J Otolaryngol Head Neck Surg. 2015;67(4):412–6.
67. Castelnuovo P, Dallan I, Pistochini A, Battaglia P, Locatelli D, Bignami M. Endonasal endoscopic repair of Sternberg's canal cerebrospinal fluid leaks. Laryngoscope. 2007;117(2):345–9.
68. Kirtane MV, Lall A, Chavan K, Satwalekar D. Endoscopic repair of lateral sphenoid recess cerebrospinal fluid leaks. Indian J Otolaryngol Head Neck Surg. 2012;64(2):188–92.
69. Alexander NS, Chaaban MR, Riley KO, Woodworth BA. Treatment strategies for lateral sphenoid sinus recess cerebrospinal fluid leaks. Arch Otolaryngol. 2012;138(5):471–8.
70. Ulu MO, Aydin S, Kayhan A, Ozoner B, Kucukyuruk B, Ugurlar D, et al. Surgical management of sphenoid sinus lateral recess cerebrospinal fluid leaks: a single neurosurgical center analysis of endoscopic endonasal minimal transpterygoid approach. World Neurosurg. 2018;118:473–82.
71. Moon JH, Kim EH, Kim SH. Various modifications of a vascularized nasoseptal flap for repair of extensive skull base dural defects. J Neurosurg. 2019;2019:1–9.
72. Harvey RJ, Sheahan PO, Schlosser RJ. Inferior turbinate pedicle flap for endoscopic skull base defect repair. Am J Rhinol Allergy. 2009;23(5):522–6.

Repair of Cerebrospinal Fluid Leaks of the Posterior Cranial Fossa

23

Carl H. Snyderman, Paul A. Gardner, and Eric W. Wang

23.1 Introduction

One of the challenges of endoscopic endonasal surgery (EES) of the skull base has been the reconstruction of dural defects. Postoperative cerebrospinal fluid (CSF) leaks are a major source of postoperative morbidity and pose the greatest risk for intracranial infection [1]. Postoperative CSF leaks also increase the risk of other complications, delay recovery, and greatly increase the cost of care. Although great progress has been made in the prevention and treatment of CSF leaks with EES, there remains a 5–10% risk of postoperative CSF leak [2]. Potential risk factors for postoperative CSF leak include patient characteristics, type and extent of pathology, size and location of surgical defect, surgical approach, reconstructive technique, and postoperative care [2, 3]. Transclival and transodontoid approaches to the posterior cranial fossa are used for a variety of conditions, extending from the posterior clinoids to the craniovertebral junction [4–7]. For endonasal approaches, the clivus is divided into unequal thirds: upper, middle, and lower. The upper clivus is situated behind the pituitary gland and extends from the posterior clinoids to the floor of the sella; it requires transposition of the pituitary gland for access [4, 5]. It is bounded by the parasellar internal carotid arteries (ICAs) and cavernous sinus laterally. The middle clivus extends from the floor of the sella to the floor of the sphenoid sinus and is bounded by the paraclival ICA and abducens nerve (interdural segment of Dorello's canal), laterally. The lower clivus extends from the floor of the sphenoid sinus to foramen magnum and is bounded by foramen lacerum and hypoglossal canals laterally.

Prevention of CSF leak remains the best strategy, avoiding an intraoperative leak when possible and performing a secure repair. In select tumor cases, the outer (periosteal) layer of the dura can be stripped with the preservation of the inner (meningeal) layer, thereby achieving clear tumor margins and avoiding a CSF leak. Dural defects of the posterior cranial fossa are among the most difficult defects to repair and present unique challenges.

There is a great diversity in reconstructive strategies and techniques among skull base surgeons. This chapter represents our current reconstructive algorithm for EES of the posterior cranial fossa based on our cumulative experience

C. H. Snyderman (✉)
Departments of Otolaryngology and Neurological Surgery, University of Pittsburgh School of Medicine, Pittsburgh, PA, USA
e-mail: snydermanch@upmc.edu

P. A. Gardner
Departments of Neurological Surgery and Otolaryngology, University of Pittsburgh School of Medicine, Pittsburgh, PA, USA
e-mail: gardpa@upmc.edu

E. W. Wang
Departments of Otolaryngology, Neurological Surgery and Ophthalmology, University of Pittsburgh School of Medicine, Pittsburgh, PA, USA
e-mail: wangew@upmc.edu

A. A. AlQahtani et al. (eds.), *CSF Rhinorrhea*, https://doi.org/10.1007/978-3-030-94781-1_23

of *trial and error* and evidence-based review of the literature [3]. There is no "one best" strategy for all patients. Reconstructive choices depend on multiple factors including patient characteristics, prior and planned therapy, available reconstructive options, available resources, and experience of the surgeon. In general, use of a vascularized flap as part of a multi-layer intradural and extradural reconstruction is preferred when available [2, 3, 8]. A variety of materials may be substituted for dura, including autologous (fascia lata, deep temporal fascia), homologous (cadaveric pericardium, dura, dermis), and allogeneic (submucosal porcine intestine) tissues.

23.2 CSF Leak Repair: Transclival Approach

Reconstruction of dural defects following a transclival approach is considered separately for upper and middle/lower clival defects. For all large defects, a multilayer reconstruction consisting of intradural and extradural grafts supplemented with adipose tissue and a vascularized flap achieves optimal results (Fig. 23.1).

23.2.1 Upper Transclival Approach

An upper transclival approach to the dorsum sellae and posterior clinoids requires interdural

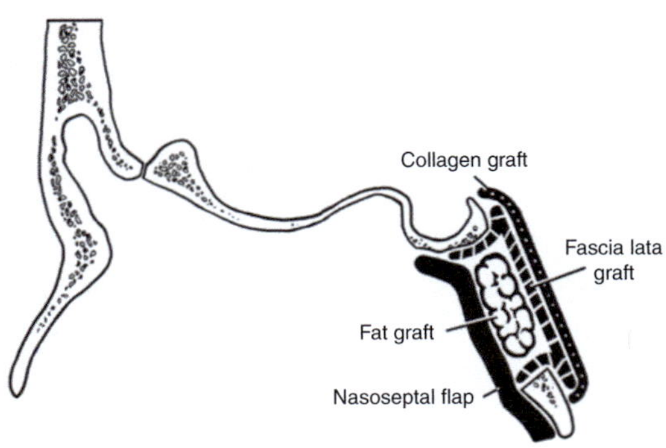

Fig. 23.1 Standard reconstruction of large clival defects includes an intradural collagen graft, an extradural fascial graft, adipose tissue graft, and a vascularized flap. The adipose tissue graft may be omitted with smaller defects, especially of the upper clivus

transposition of the pituitary gland on one or both sides [4, 5]. The bone over the parasellar ICA is usually removed and the ICA partially or completely exposed. A typical dural defect is <2 cm in greatest dimension. An intradural collagen graft is placed intradurally beyond the margins of the defect. A small extradural fascial graft (autologous or homologous) is placed extradurally overlapping the dural and bone defect. With small defects, an extradural graft is not always necessary. The pituitary gland is returned to its normal position and provides a good buttress for the fascial graft. This is then covered with a vascularized nasoseptal flap (NSF). The NSF incorporates all of the mucosa of the nasal septum sparing a 1 cm strip below the olfactory sulcus. It is typically oriented in a vertical or slightly oblique direction. Due to exposure of the cavernous ICA with pituitary transposition, rigid reconstruction with cartilage, bone or alloplastic material is not recommended. Furthermore, a vascularized NSF provides ample protection of exposed parasellar ICAs. The reconstruction is supported with morselized collagen material and either a Foley balloon catheter inflated with saline or Merocel tampons. Absorbable packing is not used for significant clival defects since it may not provide adequate support.

23.2.2 Middle/Lower Transclival Approach

Transclival approaches to the middle and lower clivus often result in a large and deep defect that extends from the floor of the sella to the lower limit of the clivus (Fig. 23.2) [6]. One or both paraclival ICAs are often exposed. A typical dural defect is 3–5 cm in greatest dimension. An intradural collagen graft is placed intradurally beyond the margins of the defect (Fig. 23.3). Ability to tuck the graft laterally may be limited by the interdural segment of the abducens nerve as it enters Dorello's canal and caution is warranted. A large extradural fascial graft (facia lata) is placed extradurally overlapping the dural and bone defect and providing

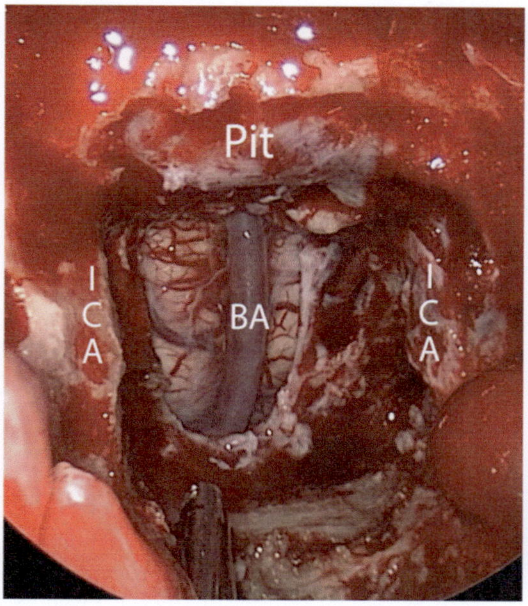

Fig. 23.2 This clival defect extends from the dorsum sella to foramen magnum. It is bounded by the pituitary (pit) gland superiorly and the paraclival internal carotid arteries (ICA) laterally. There is a large dural defect of the posterior cranial fossa with exposure of the basilar artery (BA)

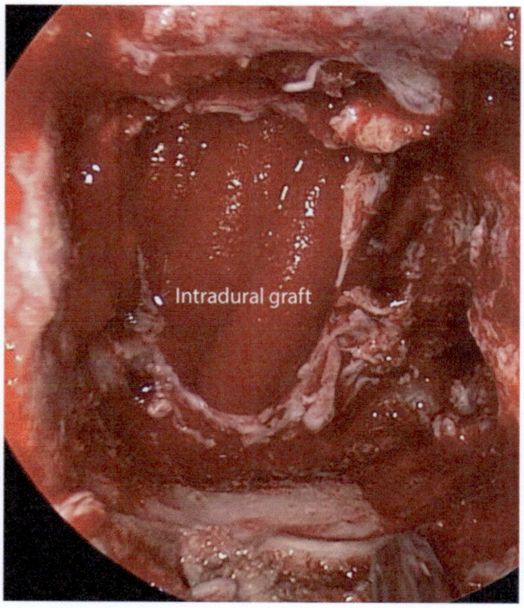

Fig. 23.3 A collagen graft (DuraMatrix, Integra Life Sciences, Stryker, Kalamazoo, Michigan) or similar material (acellular dermal graft) is placed intradurally with overlap of the dural edges

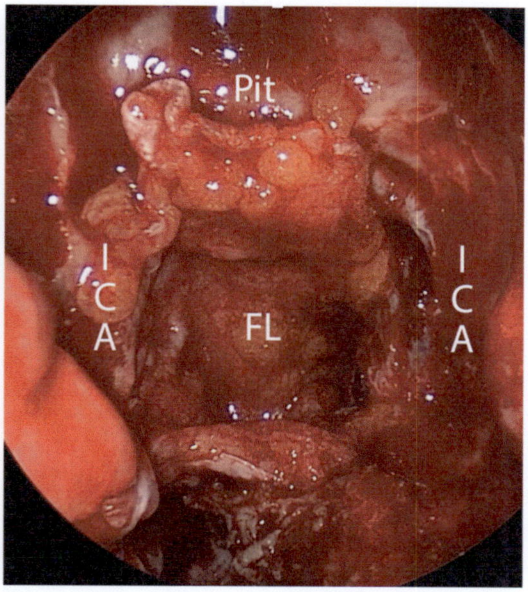

Fig. 23.4 A generous fascia lata (FL) graft provides coverage of the dural and bone defects as well as the exposed internal carotid arteries (ICA). Pit: pituitary gland

coverage of the walls of the clival defect, sella, and paraclival ICAs (Fig. 23.4). Folding of the graft invariably occurs due to the geometry of the defect, and these folds should be smoothed as much as possible. Adipose tissue harvested from the fascia lata donor site or abdomen is used to fill the clival defect in order to prevent pontine herniation (Fig. 23.5) [9]. An extended NSF that includes mucosa from the nasal floor and inferior meatus is oriented horizontally to cover the entire defect and paraclival ICAs (Fig. 23.6) [10]. It is important that the entire adipose tissue graft is covered to provide vascularization and prevent necrosis. The edges of the fascia lata graft may be exposed superiorly and inferiorly. It is also important, when accessing the lower clivus or craniovertebral junction, to separate the reconstruction from the lower nasopharynx and oropharynx to prevent CSF leak at the caudal limit of the defect which can be very difficult to repair. The surgical approach includes the design of an inferiorly based retropharyngeal (RP) mucosal flap, if not involved by tumor (Fig. 23.7) [11]. A wide,

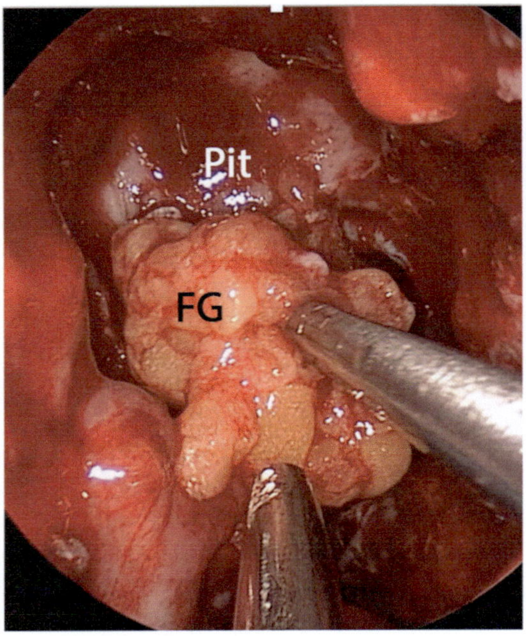

Fig. 23.5 For deep clival defects, a fat graft (FG) is interposed between the fascia lata and vascular flap to prevent pontine herniation and create a planar surface for the flap. Pit: pituitary gland

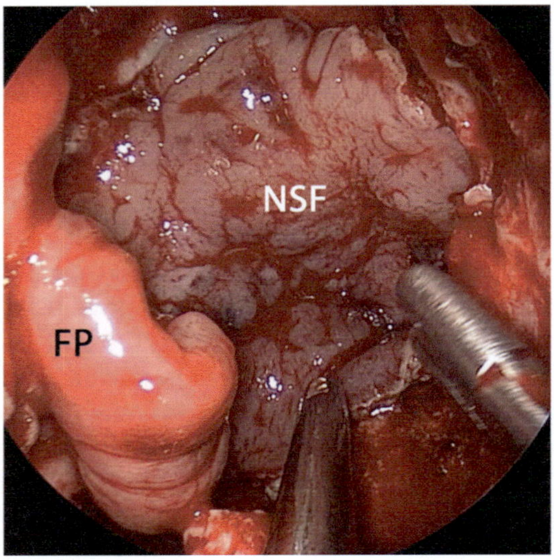

Fig. 23.6 The nasoseptal flap (NSF) or alternate vascularized flap is positioned to cover the adipose tissue and fascia lata. The flap pedicle (FP) can be folded on itself so that the larger distal part of the flap is optimally positioned

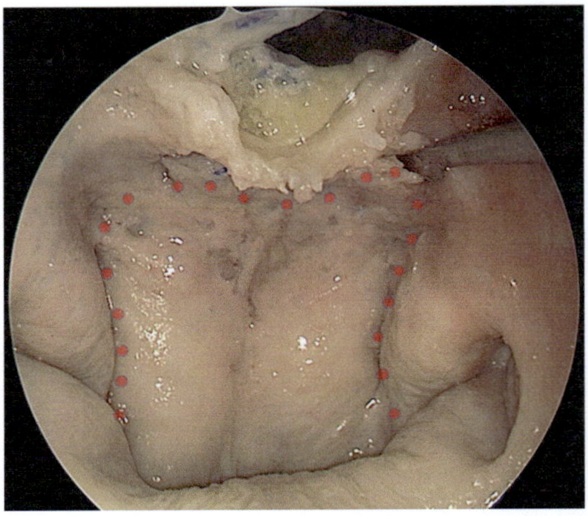

Fig. 23.7 Anatomical specimen demonstrating the outline of an inferiorly based rhinopharyngeal flap

inverted U-shaped RP flap including nasopharyngeal mucosa, muscle and even basopharyngeal fascia can be elevated with needle-tip electrocautery as far inferiorly as the anterior arch of C1 and tucked inferiorly behind the soft palate during tumor resection. For reconstruction, it is brought back up into position after the NSF is in position. It is in apposition to the inferior aspect of the nasoseptal flap and overlaps the underlying edge of the fascia lata graft. In cases of recurrent leak or large defects in obese patients, the inferior edge of the flap can even be sutured to the RP flap using a running V-Loc suture (Covidien-Medtronic, Dublin, Ireland) or similar technique [12]. Again, rigid reconstruction with cartilage, bone or alloplastic material is not recommended due to the risk of vascular injury. The vascularized NSF provides ample protection of exposed paraclival ICAs. The reconstruction is supported with morselized collagen material and Merocel tampons. A Foley balloon catheter does not provide adequate support in this region, and there is risk of migration into the oropharynx. Absorbable packing is not used for significant clival defects since it may not provide adequate support and is at risk for aspiration.

23.3 CSF Leak Repair: Transodontoid Approach

The transodontoid approach may include removal of all or part of the anterior arch of C1, the odontoid (dens) and part of the body of C2, and the anterior foramen magnum [7]. Although a CSF leak can usually be avoided in patients with basilar invagination and inflammatory pannus, removal of tumors at this level (chordoma, meningioma) may result in a significant dural defect. Reconstruction of dural defects at this level is difficult due to the lack of inferior support, and an RP flap is strongly recommended when possible. This flap is dissected and reflected inferiorly below the level of C1. Following tumor excision, a dural substitute is placed intradurally. Fascia lata is placed extradurally and extends to the edges of the mucosal defect. A small adipose tissue graft may be used to fill the defect and provide a planar surface for an NSF. In the absence of an adipose tissue graft, the defect is often too deep and limits the reach (and coverage) of the NSF. The RP flap is transposed superiorly so that it overlaps the edge of the fascia lata graft and is aligned with the NSF and can be reinforced by suturing the fascia lata or NSF to the retropharyngeal tissues or edge of the RP flap as described above [12]. The reconstruction is supported with morselized collagen material and Merocel tampons.

23.4 Limitations and Surgical Challenges

Dural defects following EES of the posterior cranial fossa are a formidable challenge for the endonasal skull base surgeon and are associated with a significant learning curve. A team-based approach is essential for problem-solving and optimal surgical technique.

Reconstructive choices depend on multiple factors including patient characteristics, prior and planned therapy, available reconstructive options, available resources, and experience of the surgeon. In general, use of a vascularized flap as part of a multi-layer intradural and extradural reconstruction is preferred when available [2, 3, 8]. A variety of materials may be substituted for dura including autologous (fascia lata, deep temporal fascia), homologous (cadaveric pericardium, dura, dermis), and allogeneic (submucosal porcine intestine) tissue. The NSF is the preferred flap for most reconstructions but may not be available due to prior surgery or tumor involvement. In revision surgeries, perfusion of the vascular pedicle can be assessed with a Doppler probe or indocyanine green fluoroscopy [13]. Alternative vascularized flaps include the lateral nasal wall (inferior turbinate) flap, temporoparietal fascial flap, and extracranial pericranial flap [14–18].

23.5 Postoperative Care

A lumbar spinal drain is placed at the time of surgery for all posterior fossa defects. A randomized trial demonstrated a significant benefit in this patient group [19]. Spinal fluid is drained at a rate of 5–10 cc/h for 72 h postoperatively. The patient's head is elevated >30° for at least 2 weeks and activities that may increase intracranial CSF pressure are avoided (straining, lifting, bending, nose blowing, etc.). In patients with obstructive sleep apnea, resumption of positive airway devices may start as early as 1–2 weeks following surgery depending on the size and extent of dural defect [20]. Pediatric patients and patients with decreased mental status are at risk of pulling on the strings and dislodging the Merocel tampons. In such patients, the strings may be trimmed short so that they do not protrude from the nose. If packing is dislodged prematurely, it may be necessary to replace the packing under endoscopic visualization at the bedside or in the operating theater. A computed tomographic (CT) scan is obtained within 24 h of surgery to assess the degree of baseline pneumocephalus and screen for hemorrhagic complications. Follow-up imaging depends on the clinical course of the patient.

Antibiotic prophylaxis continues for as long as nasal packing is in place. Nasal packing is removed under endoscopic visualization at 1 week, and minimal debridement is performed at that time. Patients are seen at intervals of 1–2 weeks over the first month until adequate healing is confirmed.

23.6 Management of Postoperative CSF Leak

Patients should be queried for rhinorrhea and postnasal drainage postoperatively. Because of their location, CSF leaks of the lower clivus may not be obvious and CSF rhinorrhea may be absent. Rather, salty taste in the back of the throat, frequent throat-clearing, or nocturnal cough may be present. Increasing pneumocephalus on postoperative imaging or a change in mental status warrant investigation for a CSF leak. In our opinion, suspected CSF leaks should be managed promptly with surgical repair to prevent intracranial infection. At revision surgery, the most common observation is non-adherence of the extradural fascia lata graft inferiorly. This may be due to displacement of the graft, a fold of the graft that is not in contact with bone, retained sinus mucosa, a hole in the graft, or increased intracranial pressure. Minor repositioning of the tissues with replacement of nasal packing is usually all that is necessary. If the site of CSF leak is not apparent, it may be necessary to completely elevate the vascular flap and inspect the entire reconstruction. Additional adipose tissue may be placed to fill any dead spaces or replace infected or necrotic tissue. Suturing of the inferior fascial edge to the retropharyngeal tissue using the V-Loc suture (Medtronic, Jacksonville, Florida) can provide a secure closure where it is needed most [12]. CSF diversion, typically in the form of lumbar drainage, is used on all revision cases. Rarely, necrosis of the vascular flap may occur [21]. The primary risk factor is revision surgery with a narrowed NSF pedicle. Rather than presenting with a CSF leak, these patients develop signs of infection and require debridement of necrotic tissue and treatment of infection. A secondary reconstruction with an alternative vascularized flap may be necessary if coverage is inadequate.

23.7 Literature Review

Although there is no consensus regarding the optimal reconstruction of dural defects with EES of the posterior fossa, review of the literature confirms the increased risk of postoperative CSF leak with transclival approaches, especially in the pediatric population [22]. In a systematic review by Soudry et al., improved results were noted for clival defects (51 patients in four studies) with the use of vascularized flaps [2]. The value of intraoperative lumbar drainage was indeterminate. Subsequent published series are generally too small to derive useful information regarding reconstruction of clival defects with the exception of a report of 136 transclival approaches for a variety of pathologies by Shkarubo et al. [23]. They described their reconstruction of dural defects using intraoperative lumbar drainage with a gasket-seal technique (fascia lata, adipose tissue, bone and cartilage, and fibrin glue) or micro-suturing of dura and fascia lata. Although the number of patients with intraoperative CSF leaks is not stated, the postoperative CSF leak rate was 6.6% overall. A recent *International Consensus Statement on Endoscopic Skull Base Surgery* revealed a 19.1% rate of reconstructive failure for a total of 299 patients with clival defects [3]. There was insufficient data for the craniocervical junction (transodontoid approaches).

23.8 Conclusion

EES of the posterior cranial fossa has extended the capabilities of the skull base surgeon but has created a need for more effective reconstructive techniques. A multi-layered reconstruction with fascial grafts, adipose tissue, and vascularized flaps allows reconstruction of even the most challenging defects and should be supplemented with CSF diversion. An evidence-based approach to skull base reconstruction fosters continuous improvement with an acceptable risk of postoperative CSF leak.

References

1. Kono Y, Prevedello DM, Snyderman CH, Gardner PA, Kassam AB, Carrau RL, Byers KE. One thousand endoscopic skull base surgical procedures demystifying the infection potential: incidence and description of postoperative meningitis and brain abscesses. Infect Control Hosp Epidemiol. 2011;32(1):77–83.
2. Soudry E, Turner JH, Nayak JV, Hwang PH. Endoscopic reconstruction of surgically created skull base defects: a systematic review. Otolaryngol Head Neck Surg. 2014;150(5):730–8.
3. Wang EW, Zanation AM, Gardner PA, Schwartz TH, Eloy JA, Adappa ND, Bettag M, Bleier BS, Cappabianca P, Carrau RL, Casiano RR, Cavallo LM, Ebert CS Jr, El-Sayed IH, Evans JJ, Fernandez-Miranda JC, Folbe AJ, Froelich S, Gentili F, Harvey RJ, Hwang PH, Jane JA Jr, Kelly DF, Kennedy D, Knosp E, Lal D, Lee JYK, Liu JK, Lund VJ, Palmer JN, Prevedello DM, Schlosser RJ, Sindwani R, Solares CA, Tabaee A, Teo C, Thirumala PD, Thorp BD, de Arnaldo Silva Vellutini E, Witterick I, Woodworth BA, Wormald PJ, Snyderman CH. ICAR: endoscopic skull-base surgery. Int Forum Allergy Rhinol. 2019;9(S3): S145–365.
4. Fernandez-Miranda JC, Gardner PA, Rastelli MM Jr, Peris-Celda M, Koutourousiou M, Peace D, Snyderman CH, Rhoton AL Jr. Endoscopic endonasal transcavernous posterior clinoidectomy with interdural pituitary transposition. J Neurosurg. 2014;121(1): 91–9.
5. Gardner PA, Snyderman CH. Endoscopic endonasal pituitary transposition approach to the superior clivus. In: Snyderman CH, Gardner PA, editors. Master techniques in otolaryngology-head and neck surgery: skull base surgery volume. Philadelphia: Wolters Kluwer; 2015. p. 357–64.
6. Gardner PA, Snyderman CH. Transclival approach to the middle and lower clivus. In: Snyderman CH, Gardner PA, editors. Master techniques in otolaryngology-head and neck surgery: skull base surgery volume. Philadelphia: Wolters Kluwer; 2015. p. 365–72.
7. Locatelli D, Karligkiotis A, Turri-Zanoni M, Canevari FR, Pozzi F, Castelnuovo P. Endoscopic endonasal approaches for treatment of craniovertebral junction tumours. Acta Neurochir Suppl. 2019;125:209–24.
8. Harvey RJ, Parmar P, Sacks R, Zanation AM. Endoscopic skull base reconstruction of large dural defects: a systematic review of published evidence. Laryngoscope. 2012;122(2):452–9.
9. Koutourousiou M, Filho FV, Costacou T, Fernandez-Miranda JC, Wang EW, Snyderman CH, et al. Pontine encephalocele and abnormalities of the posterior fossa following transclival endoscopic endonasal surgery. J Neurosurg. 2014;121(2):359–66.
10. Peris-Celda M, Pinheiro-Neto CD, Funaki T, Fernandez-Miranda JC, Gardner P, Snyderman C, et al. The extended nasoseptal flap for skull base reconstruction of the clival region: an anatomical and radiological study. J Neurol Surg B Skull Base. 2013;74(6): 369–85.
11. Champagne PO, Zenonos GA, Wang EW, Snyderman CH, Gardner PA. The rhinopharyngeal flap for reconstruction of lower clival and craniovertebral junction defects. J Neurosurg. 2021;1–9; [online ahead of print].
12. Zwagerman NT, Geltzeiler MN, Wang EW, Fernandez-Miranda JC, Snyderman CH, Gardner PA. Endonasal suturing of nasoseptal flap to nasopharyngeal fascia using the V-Loc™ wound closure device: 2-dimensional operative video. Oper Neurosurg (Hagerstown). 2019;16(2):40–1.
13. Geltzeiler M, Igami Nakassa ACI, Turner M, Setty P, Zenonos G, Hebert A, Wang E, Fernandez-Miranda J, Snyderman C, Gardner P. Evaluation of intranasal flap perfusion by intraoperative indocyanine green fluorescence angiography. Oper Neurosurg (Hagerstown). 2018;15(6):672–6; [Epub ahead of print]
14. Clavenna MJ, Turner JH, Chandra RK. Pedicled flaps in endoscopic skull base reconstruction: review of current techniques. Curr Opin Otolaryngol Head Neck Surg. 2015;23(1):71–7.
15. Choby GW, Pinheiro-Neto CD, de Almeida JR, Ruiz-Valdepeñas EC, Wang EW, Fernandez-Miranda JC, et al. Extended inferior turbinate flap for endoscopic reconstruction of skull base defects. J Neurol Surg B Skull Base. 2014;75(4):225–30.
16. Fortes FS, Carrau RL, Snyderman CH, Kassam A, Prevedello D, Vescan A, et al. Transpterygoid transposition of a temporoparietal fascia flap: a new method for skull base reconstruction after endoscopic expanded endonasal approaches. Laryngoscope. 2007;117(6):970–6.
17. Zanation AM, Snyderman CH, Carrau RL, Kassam AB, Gardner PA, Prevedello DM. Minimally invasive endoscopic pericranial flap: a new method for endonasal skull base reconstruction. Laryngoscope. 2009;119(1):13–8.
18. Gode S, Lieber S, Nakassa ACI, Wang EW, Fernandez-Miranda JC, Gardner PA, et al. Clinical experience with secondary endoscopic reconstruction of clival defects with extracranial pericranial flaps. J Neurol Surg B Skull Base. 2019;80(3):276–82.
19. Zwagerman NT, Wang EW, Shin SS, Chang YF, Fernandez-Miranda JC, Snyderman CH, Gardner PA. Does lumbar drainage reduce postoperative cerebrospinal fluid leak after endoscopic endonasal skull base surgery? A prospective, randomized controlled trial. J Neurosurg. 2018;1:1–7.
20. Choi DL, Reddy K, Weitzel EK, Rotenberg BW, Vescan A, Algird A, Sommer DD. Postoperative continuous positive airway pressure use and nasal saline rinses after endonasal endoscopic skull base surgery in patients with obstructive sleep apnea: a practice pattern survey. Am J Rhinol Allergy. 2019;33(1):51–5. https://doi.org/10.1177/1945892418804987; Epub 2018 Oct 22
21. Chabot JD, Patel C, Zwagerman N, Zenonos G, Wang E, Snyderman C, Gardner P, Fernandez-

Miranda JC. Nasoseptal flap necrosis: incidence, clinical description, and outcomes. J Neurol Surg B. 2016;77(S1):S34–5.
22. Stapleton AL, Tyler-Kabara EC, Gardner PA, Snyderman CH, Wang EW. Risk factors for cerebrospinal fluid leak in pediatric patients undergoing endoscopic endonasal skull base surgery. Int J Pediatr Otorhinolaryngol. 2017;93:163–6.
23. Shkarubo AN, Koval KV, Chernov IV, Andreev DN, Pantelevev AA. Endoscopic endonasal transclival approach to tumors of the clivus and anterior region of the posterior cranial fossa (results of surgical treatment of 136 patients). World Neurosurg. 2019;121:e246–61.

24 The Proper Use of Reconstructive Material

Karan Jolly, Shahzada K. Ahmed, and Anshul Sama

24.1 Introduction

Over the last few decades, endoscopic endonasal surgery has pushed boundaries, tackling a greater array of sinonasal, skull base and intracranial pathologies. A greater understanding of endoscopic anatomy has allowed development of new surgical corridors, enabling complex skull base resections. One of the challenges posed by this is the subsequent reconstruction required to prevent life-threatening morbidity, such as cerebrospinal fluid (CSF) leak, meningitis, intracranial abscess and pneumocephalus. Advancements in reconstructive techniques have allowed for the evolution of endoscopic skull base techniques providing adequate separation of the sinonasal and intracranial compartments. The emergence of a range of flaps and biosynthetic materials has been pivotal in this journey. In this chapter, we will discuss the use of reconstructive techniques and materials to allow for a robust skull base repair that seals the intracranial cavity from the nasal cavity.

Skull base repair requires meticulous replacement of the normal anatomical layers breached, the success of which can be measured by the absence of a postoperative CSF leak [1]. CSF leak rates following endoscopic repair have fallen significantly from 30–40% to 6.7–11.5% [1, 2]; owed to better instrumentation, endoscopic technology and surgical materials and techniques such as vascularised nasoseptal flaps [3, 4]. Modern reconstructive techniques employ a combination of synthetic dural replacement drafts, autologous free grafts, vascularised flaps and synthetic tissue glues and sealants to achieve repair [5]. Despite variations in techniques used, certain factors need to be considered in order to plan the most appropriate type of repair for each case. These include size of the defect, underlying pathology, tissue availability, flow rate of CSF, use of pre or post chemoradiotherapy and also patient and surgeon preference [6, 7]. We will aim to discuss these in an attempt to suggest optimal options for repair in different scenarios.

24.2 Materials

24.2.1 Free Autografts

Free autografts, harvested from a donor site and implanted at the site of surgery, have the benefit of being readily available with no risk of tissue reaction and can include fat, mucosa, cartilage, bone and fascia (temporalis fascia or fascia lata) [8]. Fascial grafts serve to be an excellent underlay (subdural or extradural) and are the first option in

K. Jolly · S. K. Ahmed (✉)
Department of Otolaryngology, University Hospital Birmingham, Birmingham, UK
e-mail: Kjolly@nhs.net; Shahz.ahmed@uhb.nhs.uk

A. Sama
Department of Neurosurgery, Nottingham University Hospitals Trust, Nottingham, UK
e-mail: Anshul.sama@nottingham.ac.uk

A. A. AlQahtani et al. (eds.), *CSF Rhinorrhea*, https://doi.org/10.1007/978-3-030-94781-1_24

a multilayer approach as well as an overlay graft [9]. Intracranial fat graft can be used in combination with eradicate any dead space, for example in the sellar region. This provides an adequate repair in low-flow CSF leaks and smaller defects (<1 cm) [9]. The disadvantage of these grafts is the potential morbidity related to the donor site including wound infection, haematoma, scar and seroma. Free mucosal grafts, harvested from the turbinates or nasal septum, can be placed as an overlay for additional support, taking care to place it with the mucosal surface outwards towards the nasal cavity to prevent formation of a mucocele. The use of free cartilage or bone grafts provides rigid support in defects where there is high risk of herniation, e.g. meningoencephaloceles arising from Sternberg's canal [10] and may also be used in a gasket seal configuration in smaller high flow leaks [11]. Free bone grafting is controversial, especially when postoperative radiotherapy is to be considered due to the risk of osteoradionecrosis and repair breakdown [4] (Table 24.1).

24.2.2 Synthetic Dural Grafts

Over recent years, there has been an increase in synthetic grafts that are used as dural substitutes for repair and have been used successfully during open middle and posterior fossa surgery [12, 13]. They can be used as alternatives to fascial/mucosal grafts for both intra and extra dural grafting, without additional donor site morbidity but at additional cost [8]. These grafts are often made of a collagen matrix and come in many sizes, making them useful in larger defects as a single or multilayer repair or in combination with autologous tissue. A significant number of synthetic grafts contain animal extracts such as gelatin, which should be discussed with patients prior to their use. Titanium and polydioxanone plate (PDS) have been shown to be useful for rigid support in larger defects where bone or cartilage grafting may not be feasible. PDS has been demonstrated in the repair of large anterior skull base defects to prevent brain herniation [14]. Use of synthetic grafts very much depends on surgeon preference, availability and cost implications. It is important to note, when using synthetic dural grafts, their enhancement in the early phases post-operatively can easily be confused with residual disease and radiologists should be made aware of this [15].

Table 24.1 Free autologous graft materials

Intranasal	Extranasal
Mucosa (inferior/middle turbinate/nasal floor)	Fat (adipose)
Septal mucosa	Fascia (temporalis or fascia lata)
Bone (vomer)	
Cartilage (septum)	

24.2.3 Vascularised Flaps

Vascularised flaps can be divided into intranasal and extranasal in origin, and technical details of each have been discussed other chapters of this book. By far the main workhorse of endoscopic skull base repair is the revolutionary Hadad-Bassagasteguy nasoseptal flap, first described in 2006 with several modifications since [9, 16]. Use of this flap however depends on the size of defect and availability of disease-free septal mucosa. It can be successfully used for defects anywhere, from the posterior table of the frontal sinus back to the clivus. Morbidity related to these flaps include nasal crusting and anosmia/hyposmia; however, its use encourages rapid healing [3, 11]. Studies demonstrated the use of vascularised flaps to be advantageous in larger defects measuring >3 cm and with high-flow CSF leaks, over free grafting, especially if post-operative radiotherapy is planned [2, 4, 17, 18]. Nasoseptal flap serves to be particularly useful in repair of ventral skull base lesions where CSF flow rates can be challenging [11]. A review by Harvey et al. analysing reconstructive techniques of the skull base demonstrated an overall 11.5% CSF leak rate: 15.6% with free grafts and 6.7% with vascularised flaps, respectively [2]. Providing sufficient mucosa is available, bilateral non-adjacent nasoseptal flaps can be raised to cover almost 60% of the skull base [1]. Where intranasal flaps are not possible, vascularised extranasal flaps can be utilised. These include the transfrontal pericranial flap for anterior defects and the temporoparietal fascial flap for middle and posterior fossa defects. Although very effective, these flaps have additional morbidity related to external approaches [11].

24.2.4 Absorbable Sealants and Glues

A wide range of sealants and glues are available as adjuncts to reinforce the primary reconstructive layers at the skull base. These are often applied at the end of the reconstruction again in a multilayer fashion. Commonly SURGICEL® (Ethicon Inc., New Jersey, USA) is used to provide haemostasis and a scaffold onto which further glues are applied. Fibrin-based adhesive glues such as TISSEEL® (Baxter, Illinois, USA) and Evicel® (Ethicon Inc., New Jersey, USA) are used to hold the layers in place and prevent graft migration. Fibrin sealant patches such as TachoSil® (Baxter, Illinois, USA) can also be used as an overlay over the initial duraplasty instead of nasoseptal flaps or free mucosal grafts as an additional layer of support. The nasal cavity is then typically packed with absorbable (NasoPore®, Stryker, Michigan, USA) or non-absorbable (MEROCEL®, Medtronic Xomed, Jacksonville, FL, USA) products to provide further support and haemostasis. Whilst commonly used, it is very important for surgeons to familiarise themselves with the ingredients of these products. A significant proportion of them, including synthetic dural grafts, contain traces of animal or human derivatives which may conflict with patient's religious or personal beliefs. It is therefore worth discussing the use of these adjuncts with patients prior to surgery as there are many alternatives [19].

24.2.5 Reconstructive Factors

When planning any endoscopic skull base procedure, the pre-operative CT and MRI scans must be carefully assessed to try and estimate the size and site of the defect. Depending on the underlying pathology and health of the sinonasal cavity, this can equip the surgeon with a range of potential reconstructive options.

24.3 Size and Site

The size of the defect can be measured preoperatively with the benefit of CT and MRI images. Intra-operatively, neuropatties can be used to estimate the size or more definitively a surgical paper ruler can be trimmed and held next to the defect at the skull base. The size of the defect is important for reconstruction dictating the grafts options that may be considered. To achieve a successful duraplasty where segments of dura are resected/absent, the intradural inlay graft must be 30% larger than the defect size [3] (Fig. 24.1).

A recent study looking at factors affecting the outcomes of skull base repair showed that the size and site of the defect did not affect the success of the repair [3]. This being said, the authors used different repair techniques for each of the different

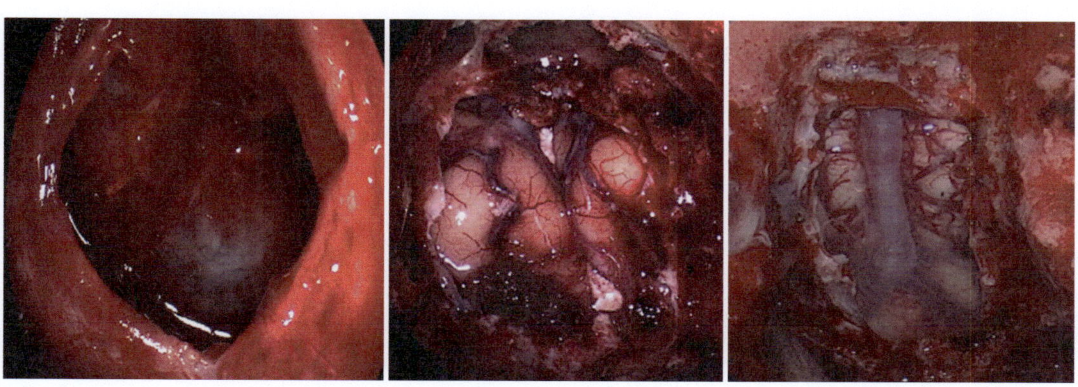

Fig. 24.1 Demonstrating sellar, cribriform and clival defects

locations based on their experience and patient factors. Heterogeneity of repair techniques between different case series in the literature makes analysis of these techniques very challenging. A well-established factor for repair strategies used at each location of the skull base is the rate of CSF flow [3, 4].

Frontal sinus, ethmoidal roof and planum sphenoidale defects require adequate access with a fronto-spheno-ethmoidectomy and can be successfully repaired with a multi-layered approach using an autologous or synthetic intradural graft 30% larger than the defect to allow adequate inlay followed by an extradural layer of the same material placed under the bony defect and finally a third overlay of free mucosal or synthetic dural graft. Small cribriform defects (<1 cm) may be repaired with one intradural and then a single extradural overlay technique using free autologous graft or synthetic dural graft. Care must be taken during extradural dissection to create a pocket for the graft as the dura is very thin in this region and can easily tear. Where there is a visible dural tear in this region, a free graft (fat, fascia or synthetic) can be tucked in as an intradural layer followed by the overlay layer for a more robust repair. Larger craniofacial resections are best repaired with a multi-layered approach, with an intracranial intradural, intracranial extradural and then an extracranial overlay. For any of these layers free fascial or synthetic dural grafts may be used with a vascularised flap preferred as the final overlay, promoting faster healing of these larger defects. Often this will be a nasoseptal flap, however in the absence of healthy mucosal flap, a pericranial flap can be used successfully. Anterior cranial fossa defects are often associated with low CSF flow and easier epidural dissection as well as having better bony support for reconstruction. In addition, the frontal lobes serve as extra support for the inlay grafts [20, 21]. However, large defects associated with brain herniation may occasionally need to be supported with a rigid repair layer as discussed earlier [14]. Figure 24.2 demonstrates a multi-layered approach to repairing an anterior cranial fossa approach with a number of different materials available. These can be used alongside a range of tissue sealants/glues and absorbable packs.

Large sellar and clival defects are also repaired with a multi-layered approach with an intradural and extradural duraplasty. A third mucosal or synthetic graft layer may be used if there is no breach of the arachnoid or a low-flow CSF leak; however, in the presence of a high-flow leak a nasoseptal flap offers better outcomes of <5% leak rates in some studies [22].

24.4 Pathology

An understanding of the pathology can serve to be useful for appropriate repair. Certain lesions are associated with higher risks of postopera-

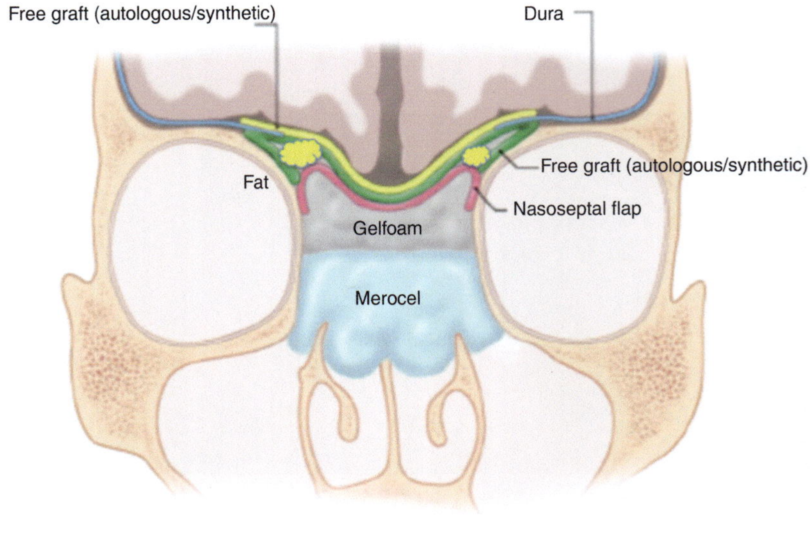

Fig. 24.2 An image demonstrating a multi-layered approach to repairing an anterior cranial fossa defect

tive CSF leak, for which vascular flaps should be considered. These include meningiomas (extensive defect with dural and arachnoid disruption), craniopharyngiomas (breach of arachnoid) and patients who are morbidly obese or with high suspicion of idiopathic intracranial hypertension (IIH). Malignant skull base lesions often require expanded approaches to gain negative resection margins and options for intranasal vascular flaps can be limited. In this case, extranasal vascular flaps may be the best option. The use of preoperative or postoperative radiotherapy is also very important, as it is associated with a higher rate of failure [16]. In these cases, the use of bone grafts or synthetic grafts are usually avoided due to higher risk of infection and extrusion [4]. Instead, vascularised flaps confer an advantage in that they withstand the effects of radiation better, resulting in a better repair rate [9].

24.5 Conclusion

Advances in endoscopic skull base reconstruction are partly owed to implementation of improved and meticulous reconstructive techniques. This being said, reconstruction can be challenging and should be planned before the day of surgery with a range of different options available. Although there is a wide degree of heterogenicity in repair techniques used between surgeons, we propose a stepwise approach. One of the most important factors for success of repair is the extent of CSF leak. Small (<1 cm) uncomplicated defects with no or low CSF leaks may be repaired with a single-layer approach, but for other defects, we recommend a multi-layered approach. We summarise our recommendations on the use of reconstructive materials for skull base repair in Table 24.2.

Table 24.2 Recommendations on the use of reconstructive materials for skull base repair

	Exposed dura or vessels with no CSF leak	Low-flow CSF leak	High-flow CSF leak
No of layers	Single	Multiple	Multiple
Intradural intracranial	No dural defect, overlay technique with: – Autologous (fascia/fat/mucosa) or – Synthetic dural graft overlay technique or – Fibrin sealant patch (Tachosil)	– Autologous (fascia/fat) or – Synthetic dural graft	– Autologous (fascia/fat) or – Synthetic dural graft
Extradural intracranial		– Autologous (fascia/fat) or – Synthetic dural graft	– Autologous (fascia/fat/bone/cartilage) or – Synthetic dural graft
Extracranial overlay		***Optional:*** – Fibrin sealant patch or – Autologous (fascia/mucosa)	***Recommended:*** – Nasoseptal flap or – Extranasal vascularised flap if nasoseptal flap not available

References

1. Soudry E, Turner JH, Nayak JV, Hwang PH. Endoscopic reconstruction of surgically created skull base defects: a systematic review. Otolaryngol Head Neck Surg. 2014;150(5):730–8.
2. Harvey RJ, Parmar P, Sacks R, Zanation AM. Endoscopic skull base reconstruction of large dural defects: a systematic review of published evidence. Laryngoscope. 2012;122(2):452–9.
3. Turri-Zanoni M, Zocchi J, Lambertoni A, Locatelli D, Castelnuovo P. Endoscopic endonasal reconstruction of anterior skull base defects: what factors really affect the outcomes? World Neurosurg. 2018;116:e436–43.
4. Gruss CL, Al Komser M, Aghi MK, Pletcher SD, Goldberg AN, McDermott M, El-Sayed IH. Risk factors for cerebrospinal leak after endoscopic skull base reconstruction with nasoseptal flap. Otolaryngol Head Neck Surg. 2014;151(3):516–21.
5. Kassam AB, Thomas A, Carrau RL, Snyderman CH, Vescan A, Prevedello D, Mintz A, Gardner P. Endoscopic reconstruction of the cranial base using a pedicled nasoseptal flap. Neurosurgery. 2008;63(1 Suppl 1):ONS44–52.
6. Zanation AM, Carrau RL, Snyderman CH, Germanwala AV, Gardner PA, Prevedello DM, Kassam AB. Nasoseptal flap reconstruction of high flow intraoperative cerebral spinal fluid leaks during endoscopic skull base surgery. Am J Rhinol Allergy. 2009;23(5):518–21.
7. Thorp BD, Sreenath SB, Ebert CS, Zanation AM. Endoscopic skull base reconstruction: a review and clinical case series of 152 vascularized flaps used for surgical skull base defects in the setting of intraoperative cerebrospinal fluid leak. Neurosurg Focus. 2014;37(4):E4.
8. Oakley GM, Christensen JM, Winder M, Teo C, Harvey RJ. Collagen matrix as an inlay in endoscopic skull base reconstruction. J Laryngol Otol. 2018;132:214–23.
9. Zanation AM, Thorp BD, Parmar P, et al. Reconstructive options for endoscopic skull base surgery. Otolaryngol Clin N Am. 2011;44(5):1201–22.
10. Zuniga MG, Turner JH, Chandra RK. Updates in anterior skull base reconstruction. Curr Opin Otolaryngol Head Neck Surg. 2016;24:75–82.
11. Hachem RA, Elkhatib A, Beer-Furlan A, Prevedello D, Carrau R. Reconstructive techniques in skull bae surgery after resection of malignant lesions: a wide array of choices. Curr Opin Orolaryngol Head Neck Surg. 2016;24:91–7.
12. Braca JA 3rd, Marzo S, Prabhu VC. Cerebrospinal fluid leakage from tegmen tympani defects repaired via the middle cranial fossa approach. J Neurol Surg B Skull Base. 2013;74:103–7.
13. Narotam PK, Qiao F, Nathoo N. Collagen matrix duraplasty for posterior fossa surgery: evaluation of surgical technique in 52 adult patients. Clinical article. J Neurosurg. 2009;111:380–6.
14. Alasousi F, Okpaleke C, Dadgostar A, Javer A. The use of polydioxanone playes for endoscopic skull base repair. Am J Rhinol Allergy. 2017;31(2):122–6.
15. Walsh E, Illing E, Riley KO, Cure J, Srubiski A, Harvey RJ, et al. Inaccurate assessments of anterior cranial base malignancy following nasoseptal flap reconstruction. J Neurol Surg B Skull Base. 2015;76:385–9.
16. Hadad G, Bassagasteguy L, Carrau RL, et al. A novel reconstructive technique after endoscopic expanded endonasal approaches: vascular pedicle nasoseptal flap. Laryngoscope. 2006;116:1882–6.
17. Cavallo LM, Messina A, Cappabianca P, Esposito F, de Divitiis E, Gardner P, Tschabitscher M. Endoscopic endonasal surgery of the midline skull base: anatomical study and clinical considerations. Neurosurg Focus. 2005;19(1):E2.
18. Eloy JA, Shukla PA, Choudhry OJ, et al. Challenges and surgical nuances in reconstruction of large planum sphenoidale tuberculum sellae defects after endoscopic endonasal resection of parasellar skull base tumors. Laryngoscope. 2013;123(6):1353–60.
19. Jolly K, Darr A, Aslanidou A, Bowyer D, Shahzada A. The intra-operative use of biological products: A multicenter regional patient perspective of a potential consenting conundrum. Clin Otolaryngol. 2019;44(5):831–5.
20. Pinheiro-Neto CD, Prevedello DM, Carrau RL, et al. Improving the design of the pedicled nasoseptal flap for skull base reconstruction: a radioanatomic study. Laryngoscope. 2007;117(9):1560–9.
21. Gardner PA, Kassam AB, Thomas A, Snyderman CH, Carrau RL, Mintz AH, Prevedello DM. Endoscopic endonasal resection of anterior cranial base meningiomas. Neurosurgery. 2008;63(1):36–52.
22. Sigler A, D'Anza B, Lobo B, Woodard T, Sindwani R. Endoscopic skull base reconstruction: an evolution of materials and methods. Otolaryngol Clin N Am. 2017;50(3):643–53.

External Approaches for Skull Base Reconstruction

25

Gustavo G. Rangel, Rafael Martinez-Perez, Daniel M. Prevedello, Ricardo L. Carrau, and Amin Kassam

25.1 Introduction

Advancements in the resection of skull base tumors often result in defects that are not amenable for primary closure. It is mandatory; however, that the closure provides a hermetic barrier between the intradural space and the sinonasal tract to avoid CSF leaks, infectious complications, and death. As such, a skull base reconstruction that achieves the following goals is of paramount importance: (1) support the brain, (2) separate the intracranial and extracranial compartments, (3) provide lining for the nasal cavity, (4) reconstruct the nasal vault and other components of the aerodigestive tract, (5) provide volume to decrease dead space, and (6) restore the cranio-maxillo-facial aesthetics. Besides the location of the defect, other factors should be considered when planning the most appropriate reconstructive technique, such as size of the defect, history of neoadjuvant therapy previous surgery or radiation therapy, high versus low-flow CSF leaking, previous surgeries or traumas, and disposition of grafts.

In order to achieve these objectives, we advocate a multidisciplinary approach for the treatment of skull base pathologies, allowing the proper management of the disease including resection of any large and complex lesions with its subsequent reconstruction and adjuvant therapy while minimizing complications. Many surgical techniques have been developed to achieve an adequate skull base reconstruction. They report varying degrees of technical complexity, approaches, feasible tissue donors, and outcomes. In this chapter, we present current techniques used after open skull base surgery exploring all available options but tailored to each case in particular. Endoscopic transnasal approaches are not included in the scope of this chapter as they will be extensively discussed by others.

G. G. Rangel
Department of Otolaryngology - Head and Neck Surgery, St. Jude Children's Hospital, University of Tennessee Health Science Center, Memphis, TN, USA

R. Martinez-Perez
Department of Neurological Surgery, Anschutz School of Medicine, University of Colorado, Aurora, CO, USA

D. M. Prevedello (✉)
Department of Neurological Surgery, The Ohio State University Wexner Medical Center, Columbus, OH, USA
e-mail: daniel.prevedello@osumc.edu

R. L. Carrau
Department of Otolaryngology-Head and Neck Surgery, The Ohio State University Wexner Medical Center, Columbus, OH, USA
e-mail: ricardo.Carrau@osumc.edu

A. Kassam
Aurora St. Luke's Medical Center, Aurora Neuroscience Innovation Institute, Milwaukee, WI, USA
e-mail: amin@neekahealth.com

A. A. AlQahtani et al. (eds.), *CSF Rhinorrhea*, https://doi.org/10.1007/978-3-030-94781-1_25

25.2 Systematic Zone-Based Approach

Few classifications have been described to better delineate the location, extent, and configuration of the surgical defects. In this sense, an optimal classification should comply with standardized nomenclature: (1) to facilitate communication among clinicians and (2) to create an algorithm that directly links the clinical decision-making with the best outcome for each case. Most of these attempts have failed to reach this kind of perfection. We prefer to use the classification developed by Irish and colleagues [1] that divides the skull base into three regions according to anatomical landmarks and tumor growth patterns. Region I includes tumors of the anterior fossa, clivus, and ventral extensions posteriorly into the foramen magnum. Region II includes tumors that arise in the lateral skull base with extension into the infratemporal and pterygopalatine fossa, involving middle cranial fossa. Region III includes lesions arising from the ear or temporal bone with extension into the posterior fossa (Fig. 25.1).

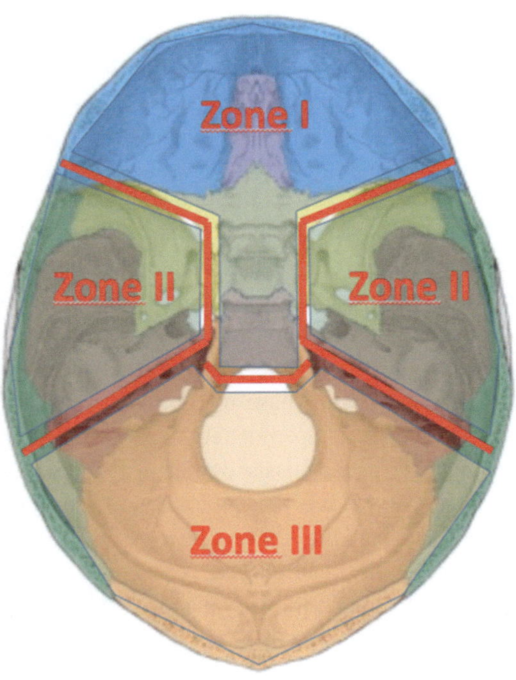

Fig. 25.1 Irish and colleagues schematic division of the zones of reconstruction

25.2.1 Anterior Skull Base (Zone I)

Tumors arising from the anterior skull base might invade both soft and hard tissues of the skull base creating a free communication between the cranial cavity and paranasal sinuses. Repair of most large defects in the anterior cranial fossa following the surgical removal of tumor or craniofacial trauma represents a challenge, given the often extensive bony and dural defects. Traditionally, surgeries for lesions located at the anterior fossa carries a significantly higher incidence of postoperative CSF leaks, that in some series account for more than one-third of cases [2]. Second, given its location, it is also important to maintain a functional sinonasal system and to achieve good cosmetic results.

As the complexity of surgical approaches and tumor removal in the anterior cranial fossa evolved, various reconstruction techniques also developed.

25.2.2 Middle Fossa Skull Base Defects (Zone II)

Temporal bone or middle fossa defects are much less frequent and have lower rates of CSF leaks. For didactic purposes, we classify temporal bony defects in anterior or petrous as such as tegmen tympani defects (Zone II) and mastoid defects as posterior (Zone III).

Tegmen tympani defects might be the potential source of cerebrospinal fluid (CSF) leakage into the mastoid and middle ear and, eventually, causing rhinorrhea given its communication through the Eustachian tube [3]. Symptoms may vary from the anterior fossa patterns, albeit unilateral nasal discharge is a common presentation, given its communication through the Eustachian tube. Other clinical manifestations include unilateral conductive hearing loss, tinnitus, imbalance, aural fullness, and meningitis. A tegmen defect is often a spontaneous idiopathic process and frequently associated with idiopathic intracranial hypertension. However, temporal bone surgery, trauma, infections, or neoplastic invasion of the skull base may play a role as well [3].

25.2.3 Posterior Fossa Defects and Posterior Petrous Bone (Zone III)

Communications between mastoid air cells and the petrous apex into the sphenoid sinus is another possible explanation for spontaneous CSF leak in a patient with tumor invasion or surgery over the posterior third of the petrous bone. One should have a high level of suspicion for this possibility when a fluid level is seen in the mastoid air cells [3].

25.3 General Concepts in External Skull Base Reconstruction

In terms of general concepts of reconstruction, flaps can be classified by:

(a) Congruity: describing the distance from the recipient to donation site (e.g., local, regional, distant).
(b) Configuration: referring to design and method of transfer (e.g., advancement, rotation, transposition, interpolation).
(c) Components: skin, muscle, fascia, and bone.
(d) Circulation: island, axial or free flap.

If aiming to repair the skull base, multiple options could be used through an open skull base approach. For this reason, a brief description of potential options will be presented.

25.3.1 Free Grafts

A free graft is considered a viable option for small defects, although its popularity for use during open skull base surgery has decreased over the recent years. Repair of large defects using free grafts may result in rates of postoperative CSF leaks of up to 40% [4]. Free grafts can be classified as autologous or heterologous.

Free autografting implies the harvesting of tissue from a donor site to be transferred and implanted in a recipient site. Regretfully, this method bears significant disadvantages. Free tissue grafts lack blood supply; therefore, they require a well-vascularized recipient bed to allow the take of the flap [5]. Local grafts are often insufficient in size or their take is incomplete, not allowing for a reliable restoration of extensive anterior skull base defects. Most commonly used free grafts include periosteum from the calvarium, fascia (temporalis fascia and fascia lata), cartilage, bone, and fat. Bone grafts are rarely used in skull base reconstruction. A relatively common indication for using bone grafts is the need for reconstruction of the orbital rim [6]. A rare but important consideration must be taken in, morbidly obese patients with obstructive sleep apnea, who may experience brain herniation through a large defect in the anterior cranial fossa [7]. Despite some benefits, bone grafts are prone to radionecrosis, which can evolve into more serious complications [5].

Heterologous free grafts, including a synthetic dura and bone substitute, might be used to cover small defects. However, this option bears significant drawbacks, as synthetic materials carry a high risk of migration, bacterial colonization, and extrusion and are costly [8, 9].

25.3.2 Local and Regional Flaps

The pedicle nasoseptal or Hadad-Bassagasteguy flap [10] is one of the most popular local options for anterior skull base (Zone I). However, its use may be limited by tumor invasion, failure of the pedicle, lack of healthy mucosa, limited reach, or size. Although still possible to harvest other flaps from the nasal vault, such as the lateral nasal wall or inferior turbinate flaps, these are less reliable choices. When a nasoseptal flap is unavailable, other less common flap options must be considered, including the Oliver palatal island, the facial artery mucosal muscular, the temporoparietal, temporalis muscle, pericranial flaps, and other variations. A full description of these techniques is offered in other chapters. In the following text, we will describe the way that these options are used in open skull base surgery.

25.3.3 Microvascular Free Flaps

Microvascular tissue transfer is useful for repairing large three-dimensional defects in the skull base [11]. Flaps could be tailored to repair bone, dura, and soft tissue defects. In these cases, a volumetric fill of dead space is obtained with high vascular quality. Size of the defect, donor site, and viability of recipient's vessels are important considerations. For skull base reconstruction purposes, the rectus abdominis musculocutaneous, radial forearm fasciocutaneous, anterolateral thigh fasciocutaneous are the most commonly used. In patients requiring bony reconstruction common choices include the radial forearm osteocutaneous flap, fibula osteocutaneous flap, and osteocutaneous scapular flap [12]. A comprehensive description of the use of free flaps for skull base reconstruction can be found in Chap. 21 (Microvascular Free flap).

25.4 External Surgical Approaches for Skull Base Reconstruction

It is necessary to preview the volume, tissue components, localization, and surrounding structures of the skull base defect. In the following section, we describe the most used external approaches and reconstruction options.

25.4.1 Subfrontal and Transbasal Approaches

A subfrontal approach is considered to be the most established external approach for anterior skull base tumors, although some modifications are commonly advocated to reach the anterior cranial fossa [13]. Reconstruction rarely requires any other supplemental approach as a subfrontal approach is usually adequate.

The surgical technique of the transbasal approach has been widely described [14]. Briefly, the skin is incised posterior to the hairline, and a coronal flap is created in a subperiosteal plane. A coronal flap is elevated anteriorly beyond the supraorbital ridges and laterally superficial to the temporalis fascia. The pericranial flap is elevated up at the end of the surgery from the galea of the coronal flap extending to be 1.5 cm distal from the supraorbital nerves and vessels. These should have been carefully identified and dissected from the supraorbital notches upon the elevation of the coronal flap and exposure of the orbital rims. The lateral and medial walls of the orbits are then exposed, dissecting the periorbita and identifying the anterior ethmoidal arteries, which are clipped or ligated to further the exposure. Osteotomies of the anterior or the anterior and posterior frontal sinus walls, together with the nasal bony frame, part of the medial wall of the orbit, and a segment of the perpendicular plate of ethmoid bone, are then performed. Once the craniotomy is completed, gentle frontal lobe retraction is applied to expose the skull base. The tumor is resected including bilateral ethmoidectomies and sphenoidectomies if indicated. Finally, the dural defect is closed either primarily or using a dural graft. Collagen matrix can be used epidurally followed by the pericranial flap that is rotated to cover the entire skull base dura. It is important to adjust the pericranium in between the dura and the roof of the orbits laterally in order to have proper support. Often an endoscope is used through the nose to confirm proper placement. Nasal packing can also be used to keep the pericranium flap in position.

25.4.1.1 Pericranial Flap

The pericranial flap is a frequent reconstruction choice after a transbasal approach (Fig. 25.2). The flap limits are the supraorbital ridges ventrally and the superior temporal line laterally [14]. Its blood supply relies on the paired supraorbital (SO) and supratrochlear (ST) vessels arising from their corresponding ipsilateral ophthalmic artery; the SO trunk emerges from its homonymous foramen and is the dominant vessel; thus, its preservation is paramount for the flap survival. However, one supraorbital artery could supply the entire flap (i.e., minimum pedicle width is 3 cm), efforts should be made to preserve both pedicles, unless the defect does not demand a full pericranial flap and base it in one pedicle will allow further rotation of the flap.

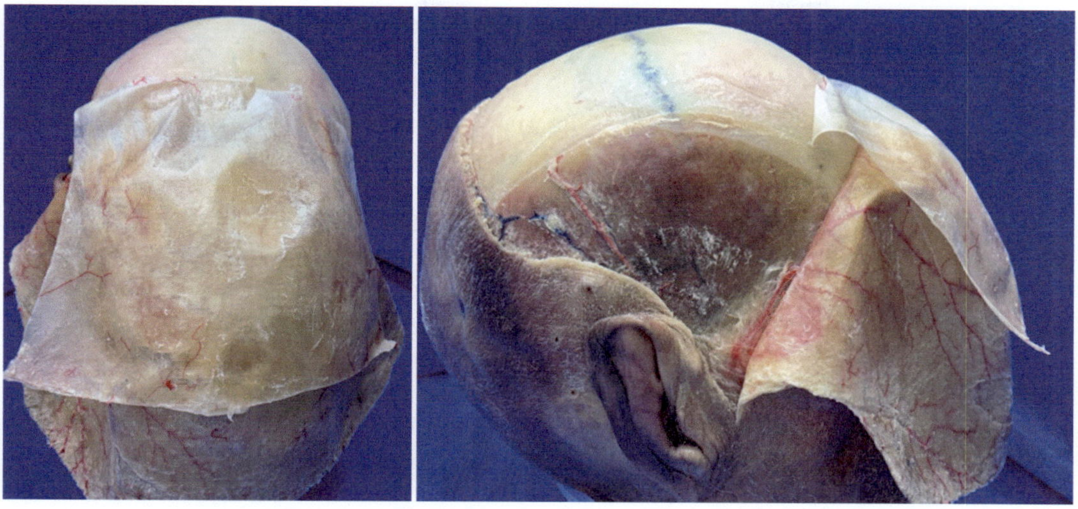

Fig. 25.2 An anteroposterior and a lateral view of a pericranial flap harvested in a cadaveric specimen

Indications and Limitations

The pericranial flap (PF) has many advantages over other options. First, the PF is easy to harvest and does not require additional incisions other than those required for the coronal flap elevation. Second, it has a significant vascular supply from the supratrochlear and supraorbital arteries, which assures its viability and healing [15]. For these reasons, the PF became the most popular for repairing defects following an open skull base resection.

Conversely, its use may be limited by prior facial trauma that could have compromised its vasculature. Its arch of rotation is restricted, which reduces the versatility of this flap [16]. Others have reported a relatively high rate of persistent CSF leak when using pericranial or galeal flap accounts, in comparison to the rest of rotational flaps [17]. However, that does not match our experience.

Key Points

1. History of previous surgery, trauma or radiation, assess facial nerve function, and full examination of the scalp, looking for incisions or wounds that could jeopardize the vascular supply.
2. Use CT to measure the distance from orbital to most distant part of the defect to preview the length of the flap.
3. Dissect the SO neurovascular bundle from the foramen by opening its inferior aspect with small osteotomes.
4. Delay the dissection of the flap until the end of the surgery. This better preserves its integrity and blood supply.
5. Confirm that at least one supraorbital pedicle is in good condition, and the flap is viable before reconstruction.
6. Avoid overstretching or twisting the flap during the replacement of the craniotomy bone grafts.
7. Fix the flap to the bone with sutures whenever is possible.

8. Consider obliterating the sphenoid sinus with fat to prevent displacement of the tip of the flap.
9. Use nasal packing to bolster the reconstruction if needed.
10. Irrigate the sinonasal corridor postoperatively with nasal saline solution to prevent and treat crusting.

25.4.2 Temporalis Muscle Flap

In 2003, Tender et al. described the use of vascularized temporalis muscle flap for successfully repairing defects along the tegmen tympani, via a subtemporal approach [18]. A few years later, in 2009, Taha and colleagues [8] used the same approach to repair a large middle fossa defect with a temporoparietal flap.

Tegmen defects often manifest by CSF leak that can present as rhinorrhea and/or otorrhea. When otorrhea is present, frequently a tympanic membrane defect is encountered and the brain may be observed herniating in the middle ear. Imaging often confirms a middle fossa meningoceles or encephaloceles (Fig. 25.3).

A temporal craniotomy centered over the preauricular line is performed. With a high-speed drill, the craniotomy is then extended inferiorly to the level of the skull base. The dura mater is gently elevated off the skull base from a lateral to a medial direction. The defect in the tegmen is identified, and the herniated brain tissue coagulated and separated from the defect. The osseous and dural defects are first sealed with the collagen membranes, and then the flap is placed between the skull base and the dura.

As in the subfrontal approach, the subtemporal approach requires some level of brain retraction, although, in contrast to the transmastoid approaches, it allows for direct access to the bone and dural defects, as well as the herniated brain. This is particularly relevant for difficult cases,

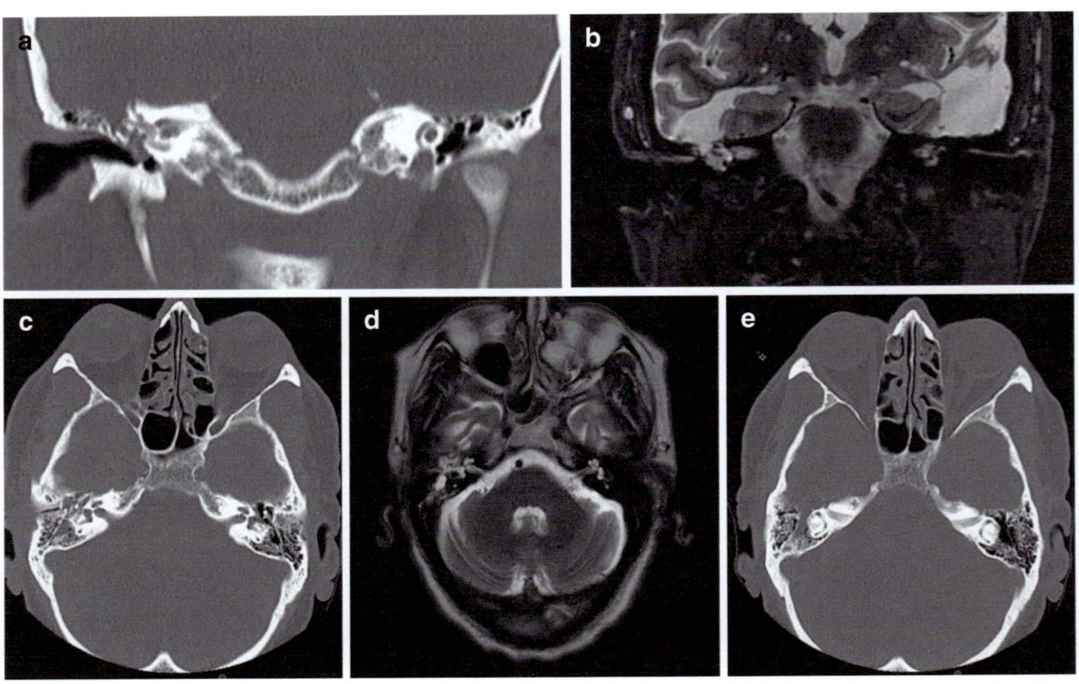

Fig. 25.3 A 67-year-old male with a 3-month history of progressively worsening headaches, right aural fullness, and conductive right hearing loss due to acquired meningocele. CT image shows a 6-mm defect within tegmen tympani (**c**) immediately lateral to the semicircular canal (**e**), complete opacification of the epitympanum and mesial tympanum and lateral displacement in the ossicular chain (**a**). In the MRI is a heterogeneous high T2 signal intensity (**d**) throughout this area which is contiguous with cystic encephalomalacia of the temporal lobe (**b**)

in which the brain herniates through the bone defect. Likewise, direct visualization allows primary close with suturing or collagen membrane plugging of the dural defect.

25.4.2.1 Temporalis Muscle Flap

The patient is positioned supine with an ipsilateral shoulder roll, and the head rotated to the contralateral side. Head might be fixed using a three-point fixing Mayfield arc. A horseshoe incision is placed with its anterior margin 1 cm in front of the pinna, and then it is curved posteriorly and inferiorly toward the mastoid tip. Hemicoronal incision could be used to expose the pericranium, aesthetic considerations should be considered for choosing the incisions, and endoscopic-assisted option shall be considered. Preauricular extension to the intertragic notch facilitates the exposure of the zygomatic root and the dissection of the pedicle flap and provides better rotation. Interlayer dissection is a convenient option to preserve facial nerve function and give room to zygomatic arch osteotomies. Careful release of the arch with further reconstruction should not impair the facial skeleton. Leaving the mid-portion of the arch attached to the masseter muscle promotes inferior retraction of the muscle and could help reconstruction. The pedicle divides in Y-shaped, anterior and posterior deep temporal artery, a branch from the internal maxillary artery (IMA), knowing that we could split the flap in two separate pedicles and then have different axes.

Indications and Limitations

The main indication for this flap is the reconstruction of the floor of the middle fossa extending to the central aspect of the skull base. It can be approached transcranial with a subtemporal craniotomy or extracranially through the infratemporal fossa (e.g., transpterygoid approach) [19]. Concerns about persistent CSF leaks and encephaloceles have been raised, although clinical results showed a low rate of these complications, even in the absence of a bone graft or titanium plates. Nonetheless, given its nature, atrophy of the muscle with loss of volume or scarring that might induce muscle retraction may lead to late postoperative CSF leaks [10]. Intraoperative use of lumbar drains is advocated by some to minimize brain retraction (see Sect. 25.6, limitations and complications of the open skull base surgery) [20].

Key Points

1. Consider situations that could impact muscle volume or blood supply (nutritional status, previous embolizations of the pedicle, effects of the adjuvant radiotherapy).
2. Serial imaging to evaluate the muscle volume and extension (MRI) and estimate skull base defect (CT).
3. Aesthetic placement of the incision (consider the hairline) not using electrocautery over hair follicles. Consider the use of endoscopy and elevators to raise the flap through a skin tunnel.
4. Start raising the temporalis muscle flap at its margins with the pericranium to use its maximum length.
5. An interfascial approach will preserve the frontal branches of the facial nerve.
6. Consider translocating the midportion of the zygomatic arch and removing the coronoid process of the mandible to enhance the flap arc of rotation. One may leave the zygomatic arch attached to the masseter muscle.
7. Consider splitting the flap vertically to gain two flaps with different axes of rotation.
8. When placing the flap, make sure it is not twisted or overstretched.
9. Use a suction drain for the temporal fossa, no compressive dressing is needed.

25.4.3 Transmastoid

Approaching a CSF leak through the mastoid is a good choice for cases in which some repair in the middle ear is needed, e.g., encephalocele or complication of a translabyrinthine approach.

Every transmastoid approach consists of full open of the mastoid air cells. Using the temporal line as a reference to dissect the middle fossa is inconsistent. Therefore, we advocate exposing the sinodural or Citelli's angle first, as it is superficial and reliably indicates the position of the middle fossa dura and sigmoid sinus. Once that is accomplished, a cutting burr is applied parallel to the middle fossa dura to open all cells in contact with the middle fossa. It is recommended to leave a thin layer of cortical bone over the dura. At this point, a thorough exam is necessary to look for dural defects or encephaloceles. The dissection of the middle fossa dura stops at the antrum. Upon opening the mastoid, one can appreciate the lateral semicircular canal (LSC) and the *aditus ad antrum* (the aperture of the epitympanic recess to the mastoid antrum). Following this dissection, it is crucial to consider that the facial nerve lies 1–2 mm ventral to the LSC, and the tip of the uncus will point to the end of the tympanic segment. At this point, the entire middle fossa interface along the mastoid bone is exposed.

CSF rhinorrhea is a major complication of the posterior fossa approach through the labyrinth. In this technique, full exposure of the sigmoid sinus and identification of the jugular bulb is performed to obtain maximum retraction of the sigmoid sinus. The mastoid segment of the facial nerve is dissected entirely, all the labyrinth bone is removed, and the endolymphatic sac is clipped (Fig. 25.4).

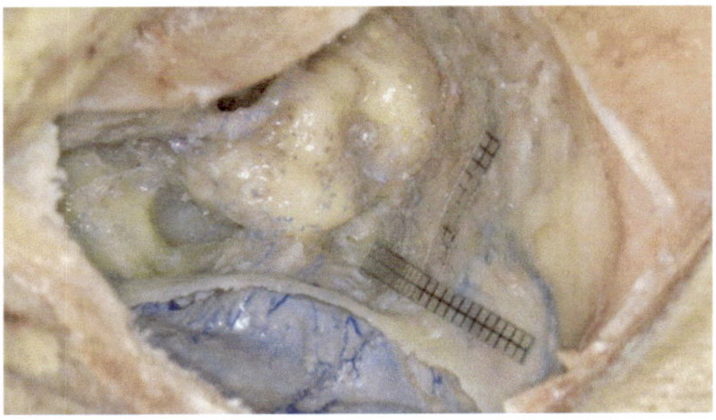

Fig. 25.4 A presigmoid transmastoid dissection emphasizing a full exposure of the tegmen mastoideum and tympani to carry a Zone II reconstruction

25.5 Combined Endoscopic Assist External Approaches

25.5.1 Temporoparietal Flap Combined with Transpterygoid Approach

In order to reconstruct skull base defects, particularly those related to the posterior aspect of Zone 1 (ventral defects), one could use vascularized temporoparietal fascia. It is elevated via a preauricular-hemicoronal incision preserving the superficial temporal artery and vein. The vascularized flap is then transferred to the sinonasal cavity through the infratemporal and pterygopalatine fossa.

Even though the flap could be harvested from either side, it is preferable to choose the side that the defect is more significant from the endonasal perspective or one where a transpterygoid approach has been completed.

Endonasal preparation—ethmoid, big antrostomy, SPA ligation, remove of full posterior and partial lateral maxillary sinus wall, and full exposure of pterygoid plates through the lateral and inferior displacement of the PPF content to create a tunnel from ITF. Pterygoid plates may be drilled over the anterior aspect to enlarge this tunnel.

Transposition—the superficial layer of the deep temporal fascia is incised, avoiding facial nerve, creating the tunnel to TPF trough infratemporal fossa. Dilators are used to develop a non-compression space for the pedicle. The flap is then passed from the external region to the sinonasal cavity and is placed covering the skull base defect.

25.5.1.1 Temporoparietal Flap

The temporoparietal flap (TPF) is often an excellent alternative to extensively cover large anterior and middle fossa defects [21]. The TPF, as a vascularized flap, offers high chances of a successful repair of a CSF leak, even after in sites with poor vascularity due to the deleterious effects of radiotherapy.

The temporal branch of the facial nerve arises from the facial nerve main trunk within the parotid gland and travels anterosuperiorly to innervate the frontalis orbicularis oculi, and corrugator supercilii [22]. Knowing its anatomy and proximity to the orbital rim is mandatory to avoid undesirable effects.

The preauricular incision could vary in shape and length combined with a hemicoronal incision similar to that needed for the temporalis muscle flap. A careful study of the various layers of the scalp is extremely useful. An incision is carried in a straight vertical line to avoid proximal damage to the superficial temporal artery (STA), judicious use of bipolar cautery is recommended to avoid alopecia by damage to the follicles. Just underneath the hair follicles one can see the temporoparietal fascia. Dissection over this plane should expose the superior temporal line, respecting the temporal branches of facial nerve that run up to 3 cm above zygomatic arch and 1.5 cm posteriorly to orbital rim (Pitanguy's line—from 5 mm below tragus to 1.5 cm above the lateral extremity of eyebrow). Of note, the facial branches are situated in the superficial temporal fat pad between the superficial temporoparietal fascia and superficial layer of the deep temporal fascia, inferiorly the flap could be extended to through a dissection of the parotid gland and the STA and vein if more rotation is needed, posteriorly the flap can be freely extended even to aponeurotic gala but taking in consideration that the edges of the flap could be ischemic if too long. A reasonable option is to follow the posterior branch of STA and ligate the anterior one, with this sparing the facial zone and utilizing wisely the surface area of the flap. After complete separation from temporal fascia, the flap is rotated based on the inferior pedicle (Fig. 25.5).

Indications and Limitations

The TPF might be used to cover defects in the anterior and middle fossa. Endoscopic-assisted approaches might be implemented, such as the transpterygoid approach [19].

Its high vascularity and thinness make it an excellent, albeit time-consuming, alternative to cover large defects not only in the temporal fossa but also at the anterior fossa. Likewise, a bipedicled flap may provide an area of up to 15 cm wide, which is more than enough to cover the entire anterior cranial fossa [23].

In cases with previous trauma or surgery of the superficial temporal artery, other approaches should be considered.

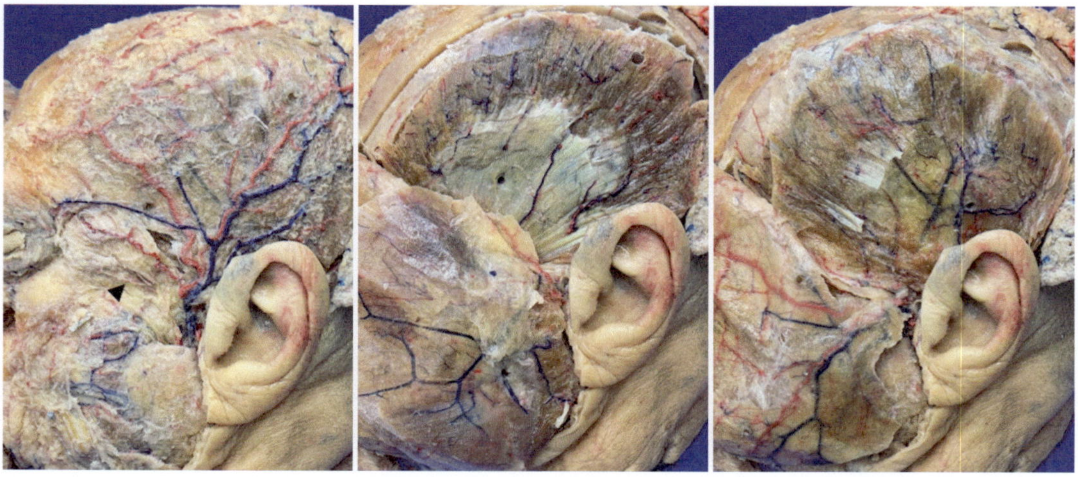

Fig. 25.5 A sequence of TPF dissection. The right dissection over superficial temporoparietal fascia (STF) shows STA pedicle and the temporal branches of the facial nerve (arrowhead), in the middle the STF fascia is reflected and is possible to see the superficial layer of deep temporal fascia covering the temporalis muscle, on the right the deep layer of the temporal fascia attached to pericranium and some fibers of the temporalis muscle

Key Points

- Damage of the hair follicles may result in alopecia, which can be avoided by dissecting the TPF from the overlying subcutaneous tissue under magnification.
- The superficial temporal artery is the main supply of the TPF. US Doppler may confirm its patency and elucidate its location when planning the incision.
- The TPF is a highly vascular flap.
- The TPF is deeply adherent to the adjacent tissues in the upper part of the dissection and close to the superior temporal line. As such, it is recommended to start the dissection near the ear where the loose areolar tissue permits to create a plane that might be followed cranially easily.
- Avoid the cauterization near its pedicle to prevent injury to its blood supply.
- One should not cross an imaginary line connecting the tragus to a point 3 cm superior and 2 cm lateral to the lateral supraorbital rim demarks an anterior line to avoid unintended injuries to the temporalis bran of the facial nerve.

25.5.2 Minimally Invasive Endoscopic Pericranial Flap [24]

In situations where a nasoseptal flap is not available for defects of the Zone 1, ventral skull base defects, a pericranial flap is a great alternative for reconstruction. The pericranial flap can be harvested via a full coronal incision or endoscopically with limited incisions.

If used for endonasal reconstruction, the flap is pedicled on one side and is harvested endoscopically through a mini coronal incision (5 cm). Skin and aponeurotic tissue are elevated from midline to temporal line using a long retractor and a scope. Careful dissection around supraorbital pedicles and Doppler localization are important to define pedicle width, usually 3 cm around the supraorbital artery. Flap transposition to the nasal cavity is prepared through 2 cm by 0.5 cm osteotomy over the nasion. Bilateral opening of the frontal recesses is completed endonasally, the flap is placed assisted by the endoscopic view and will rely upon the dura and the bone of anterior cranial fossa. The flap could reach from orbit to orbit all the way to the clivus. In order to optimize length, it is important to harvest the flap even more posterior than the coronal suture. Nose is packed to keep the flap in position. These are left in place for 5–7 days.

25.6 Microvascular Free Flaps in Open Approaches

A microvascular transfer of tissue is useful for repairing a three-dimensional defect in skull base open skull base surgery. Free microvascular tissue transfer is indicated to reconstruct complex, large, and difficult skull base defects, in cases of revision surgery and previously irradiated fields. The flap could be tailored to repair bone, dural, and soft tissue defects. By using microvascular free flaps, a volumetric fill of dead space is obtained with high vascular quality. Previous considerations are necessary such as the size of the defect, the donor site, viability of recipient's vessels.

There is a trend toward a more frequent use of free tissue transfer for the repair of the cranial base [2, 4, 25, 26]. Free flaps (FF) have some advantages over rotational flaps, as there is an increased risk of wound complications when the regional tissue has been previously irradiated or if there are plans for postoperative radiation [4]. On the other hand, these techniques usually require a qualified, trained surgeon, and it is time-consuming. Therefore, FF are, generally speaking, reserved for large defects, whenever previous or adjunctive radiation therapy has been already given or is planned to, or those defects involving several tissue layers [4].

Indications and Limitations

Free flaps are usually reserved for patients with extensive defects in which a maxillectomy is required, with or without orbital exenteration, or with large skin defects along the forehead and palpebral tissues [27]. Other authors have supported the idea of using this approach for large extensive defects, or when the regional tissue has been irradiated or there exist plans for postoperative radiation therapy.

Conversely, cosmetic results are not satisfactory in many cases. Likewise, using free pedicled flaps for repairing anterior and lateral cranial fossa defects requires longer operative times and increases the complexity of the surgery. Free flaps have, after all, a rate of complications between 10% and 50%, although higher rates of complications have been reported in series that included the most complex cases [4, 20, 27].

Key Points

1. Highly reliable method of reconstruction.
2. Consider donor site morbidity.
3. For a radial forearm flap, perform an Allen test, to ascertain adequate hand vascularization and avoid catastrophic complications.
4. Careful Doppler monitoring postoperatively.
5. Flap should be designed to fit the defect, preventing tension or kinking of the pedicle; therefore, avoiding areas of regional ischemia [12]
6. It is recommended to use the well-vascularized portion of the flap to complete a watertight seal of the dura.
7. Drain the donor site to prevent hematoma or seroma that may lead to secondary infection.
8. Prepares for alternative options.

25.7 Limitations and Complications of the External Approaches

When dealing with extensive approaches, it is essential to have an upfront discussion of potential risks and complications. It is important that the patient and all members of the teams are aware of potential complications and sequelae.

Persistent CSF leak may represent the most common major complication associated with skull base reconstruction. When combining the use of pedicled vascular flaps with a multilayer reconstruction technique and the aforementioned principles, the current literature range cites rates of postoperative CSF leaks between 5% and 10% [24]. Nonetheless, the incidence of CSF leak varies widely depending on the series reported, based on the magnitude of the defect, its location, and the approach/technique and materials used for closing the defect [16, 20, 27]. As such, recurrent CSF leaks are more frequent in the posterior fossa that anterior fossa defects, which are more frequent than in the middle cranial fossa. Pedicled flaps, despite its technical complexity, significantly reduced the rate of CSF leaks [4, 5]. Likewise, pericranial flap, despite its benefits as a versatile and mobile flap, has reported a higher incidence of infectious complications in comparison to other rotational flaps [16].

Another key factor in planning the surgical repair of a skull base defects is the planning of adjuvant therapies. As such, previously irradiated tissues or postoperative radiation therapy increase the risk of wound dehiscence and CSF leak [4, 27]. Therefore, in this setting, pedicled flaps have been advocated for several experts [4, 27].

Others consider that bony reconstruction of the skull base is necessary to prevent herniation of the cranial content [28]. However, reconstructive techniques that avoid the use of bone grafts have demonstrated a very low incidence of this complication [27]. Moreover, the use of bone grafts or implants has demonstrated an increased risk of wound dehiscences and infections [20].

The complexity of the resections and reconstructions of the lateral skull base does not allow for one ideal technique for a given defect. It is crucial for the reconstructive surgeons to evaluate all the options and use their clinical judgment to select a method that they feel would work best for the unique characteristics of each defect.

References

1. Irish JC, Gullane PJ, Gentili F, Freeman J, Boyd JB, Brown D, Rutka J. Tumors of the skull base: outcome and survival analysis of 77 cases. Head Neck. 1994;16(1):3–10.
2. Imola MJ, Sciarretta V, Schramm VL. Skull base reconstruction. Curr Opin Otolaryngol Head Neck Surg. 2003;11(4):282–90.
3. Caltabiano GA, Viglianesi A, Bellomia D, Chiaramonte R, Pero G, Chiaramonte I. Spontaneous temporal cerebrospinal fluid leak: a case report and literature review. Neuroradiol J. 2010;23(4):420–5.
4. Thompson NJ, Roche JP, Schularick NM, Chang KE, Hansen MR. Reconstruction outcomes following lateral skull base resection. Otol Neurotol. 2017;38(2):264–71.
5. Hachem RA, Elkhatib A, Beer-Furlan A, Prevedello D, Carrau R. Reconstructive techniques in skull base surgery after resection of malignant lesions: a wide array of choices. Curr Opin Otolaryngol Head Neck Surg. 2016;24(2):91–7.
6. Engle RD, Butrymowicz A, Peris-Celda M, Kenning TJ, Pinheiro-Neto CD. Split-calvarial osteopericranial flap for reconstruction following endoscopic anterior resection of cranial base. Laryngoscope. 2015;125(4):826–30.
7. Battaglia P, Turri-Zanoni M, Castelnuovo P, Prevedello DM, Carrau RL. Brain herniation after endoscopic transnasal resection of anterior skull base malignancies. Neurosurgery. 2015;11(3):457–62.
8. Taha M, Carroll T, McMahon J. Vascularized temporoparietal fascial flap for the treatment of a traumatic cerebrospinal fluid fistula in the middle cranial fossa. J Neurosurg. 2009;111(2):393–5.
9. Raffaini M, Costa P. The temporoparietal fascial flap in reconstruction of the cranio-maxillofacial area. J Cranio-Maxillofac Surg. 1994;22(5):261–7.
10. Hadad G, Bassagasteguy L, Carrau RL, Mataza JC, Kassam A, Snyderman CH, Mintz A. A novel reconstructive technique after endoscopic expanded endonasal approaches: vascular pedicle nasoseptal flap. Laryngoscope. 2006;116(10):1882–6.
11. Genden EM. Reconstruction of the head and neck: a defect-oriented approach. New York, NY: Thieme; 2012.
12. Urken ML. Multidisciplinary head and neck reconstruction: a defect-oriented approach. Lippincott Williams & Wilkins; 2012.
13. Snyderman CH, Janecka IP, Sekhar LN, Sen CN, Eibling DE. Anterior cranial base reconstruction: role of galeal and pericranial flaps. Laryngoscope. 1990;100(6):607–14.
14. Raveh J, Laedrach K, Speiser M, Chen J, Vuillemin T, Seiler R, Ebeling U, Leibinger K. The subcranial approach for fronto-orbital and anteroposterior skull-base tumors. Arch Otolaryngol Head Neck Surg. 1993;119:385–93.
15. Argenta LC, Friedman RJ, Dingman RO, Duus EC. The versatility of pericranial flaps. Plast Reconstr Surg. 1985;76(5):695–702.
16. Safavi-Abbasi S, Komune N, Archer JB, Sun H, Theodore N, James J, Little AS, Nakaji P, Sughrue ME, Rhoton AL, Spetzler RF. Surgical anatomy and utility of pedicled vascularized tissue flaps for multilayered repair of skull base defects. J Neurosurg. 2016;125(2):419–30.
17. Friedman JA, Ebersold MJ, Quast LM. Post-traumatic cerebrospinal fluid leakage. World J Surg. 2001;25(8):1062–6.
18. Tender GC, Kutz S, Awasthi D, Rigby P. Vascularized temporalis muscle flap for the treatment of otorrhea. J Neurosurg. 2003;98(5):1128–32.
19. Fortes FS, Carrau RL, Snyderman CH, Kassam A, Prevedello D, Vescan A, Mintz A, Gardner P. Transpterygoid transposition of a temporoparietal fascia flap: a new method for skull base reconstruction after endoscopic expanded endonasal approaches. Laryngoscope. 2007;117(6):970–6.
20. Hoang S, Torres MJ, Rivera AL, Litofsky NS. Middle cranial fossa approach to repair Tegmen defects with autologous or alloplastic graft. World Neurosurg. 2018;118:e10–7.
21. Davidge KM, van Furth WR, Agur A, Cusimano M. Naming the soft tissue layers of the temporoparietal region: unifying anatomic terminology across surgical disciplines. Neurosurgery. 2010;67(3):ons 120-3.
22. Poblete T, Jiang X, Komune N, Matsushima K, Rhoton AL. Preservation of the nerves to the frontalis muscle during pterional craniotomy. J Neurosurg. 2015;122(6):1274–82.
23. Krayenbühl N, Isolan GR, Hafez A, Yaşargil MG. The relationship of the fronto-temporal branches of the facial nerve to the fascias of the temporal region: a literature review applied to practical anatomical dissection. Neurosurg Rev. 2007;30(1):8–15.
24. Zanation AM, Snyderman CH, Carrau RL, Kassam AB, Gardner PA, Prevedello DM. Minimally invasive endoscopic pericranial flap: a new method for endonasal skull base reconstruction. Laryngoscope. 2009;119(1):13–8.
25. Thurnher D, Novak CB, Neligan PC, Gullane PJ. Reconstruction of lateral skull base defects after tumor ablation. Skull Base. 2007;17(01):079–88.
26. Moncrieff MD, Hamilton SA, Lamberty GH, Malata CM, Hardy DG, Macfarlane R, Moffat

DA. Reconstructive options after temporal bone resection for squamous cell carcinoma. J Plast Reconstr Aesthet Surg. 2007;60(6):607–14.
27. Gil Z, Abergel A, Leider-Trejo L, Khafif A, Margalit N, Amir A, Gur E, Fliss DM. A comprehensive algorithm for anterior skull base reconstruction after oncological resections. Skull Base. 2007;17(01): 025–37.
28. Derome PJ. The transbasal approach to tumors invading the base of the skull. Oper Neurosurg Tech. 1988;1:619–33.

Part V

Postoperative Instructions

26

Werner Hosemann and Peter Valentin Tomazic

26.1 Introduction

Any postoperative measure and monitoring strategy following closure of a frontal skull base leak is strongly dependent on the cause, size, location, and nature ("high ./. low flow") of the defect, on the chosen grafting material together with the applied technique for defect closure and also on certain other factors related to the patient's general medical condition [1, 2].

An important factor of successful skull base repair is to take proactive intraoperative measures in order to avoid healing and health problems in the subsequent clinical course (Fig. 26.1). This anticipative strategy may include preservation of mucosa and turbinate tissues as well as ensuring ventilation and drainage of dependent sinus compartments besides careful selection of local flaps and transplants for defect closure.

During the early postoperative period, medical observation and care is focused on recognizing or, better still, on avoidance of any complication and on minimizing deficits of nasal physiology besides providing on-time personal recovery and taking care of special problems like hormonal imbalance in those cases having had lesions in the pituitary region. Generally, the related recommendations and algorithms for postoperative observation and therapy differ in literature and evidence for most of the common postoperative regimens is low.

26.2 Packing of the Surgical Field and Duration of Packing

Various packing materials from resorbable materials like surgifoam, surgicell to non-resorbable gauze packing or a variety of balloons (e.g., foley catheter, rhinorapid sponges) are described in literature. Packing is used in around 60% of cases; however, large scale randomized control trials are missing to support its benefit. The same holds true for duration although many authors recommend to remove them 3–5 days after surgery. Resorbable materials are applied as support and keep grafting material in position. Balloons are used as an abutment for vascularized flaps mainly. Important considerations for packing are: (1) Not to displace the grafting material while placing the packing. (2) Insert a soft layer (e.g., surgifoam) of packing material between the graft and the remaining packing (e.g., balloon) to avoid ripping out the grafting material upon removal of packing. (3) Try to keep sinus outflow tracts open when placing resorbable material to maintain ventilation and drainage [3, 4].

W. Hosemann (✉)
Oto-Rhino-Laryngology, Head and Neck Surgery, University Hospital Greifswald, Greifswald, Germany

P. V. Tomazic
Division of General Otorhinolaryngology, Head and Neck Surgery, Medical University of Graz, Graz, Austria
e-mail: peter.tomazic@medunigraz.at

A. A. AlQahtani et al. (eds.), *CSF Rhinorrhea*, https://doi.org/10.1007/978-3-030-94781-1_26

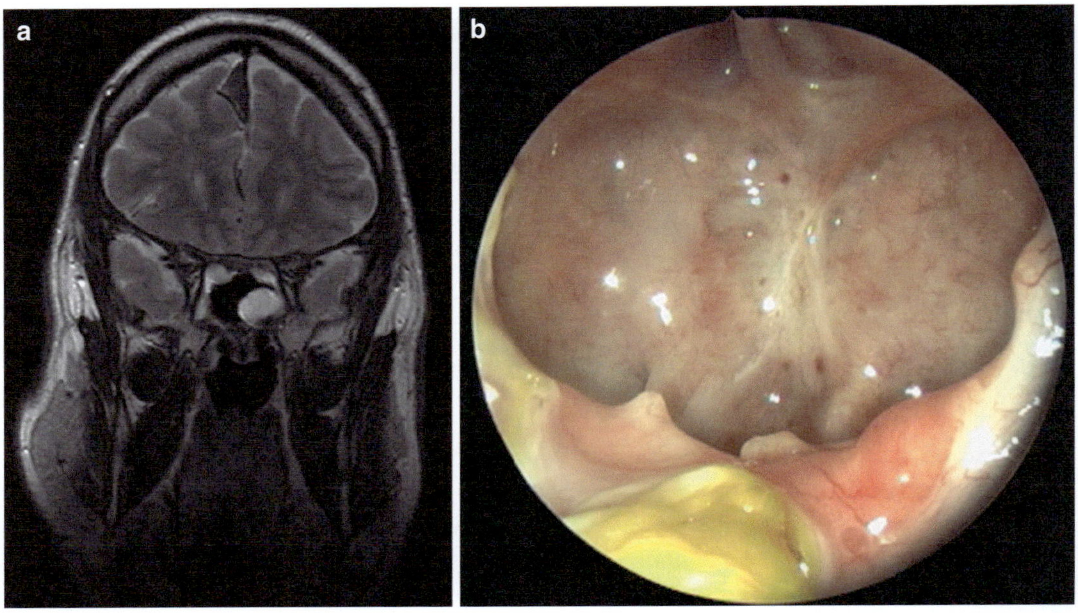

Fig. 26.1 (**a**) MRI revealing a small mucocele below the lateral parts of a nasoseptal flap after transsphenoidal surgery. (**b**) Endoscopy of the sphenoid sinus access several months later showing spontaneous resolution of the mucocele (30° endoscope)

26.3 General Postoperative Observation and Care

Immediately after skull base repair, atraumatic extubation merging with a smooth post-anesthetic recovery phase is strived for. Any delay of recovery from general anesthesia is attempted to be avoided.

Postoperative observation and treatment of patients in units for intermediate or intensive care are dependent on individual factors of the patient, the defect, and related closure techniques. Following repair of minor, clearly defined skull base defects, patients may be observed subsequently in a regular hospital ward for at least 24 h or for the time of administration of occlusive nasal packings. In contrast, those patients having had closure of big defects or patients having undergone major intradural manipulation should be supervised postoperatively in an intermediate intensive care unit (ICU) for at least 24 h monitoring vigilance, cognitive functions, motor activity and senses at defined time intervals. If felt necessary, a special ophthalmologic control is called for. A bladder catheter may be left in place overnight and removed the following day [2, 5, 6].

Lumbar drains are suggested as helpful in some publications to reduce the rate of postoperative CSF leaks after major endoscopic skull base surgery with repair of large dural defects. Other authors share the opposite view and avoid lumbar drains at all. In any case, duration of drainage is kept as short as possible [7–10].

Intake and output as well as serum and urine status (sodium, osmolarity) may be assessed and evaluated in patients after transsphenoidal interventions. Following major surgery on or nearby the pituitary gland and stalk, the pituitary–adrenal axis may be controlled by measuring the cortisol level in the morning of the second or third postoperative day and serum sodium concentration should be controlled at least once after 5–10 days. The incidence of postoperative sodium dysregulation ranges around 10% of respective major cases. As hyponatremia may occur also delayed and may show up in a nonspecific way, patients should be informed about the specific signs and symptoms. A regular endocrinologic control may be scheduled around 4–6 weeks postoperatively in appropriate cases. Hormonal substitution should be induced, if needed [11–13].

Relevant infections of the operative cavity may occur in around 1–2%. The most important risk factor is a more or less obvious postoperative CSF leak. Many infections are also causally linked with a lumbar drainage infection. Due to these facts, conspicuous nasal secretion at any time postoperatively is carefully collected and analyzed for beta$_2$-transferrin or by beta-trace protein assay in order to substantiate possible CSF leaks as timely as possible. Certain extended defects ($\geq$2 cm^2) around the sella and clivus show a higher risk of postoperative leaks also after regular closure with a nasoseptal flap. Greater care is generally required in obese patients and patients following radiotherapy [14–17].

Nasal cannulas and transnasal tubes are avoided as far as possible. Special caution is needed while inserting enteral feeding tubes transnasally—correct feeding tube placement should be documented radiographically [18].

Longer term postoperative follow-up continues until symptoms resolve and the endoscopic examination is near to normal.

26.4 Imaging (CT Brain) in Early Post-op Period

Role and timing of postoperative imaging is a matter of controversial debate in literature and is also dependent on individual factors of the patient. After long-lasting surgical interventions leading probably to a prolonged anesthetic recovery phase, CT scans are often called for as soon as possible. MRI may follow 48 h later.

Generally, a CT—or MRI—scan may be performed after major surgery on the first or second postoperative day to rule out incipient local, collateral, or intracranial complications (mostly infections, hemorrhage, accumulation of air), to control the correct position of any reconstruction material and to attest the viability of vascularized local flaps by administration of gadolinium in MRI. Immediate revision surgery may follow confirmation of impeding or actual complications. Besides, the first postoperative scans serve as a "baseline" for follow-up and may allow checking the completeness of resection. Early postoperative imaging is advised especially in tumor surgery to rule out confounding contrast enhancements by reactive granulation tissue at a later time [5, 6, 15].

Subsequent imaging is done on an individual base referring to local factors and the underlying disease. Following major surgery, an additional regular control of the findings by means of CT scan or MRI is performed around 3 months after the intervention. Some also benign tumors are scheduled for control imaging regularly after 6–12 months.

Viable vascular pedicled nasoseptal flaps have a characteristic enhanced MR imaging appearance (T1) after administration of gadolinium ("C-shaped flap" within the operative defect, "open cup appearance"). Lack of the respective enhancement may but must not indicate flap failure, risk for CSF leak, and the need of revision surgery [19–23].

Understanding the normal evolution of imaging features in the first 6 months after surgery which mirrors regular wound reaction and healing is advised for any surgeon. Secondary sinus opacities may persist even after 1 year and do often not correlate to clinical symptoms. Mucocele formation beneath naso-septal flaps may be expected in up to 3%, the range being higher in younger patients [23–27] (Fig. 26.1).

26.5 Bed Rest

As of today, no studies exist addressing bed rest after CSF leak repair. A wide range is reported in literature from 0.5 to 7 days. The empirical importance to that topic lies in the idea that patient would not displace grafting material by excess movements. Other ideas are that early patient mobilization reduces intracranial pressure and thus the rate of recurrent leakage. If bed rest is advocated, caution needs to be taken on antithrombotic measures. If the patient becomes mobilized, instructions about postoperative behavior and dos and don'ts need to be carefully addressed. Another associated factor to bed rest is length of hospital stay which also differs according to the medical system and associated costs [28].

26.6 Head Elevation

The postoperative elevation of the head follows the same principle as early mobilization in order to decrease intracranial pressure. There is no evidence in literature to support this. Since it does not cause additional burden to the patient or the personnel, it could be advocated in the postoperative course.

26.7 Deep Venous Thrombosis Prophylaxis

There is no sound evidence with regard to timing or type of medical anticoagulation in patients following skull base surgery. Generally, cautious movement and mobilization of patients is advocated after 24 h of bed rest. If neurological factors or specific drains impede autonomous mobilization and intensified nursing care cannot counterbalance this disadvantage, appropriate pharmacological regimens are called for [1, 10].

26.8 Hospital Stay

No studies exist to investigate the impact on hospital stay on success rates of endoscopic CSF leak repair, and this factor is also associated with the respective medical system and associated costs but is reported to be around 36 h [29].

26.9 Diet Restrictions

Patients are advised to have a soft and low-salt diet after CSF leak repair in addition to stool softeners and antiemetic therapy to avoid elevation of intracranial pressure through obstipation and/or vomiting. Soft diet should also decrease the risk of coughing. Moreover, food causing flatulence should be refrained from. In general, structured weight loss is recommended in obese patients to avoid recurrence.

26.10 Drug Therapy

Even minor local infection in the operative cavity may result in problems by, e.g., interfering with regular ingrowth of free tissue transplants. The recommended perioperative antibiotic regimens for prophylaxis differ in literature. Mostly i.v. antibiotic therapy is started immediately before surgery, and administration is continued for 24–48 h, followed by oral intake for 3–10 days. According to literature, cefalosporins (e.g., ceftriaxone) and vancomycin are the most frequently used drugs. Alternative pharmaceuticals are ampicillin-sulbactam, clarithromycin, aminoglycosides, or metronidazole as monotherapy or also in combination. The majority of authors promote therapy as long as any nasal packing is in place, not only to reduce the risk of toxic shock syndrome [1, 2, 6, 28, 30–32]. Two weeks postoperatively, Gentamicin is sometimes given as a nasal spray for about 2 months [33].

After major skull base surgery leading to manipulation of the pituitary gland or stalk, a prophylactic perioperative application of corticoids (e.g., 100 mg hydrocortisone) is often advised also in patients without previously defined pituitary dysfunction [1].

Sometimes antitussives, antiemetics, and antihistamines are also recommended. Stool softeners on demand may be given to avoid straining causing increases of intracranial pressure, and soft bowel regimen may be prolonged for a period of few weeks [4].

Intravenous pain medications may be given in the immediate postoperative period, being replaced by oral drugs like acetaminophen as soon as possible. Medications associated with coagulopathy or platelet dysfunction (NSAIDs) are restricted for a period of around 2 weeks.

If possible and tolerated, systolic blood pressure should be regulated to be not higher than 140 mm Hg. If an increased CSF pressure is suspected, additionally acetazolamide may be applied.

26.11 Precautions: Blowing the Nose, Lifting Heavy Objects, Leaning Forward, Sneezing, Coughing, Vomiting, Constipation, Physical Activity

Usually, certain rules of activity restriction are followed after skull base reconstruction—the level of stringency depends on the size of the skull base defect, type of repair, and individual biologic factors of the patient. Any patient is instructed to avoid maneuvers that may lead to inadequate intracranial pressure increase like heavy lifting, strenuous activity, and bearing down. The same holds true for pressure rise within the nasopharynx in conjunction with nose blowing, Valsalva maneuver, or sneezing—if it is inevitable, the latter should be done with the mouth open. Using straws for drinking should be avoided as negative nasopharyngeal pressure may result. These rules are maintained for up to 4 weeks [1, 2].

Tobacco use is generally restricted as smoking is a predictor of bad outcome concerning nasal physiology.

26.12 OSA Patients and CPAP

For patients with CSF leak repair, postoperative CPAP could cause displacement of grafts, recurrent leak, and pneumatocephalus internus. Many surgeons thus recommend to refrain from CPAP use postoperatively, but no studies are present to validate the timeline of resuming CPAP therapy. The recommendations thus are based on surveys by the NSABS and 91.4% of surgeons recommend pausing CPAP for low-flow intraoperative CSF leak and 92.2% for high-flow intraoperative CSF leak. At least 2 weeks of restrictions was recommended by the majority of surgeons in case of a low-flow intraoperative CSF leak (81.1%) or high-flow intraoperative CSF leak (87.9%) [34]. A more recent survey evaluated the timeline in more detail where in the presence of a small CSF leak, the mean duration would be 14.3 days (median, 14; SD, 9.8) and 20.7 days (median, 21; SD, 11.8) in the presence of a larger leak [35].

26.13 Air Travel

Small case studies have reported the association between recurrent CSF leak and/or pneumatocephalus following air travel after surgery. Again, there is no evidence what the optimal time interval between surgery and air travel is. The NSABS survey reported that 87% of surgeons recommended restrictions of at least 1 week with low-flow leaks and 81% recommended at least 2 weeks after high-flow leaks [34].

26.14 Sports and Heavy Duty Jobs

In animal studies, a sixfold increase of normal intracranial pressure was reached before porcine grafts failed [36] or 274–1048 cm H_2O, respectively, using various closure techniques which is a fivefold difference [37]. No human studies exist investigating the strength of grafts and their resistance to elevated intracranial pressure or the time interval to complete healing in and restitution of the integrity at skull base. However, the variability in in vivo animal studies is high and thus the time and extent of resumption of sports and heavy duty jobs should be critically evaluated. The principle is the same as in most recommendations that physical activity can lead to elevated intracranial pressure or mechanical forces leading to dislodging of grafts and recurrent leakage. Since most recommendations go toward a 1–2 week pause of activities, the time to resume more strenuous physical activity should be longer especially in contact sports or lifting of heavy items. Despite the fact of delayed CSF leak recurrence, the majority recurs within 2 weeks after primary surgery, thus a 4 weeks restriction seems feasible, but resumption of strenuous activities should definitely be preceded by nasal endoscopic follow-up [38].

26.15 Time Interval to Return to Normal Activity

Neville et al. showed that patients could artificially increase their CSF pressures by greater than 25 cm H_2O from a mean resting pressure of 14.6 cm H_2O to a mean pressure of 32.3 cm H_2O by applying the Valsalva maneuver [39]. No data exists as to what pressures early postoperative grafts are able to withstand changes but given the range of increasing intracranial pressure simply by the Valsalva maneuver patients should be informed thoroughly to avoid any pressure raising activity that may appear to be trivial like defecation, sexual activity, or lifting groceries. As for driving or starting to work, recommendations are to wait 1–2 weeks, respectively [34].

26.16 Postoperative Nasal Physiology and Local Nasal Care

The specific benefit of intensive and systematic intranasal debridement is often questioned in literature. Nevertheless, certain practical rules of local care may show benefits as well for patient's comfort as for the objective progress of local wound healing.

Postoperative nasal care is deliberately reduced during in the first days after removal of nasal packing. Generally, in this first phase of local nasal care, the major (inferior) intranasal airways are cautiously cleaned at least once a day to restore general nasal breathing and comfort. Local transplants at the skull base and also their specific covering with dissolvable packing remnants and crusts are not touched at all in this phase to avoid dislocation. Mist humidification is advised [1, 2].

Around 5 days later, the second phase of local care follows. Local care is extended and intensified as required according to endoscopic findings and patient's complaints. Any obstructing crust should be removed as long as no force is transferred to the area of skull base repair by that act. This area of grafting is not directly manipulated, and adherent crusts are left in place until they begin to separate spontaneously, usually within 2–6 weeks postoperatively. The patient is seen frequently with an individual but regular timetable. Proper healing is checked and any early sign of complication like local infection, CSF leak, or dislocation of transplants is looked for. Silastic splints covering a "reverse flap" on the nasal septum are removed after 10 days. For children who do not tolerate regular follow-up, also planned surgical debridement under general anesthesia may be considered.

Saline spray (0.9%) administration is started after removal of nasal packings. Antibiotic ointments may be introduced under endoscopic control especially into frontal sinuses following type 3 surgery. Saline irrigations are allowed 1–2 weeks postoperatively (e.g., twice a day) to wash out crusts, blood clots, and debris—this "nasal doushing" becomes the most important part of long-term local care [2].

Follow-up visits are scheduled at a later stage less frequently until nasal physiology is restored. A special training of olfaction may be advised in appropriate cases, structural integrity of the olfactory tract provided.

Following minor surgery, uneventful local healing leading to minor discomfort only may be expected. The most common postoperative complain usually is nasal crusting.

After major endonasal skull base surgery, the time-course of restrictions in nasal comfort usually is underestimated—nevertheless, the majority of patients shows a good QOL after 6 months. Postnasal drip and thick nasal discharge improve over 6–9 months [40–48] (Fig. 26.2).

The postoperative increase of intranasal space has no inevitable impact on the QOL; symptoms of an "empty nose" develop in exceptional cases only. Mucociliary clearance needs time to recover. The same holds true also for the olfactory sense in those cases with missing structural deficits. Younger patients suffer often more and longer; average postoperative QOL is also worse in patients aged ≥55 years [49–51].

Increased sinus opacification on postoperative imaging is generally noted after major surgery and may require continued follow-up and also specific management. The skull base does not

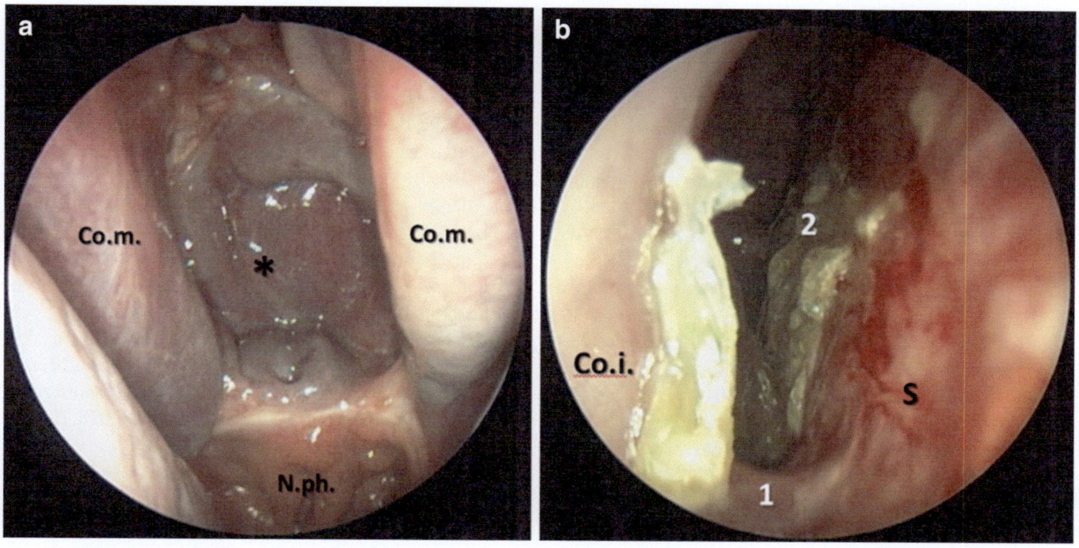

Fig. 26.2 (**a**) View into the posterior common nasal cavity after raise of a nasoseptal flap and also a reverse flap. Uneventful healing of the nasoseptal flap (*) in the posterior transsphenoidal surgical corridor. Mucosal function is normal. Co.m.: middle turbinate of both sides; N.ph.: nasopharynx (30° endoscope). (**b**) View into the anterior right nasal cavity after raise of a nasoseptal flap and secondary defect closure applying a reverse flap. Impaired nasal physiology revealing septoturbinal synechia (1) and major crusting (2). Co.i.: inferior turbinate; S: nasal septum (30° endoscope)

tend to slip down into the nasal cavity even after extensive reconstruction using exclusively soft tissues [47, 52].

Long-time nasal sequelae following major surgery applying nasoseptal flaps may result out of secondary septal perforation and local tissue necrosis leading, e.g., to nasal dorsum collapse. Other lasting complaints refer to anosmia or hyposmia, intranasal synechia or nasal valve failure. Secondary Meningitis or CSR leaks are reported with an incidence of 1–7% after major surgery [53–55].

26.17 Postoperative Adjuvant Radiotherapy in Malignant Tumors

Success and stability of skull base reconstruction are generally not endangered by necessary adjuvant or neoadjuvant radiotherapy and chemotherapy. Nevertheless, anticipating postoperative adjunctive therapy during the process of intraoperative selection of techniques for skull base reconstruction is advised, and preference of vascularized flaps is advocated. Delayed crop up of CSF leaks seems to be rare. Adjuvant therapy is scheduled and definitively started according to actual findings at follow-up visits about 6 weeks after major surgery. Patients have to be informed that postoperative radiotherapy is associated with significant reduction of the quality of life due to, e.g., increased crusting, bacterial overgrowth, and odor. Follow-up visits based on endoscopy are scheduled every 2 months during the first year, every 3 months for the second year, every 6 months until the fifth year, and then once a year. Clinical examinations are supplemented by control imaging in a different time grid [56–59].

References

1. Ramakrishnan VR, Waziri A. Postoperative care following skull base reconstruction. Adv Otorhinolaryngol. 2013;74:138–47.
2. Tien DA, Stokken JK, Recinos PF, Woodard TD, Sindwani R. Comprehensive postoperative management after endoscopic skull base surgery. Otolaryngol Clin N Am. 2016;49(1):253–63.

3. Hegazy HM, Carrau RL, Snyderman CH, Kassam A, Zweig J. Transnasal endoscopic repair of cerebrospinal fluid rhinorrhea: a meta-analysis. Laryngoscope. 2000;110(7):1166–72.
4. Oakley GM, Orlandi RR, Woodworth BA, Batra PS, Alt JA. Management of cerebrospinal fluid rhinorrhea: an evidence-based review with recommendations. Int Forum Allergy Rhinol. 2016;6(1):17–24.
5. Freyschlag CF, Gruber R, Bauer M, Grams AE, Thomé C. Routine postoperative computed tomography is not helpful after elective craniotomy. World Neurosurg. 2019;122:e1426–31.
6. Hosemann W, Schroeder HW. Comprehensive review on rhino-neurosurgery. GMS Curr Top Otorhinolaryngol Head Neck Surg. 2015;14:Doc01.
7. Casiano RR, Jassir D. Endoscopic cerebrospinal fluid rhinorrhea repair: is a lumbar drain necessary? Otolaryngol Head Neck Surg. 1999;121(6):745–50.
8. Horowitz G, Fliss DM, Margalit N, Wasserzug O, Gil Z. Association between cerebrospinal fluid leak and meningitis after skull base surgery. Otolaryngol Head Neck Surg. 2011;145(4):689–93.
9. Ransom ER, Palmer JN, Kennedy DW, Chiu AG. Assessing risk/benefit of lumbar drain use for endoscopic skull-base surgery. Int Forum Allergy Rhinol. 2011;1(3):173–7.
10. Zwagerman NT, Wang EW, Shin SS, Chang YF, Fernandez-Miranda JC, Snyderman CH, Gardner PA. Does lumbar drainage reduce postoperative cerebrospinal fluid leak after endoscopic endonasal skull base surgery? A prospective, randomized controlled trial. J Neurosurg. 2018;1:1–7.
11. Ausiello JC, Bruce JN, Freda PU. Postoperative assessment of the patient after transsphenoidal pituitary surgery. Pituitary. 2008;11(4):391–401.
12. Constantinidis J, Konstantinidis I. Avoiding complications in endoscopic skull base surgery. Curr Opin Otolaryngol Head Neck Surg. 2017;25(1):79–85.
13. Hussain NS, Piper M, Ludlam WG, Ludlam WH, Fuller CJ, Mayberg MR. Delayed postoperative hyponatremia after transsphenoidal surgery: prevalence and associated factors. J Neurosurg. 2013;119(6):1453–60.
14. Gruss CL, Al Komser M, Aghi MK, Pletcher SD, Goldberg AN, McDermott M, El-Sayed IH. Risk factors for cerebrospinal leak after endoscopic skull base reconstruction with nasoseptal flap. Otolaryngol Head Neck Surg. 2014;151(3):516–21.
15. Nunes RH, Abello AL, Zanation AM, Sasaki-Adams D, Huang BY. Imaging in endoscopic cranial Skull Base and pituitary surgery. Otolaryngol Clin N Am. 2016;49(1):33–62.
16. Kono Y, Prevedello DM, Snyderman CH, Gardner PA, Kassam AB, Carrau RL, Byers KE. One thousand endoscopic skull base surgical procedures demystifying the infection potential: incidence and description of postoperative meningitis and brain abscesses. Infect Control Hosp Epidemiol. 2011;32(1):77–83.
17. Ogiwara T, Nagm A, Hasegawa T, Hanaoka Y, Ichinose S, Goto T, Hongo K. Pitfalls of skull base reconstruction in endoscopic endonasal approach. Neurosurg Rev. 2019;42(3):683–9.
18. Hanna AS, Grindle CR, Patel AA, Rosen MR, Evans JJ. Inadvertent insertion of nasogastric tube into the brain stem and spinal cord after endoscopic skull base surgery. Am J Otolaryngol. 2012;33(1):178–80.
19. Adappa ND, Learned KO, Palmer JN, Newman JG, Lee JY. Radiographic enhancement of the nasoseptal flap does not predict postoperative cerebrospinal fluid leaks in endoscopic skull base reconstruction. Laryngoscope. 2012;122(6):1226–34.
20. Chabot JD, Patel CR, Hughes MA, Wang EW, Snyderman CH, Gardner PA, Fernandez-Miranda JC. Nasoseptal flap necrosis: a rare complication of endoscopic endonasal surgery. J Neurosurg. 2018;128(5):1463–72.
21. Jyotirmay H, Saxena SK, Ramesh AS, Nagarajan K, Bhat S. Assessing the viability of Hadad flap by postoperative contrast-enhanced magnetic resonance imaging. J Clin Diagn Res. 2017;11(6):MC01–3.
22. Kang MD, Escott E, Thomas AJ, Carrau RL, Snyderman CH, Kassam AB, Rothfus W. The MR imaging appearance of the vascular pedicle nasoseptal flap. AJNR Am J Neuroradiol. 2009;30(4):781–6.
23. Learned KO, Adappa ND, Lee JY, Newman JG, Palmer JN, Loevner LA. MR imaging evolution of endoscopic cranial defect reconstructions using nasoseptal flaps and their distinction from neoplasm. AJNR Am J Neuroradiol. 2014;35(6):1182–9.
24. Bleier BS, Wang EW, Vandergrift WA 3rd, Schlosser RJ. Mucocele rate after endoscopic skull base reconstruction using vascularized pedicled flaps. Am J Rhinol Allergy. 2011;25(3):186–7.
25. Karligkiotis A, Meloni F, Herman P, Castelnuovo P. How to avoid mucocele formation under pedicled nasoseptal flap. Am J Otolaryngol. 2014;35(4):546–7.
26. Vaezeafshar R, Hwang PH, Harsh G, Turner JH. Mucocele formation under pedicled nasoseptal flap. Am J Otolaryngol. 2012;33(5):634–6.
27. Walsh E, Illing E, Riley KO, Cure J, Srubiski A, Harvey RJ, Woodworth BA. Inaccurate assessments of anterior Cranial Base malignancy following Nasoseptal flap reconstruction. J Neurol Surg B Skull Base. 2015;76(5):385–9.
28. Lund VJ, Stammberger H, Nicolai P, Castelnuovo P, Beal T, Beham A, Bernal-Sprekelsen M, Braun H, Cappabianca P, Carrau R, Cavallo L, Clarici G, Draf W, Esposito F, Fernandez-Miranda J, Fokkens W, Gardner P, Gellner V, Hellquist H, Hermann P, Hosemann W, Howard D, Jones N, Jorissen M, Kassam A, Kelly D, Kurschel-Lackner S, Leong S, McLaughlin N, Maroldi R, Minovi A, Mokry M, Onerci M, Ong YK, Prevedello D, Saleh H, Sehti DS, Simmen D, Snyderman C, Solares A, Spittle M, Stamm A, Tomazic P, Trimarchi M, Unger F, Wormald PJ, Zanation A. European Rhinologic Society Advisory Board on Endoscopic Techniques in the Management of Nose, Paranasal Sinus and Skull Base Tumours. European position paper on endoscopic management of tumours

of the nose, paranasal sinuses and skull base. Rhinol Suppl. 2010;22:1–143.
29. Yadav YR, Parihar V, Janakiram N, Pande S, Bajaj J, Namdev H. Endoscopic management of cerebrospinal fluid rhinorrhea. Asian. J Neurosurg. 2016;11(3): 183–93.
30. Carrau RL, Snyderman C, Janecka IP, Sekhar L, Sen C, D'Amico F. Antibiotic prophylaxis in cranial base surgery. Head Neck. 1991;13(4):311–7.
31. Hasegawa H, Shin M, Kondo K, Saito N. Reconstruction of dural defects in endoscopic transnasal approaches for intradural lesions using multilayered fascia with a pressure-control spinal drainage system. World Neurosurg. 2018;114:e1316–24.
32. Johans SJ, Burkett DJ, Swong KN, Patel CR, Germanwala AV. Antibiotic prophylaxis and infection prevention for endoscopic endonasal skull base surgery: our protocol, results, and review of the literature. J Clin Neurosci. 2018;47:249–53.
33. Brown SM, Anand VK, Tabaee A, Schwartz TH. Role of perioperative antibiotics in endoscopic skull base surgery. Laryngoscope. 2007;117(9):1528–32.
34. Roxbury CR, Lobo BC, Kshettry VR, D'Anza B, Woodard TD, Recinos PF, Snyderman CH, Sindwani R. Perioperative management in endoscopic endonasal skull-base surgery: a survey of the North American Skull Base Society. Int Forum Allergy Rhinol. 2018;8(5):631–40.
35. Choi DL, Reddy K, Weitzel EK, Rotenberg BW, Vescan A, Algird A, Sommer D, D. Postoperative continuous positive airway pressure use and nasal saline rinses after endonasal endoscopic skull base surgery in patients with obstructive sleep apnea: a practice pattern survey. Am J Rhinol Allergy. 2019;33(1): 51–5.
36. de Almeida JR, Morris A, Whyne CM, James AL, Witterick IJ. Testing biomechanical strength of in vitro cerebrospinal fluid leak repairs. J Otolaryngol Head Neck Surg. 2009;38:106–11.
37. Fandino M, Macdonald K, Singh D, Whyne C, Witterick I. Determining the best graft-sealant combination for skull base repair using a soft tissue in vitroporcine model. Int Forum Allergy Rhinol. 2013;3:212–6.
38. Naunheim MR, Sedaghat AR, Lin DT, Bleier BS, Holbrook EH, Curry WT, Gray ST. Immediate and delayed complications following endoscopic Skull Base surgery. J Neurol Surg B Skull Base. 2015;76(5):390–6.
39. Neville L, Egan RA. Frequency and amplitude of elevation of cerebrospinal fluid resting pressure by the Valsalva maneuver. Can J Ophthalmol. 2005;40: 775–7.
40. Awad AJ, Mohyeldin A, El-Sayed IH, Aghi MK. Sinonasal morbidity following endoscopic endonasal skull base surgery. Clin Neurol Neurosurg. 2015;130: 162–7.
41. Balaker AE, Bergsneider M, Martin NA, Wang MB. Evolution of sinonasal symptoms following endoscopic anterior skull base surgery. Skull Base. 2010;20(4):245–51.
42. Bedrosian JC, McCoul ED, Raithatha R, Akselrod OA, Anand VK, Schwartz TH. A prospective study of postoperative symptoms in sinonasal quality-of-life following endoscopic skull-base surgery: dissociations based on specific symptoms. Int Forum Allergy Rhinol. 2013;3(8):664–9.
43. de Almeida JR, Snyderman CH, Gardner PA, Carrau RL, Vescan AD. Nasal morbidity following endoscopic skull base surgery: a prospective cohort study. Head Neck. 2011;33(4):547–51.
44. de Almeida JR, Witterick IJ, Gullane PJ, Gentili F, Lohfeld L, Ringash J, Thoma A, Vescan AD. Physical morbidity by surgical approach and tumor location in skull base surgery. Head Neck. 2013;35(4):493–9.
45. Little AS, Kelly D, Milligan J, Griffiths C, Prevedello DM, Carrau RL, Rosseau G, Barkhoudarian G, Otto BA, Jahnke H, Chaloner C, Jelinek KL, Chapple K, White WL. Predictors of sinonasal quality of life and nasal morbidity after fully endoscopic transsphenoidal surgery. J Neurosurg. 2015;122(6):1458–65.
46. Pant H, Bhatki AM, Snyderman CH, Vescan AD, Carrau RL, Gardner P, Prevedello D, Kassam AB. Quality of life following endonasal skull base surgery. Skull Base. 2010;20(1):35–40.
47. Riley CA, Tabaee A, Conley L, Amine M, Soneru CP, Anand VK, Schwartz TH. Long-term sinonasal outcomes after endoscopic skull base surgery with nasoseptal flap reconstruction. Laryngoscope. 2019;129(5):1035–40.
48. Seo MY, Nam DH, Kong DS, Lee JJ, Ryu G, Kim HY, Dhong HJ, Chung SK, Lee KE, Hong SD. Quality of life after extended versus transsellar endoscopic skull base surgery from 767 patients. Laryngoscope. 2019;129(6):1318–24.
49. Alobid I, Enseñat J, Mariño-Sánchez F, de Notaris M, Centellas S, Mullol J, Bernal-Sprekelsen M. Impairment of olfaction and mucociliary clearance after expanded endonasal approach using vascularized septal flap reconstruction for skull base tumors. Neurosurgery. 2013;72(4):540–6.
50. McCoul ED, Patel AS, Bedrosian JC, Anand VK, Schwartz TH. Intranasal cross-sectional area and quality of life changes following endoscopic transsphenoidal skull base surgery. Int Forum Allergy Rhinol. 2015;5(12):1124–8.
51. Jones SH, Iannone AF, Patel KS, Anchouche K, Raza SM, Anand VK, Schwartz TH. The impact of age on long-term quality of life after endonasal endoscopic resection of skull base meningiomas. Neurosurgery. 2016;79(5):736–45.
52. Eloy JA, Shukla PA, Choudhry OJ, Singh R, Liu JK. Assessment of frontal lobe sagging after endoscopic endonasal transcribriform resection of anterior skull base tumors: is rigid structural reconstruction of the cranial base defect necessary? Laryngoscope. 2012;122(12):2652–7.
53. Conger A, Zhao F, Wang X, Eisenberg A, Griffiths C, Esposito F, Carrau RL, Barkhoudarian G, Kelly DF. Evolution of the graded repair of CSF leaks and skull base defects in endonasal endoscopic tumor sur-

gery: trends in repair failure and meningitis rates in 509 patients. J Neurosurg. 2018;130:861–75.
54. Dolci RLL, Miyake MM, Tateno DA, Cançado NA, Campos CAC, Dos Santos ARL, Lazarini PR. Postoperative otorhinolaryngologic complications in transnasal endoscopic surgery to access the skull base. Braz J Otorhinolaryngol. 2017;83(3):349–55.
55. Lavigne P, Faden DL, Wang EW, Snyderman CH. Complications of nasoseptal flap reconstruction: a systematic review. J Neurol Surg B Skull Base. 2018;79(Suppl 4):S291–9.
56. Alves MV, Roberts D, Levine NB, DeMonte F, Hanna EY, Kupferman ME. Impact of chemoradiotherapy on CSF leak repair after skull base surgery. J Neurol Surg B Skull Base. 2014;75(5):354–7.
57. Castelnuovo P, Lepera D, Turri-Zanoni M, Battaglia P, Bolzoni Villaret A, Bignami M, Nicolai P, Dallan I. Quality of life following endoscopic endonasal resection of anterior skull base cancers. J Neurosurg. 2013;119(6):1401–9.
58. Perry A, Graffeo CS, Copeland WR 3rd, Van Abel KM, Carlson ML, Pollock BE, Link MJ. Delayed cerebrospinal fluid rhinorrhea after gamma knife radiosurgery with or without preceding transsphenoidal resection for pituitary pathology. World Neurosurg. 2017;100:201–7.
59. Turri-Zanoni M, Zocchi J, Lambertoni A, Giovannardi M, Karligkiotis A, Battaglia P, Locatelli D, Castelnuovo P. Endoscopic endonasal reconstruction of anterior skull base defects: what factors really affect the outcomes? World Neurosurg. 2018;116:e436–43.

Surgical Complications of Skull Base Reconstruction

27

Aldo Stamm, Eduardo Vellutini, and Camila Dassi

27.1 Prevention of Complications

Complex neurovascular structures that involve the skull base (SB) make it a surgically challenging region. Complications involving the SB are potentially catastrophic and should be taken into account, when considering the surgical indication [1].

In order to avoid complications, otolaryngologists and neurosurgeons must be properly trained in endoscopic skull base surgery. The challenges involving a three- or four-handed endoscopic surgery are broader when compared with a standard endoscopic sinonasal procedure. A graduated exposure to increasingly complex cases is vital, in order to achieve satisfactory expertise before facing extended endoscopic approaches [2].

Familiarity with the anatomic region and the specific techniques involving each area of the skull base is the keystone of a successful procedure. Surgical planning including review of preoperative images, multidisciplinary tumor meetings, anticipation of outcomes and complications, and detailing of the instruments necessary for the procedure are crucial to surgical success. Further, detailed planning for the reconstruction of the defect, especially if there is a large defect, is paramount [3–6].

During the operation, cautious dissection and identification of the anatomical structures along with minimal trauma to the neurovascular components are key principles that will lead to a favorable outcome [7–9].

27.2 Early Complications

27.2.1 Injury of Ethmoidal Arteries

Nasal cavity mucosa is the most common source of bleeding, both intraoperatively and postoperatively. The donor area site of the nasoseptal flap and the flap itself are common causes of perioperative oozing and postoperative epistaxis. Measures such as pre-packing the nose with neuropatties soaked in cocaine-epinephrine solution, infiltration of the mucosa with 1:100,000 epinephrine solution, meticulous manipulation of the nasal mucosa, warm saline irrigation, and electrocautery are effective options to control the mucosal bleeding during the procedure [10].

Supplementary Information The online version contains supplementary material available at [https://doi.org/10.1007/978-3-030-94781-1_27].

A. Stamm (✉)
Department of Otolaryngology, Complexo Hospitalar Edmundo Vasconcelos (HPEV), São Paulo, Brazil

E. Vellutini
Neurosciences coordinator, Hospital Alemão Oswaldo Cruz, São Paulo, Brazil

C. Dassi
Department of Otolaryngology, Complexo Hospitalar Edmundo Vasconcelos (HPEV), São Paulo, Brazil

Division of Rhinology, Department of Otolaryngology, Auckland City Hospital, Auckland, New Zealand

A. A. AlQahtani et al. (eds.), *CSF Rhinorrhea*, https://doi.org/10.1007/978-3-030-94781-1_27

Regarding arterial bleeding in the sinonasal cavity, care should be taken with the sphenopalatine artery and anterior and posterior ethmoidal arteries. During a transethmoid, transpterygoid, or transcribiform approach, careful identification of the arteries and their preemptive cauterization or ligation is recommended [10, 11].

In case of accidental injury to the anterior or posterior ethmoidal artery, complications such as severe hemorrhage, orbital hematoma, and CSF leak can occur. Active bleeding must be promptly controlled with bipolar cautery and close observation of the orbit is mandatory [12]. In some cases of posterior ethmoidal artery injury, drilling of the bony coverage of the artery may be necessary. If satisfactory endoscopic control of the bleeding cannot be achieved, an external approach through a Lynch incision is recommended for more proximal control of the artery. The anterior ethmoidal artery lies approximately 22–25 mm posterior to the anterior lacrimal crest while the posterior ethmoidal artery lies around 12–15 mm posterior to the anterior ethmoidal artery [10, 13].

27.2.2 Cranial Nerve Morbidity

A pedicled vascularized flap is the most common technique used on a multilayered reconstruction of the skull base. They are frequently associated with free fat grafts, fascia lata graft, and alloplastic materials [14].

One must consider the size of the free fat graft. Large grafts may result in the compression of the optic chiasm or optic nerves resulting in visual deterioration [15]. This is most likely to be seen after extensive drilling of the optic canal during tuberculum sellae meningioma resection.

Likewise, a "gasket seal" technique for skull base reconstruction usually results in a watertight closure of the defect and is also related to low rates of postoperative CSF leak [16]. Damage to the optic and abducens (II and VI) nerves may occur when there is a skull base defect with narrow or unstable bony rims in association with a large-sized piece of cartilage or bone used for the "Gasket-seal."

27.2.3 Mucosal Flap Necrosis

Mucosal flap necrosis is a rare complication of vascularized reconstructions. The nasoseptal flap is based upon blood supply from the nasoseptal artery and may undergo ischemic necrosis if the pedicle is injured [17].

Long surgical procedures may lead to the flap's death when surgical instruments constantly retract its pedicle. Special care should be taken during transclival, cranial-vertebral junction and transpterygoid approaches, so as to avoid inadvertent manipulation of the flap [17]. Further, narrow pedicles as a result of reoperations or technical problems while harvesting the flap may be risk factors for the nasoseptal flap necrosis (Video 27.1).

Once this complication is identified, a revision surgery should be performed.

27.2.4 Surgical Site Infection

Surgical site infections (SSIs) are infections that occur in the wound produced during an invasive surgical procedure. Meningitis, intracranial abscess, and osteomyelitis are rare but notable complications related to skull base surgery [18].

In order to avoid SSI, perioperative antibiotics are commonly used. However, the impact of it on infectious rates is unclear and the routine use of prophylactic antibiotics in endoscopic skull base surgery is also highly debated [19–21].

Besides the fact that there are no current formal recommendations for perioperative antibiotic use in skull base surgery, and regimens vary greatly across institutions, we believe that this practice might avoid infectious complications.

In our practice, we usually use an intravenous first-generation cephalosporin during anesthetic induction for all endoscopic skull base procedures and re-dosing is used on procedures that last more than 6 h. When non-absorbable packing is placed, intravenous cephalosporins are prescribed during the first 48 h, or until the packing is removed, this being followed by 7 days of oral antibiotics. If there is no nasal packing, an oral second-generation antibiotic is prescribed on a 7-day course in order to avoid acute sinusitis and extensive crusting.

27.2.5 Injury of Descending Palatine Nerve and Vidian Nerve During Access to Stemberg's Canal Defect

Sternberg's canal is a result of an incomplete fusion of different components of the sphenoid bone during intrauterine and childhood development. It forms a lateral craniopharyngeal canal, which connects the middle cranial fossa and the sphenoidal sinus. This extremely rare malformation can lead to CSF rhinorrhea, meningocele, or encephalocele [22–24].

Surgical management of CSF leaks of the lateral wall of the sphenoid sinus is challenging. Transcranial and endonasal endoscopic approaches have been effectively used in order to treat this condition, and the route to be chosen is based on the surgical team experience and on how far lateral the defect is. Regardless of its surgical complexity and its potential complications, a transethmoidal–pterygoidal–sphenoidal approach is an useful option for treating CSF leaks of the lateral [25].

When undertaking the transpterygoid approach, neural and vascular complications are the most significant. Vidian nerve injury can result in a decreased tear production that can lead to keratoconjunctivitis sicca. Another major neural complication is injury to the descending palatine nerve during the pterygopalatine fossa dissection resulting in palatal hypoesthesia. Furthermore, the infraorbital and maxillary (V2) nerves can be injured during this approach. Vascular complications encompass injury to the carotid artery and internal maxillary artery [26].

Accurate knowledge of the anatomy surrounding Sternberg's canal is the key to avoid vascular and neural complications when managing CSF leaks in this area.

27.2.6 Early Complications of Postoperative CSF Leaks

27.2.6.1 Chemical or Infectious Meningitis/Encephalitis

Meningitis is a potentially life-threatening complication of endoscopic skull base surgery that occurs in less than 5% of all cases [27]. It is mostly related to failure of the reconstruction and persistent CSF leak [28]. The overall CSF leak rate when vascularized flaps are used for the repair of the skull base defect can be up to 6%, higher rates are related to free mucosal grafts reconstructions [29, 30].

Whether infectious or chemical in nature, meningitis commonly presents with fever, headache, malaise, altered mental status and meningismus. While true bacterial meningitis must be diagnosed and promptly treated with antibiotics, chemical meningitis requires immediate treatment with steroids [27, 31].

Chemical meningitis results from irritation of the meninges with triggers such as physical manipulation, blood, foreign materials, bone dust and rupture of cystic lesions as in craniopharyngiomas and cholesterol granulomas [27, 31, 32]. The inflammatory-induced response can further lead to cerebrovascular vasospasm, thromboembolic events, and death.

With a similar presentation profile, differentiation between bacterial and chemical meningitis is challenging, and it is usually based on laboratorial findings. CSF culture growth of an infectious agent would diagnose infectious meningitis; however, sterile cultures do not exclude it especially when empiric antibiotics are prescribed before the collection of the samples. When suspected, patients with low-grade fevers, normal CSF glucose, low CSF lactate, and mild serum leukocytosis are most likely to have aseptic meningitis [27].

Nonetheless, infectious meningitis must be promptly treated to avoid potentially devastating outcomes. At initial presentation, it is hard to distinguish from chemical meningitis, it is recommended that all patients be empirically treated with antibiotics. The treatment may be discontinued after 72 h of sterile CSF cultures in cases where the harms of long-term antibiotics are greater than the dangers of bacterial meningitis [27, 31]. If there is a high suspicion of aseptic meningitis but no laboratory evidence, steroids can be added to the treatment regimen.

27.2.6.2 Pneumocephalus

While slow reabsorption of intracranial air is expected following a skull base surgery, a tension pneumocephalus (TP) is caused by a one-way passage of air through the dural defect (Fig. 27.1). Consequently, the air expansion into the intracranial space may result in increased intracranial pressure, extra-axial compression of brain parenchyma, and eventual fatal brainstem herniation.

The "Mount Fuji" sign on a CT scan is a classic find of a TP and consists of hypoattenuating subdural air that compresses and separates the frontal lobes [33].

Suspected TP necessitates prompt surgical release of the trapped air and a new and reinforced reconstruction of the skull base defect. Supplemental oxygen and strict maintenance of the blood pressure are important adjuvants to surgical treatment to maintain parenchymal perfusion [34].

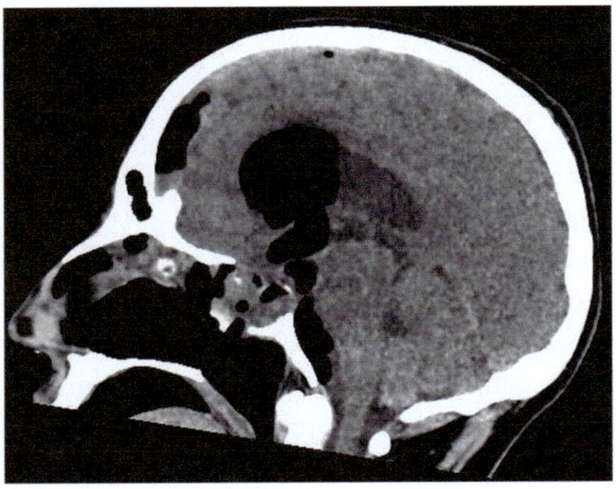

Fig. 27.1 Sagittal CT scan showing failure of the reconstruction of the skull base and subsequent pneumocephalus after 30 days of a re-do operation for pituitary adenoma

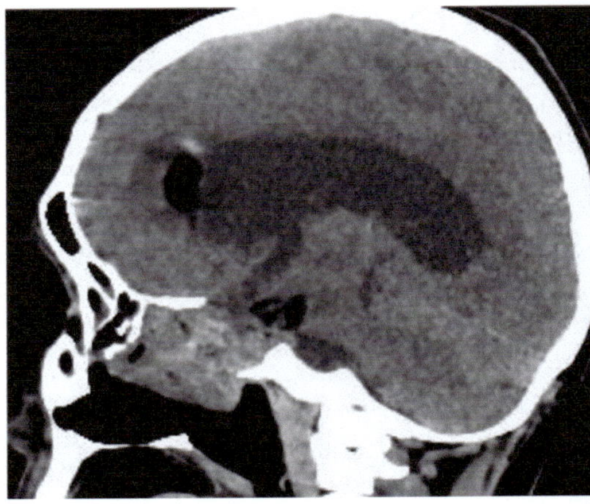

Fig. 27.2 Sagittal CT scan showing hydrocephalus after 62 days of skull base repair with a microvascular flap

27.2.6.3 Hydrocephalus

Hydrocephalus is a result of an imbalance between production and absorption of CSF that leads to distension of the ventricular system of the brain. Hydrocephalus has a range of incidence from 0.1% to 5.9% [35–37]. Prior craniotomy, prior radiation therapy, and postoperative CSF infection were also associated with an increased risk of developing hydrocephalus (Fig. 27.2).

Causes of hydrocephalus are numerous; however, neurosurgical procedures, especially those that involve opening of the ventricular system are more likely to complicate with hydrocephalus. Headache, disturbance of consciousness, nausea, vomiting, and psychomotor slowing are the main signs and symptoms related to this complication [38].

The occurrence of hydrocephalus after neurosurgical operations usually requires implantation of an external ventricular drain in the acute phase for the stabilization of intracranial pressure. Some patients will need permanent treatment, which is usually achieved with an implantation of a ventriculoperitoneal shunt [38].

27.3 Late Complications

27.3.1 Brain Herniation

A very unusual complication of endoscopic cranial resections, frontal lobe herniation seems

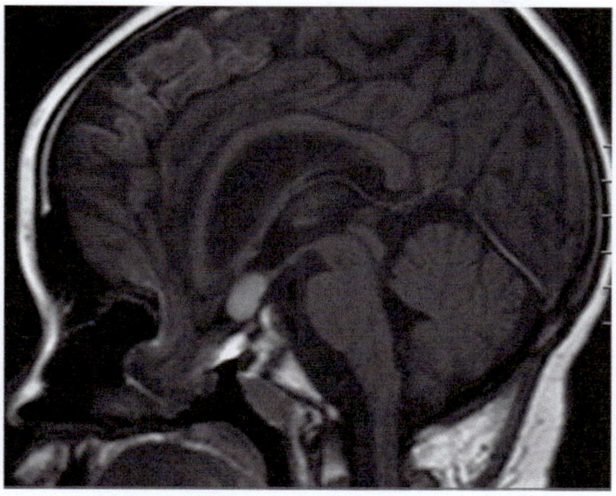

Fig. 27.3 Sagittal T1 MRI showing a 7-year-old patient with brain herniation through the skull base defect after a transplanum approach for craniopharyngioma

to be more related to the presence of increased intracranial pressure than to the size of the anterior skull base defect, surgical technique, and type of reconstruction (Fig. 27.3).

During the preoperative assessment for expanded endoscopic anterior skull base resection, clinical and radiological assessment for undiagnosed intracranial hypertension is especially recommended in patients with obesity and history of obstructive sleep apnea [39].

In high-risk patients, weight loss, sodium restriction, and acetazolamide may decrease the risk of long-term failure of anterior skull base reconstruction.

During the surgery, multilayered non-rigid reconstruction of the defect is paramount for a favorable outcome and will be enough in the vast majority of cases [40]. External transcranial approach may be considered in cases of repeated-failure of the reconstruction [39].

27.3.2 Anosmia/Hyposmia

Olfactory complications following skull base reconstruction have been the target of several studies in recent years. Although the results are controversial, the majority of them have suggested a direct relationship between the utilization of a vascularized nasoseptal flap and possible worsening of hyposmia and anosmia [41–44].

There is evidence that preserving normal sinonasal mucosa by limiting the disruption along the nasal cavity, avoiding middle turbinate resection, preserving the olfactory strip, and reducing the utilization of nasoseptal flaps may lessen postoperative morbidity related to nasal symptoms and improve rates of olfactory dysfunction [45–47].

27.3.3 Septal Perforation After Graft or Flap

Perforation develops in 14% of cases and may develop from septal cartilage necrosis as a result of the decreased vascular supply to the contralateral septal mucosa [48, 49]. The main finding related to septal perforations is mild crusting, which can be managed, in the majority of the cases, with nasal saline irrigation [48].

An interesting alternative to the conventional posterior septectomy that results in a posterior septal perforation is harvesting the nasoseptal flap from one side of the nasal septum while the mucosa from the contralateral side is completely preserved. A conventional hemitransfixion incision is performed on the contralateral side allowing the binostril approach. As with a conventional septoplasty, the hemitransfixion incision is sutured at the end of the procedure and the posterior septal perforation is avoided [50–53].

Careful preservation of the contralateral posterior nasoseptal artery, avoidance of mucosal trauma and intermittent releasing of the pressure against the nasal valve area with scopes seem to be helpful maneuvers that can preserve blood supply and potentially decrease septal complications [48, 49].

27.3.4 Donor Site Morbidity

Donor site morbidity is an important consideration in the overall decision-making algorithm for skull base reconstruction.

27.3.4.1 Anterolateral Thigh

Free tissue transfer from the thigh provides well-vascularized composite tissue options for reconstructing the skull base. Main complications related to lateral thigh free flaps are hematomas (0.9%), seromas (2%), wound dehiscence (3.8%), protracted pain for longer than 6 months (2.6%), paresthesia (33%), and musculoskeletal dysfunction (3.4%) [54, 55].

27.3.4.2 Temporoparietal Flap

The temporoparietal fascia flap (TPFF) is a useful tool for the reconstruction of large skull base defects such as resected dura or uncovered internal carotid arteries. It is usually indicated when local pedicled flaps are no longer available. Risks of alopecia, wound-healing problems, and injury of the frontal branch of the facial nerve must be taken in consideration when choosing this type of reconstruction [56].

Damage to the frontal branch of the facial (VII) nerve is always of concern among surgeons and to minimize the risk, it is recommended that the dissection remain deep to the fat pad that separates the superficial and deep layers of the temporal fascia [56].

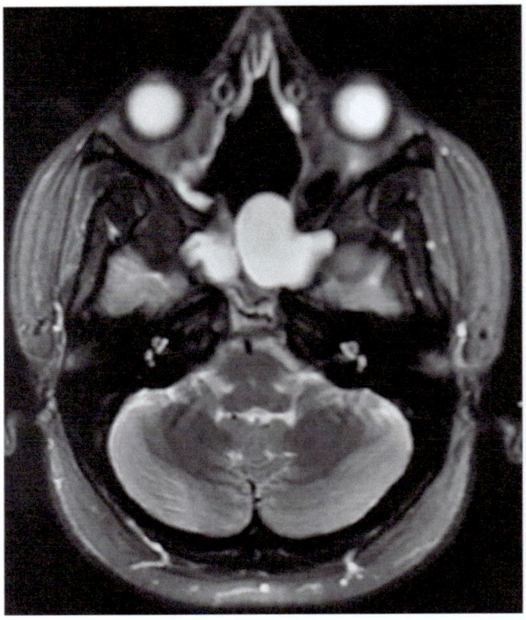

Fig. 27.4 Axial T2 MRI showing a sphenoid mucocele on the reconstruction site. Incidental finding during a 3 months postoperative follow-up after a clival chordoma resection

27.3.4.3 Pericranial Flap

The pericranial flap (PF) is an older but still pertinent option to reconstruct the skull base defect after endoscopic endonasal approaches. Regarding the indication, a PF can substitute a vascularized nasoseptal flap in cases where the latter is not available [57].

The morbidity related to the donor area of the pericranial flap is generally mild with scalp edema, pain and hematoma as the main complications. Hematoma is usually avoided by using a suction drain for 1 day [57].

27.3.5 Paranasal Sinus Mucocele

During the past two decades, vascularized flaps have been the workhorse for the reconstruction of skull base defects. As this method involves a possible insert of the tissue over normal mucosa, mucocele formation must be monitored for during long-term postoperative care (Fig. 27.4).

To minimize mucocele formation, cautious stripping of the sphenoid sinus mucosa adjacent to the defect is recommended. It is usually unavoidable to have some degree of mucosa remaining under the flap but despite this, the rates of mucocele formation after skull base reconstruction are usually lower than expected [58].

A short-term risk of 3.6% was found in patients in which aggressive mucosal stripping was avoided [58] although some authors have reported rates of between 0% and 8% [58, 59]. The pediatric population is thought to be at particular risk for this type of complication with incidence reported as high as 25% [41].

In cases that complicate with mucocele formation during long-term follow-up after skull base reconstruction, surgical treatment is usually required.

References

1. Chaaban MR, Woodworth BA. Complications of skull base reconstruction. Adv Otorhinolaryngol. 2013;74:148–62.
2. Nogueira JF, Stamm A, Vellutini E. Evolution of endoscopic skull base surgery, current concepts,

and future perspectives. Otolaryngol Clin N Am. 2010;43(3):639–52.
3. Harvey RJ, Nogueira JF, Schlosser RJ, Patel SJ, Vellutini E, Stamm AC. Closure of large skull base defects after endoscopic transnasal craniotomy. Clinical article. J Neurosurg. 2009;111(2):371–9.
4. Stamm AC, Pignatari SSN, Vellutini E. Transnasal endoscopic surgical approaches to the clivus. Otolaryngol Clin N Am. 2006;39(3):639–56, xi
5. Vellutini Ede AS, Balsalobre L, Hermann DR, Stamm AC. The endoscopic endonasal approach for extradural and intradural clivus lesions. World Neurosurg. 2014;82(6 Suppl):S106–15.
6. Stamm AC, Balsalobre L, Hermann D, Chisholm E. Endonasal endoscopic approach to clival and posterior fossa chordomas. Oper Tech Otolaryngol Head Neck Surg. 2011;22(4):274–80.
7. Beer-Furlan A, Vellutini EAS, Balsalobre L, Stamm AC. Endoscopic endonasal approach to ventral posterior fossa meningiomas: from case selection to surgical management. Neurosurg Clin N Am. 2015;26(3):413–26.
8. Mangussi-Gomes J, Beer-Furlan A, Balsalobre L, Vellutini EAS, Stamm AC. Endoscopic endonasal management of skull base chordomas: surgical technique, nuances, and pitfalls. Otolaryngol Clin N Am. 2016;49(1):167–82.
9. Stamm AM. Transnasal endoscopy-assisted skull base surgery. Ann Otol Rhinol Laryngol. 2006;115(9_suppl):45–53.
10. Vaz-Guimaraes F, Su SY, Fernandez-Miranda JC, Wang EW, Snyderman CH, Gardner PA. Hemostasis in endoscopic endonasal skull base surgery. J Neurol Surg Part B Skull Base. 2015;76(4):296–302.
11. Halderman AA, Sindwani R, Woodard TD. Hemorrhagic complications of endoscopic sinus surgery. Otolaryngol Clin N Am. 2015;48(5):783–93.
12. Welch KC, Palmer JN. Intraoperative emergencies during endoscopic sinus surgery: CSF leak and orbital hematoma. Otolaryngol Clin N Am. 2008;41(3):581–96, ix–x
13. El-Fiki M. Surgical anatomy for control of ethmoidal arteries during extended endoscopic endonasal or microsurgical resection of vascular anterior skull base meningiomas. World Neurosurg. 2015;84(6):1532–5.
14. Sigler AC, D'Anza B, Lobo BC, Woodard TD, Recinos PF, Sindwani R. Endoscopic skull base reconstruction: an evolution of materials and methods. Otolaryngol Clin N Am. 2017;50(3):643–53.
15. Jho HD. Endoscopic endonasal approach to the optic nerve: a technical note. Minim Invasive Neurosurg. 2001;44(4):190–3.
16. Garcia-Navarro V, Anand VK, Schwartz TH. Gasket seal closure for extended endonasal endoscopic skull base surgery: efficacy in a large case series. World Neurosurg. 2013;80(5):563–8.
17. Chabot JD, Patel CR, Hughes MA, Wang EW, Snyderman CH, Gardner PA, et al. Nasoseptal flap necrosis: a rare complication of endoscopic endonasal surgery. J Neurosurg. 2018;128(5):1463–72.
18. Carrau RL, Snyderman C, Janecka IP, Sekhar L, Sen C, D'Amico F. Antibiotic prophylaxis in cranial base surgery. Head Neck. 1991;13(4):311–7.
19. Brown SM, Anand VK, Tabaee A, Schwartz TH. Role of perioperative antibiotics in endoscopic skull base surgery. Laryngoscope. 2007;117(9):1528–32.
20. Wannemuehler TJ, Rabbani CC, Burgeson JE, Illing EA, Walgama ES, Wu AW, et al. Survey of endoscopic skull base surgery practice patterns among otolaryngologists. Laryngoscope Investig Otolaryngol. 2018;3(3):143–55.
21. Johans SJ, Burkett DJ, Swong KN, Patel CR, Germanwala AV. Antibiotic prophylaxis and infection prevention for endoscopic endonasal skull base surgery: our protocol, results, and review of the literature. J Clin Neurosci. 2018;47:249–53.
22. Bendersky DC, Landriel FA, Ajler PM, Hem SM, Carrizo AG. Sternberg's canal as a cause of encephalocele within the lateral recess of the sphenoid sinus: a report of two cases. Surg Neurol Int. 2011;2:171.
23. Barañano CF, Curé J, Palmer JN, Woodworth BA. Sternberg's canal: fact or fiction? Am J Rhinol Allergy. 2009;23(2):167–71.
24. Tabaee A, Anand VK, Cappabianca P, Stamm A, Esposito F, Schwartz TH. Endoscopic management of spontaneous meningoencephalocele of the lateral sphenoid sinus. J Neurosurg. 2010;112(5):1070–7.
25. Castelnuovo P, Dallan I, Pistochini A, Battaglia P, Locatelli D, Bignami M. Endonasal endoscopic repair of Sternberg's canal cerebrospinal fluid leaks. Laryngoscope. 2007;117(2):345–9.
26. Tami TA. Surgical management of lesions of the sphenoid lateral recess. Am J Rhinol. 2006;20(4):412–6.
27. Chen JX, Alkire BC, Lam AC, Curry WT, Holbrook EH. Aseptic meningitis with craniopharyngioma resection: consideration after endoscopic surgery. J Neurol Surg Rep. 2016;77(4):e151–5.
28. Conger A, Zhao F, Wang X, Eisenberg A, Griffiths C, Esposito F, et al. Evolution of the graded repair of CSF leaks and skull base defects in endonasal endoscopic tumor surgery: trends in repair failure and meningitis rates in 509 patients. J Neurosurg. 2018;130(3):861–75.
29. Harvey RJ, Parmar P, Sacks R, Zanation AM. Endoscopic skull base reconstruction of large dural defects: a systematic review of published evidence. Laryngoscope. 2012;122(2):452–9.
30. Stamm AC, Vellutini E, Harvey RJ, Nogeira JF, Herman DR. Endoscopic transnasal craniotomy and the resection of craniopharyngioma. Laryngoscope. 2008;118(7):1142–8.
31. Sanchez GB, Kaylie DM, O'Malley MR, Labadie RF, Jackson CG, Haynes DS. Chemical meningitis following cerebellopontine angle tumor surgery. Otolaryngol Head Neck Surg. 2008;138(3):368–73.
32. MacKeith SA, Soledad-Juarez M, Tiberti L, Orfila D. Recurrent aseptic meningitis as a rare but important presentation of congenital petrous apex cholesteatoma: the value of appropriate imaging. BMJ

Case Rep. 2014;2014:bcr2013010390. https://doi.org/10.1136/bcr-2013-010390.
33. Vanhoenacker FM, Herz R, Vandervliet EJ, Parizel PM. The Mount Fuji sign in tension pneumocephalus. JBR-BTR. 2008;91(4):175.
34. Schirmer CM, Heilman CB, Bhardwaj A. Pneumocephalus: case illustrations and review. Neurocrit Care. 2010;13(1):152–8.
35. Kasemsiri P, Carrau RL, Prevedello DM, Ditzel Filho LF, de Lara D, Otto BA, et al. Indications and limitations of endoscopic skull base surgery. Future Neurol. 2012;7(3):263–77.
36. Teshima M, Shinomiya H, Otsuki N, Kimura H, Taniguchi M, Hashikawa K, et al. Complications in salvage surgery for nasal and paranasal malignant tumors involving the skull base. J Neurol Surg Part B Skull Base. 2018;79(3):224–8.
37. Burkhardt J-K, Zinn PO, Graenicher M, Santillan A, Bozinov O, Kasper EM, et al. Predicting postoperative hydrocephalus in 227 patients with skull base meningioma. Neurosurg Focus. 2011;30(5):E9.
38. Mostofi K, Samii M. Secondary communicating hydrocephalus management by implantation of external ventricular shunt and minimal gradual increase of cerebrospinal fluid pressure. Asian J Neurosurg. 2017;12(2):194–8.
39. Battaglia P, Turri-Zanoni M, Castelnuovo P, Prevedello DM, Carrau RL. Brain herniation after endoscopic transnasal resection of anterior skull base malignancies. Neurosurgery. 2015;11(Suppl 3):457–62; discussion 462
40. Eloy JA, Shukla PA, Choudhry OJ, Singh R, Liu JK. Assessment of frontal lobe sagging after endoscopic endonasal transcribriform resection of anterior skull base tumors: is rigid structural reconstruction of the cranial base defect necessary? Laryngoscope. 2012;122(12):2652–7.
41. Awad AJ, Mohyeldin A, El-Sayed IH, Aghi MK. Sinonasal morbidity following endoscopic endonasal skull base surgery. Clin Neurol Neurosurg. 2015;130:162–7.
42. Gallagher MJ, Durnford AJ, Wahab SS, Nair S, Rokade A, Mathad N. Patient-reported nasal morbidity following endoscopic endonasal skull base surgery. Br J Neurosurg. 2014;28(5):622–5.
43. de Almeida JR, Snyderman CH, Gardner PA, Carrau RL, Vescan AD. Nasal morbidity following endoscopic skull base surgery: a prospective cohort study. Head Neck. 2011;33(4):547–51.
44. Dolci RLL, Miyake MM, Tateno DA, Cançado NA, Campos CAC, Dos Santos ARL, et al. Postoperative otorhinolaryngologic complications in transnasal endoscopic surgery to access the skull base. Braz J Otorhinolaryngol. 2017;83(3):349–55.
45. Griffiths CF, Cutler AR, Duong HT, Bardo G, Karimi K, Barkhoudarian G, et al. Avoidance of postoperative epistaxis and anosmia in endonasal endoscopic skull base surgery: a technical note. Acta Neurochir. 2014;156(7):1393–401.
46. Thompson CF, Suh JD, Liu Y, Bergsneider M, Wang MB. Modifications to the endoscopic approach for anterior skull base lesions improve postoperative sinonasal symptoms. J Neurol Surg Part B Skull Base. 2014;75(1):65–72.
47. Thompson CF, Kern RC, Conley DB. Olfaction in endoscopic sinus and skull base surgery. Otolaryngol Clin N Am. 2015;48(5):795–804.
48. Soudry E, Psaltis AJ, Lee KH, Vaezafshar R, Nayak JV, Hwang PH. Complications associated with the pedicled nasoseptal flap for skull base reconstruction. Laryngoscope. 2015;125(1):80–5.
49. Rowan NR, Wang EW, Gardner PA, Fernandez-Miranda JC, Snyderman CH. Nasal deformities following nasoseptal flap reconstruction of skull base defects. J Neurol Surg Part B Skull Base. 2016;77(1):14–8.
50. Stamm AC, Pignatari S, Vellutini E, Harvey RJ, Nogueira JF. A novel approach allowing binostril work to the sphenoid sinus. Otolaryngol Head Neck Surg. 2008;138(4):531–2.
51. Takemura M, Fujimoto Y, Kobayashi T, Komori M, Stamm AC, Vellutini E, et al. A modified combined transseptal/transnasal binostril approach for pituitary lesions in patients with a narrow nasal space: technical note. Neurol Med Chir (Tokyo). 2014;54(8):622–8.
52. Fujimoto Y, Balsalobre L, Santos FP, Vellutini E, Stamm AC. Endoscopic combined "transseptal/transnasal" approach for pituitary adenoma: reconstruction of skull base using pedicled nasoseptal flap in 91 consecutive cases. Arq Neuropsiquiatr. 2015;73(7):611–5.
53. Nogueira JF, Woodworth BA, Stamm A, Silva ML. A primary clival defect: endoscopic binostril approach with nasal septal flap closure and preservation of septal integrity. Ear Nose Throat J. 2019;98(5):E24–6.
54. Lakhiani C, DeFazio MV, Han K, Falola R, Evans K. Donor-site morbidity following free tissue harvest from the thigh: a systematic review and pooled analysis of complications. J Reconstr Microsurg. 2016;32(5):342–57.
55. Knott PD, Seth R, Waters HH, Revenaugh PC, Alam D, Scharpf J, et al. Short-term donor site morbidity: a comparison of the anterolateral thigh and radial forearm fasciocutaneous free flaps. Head Neck. 2016;38(Suppl 1):E945–8.
56. Veyrat M, Verillaud B, Herman P, Bresson D. How I do it. The pedicled temporoparietal fascia flap for skull base reconstruction after endonasal endoscopic approaches. Acta Neurochir. 2016;158(12):2291–4.
57. Zanation AM, Snyderman CH, Carrau RL, Kassam AB, Gardner PA, Prevedello DM. Minimally invasive endoscopic pericranial flap: a new method for endonasal skull base reconstruction. Laryngoscope. 2009;119(1):13–8.
58. Bleier BS, Wang EW, Vandergrift WA, Schlosser RJ. Mucocele rate after endoscopic skull base reconstruction using vascularized pedicled flaps. Am J Rhinol Allergy. 2011;25(3):186–7.
59. Husain Q, Sanghvi S, Kovalerchik O, Shukla PA, Choudhry OJ, Liu JK, et al. Assessment of mucocele formation after endoscopic nasoseptal flap reconstruction of skull base defects. Allergy Rhinol (Providence). 2013;4(1):e27–31.

Failure of CSF Leak Repair

28

Jacob Friedman, Bobby A. Tajudeen, and Pete S. Batra

28.1 Introduction

Endonasal endoscopic repair of cerebrospinal fluid (CSF) leaks is well established as the standard of care for defects of the anterior skull base. Studies from the last 30 years of accrued experience with endoscopic techniques have consistently demonstrated success rates of approximately 90% for primary repairs and 97% or higher when secondary repairs are considered [1–6]. The low rate of failure combined with the reduced morbidity of minimally invasive techniques has led to the preference for endoscopic procedures over traditional open rhinological approaches or neurosurgical repairs involving craniotomy. Despite the proven advantages of endoscopic repair, its true failure rate is likely underestimated in the literature due to publication bias, and when failures do occur, they lead to an increased risk of meningitis, pneumocephalus, and ensuing neurologic complications necessitating further surgery [5, 7]. Therefore, it is crucial to evaluate and discuss the causes of leak recurrence. Numerous studies have undertaken this task or commented on it, but thorough investigation has only partially elucidated the causes of endoscopic CSF leak repair failure.

J. Friedman · B. A. Tajudeen · P. S. Batra (✉)
Department of Otorhinolaryngology – Head and Neck Surgery, Rush Center for Skull Base and Pituitary Surgery, Rush University Medical Center, Chicago, IL, USA
e-mail: jacob_j_friedman@rush.edu; bobby_tajudeen@rush.edu; Pete_Batra@rush.edu

Factors that may impact the success of endoscopic repair are wide-ranging and fall into several categories (Table 28.1). These broadly include patient demographics and comorbidities,

Table 28.1 Factors that may impact CSF leak repair success

Patient demographics and comorbidities • Age, sex, smoking, BMI • ICP/BIH • DM, HTN
Etiology • Traumatic – Iatrogenic – Non-iatrogenic • Spontaneous
Site • Anatomic location, shape, size • Presence of malignancy • Presence of meningocele or encephalocele • Exposure to radiation
Variations in repair technique • Degree of leak exposure and visualization • Repair composition – Pedicled flap vs. free graft – Simple vs. composite – Underlay vs. overlay – Fat graft – Glues or synthetic materials
Adjunctive techniques or treatments • Intrathecal fluorescein • Nasal packing • Lumbar drain • Diuretics • Ventriculoperitoneal shunt

BMI body mass index, *ICP* intracranial pressure, *BIH* benign intracranial hypertension, *DM* diabetes mellitus, *HTN* hypertension

A. A. AlQahtani et al. (eds.), *CSF Rhinorrhea*, https://doi.org/10.1007/978-3-030-94781-1_28

features specific to the CSF etiology, severity, or anatomic characteristics, and variations in repair technique.

28.2 Patient Factors

28.2.1 BMI

Several large studies looking at data from a wide array of CSF leak types observed no association of repair failure with demographic data such as age or sex [1, 4, 6]. In these studies, no association with BMI was observed; however, in analysis of certain CSF leak subgroups, there is considerable evidence that elevated BMI does play a role in leak development and recurrence.

Elevated BMI is associated with the de novo development of spontaneous CSF rhinorrhea and may have a causative role in its development [8]. One proposed mechanism purports that increased intraabdominal pressure from central obesity raises intrathoracic pressure and impedes cardiac venous return. This, in turn, causes increased intracranial venous pressure and decreased CSF resorption at the arachnoid villi. In the context of susceptible skull base anatomy, this elevated pressure may result in herniation of meninges and dural defect over time through which CSF begins to leak. For these reasons, elevated BMI and elevated intracranial pressure (ICP) are theorized as potential risk factors for leak recurrence after successful repair.

Considerable evidence that BMI plays a role in repair failure arises from several studies. Basu et al. analyzed a group of eight patients with spontaneous leaks. In this group, only the patient with the highest BMI (>45 kg/m^2) suffered recurrence, and in fact, recurred despite a second repair. In their group of 11 patients with leaks sustained during transcranial procedures or during endoscopic skull base surgery, two patients with the highest BMI suffered recurrence in addition to several others. Sample size and the effect of confounders in this study limit the inferences that can be drawn from this data, but the subgroup analysis performed in this study is unique, and their findings suggest the possibility that BMI is a meaningful risk factor whose effect can be measured when the correct subgroup is analyzed [2]. This effect was more clearly observed in a very large study of CSF leaks after sellar surgery. Analysis of 1163 patients demonstrated the association of higher BMI with failure of intraoperative CSF leak repair; however, the magnitude of this effect was not overwhelming (OR = 1.055) [9]. In two other large studies with a high proportion of large skull base defects, BMI had a stronger association with leak recurrence. In one of these series, a review of 615 patients who underwent endoscopic skull base surgery reported that postoperative leaks occurred in 19% of obese patients compared to 12% in the non-obese group (OR = 1.75) [10, 11]. Higher BMI is associated with leak repair failure; its effects are most apparent in the subset of larger skull base defects, and possibly at the extremes of obesity.

28.2.2 Elevated ICP

As discussed, elevated ICP is suspected to play a role in the development of spontaneous CSF leaks [8]. Its role as a risk factor for recurrence after leak repair is well supported in the literature. In one study of 53 cases, all patients with elevated ICP, as measured by CSF opening pressure, experienced recurrence of leak after repair, and these represented 100% of recurrences (3 out of 53 cases) [12]. Similarly, in another study of 97 cases, seven of eight total recurrences had elevated ICP as evidenced by an empty sella, skull base erosions, hydrocephalus, prior diagnosis of intracranial hypertension (ICH), or presence of intracranial AVM. Additionally, the finding that postoperative vomiting is associated with recurrence is likely attributable to the transient elevation in ICP during emesis [10].

28.2.3 Other Factors

General risks of neurosurgical non-healing, such as prolonged steroid usage, failure despite multiple attempts at closure, and ongoing chemotherapy or radiotherapy, should also be taken into consideration, but no association has been established between surgical failure and these concomitant factors [2, 12, 13].

28.3 Etiology

CSF leaks result from a wide range of pathologies (Table 28.2). Characteristics of each etiology may make surgical failure more or less likely. Classically, spontaneous leaks have been singled out as a subset more likely to recur after repair, but many other features of leak etiology and the particulars of size and location should be considered for their impact on the likelihood of recurrence.

Several larger studies surveying an array of leak types did not find the etiology of the CSF leak to be an independent predictor of failure [1, 3, 4, 6]. However, more focused studies have demonstrated an association between spontaneous leaks and recurrence in the context of elevated ICP, and higher failure rates have been seen with the repair of iatrogenic leaks resulting following skull base surgery [2, 14, 15].

28.3.1 Iatrogenic Leaks

CSF leaks resulting from endoscopic sinus surgery (ESS) are common and discussed frequently in the literature. Common sites for leak after ESS are the lateral lamella of the cribriform plate and the posterior ethmoid roof, especially in the context of decreased skull base height [16]. Though the size of these defects can vary, they tend to be small and do not communicate with a cisternal space. Generally, these repairs are considered straightforward, and the rate of successful repair is reliably high when managed appropriately. If a leak is observed intraoperatively, it is recommended that repair be undertaken at that time [1, 2, 17].

Table 28.2 Causes of CSF leak

Traumatic • Iatrogenic – Endoscopic sinus surgery – Endoscopic skull base surgery – Transcranial skull base surgery • Non-iatrogenic – Closed or blunt trauma – Penetrating trauma
Spontaneous • Elevated ICP – Obstructive – Non-obstructive • Inflammatory erosion • Neoplastic erosion • Congenital skull base defect • Idiopathic

Patients with leaks resulting from transcranial procedures are identified as a distinct population with high risk for endoscopic repair failure. In one analysis of patients with leaks sustained during transcranial procedures or during endoscopic skull base resection, 46% (5/11) suffered recurrence, compared with 8% recurrence after repairs for spontaneous leaks or leaks after endoscopic sinus surgery. This disparity is attributed to difficulty visualizing the dural defect in these circumstances, as it tended to be out of view from an endoscopic approach or did not appear directly opposite the bony opening through which the leak flowed. Leak recurrence was reported in 4/4 cases in which the dural defect was not directly visualized [2].

Patients who have undergone endoscopic resection of intradural pathology along the skull base comprise another population with iatrogenic leaks at high risk for recurrence after primary repair [2]. In this group, large defects, leaks communicating with a cisternal space, and leaks at the posterior base of skull are features that portend recurrence [16]. The effect of other risk factors such as BMI and the use of non-pedicled flaps is also more pronounced in this group [11].

28.3.2 Non-Iatrogenic Traumatic Leaks

Among patients with non-iatrogenic traumatic leaks, special consideration must be given to high-velocity penetrating trauma of the skull base. This type of injury can shatter the skull base with multiple small fractures radiating from the primary point of penetrative trauma. In a case of a gunshot wound penetrating the cribriform area, Castelnuovo reports a surgical failure attributed to numerous microleaks in the area of the trauma. Revision with a large amount of abdominal fat ultimately controlled the leak [3]. More typical traumatic leaks can often be treated conservatively with bed rest, head-of-bed elevation, and activity precautions with the option of a lumbar drain if these measures prove insufficient [18]. Some question the adequacy of this approach in light of a 29% rate of subsequent meningitis; they advocate consideration of a proactive endoscopic repair for these patients to minimize long-term risk of ascending intracranial infectious complications [1, 2].

28.3.3 Spontaneous Leaks

Spontaneous CSF leaks have been considered a unique population prone to recurrence after repair by any means, endoscopic or otherwise [19]. Published recurrence rates in this group range widely from 20% to over 80%, including recurrence at the primary site and late recurrence at a different location [4, 12, 19–21]. Evolution in our understanding of spontaneous leaks has led to the description of its association with elevated ICP and the development of updated management algorithms for these patients. In 56 patients with spontaneous leaks treated initially with surgical repair and then stratified to receive adjunctive diuretics or CSF shunting, an 11% recurrence rate was reported [22]. Others reported a comparable recurrence rate of 13% employing a similar management algorithm, and in recent literature as many as 93% of spontaneous leaks thus treated remained closed after primary repair [23, 24].

28.4 Site of CSF Leak

Although large-scale systematic review has not borne out an association between the anatomic site of a leak and risk of recurrence, a case-by-case analysis by Castelnuovo et al. of 24 published cases of recurrence and four of their own revealed that difficulty repairing a leak in the superior or lateral sphenoid sinus is noted by several authors as a reason for surgical failure [3, 5]. Others who have noted this difficulty advocate a transpterygoid approach to achieve adequate exposure of leaks in the lateral pterygoid recess of the sphenoid sinus [16, 18].

The posterior skull base is prone to leaks in the area of the clivus due to skull base surgery. The pontine cistern lies posterior to the clivus and can be the source of a formidable CSF leak. Leaks communicating with the subarachnoid cisterns are termed “high-flow,” and such defects demand meticulous closure. The higher risk of failure has led experts to advocate multilayered repair in conjunction with a pedicled flap, such as nasoseptal flap [11, 16]. The high rate of repair failure for defects after resection of craniopharyngioma and tumors with intraventricular extension is likely explained by their tendency to produce high-flow leaks [9].

In skull base surgery, the presence and characteristics of tumor tissue introduces an additional element that may complicate repair. Recurrence of CSF leak is more likely after resection of pituitary adenomas larger than 4 cm [14]. The larger defects created in these operations may also predispose toward leak repair failure; leaks are more likely to occur after repair of 6 cm^2 defect than after repairs of 3 cm^2 defect [11]. Size smaller than 4 cm likely has no measurable effect [12]. Residual tumor at the site of the leak is an obstacle, but not a contraindication to repair attempts. Basu reports successful repair of three of four leaks with residual tumor present at the leak site, and even adjuvant radiation has not been found to preclude successful repair [2, 25].

The presence of meningocele or encephalocele has not been observed to have an association with surgical failure [6].

Despite the reliability of endoscopic repair in most cases, it is imperative to consider the features of CSF leaks for which an open or combined approach would be more appropriate than an endoscopic-only repair. Such circumstances include but are not limited to the need for frontal sinus obliteration or cranialization, leaks of the extreme lateral or superior aspect of the frontal sinus, the presence of a large encephalocele with incorporated intracranial vessel, and massive skull base defects. This is especially true when a revision procedure is being considered in these difficult scenarios [16, 18].

28.5 Technique

Over the years, the choice between a pedicled flap or a free graft, use of bone or cartilage in the repair, overlay or underlay techniques, or reinforcement with fibrin glue have all been shown to have comparable efficacy in experienced hands [6, 12]. Certain special cases, such as reconstruction after endoscopic resection of intradural pathologies benefit from the use of a pedicled flap, but its superiority is not demonstrated in all circumstances [3, 11]. So long as sound technique is maintained, the method of repair should be tailored to the individual circumstance using the wide array of repair methods that have all been proven successful over the years.

The most important issues of repair technique are adequate exposure of the leak site, meticulous preparation of the graft bed to ensure tight adhesion of the repair, and clearly visualization of the dural defect. Dural defects that are repaired without being visualized will recur with near certainty [2, 16]. Individual failures have been attributed to inadequate preparation of marginal mucosa, underestimating 5 mm of tissue shrinkage in the postoperative period, overly conservative technique precluding exposure of the dural defect, and forgoing a bone graft or craniotomy in a larger (20 mm) defect [3].

28.6 Adjunctive Management

In an effort to reduce surgical failures, comprehensive management of CSF leaks has expanded to include the use of several adjunctive procedures, techniques, and medical treatments.

Intrathecal fluorescein can provide accurate, real-time visual localization of the CSF leak, which is a prerequisite to consistently successful repair (Fig. 28.1). Fluorescein also enables intraoperative confirmation of watertight closure

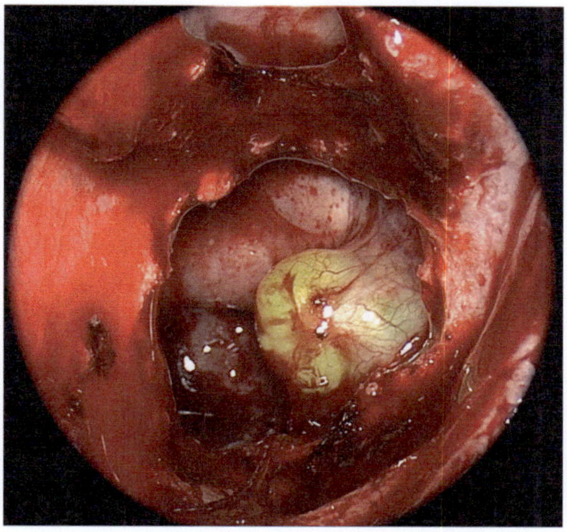

Fig. 28.1 Endoscopic view with 0-degree scope demonstrates left lateral sphenoid meningocele with fluorescein-stained CSF

which can be further tested with careful utilization of a Valsalva maneuver [26]. The FDA has not approved the use of fluorescein in this manner, and reported adverse effects include seizures, radicular symptoms, and transient paresis. However, concerns about the safety of fluorescein have been mitigated by safe experience with slow instillation of dilute concentrations of the dye; 0.1 ml of 10% fluorescein is mixed in 10 cc of patient's CSF and instilled at 1 cc/min over 10 min [27]. Nevertheless, the patient must be appropriately counseled, consented, and monitored for adverse effects.

The placement of a lumbar drain enables ongoing control of pressure by active CSF diversion, along with enabling the administration of intrathecal fluorescein. Whether the use of a lumbar drain has an effect on the success of leak repair has been vigorously debated in the literature. Casiano et al. demonstrated that lumbar drain use is not essential in the repair of leaks up to 3 cm, and others have published similar findings; however, in a randomized controlled trial assessing the use of lumbar drain in endoscopic skull base surgery, risk of post-op leak in the lumbar drain group was only 8% compared to 21% without a drain [15, 28]. The best interpretation of available evidence is that use of a lumbar drain does not provide significant benefit in smaller leaks, but it may be instrumental in diverting CSF to increase the success of repair in large or high-flow leaks.

The lumbar drain also serves diagnostic utility in patients with elevated CSF pressures. Identifying and managing elevated ICP in the context of spontaneous leaks is especially crucial, as this may be the causative factor in surgical failure or leak recurrence. Besides perioperative lumbar drainage, these patients can require long-term medical therapy or surgical measures to achieve lifelong control of ICH. Classic long-term interventions include acetazolamide and ventricular shunting. Recent literature has described venous sinus stenting in patients with ICH and associated venous sinus stenosis and surgical or non-surgical weight loss in obese patients [29, 30]. The precise indications for these newer interventions are still under scrutiny, and their effectiveness in preventing recurrent CSF leak remains unproven.

The introduction of treatment algorithms employing the use of lumbar drains, acetazolamide, or ventriculoperitoneal shunt in the context of ICH initially improved the success rate of repair for spontaneous leaks from less than 80% to about 90% (Fig. 28.2) [22, 23]. Follow-up studies assessing this approach show even better

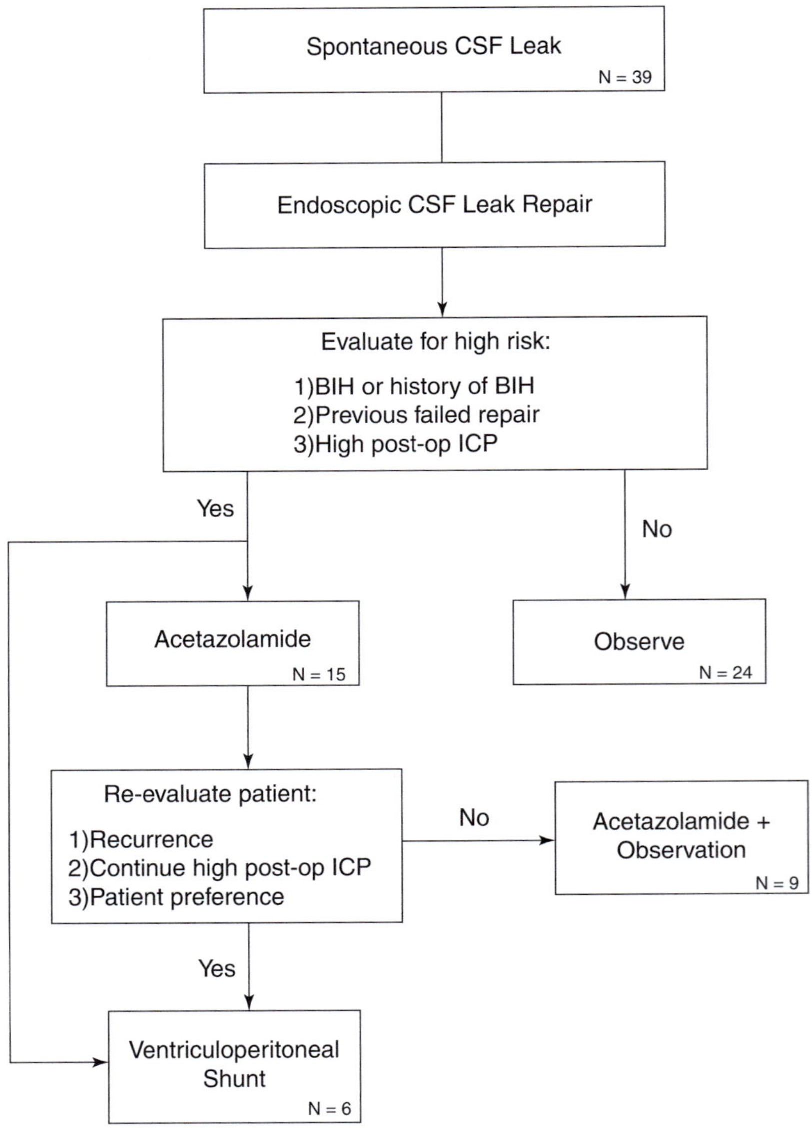

Fig. 28.2 Seth et al. [23] employed this algorithm to achieve high rates of success after repair of spontaneous CSF leaks

results with 93% primary and 100% secondary success [24]. Studies of long-term follow-up in these patients will reveal to what extent these measures suffice to mitigate recurrence.

In order to avoid transient elevations in ICP unrelated to underlying ICH, it is also important to discuss with the anesthesia team a proactive plan for prophylactic management of "bucking" on emergence and postoperative nausea and vomiting [10]. Strict bed rest with head of bed elevation for 24–48 h and activity restriction in the postoperative period are common to many protocols and are intuitive measures to maintain stable ICP.

The use of these adjunctive approaches and the various techniques for leak repair are integrated and applied in the Cornell closure algorithm. This algorithm categorizes leaks by etiology and severity to define a graded approach to repair. Small extradural or intrasellar pathologies are managed with absorbable materials and dural sealant glue while large defects, pathologies beyond the sella, and spontaneous leaks are treated with multilayer closure including pedicled nasoseptal flaps and lumbar drain placement [31].

28.7 Recurrence

Rhinorrhea in the immediate or late post-op period should raise suspicion for recurrence of CSF leak. This may represent failure at the site of repair or recurrence at another site. In the population of patients with spontaneous leaks and late recurrence, a new leak site should be considered and may be due to under-managed ICH.

The differential diagnosis for rhinorrhea in post-repair patients should certainly entertain suspicion for leak recurrence, but other causes should also be considered. These include postoperative drainage of mucus or irrigation fluid and rhinorrhea of allergic or nonallergic rhinitis. The diagnostic workup does not differ significantly from rhinorrhea in other posttraumatic patients. Physical examination should include a Dandy maneuver, nasal endoscopy, otoscopy, and, if available, visual inspection of fluid stain for a halo sign. Fluid should be sent immediately for the detection of ß2-transferrin. The presence of glucose in the rhinorrhea fluid is a traditional sign of CSF leak; however, it is an unreliable indicator given the presence of reducing substances in mucus and should not serve as the basis of establishing diagnosis. If CSF rhinorrhea is confirmed or highly suspected, imaging should be undertaken with high-resolution computed tomography. Contrast-enhanced magnetic resonance imaging cisternography can often be helpful as well. Ultimately, some leaks may not be localized on imaging. In these cases, intrathecal fluorescein with intraoperative nasal endoscopy represents the best method for identifying the leak site.

If a recurrent leak is confirmed in the immediate postoperative period, intervention should not be delayed. Late recurrence requires timely, but not emergent, attention. The underlying reason for recurrence must be considered in order to determine the appropriate course of action. In a case of persistent ICH, acetazolamide or a VP shunt may be indicated with conservative management and observation of the leak site. If concerns about the adequacy of the initial repair are harbored, revision surgery should be considered and carefully planned. If features of the leak pose significant challenges to endoscopic repair, then combined, open, or transcranial approaches should now be considered.

28.8 Conclusion

Endoscopic repairs of CSF leaks are reliably successful and have become increasingly so in recent years [10]. Poorer success rates in patients with spontaneous leaks led to the discovery of its epidemiologic associations with elevated BMI and increased ICP [32]. Elevated BMI plays a role in the recurrence of large or high-flow leaks, and ICH was observed to be a risk factor for recurrence in all leak types. Updated management algorithms that address underlying elevated ICP have demonstrated improved success rates.

Accrued experience with numerous methods and approaches has yielded an abundance of effective surgical techniques for the endoscopic repair of CSF leaks in the anterior and posterior skull base as long as certain fundamental principles are observed:

1. The source of the leak must be clearly visualized with an endoscopic approach appropriate for achieving optimal exposure.
2. The margins of the skull base defect must be meticulously prepared, exposing underlying bone to facilitate tight graft adhesion.
3. Grafts should be oversized to allow for shrinkage.
4. The repair of large or high-flow leaks should be multilayered, include a pedicled flap, and consider employing the use of a lumbar drain.
5. Underlying elevated ICP should be identified and addressed medically or surgically to decrease the risk of leak recurrence.

If these principles cannot be achieved, combined, open, or transcranial approaches may be required in select cases.

Conflict of Interest JF: No conflict of interest. No financial disclosures.

BAT: Advanced Rx (research grant).

References

1. Banks CA, Palmer JN, Chiu AG, O'Malley BW, Woodworth BA, Kennedy DW. Endoscopic closure of CSF rhinorrhea: 193 cases over 21 years. Otolaryngol Head Neck Surg. 2009;140(6):826–33.
2. Basu D, Haughey BH, Hartman JM. Determinants of success in endoscopic cerebrospinal fluid leak repair. Otolaryngol Head Neck Surg. 2006;135(5):769–73.
3. Castelnuovo P, Mauri S, Locatelli D, Emanuelli E, Delu G, Di Giulio G. Endoscopic repair of cerebrospinal fluid rhinorrhea: learning from our failures. Am J Rhinol. 2001;15(5):333–42.
4. Mirza S, Thaper A, McClelland L, Jones NS. Sinonasal cerebrospinal fluid leaks: management of 97 patients over 10 years. Laryngoscope. 2005;115(10):1774–7.
5. Psaltis AJ, Schlosser RJ, Banks CA, Yawn J, Soler ZM. A systematic review of the endoscopic repair of cerebrospinal fluid leaks. Otolaryngol Head Neck Surg. 2012;147(2):196–203.
6. Hegazy HM, Carrau RL, Snyderman CH, Kassam A, Zweig J. Transnasal endoscopic repair of cerebrospinal fluid rhinorrhea: a meta-analysis. Laryngoscope. 2000;110(7):1166–72.
7. Horowitz G, Fliss DM, Margalit N, Wasserzug O, Gil Z. Association between cerebrospinal fluid leak and meningitis after Skull Base surgery. Otolaryngol Head Neck Surg. 2011;145(4):689–93.
8. Schlosser R, Wilensky EM, Grady MS, Bolger WE. Elevated intracranial pressures in spontaneous cerebrospinal fluid leaks. Am J Rhinol. 2003;17(4):191–5.
9. Karnezis TT, Baker AB, Soler ZM, Wise SK, Rereddy SK, Patel ZM, et al. Factors impacting cerebrospinal fluid leak rates in endoscopic sellar surgery. Int Forum Allergy Rhinol. 2016;6(11):1117–25.
10. Conger A, Zhao F, Wang X, Eisenberg A, Griffiths C, Esposito F, et al. Evolution of the graded repair of CSF leaks and skull base defects in endonasal endoscopic tumor surgery: trends in repair failure and meningitis rates in 509 patients. J Neurosurg. 2018;130(3):861–75.
11. Fraser S, Gardner PA, Koutourousiou M, Kubik M, Fernandez-Miranda JC, Snyderman CH, et al. Risk factors associated with postoperative cerebrospinal fluid leak after endoscopic endonasal skull base surgery. J Neurosurg. 2018;128(4):1066–71.
12. Zweig JL, Carrau RL, Celin SE, Schaitkin BM, Pollice PA, Snyderman CH, et al. Endoscopic repair of cerebrospinal fluid leaks to the sinonasal tract: predictors of success. Otolaryngol Head Neck Surg. 2000;123(3):195–201.
13. Krishnan K, Müller A, Hong B, Potapov A, Schackert G, Seifert V, et al. Complex wound-healing problems in neurosurgical patients: risk factors, grading and treatment strategy. Acta Neurochir. 2012;154(3):541–54.
14. Han, Zong-Li|He, Dong-Sheng|Mao, Zhi-Gang|Wang, Hai-Jun. Cerebrospinal fluid rhinorrhea following trans-sphenoidal pituitary macroadenoma surgery: experience from 592 patients. Clin Neurol Neurosurg. 2008;110(6):570–9.
15. Zwagerman NT, Wang EW, Shin SS, Chang Y, Fernandez-Miranda JC, Snyderman CH, et al. Does lumbar drainage reduce postoperative cerebrospinal fluid leak after endoscopic endonasal skull base surgery? A prospective, randomized controlled trial. J Neurosurg. 2018;1–7.
16. Batra P. Endoscopic evaluation and treatment of CSF leaks. In: Johnson J, Rosen C, editors. Bailey's head and neck surgery - otolaryngology. 5th ed. Baltimore, MD: Lippincott Williams & Wilkins; 2014. p. 662–74.
17. Prosser JD, Vender JR, Solares CA. Traumatic cerebrospinal fluid leaks. Otolaryngol Clin North Am. 2011;44(4):857–73.
18. Lindstrom DR, Toohill RJ, Loehrl TA, Smith TL. Management of cerebrospinal fluid rhinorrhea: the Medical College of Wisconsin experience. Laryngoscope. 2004;114(6):969–74.
19. Hubbard JL, McDonald TJ, Pearson BW, Laws ER Jr. Spontaneous cerebrospinal fluid rhinorrhea: evolving concepts in diagnosis and surgical management based on the Mayo Clinic experience from 1970 through 1981. Neurosurgery. 1985;16(3):314–21.
20. Schlosser RJ, Woodworth BA, Wilensky EM, Grady MS, Bolger WE. Spontaneous cerebrospinal fluid

leaks: a variant of benign intracranial hypertension. Ann Otol Rhinol Laryngol. 2006;115(7):495–500.
21. Schick B, Ibing R, Brors D, Draf W. Long-term study of endonasal duraplasty and review of the literature. Ann Otol Rhinol Laryngol. 2001;110(2):142–7.
22. Woodworth BA, Prince A, Chiu AG, Cohen NA, Schlosser RJ, Bolger WE, et al. Spontaneous CSF leaks: a paradigm for definitive repair and management of intracranial hypertension. Otolaryngol Head Neck Surg. 2008;138(6):715–20.
23. Seth R, Rajasekaran K III, Luong A, Benninger MS, Batra PS. Spontaneous CSF leaks: factors predictive of additional interventions. Laryngoscope. 2010;120(11):2141–6.
24. Chaaban MR, Illing E, Riley KO, Woodworth BA. Spontaneous cerebrospinal fluid leak repair: a five-year prospective evaluation. Laryngoscope. 2014;124(1):70–5.
25. Alves MVO, Roberts D, Levine NB, DeMonte F, Hanna EY, Kupferman ME. Impact of chemoradiotherapy on CSF leak repair after skull base surgery. J Neurol Surg B Skull Base. 2014;75(5):354–7.
26. Seth R, Rajasekaran K, Benninger MS, Batra PS. The utility of intrathecal fluorescein in cerebrospinal fluid leak repair. Otolaryngol Head Neck Surg. 2010;143(5):626–32.
27. Senior BA, Jafri K, Benninger M. Safety and efficacy of endoscopic repair of CSF leaks and Encephaloceles: a survey of the members of the American Rhinologic Society. Am J Rhinol. 2001;15(1):21–6.
28. Casiano RR, Jassir D. Endoscopic cerebrospinal fluid rhinorrhea repair: is a lumbar drain necessary? Otolaryngol Head Neck Surg. 1999;121(6):745–50.
29. Manfield JH, Yu KK, Efthimiou E, Darzi A, Athanasiou T, Ashrafian H. Bariatric surgery or non-surgical weight loss for idiopathic intracranial hypertension? A systematic review and comparison of meta-analyses. Obes Surg. 2016;27(2):513–21.
30. Fargen KM, Liu K, Garner RM, Greeneway GP, Wolfe SQ, Crowley RW. Recommendations for the selection and treatment of patients with idiopathic intracranial hypertension for venous sinus stenting. J NeuroInterv Surg. 2018;10(12):1203–8.
31. Patel KS, Komotar RJ, Szentirmai O, Moussazadeh N, Raper DM, Starke RM, et al. Case-specific protocol to reduce cerebrospinal fluid leakage after endonasal endoscopic surgery. J Neurosurg. 2013;119(3):661–8.
32. Schlosser RJ, Wilensky EM, Grady MS, Palmer JN, Kennedy DW, Bolger WE. Cerebrospinal fluid pressure monitoring after repair of cerebrospinal fluid leaks. Otolaryngol Head Neck Surg. 2004;130(4):443–8.

29 Role of Lumbar Drain in CSF Leak Management

Stephanie H. Chen, Jean Anderson Eloy, and Jacques J. Morcos

29.1 Introduction

Cerebrospinal fluid (CSF) leaks (spontaneous, traumatic, or secondary to surgical procedures) result in an open communication of the sterile subarachnoid space with the outside world. This can have catastrophic consequences, such as meningitis, empyema, or abscess formation, which can lead to significant morbidity and mortality [1, 2]. Other complications of continuous CSF leakage include relentless orthostatic headaches and subdural hematomas. Lumbar drains have been used for the prevention of postoperative CSF leaks, management of delayed postoperative CSF leaks, and treatment of spontaneous and traumatic CSF leaks. In this chapter, we will review some of the basic concepts related to lumbar drains for the management of CSF rhinorrhea, discuss the available literature, and provide some of the personal preferences and recommendations from the authors' experiences.

S. H. Chen · J. J. Morcos (✉)
Department of Neurosurgery, University of Miami Miller School of Medicine, Miami, FL, USA
e-mail: JMorcos@med.miami.edu

J. A. Eloy
Department of Otolaryngology, Rutgers New Jersey Medical School, Newark, NJ, USA

29.2 Concept and Role of Lumbar Drain in CSF Leak

Approximately 70–80% of CSF is formed by the choroid plexuses in the lateral, third, and fourth ventricles at a rate of 0.35 ml/min (350–500 ml/day) [3]. CSF circulates from choroid plexus, through the ventricles, to the cisterna magna, basal cisterns, subarachnoid space, eventually draining into the dural venous sinuses. In cases of normal physiology, the pressure of the CSF spaces drives fluid through the resistance of the CSF channels and the resistance of the villi. However, a disruption in the barrier between the anterior and middle cranial fossa and sinonasal cavity creates a lower resistance pathway and greater pressure gradient as the sinonasal compartment is at atmospheric pressure. Subsequently, the CSF follows basic fluid principles, following the channel of least resistance, resulting in CSF rhinorrhea.

Lumbar drains (LD) are small flexible plastic tubes (Fig. 29.1) that are introduced into the lumbar subarachnoid space in order to provide an alternate CSF pathway utilizing gravity. CSF drains into the LD, bypassing the intranasal fistula, thus allowing time for the natural healing and scarring of the defect. LDs are the second line of treatment for CSF leaks after maximal medical management with head of bed at ≥30°, routine use of stool softeners, and avoidance of straining/Valsalva maneuvers. The rates of successful obliteration of CSF leaks with LDs is

A. A. AlQahtani et al. (eds.), *CSF Rhinorrhea*, https://doi.org/10.1007/978-3-030-94781-1_29

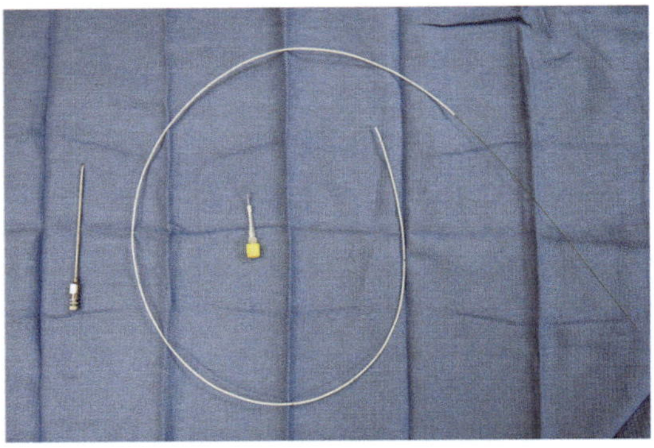

Fig. 29.1 Lumbar drain with wire, 14G Tuohy needle and cap

dependent on the etiology and location. Alternatively, LDs can be placed prophylactically prior to surgery for multiple reasons including decompression of CSF spaces, high probability of post-op CSF leak, or injection of intrathecal fluorescein to localize CSF fistulas.

29.3 The Use of Lumbar Drain in CSF Leak

CSF rhinorrhea from non-iatrogenic trauma is associated with 2% of all head traumas and 12–30% of skull base fractures [4]. The majority of CSF leaks from closed head injury resolve with conservative management. Bell et al. reported that 85% of 34 cases resolved with nonsurgical treatment over a period of 10 days, while the addition of CSF diversion with an LD only increased success rate to 90% [5]. Similarly, Mincy et al. reported spontaneous closure in 68% of posttraumatic CSF fistulas within 48 h of injury and 85% within 1 week [6]. While Albu et al. suggest that initial LD insertion may decrease length of CSF leak time (4.83 ± 1.88 vs. 7.03 ± 2.02 days, $p < 0.0001$), there was no difference in meningitis rates [7]. Thus, CSF diversion for traumatic CSF leaks is typically reserved for patients who initially fail bed rest, head elevation, and strict CSF rhinorrhea precautions [5, 8]. Surgical repair is reserved for patients who fail conservative management or experience neurologic deterioration.

Spontaneous skull base CSF leaks are often associated with sustained intracranial hypertension [9, 10]. Thus, conservative management with nonsurgical management and temporary CSF diversion is often associated with a higher risk of failure [11]. Surgical treatment through an endoscopic endonasal approach is most commonly used for anterior skull base leaks while middle cranial fossa approaches are used for lateral temporal bone leaks. Routine LD use is more common in anterior skull base repairs than lateral skull base repairs [11]. Advantages of LD placement with surgery include the use of intraoperative fluorescein to localize the site of the leak with endoscopy and measurement of postoperative intracranial pressures. While many authors continue the LD for 2–5 days after anterior skull base repairs, multiple series and meta-analyses suggest that LD use does not influence the overall success or failure of the anterior skull base repair [11–13]. Taking into consideration the risks of LD, increased financial costs, and increased length of hospital stays, judicious use of LD is recommended [14].

Delayed postoperative CSF leak is the most common serious complication of anterior skull base procedures. The rates of CSF leaks associated with transsphenoidal surgery are 3–6% [15, 16]. LD placement or large volume lumbar punctures are widely accepted strategies in managing delayed postoperative CSF leaks. In one series of 1002 patients who underwent endoscopic transsphenoidal surgery, 69% (18/26) of patients with postoperative CSF leaks resolved with lumbar drainage or puncture alone, whereas 31% (8/26) required additional surgery [15]. Similarly in patients with a CSF leak after lateral skull base procedures, 76% (48/63) resolved with lumbar drainage while 24% (15/63) required revision surgery [17]. Thus, in the senior author's practice, postoperative CSF leaks are managed initially with lumbar drainage. Persistent or recurrent CSF leaks after lumbar drainage are treated with revision operation.

29.4 Indications for Lumbar Drain Placement in Skull Base Surgery

Lumbar drains are sometimes inserted prior to skull base surgery. For open transcranial skull base procedures, preoperative LD serves to decompress CSF spaces and improve access to the tumor and skull base. This is of particular importance in procedures where CSF cisterns cannot be accessed early on. We primarily consider LD placement for subtemporal, interhemispheric, and bifrontal transcranial approaches (Fig. 29.2a, b, c). For endoscopic endonasal skull base procedures, LD allows for injection of fluorescein to detect occult CSF leaks. The LD is only maintained postoperatively in cases where the air sinuses have been violated and there is a high concern for CSF fistula.

The rate of CSF leaks after skull base surgery ranges from 3% to 40% with the highest rates associated with endoscopic endonasal surgery (EES) [14–16, 18, 19]. CSF leaks associated with skull base reconstructions are distinct from spontaneous or traumatic CSF leaks in that they more frequently involve large dural defects and "high-flow leaks" as defined as one that violates a ventricle or cistern [20]. In contrast, "low-flow leaks" are defined as those that occur with dural opening but do not involve the ventricle or an arachnoid cistern. It has been demonstrated that LDs are not required for routine CSF leak repair or for skull base reconstructions with low-flow CSF leaks [20–22].

LDs are often used in the perioperative period of large EES skull base reconstructions to reduce intracranial pressure and stress on the repair. However, with the increased use of vascularized pedicled flaps for skull base reconstruction, the routine use of LDs for high-flow leaks has also been questioned. A number of retrospective EES series found increased risks of perioperative morbidity without a significant decrease in CSF leak rate with LD use [19, 23–26]. Similarly, a meta-analysis of six retrospective studies including 153 cases reported no significant benefit of lumbar drainage in reducing postoperative CSF leak recurrence (OR: 2.67, 95% CI: 0.64–11.10) in patients undergoing skull base resections [27]. However, there is significant heterogeneity in the literature in the definition of high-flow CSF leaks as well as size and location of the defects. Zwagerman et al. performed a prospective randomized controlled trial evaluating the use of perioperative LD for "high-flow CSF leaks" defined as a large dural defect ≥ 1 cm^2, extensive arachnoid dissection, and/or opening into the ventricle or cistern. The authors randomized 187 patients to either LD at 10 ml/h for 72 h after completion of surgery or no drainage. They found

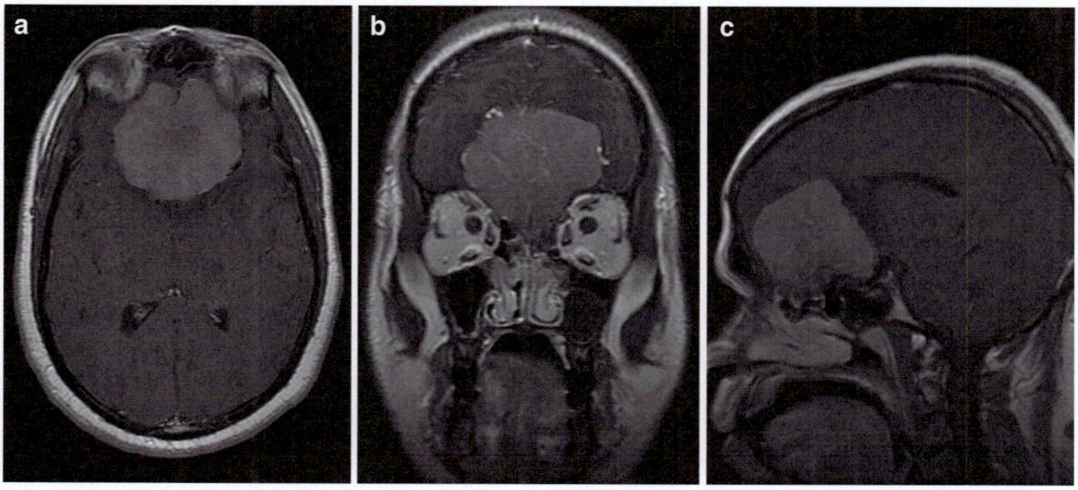

Fig. 29.2 Olfactory groove meningioma requiring bicoronal craniotomy with preoperative lumbar drain placement for CSF decompression

that the postoperative LD cohort had an 8.2% rate of CSF leak compared to 21.2% in the control group (OR 3.0, 95% CI: 1.2–7.6, p = 0.017). Furthermore, in a subgroup analysis, LD resulted in lower postoperative CSF leaks in patients with anterior and posterior fossa defects, but no difference in the suprasellar/sellar group [28].

In conclusion, we reserve the use of perioperative LDs in skull base procedures:

1. For CSF decompression in cases where early access to the cisterns is not possible.
2. To permit the use of intraoperative intrathecal fluorescein.
3. For high-flow CSF leaks with large dural defects.

29.5 Contraindications of LD in Skull Base Surgery

LD placement is a relative contraindication prior to skull base surgery in patients with obstructive hydrocephalus. In cases of large tumors with significant mass effect, decreasing CSF pressure in the spinal canal by lumbar drainage can cause CSF and brain mass to herniate downwards. Thus, in these cases, if early CSF drainage is needed from the LD to access the tumor, an external ventricular drain may be preferred. If an LD is used, care must be taken to prevent large volume CSF egress during insertion of the LD, and CSF should be removed slowly. Further contraindications to LD placement include coagulopathy (INR > 1.4) and thrombocytopenia (platelet count <50,000) to avoid spinal hematoma as well as local skin infection near the site of the drain due to the risk of contaminating CSF.

29.6 LD Procedure, Precautions and Patient's Instructions

29.6.1 Equipment (Fig. 29.3a)

1. Lumbar Access Kit (14 G Tuohy needle, catheter, connectors, sterile drapes, chloroprep sticks).
2. Lumbar drain collection bag.
3. Lidocaine 1% with epinephrine and 25G needle for injection.
4. Mastisol, tegaderm.
5. Sterile gloves, gown, mask, hat.

29.6.2 Procedure

1. Position patient in lateral decubitus position (or sitting) with knees tucked into chest and neck flexed (fetal position) to facilitate opening of the interlaminar space.
2. Widely prep and drape the patient in sterile fashion. Prepare tray and drain.
3. Approximate the L4-5 (L3-4) interlaminar space at the intersection of the spinous processes and top of the iliac crest (Fig. 29.3b).
4. Anesthetize the skin, tract, and interspinous ligament if necessary.
5. The Tuohy needle is inserted with the bevel facing up at a 60-degree angle to the skin into the interspinous space until the dura is penetrated (Fig. 29.3c).
6. Orient the bevel cranially and remove the needle stylet.
7. If CSF is obtained, thread the lumbar drain catheter over the wire into the Tuohy needle to at the 15–20 cm mark (Fig. 29.3d).
8. If the catheter cannot be advanced, withdraw the needle slightly or angle the needle more. NEVER PULL BACK ON THE CATHETER as this can cause shearing off of the catheter tip inside the thecal sac.
9. Remove the needle over the drain and the wire inside the catheter while maintaining the catheter position. Cap the catheter.
10. Mastisol around the site, spiral drain around on the mastisol, cover with tegaderm, ± suture drain at insertion site and connect the catheter to the drainage bag (Fig. 29.4).

29.6.3 Management

There are two primary protocols for managing LDs: draining at specific level or draining a specific volume per unit time. In the former, the

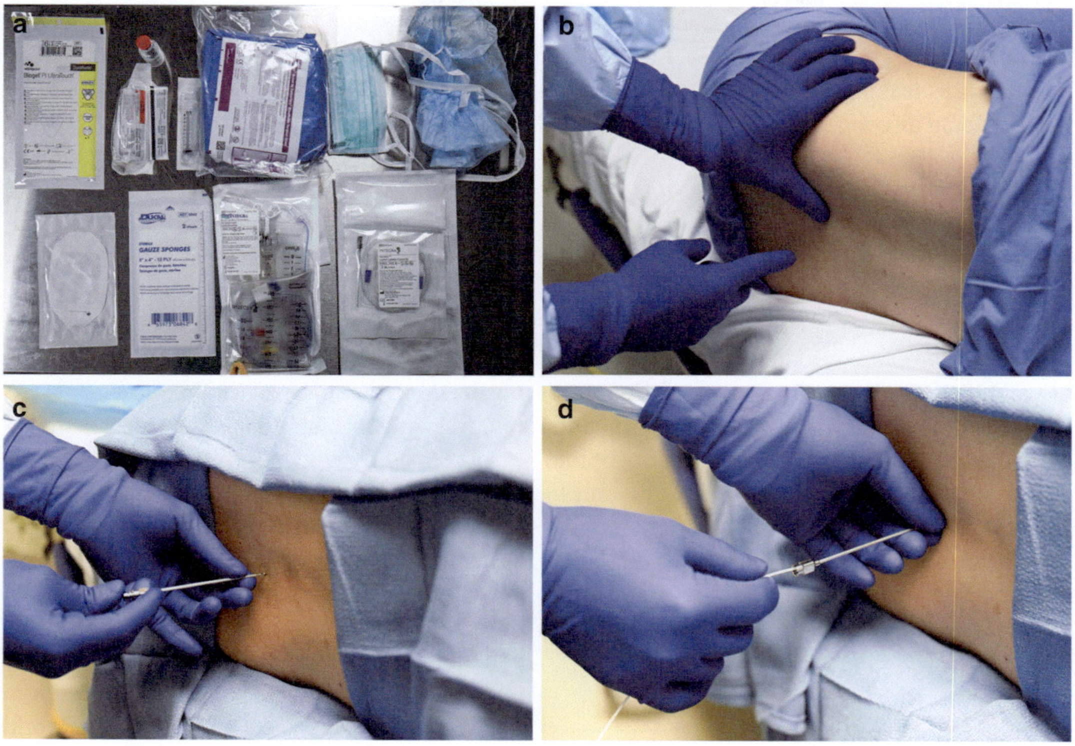

Fig. 29.3 (**a**) Equipment needed for lumbar drain placement. (**b**) Approximate L4–5 interlaminar space by palpating top of the iliac crest and spinous process. (**c**) Insert Tuohy needle at a 60-degree angle. (**d**) Thread lumbar drain catheter over the wire into the Tuohy needle until the 15–20 cm mark on the lumbar drain

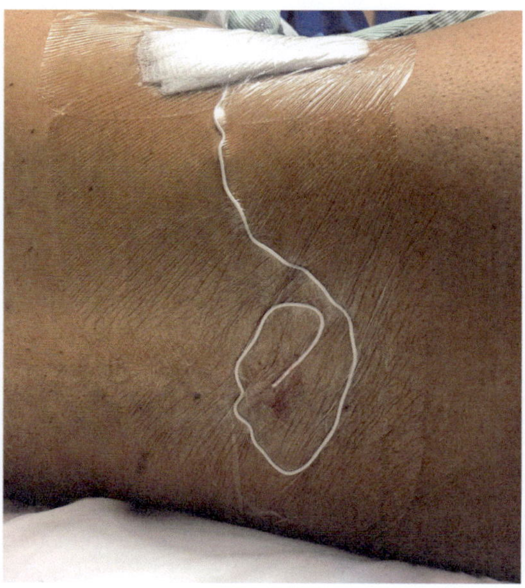

Fig. 29.4 Lumbar drain spiraled on the back with clear tegaderm dressing. All connectors and plastic portions should be padded with gauze. Inform patients to keep clean and intact

drain can be placed at a specific level in relation to the tragus and CSF will drain continuously. However, to avoid over- or under-drainage, the drain must be frequently adjusted based on the patient's position, which can be laborious and prone to error. We prefer intermittent hourly volume of drainage (10–15 cc/h). The drain is intermittently clamped once the desired volume has been drained.

29.6.4 Precautions

Thorough preparation and instructions regarding LD care should be provided to the patient prior to the procedure. Patients should notify nursing staff when changing positions or getting out of bed so that the drain can be clamped and leveled if necessary. The sterile dressing should remain intact at all times, and neither the patient nor their family should touch the drain. Finally, the patient should be educated on warning signs including severe headaches, confusion, nausea, fever, pain, incontinence, leaking of fluid around the drain site, or tubing disconnection.

29.6.5 Removal

At the time of removal, the dressing should be removed under sterile conditions. Prep the drain site with chloroprep or iodine prep. Remove the LD and confirm that the catheter is fully intact with black dot at the tip. It is a good practice to place the patient again in the fetal position for the drain removal, to facilitate opening of the interlaminar space and minimizing the risk of the catheter "snapping" due to pinching. Suture the insertion site with a dissolvable 4–0 monocryl suture. Apply a sterile dressing and have the patient remain flat in bed for 1 h.

29.7 Complications of LD

The most feared complication of LDs is a *brain herniation syndrome* (uncal, subfalcine, tonsillar) due to excess CSF drainage. In one case-matched study, there was a 10% rate of brain herniation syndrome in patients who underwent craniotomy with LDs in contrast to 3.3% of patients with craniotomy alone [29]. Signs of herniation include deterioration of consciousness, oculomotor palsy, respiratory distress, and decorticate or decerebrate rigidity. Treatment of over-drainage includes immediately clamping the drain and placing the patient in Trendelenburg position. If herniation is suspected, preservative-free 0.9% normal saline can be slowly injected into the LD.

Similarly, there are rare cases of persistent pneumocephalus in which lumbar drainage can lead to suctioning of the air through an anterior skull base defect. Failure to recognize this phenomenon can result in acute neurologic deterioration and infection. Treatment involves clamping the LD and repeat operation with skull base reconstruction using a multilayer vascularized flap is possible.

Another serious complication of LD placement is *infection* and meningitis. There is a 3–7% risk of infection with LD placement [30]. As there is no level I evidence regarding duration or CSF sampling of LDs, there remains significant heterogeneity in practice among physicians. It is known that both longer duration of catheterization (>4 days) and CSF leak at site of puncture are independent risk factors for infection [30, 31]. Thus, in our practice LDs are maintained for 3–5 days only and surveillance CSF samples are obtained at the time of drain placement and removal. Any leaking around the catheter should be prevented by stitching the drain, and leaking into non-sterile areas should prompt consideration for drain removal. Prolonged prophylactic systemic antibiotics (PPSA) also remain controversial for LDs. Lewis et al. found no significant difference in incidence of LD infections after discontinuing their institutional protocol for daily CSF testing and PPSA [32]. Guidelines from numerous medical societies including the World Health Organization, the American Society of Health-System Pharmacists, the Infectious Diseases Society of America, the Surgical Infection Society, and the Society for Healthcare Epidemiology of America state insufficient evidence to support use of antibiotics and advocate against the routine use of PPSA [33, 34].

The most common side effects of CSF drainage include *headaches, dizziness, and nausea.* These symptoms may be alleviated by caffeine, salt, acetaminophen, and antiemetics. However, if the symptoms are severe, this may indicate over-drainage. Care should be taken to ensure that the LD is leveled appropriately the patient's position and the LD should be clamped when the patient is standing. Finally, if symptoms persist after the drain is removed, this may indicate a *spinal fluid leak* and a blood patch can be performed to seal the leak.

Occasionally, the catheter can irritate a nerve root in the lumbar space leading to brief shooting *leg or back pain.* Redirecting the catheter at the time of insertion or having the patient reposition their body typically alleviates the pain. There are rarely sustained radicular or back symptoms after drain removal [35]. Patients with persistent back pain and neurologic findings such as weakness, sensory loss, or incontinence require urgent assessment for spinal hematoma. While rare, spinal magnetic resonance imaging should be performed, and surgical intervention with a laminectomy and hematoma evacuation should be performed emergently in the presence of neurologic symptoms to prevent permanent neurologic deficits.

References

1. Daly DT, et al. Extracranial approaches to the repair of cerebrospinal fluid rhinorrhea. Ear Nose Throat J. 1992;71(7):311–3.
2. Marentette LJ, Valentino J. Traumatic anterior fossa cerebrospinal fluid fistulae and craniofacial considerations. Otolaryngol Clin N Am. 1991;24(1):151–63.
3. Marmarou A, Beaumont A. Physiology of the Cerebrospinal Fluid and Intracranial Pressure. In: Youmans JR, Winn HR, editors. Youmans neurological surgery. Philadelphia, PA: Saunders; 2011. p. 169–82.
4. Eljamel MS. Fractures of the middle third of the face and cerebrospinal fluid rhinorrhoea. Br J Neurosurg. 1994;8(3):289–93.
5. Bell RB, et al. Management of cerebrospinal fluid leak associated with craniomaxillofacial trauma. J Oral Maxillofac Surg. 2004;62(6):676–84.
6. Mincy JE. Posttraumatic cerebrospinal fluid fistula of the frontal fossa. J Trauma. 1966;6(5):618–22.
7. Albu S, Florian IS, Bolboaca SD. The benefit of early lumbar drain insertion in reducing the length of CSF leak in traumatic rhinorrhea. Clin Neurol Neurosurg. 2016;142:43–7.
8. Kirtane MV, Gautham K, Upadhyaya SR. Endoscopic CSF rhinorrhea closure: our experience in 267 cases. Otolaryngol Head Neck Surg. 2005;132(2):208–12.
9. Chaaban MR, et al. Spontaneous cerebrospinal fluid leak repair: a five-year prospective evaluation. Laryngoscope. 2014;124(1):70–5.
10. Schlosser RJ, et al. Elevated intracranial pressures in spontaneous cerebrospinal fluid leaks. Am J Rhinol. 2003;17(4):191–5.
11. Lobo BC, Baumanis MM, Nelson RF. Surgical repair of spontaneous cerebrospinal fluid (CSF) leaks: a systematic review. Laryngoscope Investig Otolaryngol. 2017;2(5):215–24.
12. Casiano RR, Jassir D. Endoscopic cerebrospinal fluid rhinorrhea repair: is a lumbar drain necessary? Otolaryngol Head Neck Surg. 1999;121(6):745–50.
13. Hegazy HM, et al. Transnasal endoscopic repair of cerebrospinal fluid rhinorrhea: a meta-analysis. Laryngoscope. 2000;110(7):1166–72.
14. Caggiano C, Penn DL, Laws ER Jr. The role of the lumbar drain in endoscopic endonasal skull base surgery: a retrospective analysis of 811 cases. World Neurosurg. 2018;117:e575–9.
15. Strickland BA, et al. Identification and repair of intraoperative cerebrospinal fluid leaks in endonasal transsphenoidal pituitary surgery: surgical experience in a series of 1002 patients. J Neurosurg. 2018;129(2):425–9.
16. Gardner PA, et al. Endoscopic endonasal resection of anterior cranial base meningiomas. Neurosurgery. 2008;63(1):36–52; discussion 52-4
17. Allen KP, et al. Lumbar subarachnoid drainage in cerebrospinal fluid leaks after lateral skull base surgery. Otol Neurotol. 2011;32(9):1522–4.
18. Fraser S, et al. Risk factors associated with postoperative cerebrospinal fluid leak after endoscopic endonasal skull base surgery. J Neurosurg. 2018;128(4):1066–71.
19. Ivan ME, et al. Risk factors for postoperative cerebrospinal fluid leak and meningitis after expanded endoscopic endonasal surgery. J Clin Neurosci. 2015;22(1):48–54.
20. Patel MR, et al. How to choose? Endoscopic skull base reconstructive options and limitations. Skull Base. 2010;20(6):397–404.
21. Stokken J, et al. The utility of lumbar drains in modern endoscopic skull base surgery. Curr Opin Otolaryngol Head Neck Surg. 2015;23(1):78–82.
22. Dehdashti AR, et al. Endoscopic endonasal reconstruction of skull base: repair protocol. J Neurol Surg B Skull Base. 2016;77(3):271–8.
23. Eloy JA, et al. Efficacy of the pedicled nasoseptal flap without cerebrospinal fluid (CSF) diversion for repair of skull base defects: incidence of postoperative CSF leaks. Int Forum Allergy Rhinol. 2012;2(5):397–401.
24. Garcia-Navarro V, Anand VK, Schwartz TH. Gasket seal closure for extended endonasal endoscopic skull base surgery: efficacy in a large case series. World Neurosurg. 2013;80(5):563–8.
25. Ransom ER, et al. Assessing risk/benefit of lumbar drain use for endoscopic skull-base surgery. Int Forum Allergy Rhinol. 2011;1(3):173–7.
26. D'Anza B, et al. Role of lumbar drains in contemporary endonasal skull base surgery: meta-analysis and systematic review. Am J Rhinol Allergy. 2016;30(6):430–5.
27. Ahmed OH, et al. Efficacy of perioperative lumbar drainage following endonasal endoscopic cerebrospinal fluid leak repair. Otolaryngol Head Neck Surg. 2017;156(1):52–60.
28. Zwagerman NT, et al. Does lumbar drainage reduce postoperative cerebrospinal fluid leak after endoscopic endonasal skull base surgery? A prospective, randomized controlled trial. J Neurosurg. 2018;1–7.
29. Motoyama Y, et al. Risk of brain herniation after craniotomy with lumbar spinal drainage: a propensity score analysis. J Neurosurg. 2018;1–11.

30. Schade RP, et al. Bacterial meningitis caused by the use of ventricular or lumbar cerebrospinal fluid catheters. J Neurosurg. 2005;102(2):229–34.
31. Liang H, et al. Risk factors for infections related to lumbar drainage in spontaneous subarachnoid hemorrhage. Neurocrit Care. 2016;25(2):243–9.
32. Lewis A, Rothstein A, Pacione D. Results of a quality improvement initiative reassessing an institutional lumbar drain infection prevention protocol. J Neurosurg Spine. 2018;29(1):54–8.
33. Allegranzi B, et al. New WHO recommendations on intraoperative and postoperative measures for surgical site infection prevention: an evidence-based global perspective. Lancet Infect Dis. 2016;16(12):e288–303.
34. Bratzler DW, et al. Clinical practice guidelines for antimicrobial prophylaxis in surgery. Am J Health Syst Pharm. 2013;70(3):195–283.
35. Evans RW. Complications of lumbar puncture. Neurol Clin. 1998;16(1):83–105.

30 Long-Term Follow-Up Strategy

Islam R. Herzallah and Mona Ashoor

30.1 Introduction

Endoscopic endonasal repair of CSF rhinorrhea has become the standard method of practice for skull base defects, with excellent prognosis and success rate by means of improved surgical techniques and advancement in surgical instrumentation. Nevertheless, in order to maintain the success of the skull base repair, it is imperative that the postoperative follow-up course is equally taken into attention to maintain the repair integrity and reduce complications such as recurrent CSF leak and meningitis. Despite the importance of postoperative management and long-term follow-up in the ultimate success of the endoscopic technique, there is generally lack of evidence on the "optimal postoperative care" [1]. Hence, many of the postoperative strategies covered in this chapter are protocols applied in our own practice or described by different experts.

I. R. Herzallah (✉)
Otolaryngology - Head & Neck Surgery Departments, Faculty of Medicine, Zagazig University, Zagazig, Egypt

M. Ashoor
Department of Otolaryngology Head and Neck Surgery, King Fahad Hospital of the University, Al Khobar, Saudi Arabia

Department of Otolaryngology Head and Neck Surgery, College of Medicine, Imam Abdulrahman Bin Faisal University, Dammam, Saudi Arabia
e-mail: mashoor@iau.edu.sa

30.2 Intraoperative Considerations

Several intraoperative measures are important for a smooth postoperative course. Patency of exposed sinus ostia should be ensured at the end of surgery. Similarly, middle meatal patency is to be maintained by adequate middle turbinate medialization if the turbinate was not already removed or utilized as a flap. Covering the repaired defect area with a mucosal graft or a flap, as applicable, avoids extensive crust formation and promotes healing. It is important to avoid covering the sinonasal mucosa with the graft or the flap to avoid mucocele formation, which has been reported in up to 8% of cases after endoscopic skull base reconstruction [2].

We usually place a dissolvable hemostatic packing (e.g., Surgicel Fibrillar, Ethicon) to seal the edges of the graft, hold it against the underlying bone, and promote inflammatory reaction and healing at the same time. The surgeon may also apply some tissue sealant (e.g., Duraseal, Medtronic) to further seal the edges of the defect and help holding the graft against the bone, although some authors have advocated that tissue sealant may be redundant and an unnecessary expense [3]. We then routinely apply several pieces of Gelfoam over the repair before placing a fixing piece of non-absorbable packing (e.g., Merocel, Medtronic) at the end to bolster the repair and ensure minimal mobilization of the graft. If possible, we place the Merocel while

A. A. AlQahtani et al. (eds.), *CSF Rhinorrhea*, https://doi.org/10.1007/978-3-030-94781-1_30

maintaining at least a partially patent nasal airway for patient's comfort. The Merocel is usually removed around the sixth postoperative day. Alternative methods of fixation include Foley's catheter balloon or cut glove finger with a piece of Merocel inside. It has to be noted, however, that there is no evidence to support better outcome with the use of nasal packing after endoscopic CSF leak repair, neither that favors one packing method over the other, and thus further research is required in this area [4].

30.3 Immediate Postoperative Care and ICU Management

Following endoscopic CSF leak repair, most patients can be admitted to the neurologic nursing floor or the specialized surgery unit. Patients with large skull base defects, meningoencephaloceles, significant intraoperative manipulations, or complex defects are admitted to a monitored neurologic intensive care unit. Head is generally kept elevated for 30°. It is advisable to maintain systolic blood pressure below 140 mmHg. Breathing from a nasal cannula should be avoided to minimize the risk of pneumocephalus and to decrease nasal dryness. Alternatively, breathing from a face tint with humidification is allowed. Urinary catheter is kept overnight and removed on the first postoperative morning to encourage ambulation. Unless the patient has signs or symptoms suggestive of potential complications (e.g., severe headache, rhinorrhea, or altered mental status), routine postoperative computed tomography after uncomplicated endoscopic skull base surgery seems to be unnecessary [5].

The use of lumbar drain in the postoperative setting remains controversial and depends on several factors, and this topic is discussed extensively elsewhere in this book. In summary, the available evidence suggests that routine placement of lumbar drains does not contribute to successful outcome [4, 6]. Additionally, using lumbar drains appears to lengthen hospital stay and incur unnecessary costs and potential complications such as pneumocephalus, persistent CSF leak from the dural puncture, meningitis, and brain herniation [4]. However, placing a lumbar drain in cases of spontaneous CSF rhinorrhea can provide useful information regarding intracranial hypertension, which should be managed appropriately to improve success rate in such cases [7–9]. Lumbar drainage was also shown to reduce postoperative CSF leak after endoscopic endonasal skull base surgery for high-flow leaks defined as those with dural defect greater than 1 cm^2 with extensive arachnoid dissection, and/or dissection into a ventricle or cistern [10].

30.4 Early Postoperative Care

Following endoscopic closure of skull base defects, it is crucial to communicate with the patient to reinforce postoperative instructions to help avoid significant increase in CSF pressure for the early postoperative period. This includes avoiding leaning forward, straining, drinking from a straw, or heavy lifting. Patients are also instructed to avoid nose blowing and to maintain an open mouth whenever sneezing. Soft bowel regimen is also prescribed. We typically ask patients to continue on postoperative instructions for 6 weeks. However, because of insufficient evidence, human clinical studies are required to clarify if and how long restricted activity is necessary postoperatively [4]. Similarly, research is required to determine when patients can safely tolerate the CSF pressure changes associated with air travel or with continuous positive airway pressure (CPAP) treatment [4].

In addition to the intraoperative antibiotic, further antibiotic prophylaxis with anti-staphylococcal coverage is continued for the duration the non-absorbable pack is left in the nose to reduce the risk of toxic shock syndrome. Starting from the first or second postoperative day, saline nasal spray is gently installed 3–4 times daily. Local ointment can also be applied repeatedly to help minimize nasal crusting. Merocel pack is left in place for around 6 days and then smoothly removed after gentle saline irrigation. Serial endoscopic debridement are

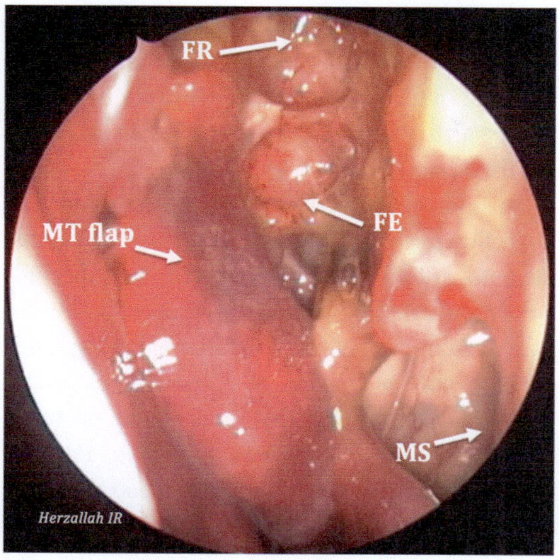

Fig. 30.1 Endoscopic view at 5 weeks post endoscopic repair of left cribriform defect CSF rhinorrhea using inlay–onlay technique with middle turbinate (*MT*) flap. *FR* frontal recess; *MS* maxillary sinus; *FE* fovea ethmoidalis

also carefully performed in the clinic to remove anterior nasal crusting and help maintain patent nasal airway, while avoiding debridement close to the repaired skull base defect for around 5–6 weeks to prevent healing disturbance and graft displacement. By this time, meticulous debridement can be performed over the repaired area, and the mucosal graft or flap is expected to be visualized incorporating into the surrounding tissues (Fig. 30.1).

30.5 Special Considerations in Patients with Spontaneous CSF Rhinorrhea

Several studies have shown that spontaneous CSF rhinorrhea is associated with idiopathic intracranial hypertension (IIH) in most cases [9, 11–13]. Unless properly diagnosed and treated, IIH can result in 25–87% recurrence rate of CSF rhinorrhea [7, 11], compared to less than 10% in patients without IIH [14].

Preoperative measurement of CSF pressure would be of limited value since the already present leak decreases the CSF pressure [15]. On the other hand, postoperative measurement can detect intracranial hypertension if the appropriate protocol is implemented. To do so, a lumbar drain is placed at the time of graft placement; the drain is opened to maintain drainage at 5–10 mL/h. On postoperative day 2, the three-way stopcock attached to the lumbar drain system is turned to the off position to clamp the drain. About 3–4 h is allowed to pass to replenish the patient's CSF volume, and then a standardized pressure transducer is connected to measure the CSF pressure before removal of the lumbar drain [9]. CSF pressure should be measured at three separate occasions during the day [7]. Some authors have highlighted the importance of continuous CSF pressure monitoring with lumber drain in place using a pressure monitoring system [8]. Such continuous monitoring takes into account intracranial pressure (ICP) changes due to patient positioning or physiologic CSF pressure fluctuation overnight, and thus can detect transient abnormal pressure elevations, e.g., in patients with obstructive sleep apnea [8, 16].

Patients with elevated CSF pressure (>25 H_2O) should undergo a proper management protocol [7, 9]. Initially, we recommend acetazolamide 500 mg twice daily, along with a weight reduction regimen. If ICP remains above 25 cm H_2O despite acetazolamide, addition of furosemide or changing to topiramate may be considered [7]. Patients who continue to have elevated CSF pressure or papilledema should undergo optic nerve fenestration or some sort of CSF diversion, e.g., ventriculo-peritoneal shunt (VPS) [7].

Serial postoperative neuro-ophthalmologic evaluations of patients should be performed. It is possible that patients could develop worsening vision after repair. In one study, 7% of patients were reported to have papilledema after closure of CSF rhinorrhea and 25% were found to have visual field defects as well [17]. Patients may also develop headache and tinnitus as signs of IIH.

30.6 Frequency and Length of Follow-Up After CSF Leak Repair

The aim of the postoperative follow-up after CSF leak repair is to ensure complete healing of the surgical site, cessation of the CSF leak, resolution of the underlying etiology, and absence of complications. It is well established that most etiologies of CSF leaks (i.e., neoplastic, iatrogenic, and traumatic) have low recurrence rates of <10%. However, spontaneous CSF leaks are known to have higher rates in the range of 25–87% [7, 11, 18]. Hence, the long-term follow-up will depend on the patient and the underlying pathology causing the CSF rhinorrhea.

After the serial evaluation and debridement stated earlier, further follow-up visits will depend on the endoscopic status of the nasal cavity, the aim should be reaching an endoscopic view with no crusting, well-incorporated graft margins, healed nasal mucosa, and no CSF leak (Fig. 30.2). There is still no consensus on the exact timing of postoperative follow-up after CSF leak repair. In a retrospective analysis by Castelnuovo et al. of 31 patients treated by the endoscopic approach for CSF rhinorrhea repair, the follow-up consisted of endoscopic evaluations every 3 months for the first year followed by twice yearly until the fifth year [19].

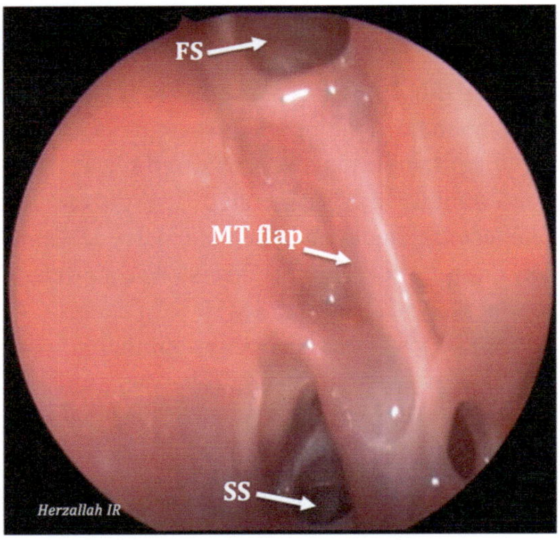

Fig. 30.2 Endoscopic view 1 year post endoscopic repair of left fovea ethmoidalis CSF rhinorrhea using inlay–onlay technique with middle turbinate (*MT*) flap. *FS* frontal sinus; *SS* sphenoid sinus

In a prospective cohort study of nasal morbidity following skull base surgery in 63 patients, the authors found that the most common morbidity is nasal crusting, which was present in 98% of patients with nearly 50% of patients having moderate to severe crusting at 1 month postoperatively. The median time to absence of nasal crusting in this cohort was 101 days. Patients who had a more complex approach had a significantly longer time to be free of nasal crusting compared with a simple approach (105 vs. 93 days). The median time for re-mucosalization in patients with nasoseptal flap (NSF) was 89 days (95% CI, 72.7–105.3) [20]. It is important to understand the timeline of these changes in order to educate patients about the expected postoperative course, as well as for timing of postoperative follow-up visits. In a literature review, the incidence of mucocele formation post endoscopic skull base reconstruction has been reported to be 8% [2]. Hence, patients should also be monitored postoperatively for signs and symptoms suggestive of mucocele formation.

A meta-analysis of complications post repair of a cerebrospinal fistula revealed a very low incidence of surgical complications such as meningitis (0.3%), brain abscess (0.9%), subdural hematoma (0.3%), smell disorders (0.6%), and headache (0.3%) [21]. Similar results were found in a survey of the members of the American Rhinologic Society for the safety and efficacy of endoscopic repair of CSF leaks and encephaloceles; it was found that 2.5% of 522 patients surgically managed for CSF fistula suffered a complication, the most common being meningitis at 1.1% [22]. This indicates that postoperative complications are rare and probably close lifelong follow-up might not be necessary, in contrast to the transcranial approach for CSF rhinorrhea repair where delayed meningitis has been reported and patient follow-up is recommended to be life-long.

30.7 Methods of Surveillance

30.7.1 Clinically

Detailed history should be taken from the patient at every postoperative visit, focusing on symptoms suggesting recurrent CSF rhinorrhea such as unilateral watery rhinorrhea, also symptoms of sinusitis/sinus mucocele as a complication of sinus drainage obstruction, and symptoms suggestive of increase intracranial pressure such as headache and blurred vision. This should be followed by an endoscopic nasal examination, utilizing rigid angled scopes (30°, 45°) to evaluate the reconstruction site, focusing on complete mucosal healing, no crusting, inflammation, patent sinus outflow tracts, and no CSF leak.

30.7.2 Postoperative Imaging

There is still no consensus on the method and timing of imaging after endoscopic skull base surgery; some authors advocated to perform a postoperative computed tomographic scan on day 1 postop in order to obtain a baseline image and to identify any complications that may not have early neurological signs but might have serious long-term complications (such as subdural hematomas and early tension pneumocephalus) [23]. However, as stated earlier in this chapter, recent evidence suggests that routine postoperative computed tomography after uncomplicated endoscopic skull base surgery seems to be unnecessary, unless the patient has signs or symptoms suggestive of potential complications (e.g., severe headache, rhinorrhea, or altered mental status) [5].

Subsequent imaging is individualized and performed based on factors such as underlying pathology and extent of tumor resection obtained (gross total vs. subtotal resection). For benign pathology, this is anywhere between 6 and 12 months, whereas imaging is performed sooner and more frequently for malignancies [1]. Figure 30.3 shows a sinus CT scan performed 1 year after successful repair of left CSF rhinorrhea.

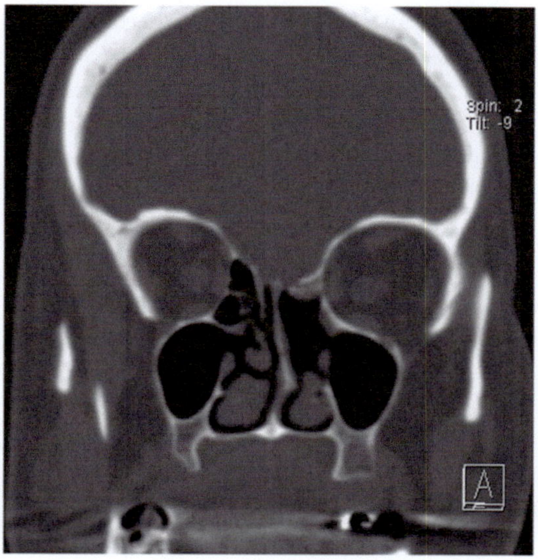

Fig. 30.3 Computed tomography of paranasal sinuses one-year post endoscopic repair of left CSF rhinorrhea using inlay–onlay technique with middle turbinate (*MT*) flap

When repair of a defect is near a sinus outflow tract, there is a risk of obstruction of the normal sinus drainage, which may lead to a mucocele formation. In such cases, a postoperative follow-up with CT scanning is appropriate to rule out the development of a mucocele when there is concern for obstruction and a pre-knowledge of the surgical procedure that was near a sinus outflow tract.

Postoperative MRI is usually done for cases in which there is concern for residual disease and to better delineate the surround structures such as dura and cranial nerves.

30.7.3 Neuro-Ophthalmological Evaluation

Patients presenting with headache or visual field disturbances after CSF leak repair, or in whom IIH is suspected as a cause of the leak, should have a neuro-ophthalmological evaluation to assess for increased ICP. In a series of 28 patients who received neuro-ophthalmologic evaluations postoperatively, two (7%) patients had papilledema and seven (25%) developed visual field defects which was due to an increase in mean CSF pressures [17].

Patients with active CSF leaks due to increased ICP usually do not present with papilledema before the surgical repair. Aaron et al. [24] examined the presence of preoperative papilledema in spontaneous CSF leaks of 16 patients, none were found to have papilledema. Once the CSF leak has been repaired without attempting to normalize the high ICP, these patients may present with postoperative papilledema. This might be explained by the hypothesis that the leak acts as a release valve reducing the incidence of papilledema [25]. Thus, it is a possibility that patients may develop worsening vision after repair.

30.7.4 Quality of Life (QOL) Assessment

QOL assessment provides important information regarding the surgical outcome of endoscopic skull base reconstruction surgery and the associated sinonasal morbidity. Numerous QOL questionnaires have been proposed for endoscopic skull base surgery outcome assessment and sinonasal morbidity postoperative. Examples of QOL forms include: Rhinosinusitis Outcome Measure (RSOM)-31 [26], Short Form-36 (SF-36) [27], Anterior Skull Base Questionnaire [27], Anterior Skull Base Nasal Inventory-12 [28], Sinonasal Outcome Test (SNOT)-20 [29], and SNOT-22 [30, 31].

Initial QOL scores are the lowest during the early months postoperatively, which gradually normalizes after 3–9 months postoperative [28–32]. More extended surgery (such as NSF) will lead to lower QOL scores, poorer SF-36, and RSOM-31 scores at 3 months after surgery [26, 27].

Olfactory outcome after endoscopic skull base surgery shows contradictory results in literature. Some patients have stated the return of olfaction sense back to normal several months postoperatively, despite surgical resection of the olfactory neuroepithelium lining the cribriform plate, superior turbinate, superior septum, and in some areas of the middle turbinate during endoscopic skull base surgery [33–35]. In contrast, other studies have documented a permanent decrease in smell function post endoscopic skull base surgery, the degree of olfactory loss corresponded to the extent of the surgical approach [36, 37]. Indeed, whenever applicable, the surgeon should make every effort to avoid unnecessary resection of the olfactory epithelium, including designing NSF with proper preservation of superior olfactory strip to reduce the risk of permanent hyposmia [38].

30.7.5 Other Methods of Surveillance

β2-Transferrin testing and fluorescein nasal endoscopic evaluation are performed only when suggested by the clinical suspicion of recurrence, as in cases of recurrent rhinorrhea or meningitis [19].

References

1. Tien DA, Stokken JK, Recinos PF, Woodard TD, Sindwani R. Comprehensive postoperative management after endoscopic skull base surgery. Otolaryngol Clin N Am. 2016 Feb;49(1):253–63.
2. Awad AJ, Mohyeldin A, El-Sayed IH, Aghi MK. Sinonasal morbidity following endoscopic endonasal skull base surgery. Clin Neurol Neurosurg. 2015;130:162–7.
3. Eloy JA, Choudhry OJ, Friedel ME, Kuperan AB, Liu JK. Endoscopic nasoseptal flap repair of skull base defects: is addition of a dural sealant necessary? Otolaryngol Head Neck Surg. 2012;147(1):161–6.
4. Oakley G, Orlandi R, Woodworth B, Batra P, Alt J. Management of cerebrospinal fluid rhinorrhea: an evidence-based review with recommendations. Int Forum Allergy Rhinol. 2015;6(1):17–24.
5. Nadimi S, Caballero N, Carpenter P, Sowa L, Cunningham R, Welch K. Immediate postoperative imaging after uncomplicated endoscopic approach to the anterior skull base: is it necessary? Int Forum Allergy Rhinol. 2014;4(12):1024–9.
6. Albu S, Emanuelli E, Trombitas V, Florian I. Effectiveness of lumbar drains on recurrence rates in endoscopic surgery of cerebrospinal fluid leaks. Am J Rhinol Allergy. 2013;27(6):e190–4.
7. Campbell R, Farquhar D, Zhao N, Chiu A, Adappa N, Palmer J. Cerebrospinal fluid rhinorrhea secondary to idiopathic intracranial hypertension: long-term outcomes of endoscopic repairs. Am J Rhinol Allergy. 2016;30(4):294–300.

8. Reh D, Gallia G, Ramanathan M, Solomon D, Moghekar A, Ishii M, et al. Perioperative continuous cerebrospinal fluid pressure monitoring in patients with spontaneous cerebrospinal fluid leaks: presentation of a novel technique. Am J Rhinol Allergy. 2010;24(3):238–43.
9. Woodworth B, Prince A, Chiu A, Cohen N, Schlosser R, Bolger W, et al. Spontaneous CSF leaks: a paradigm for definitive repair and management of intracranial hypertension. Otolaryngol Head Neck Surg. 2008;138(6):715–20.
10. Zwagerman N, Wang E, Shin S, Chang Y, Fernandez-Miranda J, Snyderman C, et al. Does lumbar drainage reduce postoperative cerebrospinal fluid leak after endoscopic endonasal skull base surgery? A prospective, randomized controlled trial. J Neurosurg. 2018;1:1–7.
11. Schlosser R, Wilensky E, Grady M, Bolger W. Elevated intracranial pressures in spontaneous cerebrospinal fluid leaks. Am J Rhinol. 2003;17(4):191–5.
12. Schlosser R, Wilensky E, Grady M, Palmer J, Kennedy D, Bolger W. Cerebrospinal fluid pressure monitoring after repair of cerebrospinal fluid leaks. Otolaryngol Head Neck Surg. 2004;130(4):443–8.
13. Schlosser R, Woodworth B, Wilensky E, Grady M, Bolger W. Spontaneous cerebrospinal fluid leaks: a variant of benign intracranial hypertension. Ann Otol Rhinol Laryngol. 2006;115(7):495–500.
14. Harvey R, Parmar P, Sacks R, Zanation A. Endoscopic skull base reconstruction of large dural defects: a systematic review of published evidence. Laryngoscope. 2012;122(2):452–9.
15. Ramakrishnan V, Suh J, Chiu A, Palmer J. Reliability of preoperative assessment of cerebrospinal fluid pressure in the management of spontaneous cerebrospinal fluid leaks and encephaloceles. Int Forum Allergy Rhinol. 2011;1(3):201–5.
16. LeVay A, Kveton J. Relationship between obesity, obstructive sleep apnea, and spontaneous cerebrospinal fluid Otorrhea. Laryngoscope. 2008;118(2):275–8.
17. Jiang Z, McLean C, Perez C, Barnett S, Friedman D, Tajudeen B, et al. Surgical outcomes and postoperative Management in Spontaneous Cerebrospinal Fluid Rhinorrhea. J Neurol Surg B Skull Base. 2018;79(02):193–9.
18. Pérez M, Bialer O, Bruce B, Newman N, Biousse V. Primary spontaneous cerebrospinal fluid leaks and idiopathic intracranial hypertension. J Neuroophthalmol. 2013;33(4):327–34.
19. Castelnuovo P, Mauri S, Locatelli D, Emanuelli E, Delù G, Di Giulio G. Endoscopic repair of cerebrospinal fluid rhinorrhea: learning from our failures. Am J Rhinol. 2001;15(5):333–42.
20. de Almeida J, Snyderman C, Gardner P, Carrau R, Vescan A. Nasal morbidity following endoscopic skull base surgery: a prospective cohort study. Head Neck. 2010;33(4):547–51.
21. Hegazy H, Carrau R, Snyderman C, Kassam A, Zweig J. Transnasal endoscopic repair of cerebrospinal fluid rhinorrhea: a meta-analysis. Laryngoscope. 2000;110(7):1166–72.
22. Senior B, Jafri K, Benninger M. Safety and efficacy of endoscopic repair of CSF leaks and encephaloceles: a survey of the members of the American Rhinologic Society. Am J Rhinol. 2001;15(1):21–5.
23. Carrau R, Weissman J, Janecka I, Snyderman C, Curtin H, Sekhar L, et al. Computerized tomography and magnetic resonance imaging following cranial base surgery. Laryngoscope. 1991;101(9):951–9.
24. Aaron G, Vaphiades M, Riley K, Doyle J, Woodworth B. Increased intracranial pressure in spontaneous CSF leak patients is not associated with papilledema. Otolaryngol Head Neck Surg. 2014;151(1_suppl):P121.
25. Aaron G, Doyle J, Vaphiades M, Riley K, Woodworth B. Increased intracranial pressure in spontaneous CSF leak patients is not associated with papilledema. Otolaryngol Head Neck Surg. 2014;151(6):1061–6.
26. Alobid I, Enseñat J, Mariño-Sánchez F, Rioja E, de Notaris M, Mullol J, et al. Expanded Endonasal approach using vascularized septal flap reconstruction for Skull Base tumors has a negative impact on sinonasal symptoms and quality of life. Am J Rhinol Allergy. 2013;27(5):426–31.
27. Abergel A. Comparison of quality of life after Transnasal endoscopic vs open Skull Base tumor resection. Arch Otolaryngol Head Neck Surg. 2012;138(2):142.
28. Little A, Kelly D, Milligan J, Griffiths C, Prevedello D, Carrau R, et al. Predictors of sinonasal quality of life and nasal morbidity after fully endoscopic transsphenoidal surgery. J Neurosurg. 2015;122(6):1458–65.
29. Balaker A, Bergsneider M, Martin N, Wang M. Evolution of Sinonasal symptoms following endoscopic anterior skull base surgery. Skull Base. 2010;20(04):245–51.
30. Pant H, Bhatki A, Snyderman C, Vescan A, Carrau R, Gardner P, et al. Quality of life following endonasal skull base surgery. Skull Base. 2010;20(01):035–40.
31. Zimmer LA, Shah O, Theodosopoulos PV. Short-term quality-of-life changes after endoscopic pituitary surgery rated with SNOT-22. J Neurol Surg B Skull Base. 2014;75(04):288–92.
32. Kirkman M, Borg A, Al-Mousa A, et al. Quality-of-life after anterior skull base surgery a systematic review. J Neurol Surg B Skull Base. 2014;75(2):73–89.
33. Hart C, Theodosopoulos P, Zimmer L. Olfactory changes after endoscopic pituitary tumor resection. Otolaryngol Head Neck Surg. 2010;142(1):95–7.
34. Kim S, Park K, Khalmuratova R, Lee H, Jeon S, Kim D. Clinical and histologic studies of olfactory outcomes after nasoseptal flap harvesting. Laryngoscope. 2013;123(7):1602–6.
35. Bedrosian J, McCoul E, Raithatha R, Akselrod O, Anand V, Schwartz T. A prospective study of postoperative symptoms in sinonasal quality-of-life following endoscopic skull-base surgery: dissociations based on specific symptoms. Int Forum Allergy Rhinol. 2013;3(8):664–9.

36. Tam S, Duggal N, Rotenberg B. Olfactory outcomes following endoscopic pituitary surgery with or without septal flap reconstruction: a randomized controlled trial. Int Forum Allergy Rhinol. 2012;3(1):62–5.
37. Georgalas C, Badloe R, van Furth W, Reinartz S, Fokkens W. Quality of life in extended endonasal approaches for skull base tumours. Rhinology journal. 2012;50(3):255–61.
38. Upadhyay S, Buohliqah L, Dolci R, Otto B, Prevedello D, Carrau R. Periodic olfactory assessment in patients undergoing skull base surgery with preservation of the olfactory strip. Laryngoscope. 2017;127(9):1970–5.
39. Ransom E, Palmer J, Kennedy D, Chiu A. Assessing risk/benefit of lumbar drain use for endoscopic skull-base surgery. Int Forum Allergy Rhinol. 2011;1(3):173–7.

Cerebrospinal Fluid Rhinorrhea in Children

31

Chadi A. Makary, Habib G. Zalzal,
and Hassan H. Ramadan

31.1 Introduction to Pediatric Cerebrospinal Fluid Leaks

Rhinorrhea, or excess mucous within the nasal passage, in children is one of the most common complaints associated with allergy and sinonasal disease. Typically, the condition is self-limiting, as once the nasal membrane mucosa stops producing excess secretions, then rhinorrhea will cease accumulation within the nasal cavity [1]. Differential diagnosis of rhinorrhea is vast, and in children, the most common etiology is infectious or allergic rhinitis. Rare, but more concerning, causes of rhinorrhea do include congenital abnormalities resulting in obstruction and drainage (such as nasal masses) or cerebrospinal fluid (CSF) leakage [1].

CSF leaks occur from an aberrant communication between the subarachnoid space and the sinuses of the nose and/or temporal bone. CSF rhinorrhea, which specifically is drainage of CSF fluid within the nasal cavity, may occur due to an osseous defect of the cranial skull base within the paranasal sinuses, or temporal bone with drainage down the eustachian tube, due to disruption within the dura mater and arachnoid meningeal layer [2]. Defects within the brain barrier resulting in CSF rhinorrhea are particularly concerning in children due to the potential for meningitis, pneumocephalus, and other neurologic complications. This chapter will describe the most common causes of CSF rhinorrhea in children, in addition to diagnostic steps and optimal treatment strategies for repairing a CSF leak.

31.2 Etiology and Pathophysiology

CSF rhinorrhea in children is uncommon and differs from its adult counterpart in multiple aspects. Etiologies of pediatric CSF leak are varied as are the approaches for surgical repairs. Congenital skull base defects constitute a large portion of pediatric CSF leaks, specifically up to 69% of the cases, while other etiologies such as accidental or iatrogenic trauma are around 30% of the cases [3].

31.2.1 Congenital Etiology

Congenital skull base defects are a rare finding resulting in the development of meningoceles (meninges only) or meningoencephaloceles (meninges and brain material). The incidence of these defects is about 1 in 4000–5000 live births

The authors deny any conflict of interests or funding sources associated with this chapter.

C. A. Makary · H. G. Zalzal · H. H. Ramadan (✉)
Department of Otolaryngology-Head and Neck Surgery, West Virginia University School of Medicine, Morgantown, WV, USA
e-mail: hramadan@hsc.wvu.edu

A. A. AlQahtani et al. (eds.), *CSF Rhinorrhea*, https://doi.org/10.1007/978-3-030-94781-1_31

[4, 5]. Location of the skull base defect in relation to the fronticulus frontalis, prenasal space, and foramen cecum and extent of herniation determine the type of nasal meningoencephaloceles. These can be classified as occipital, sincipital or frontonasal, basal, convexity, or atretic (Fig. 31.1). Occipital meningoencephaloceles are the most common (75%) and are outside the scope of discussion in this chapter. Sincipital defects occur at various locations between the nasal bones and foramen cecum and result in meningoencephaloceles at various locations in the glabella, lateral to the nose or into the orbit.

Basal defects and herniations can be divided into transethmoidal (intranasal), sphenoethmoidal (nasopharynx), transphenoidal (nasopharynx), and sphenomaxillary (pterygopalatine fossa) meningoencephaloceles [6]. Intranasal congenital meningoencephaloceles can present in a variety of symptoms (Fig. 31.2). Incidental nasal mass is the most common presentation early in life [3]. Nasal masses can lead to nasal obstruction and nasal discharge, particularly in infants due to obligate nasal breathing. Nasal obstruction can lead to spells of cyanosis relieved by mouth opening and can affect the ability of the infant to feed resulting in failure to thrive. Other presenting symptoms include spontaneous unilateral or bilateral clear CSF rhinorrhea, and acute or recurrent meningitis [7]. In a 2015 study looking at skull base defects in pediatric patients, 52% of kids presented with active CSF rhinorrhea, 6% had history of meningitis, and 52% complained of nasal obstruction [3]. A different 2010 study also showed that nasal obstruction was the presenting symptom of 50% of children with anterior skull base defects [8].

31.2.2 Traumatic Etiology

Traumatic CSF leak is the second most common etiology of CSF leak in children. It can be further divided into accidental and iatrogenic [9]. Accidental head trauma results in fractures of the skull base, which leads to CSF leakage that can present acutely or delayed. Fractures are not limited to the intranasal cavity, as temporal bone fractures can also lead to leakage of CSF into the middle ear space which subsequently drains through the eustachian tube and can also present as rhinorrhea. In either case, patients will present with clear rhinorrhea following their known trauma.

Iatrogenic skull base defects in children occur following endoscopic sinus surgery (ESS) for chronic rhinosinusitis (CRS) (Fig. 31.3) or following resection of skull base tumors. The rate of CSF leak during ESS for pediatric CRS can be as low as 0.6% [10]. These leaks are and should be repaired directly when recognized during the surgery. The incidence of CSF leak following endoscopic endonasal resection of skull base tumors in children is higher and can be up to 54%, depending on the tumor pathology and size [11].

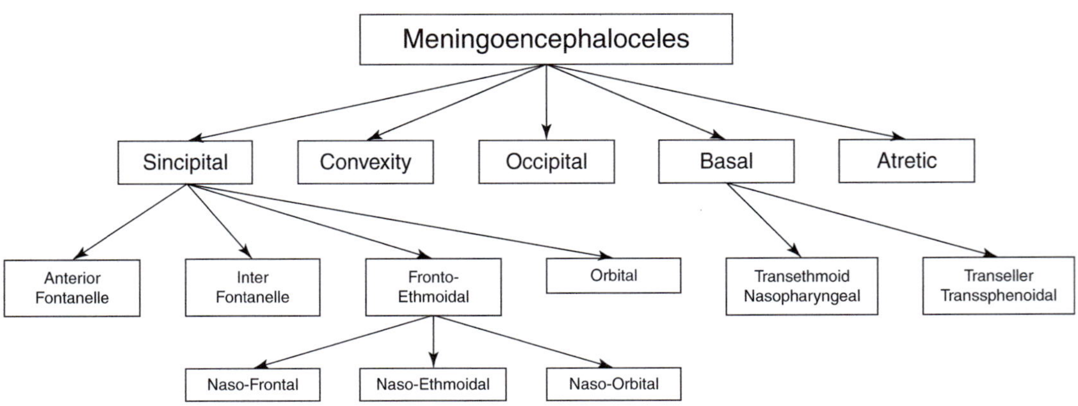

Fig. 31.1 Anatomical locations for congenital meningoencephaloceles. From a rhinologic standpoint, CSF leak repair commonly involves treatment of a sincipital or basal encephaloceles and their specific subsites shown in the flowchart

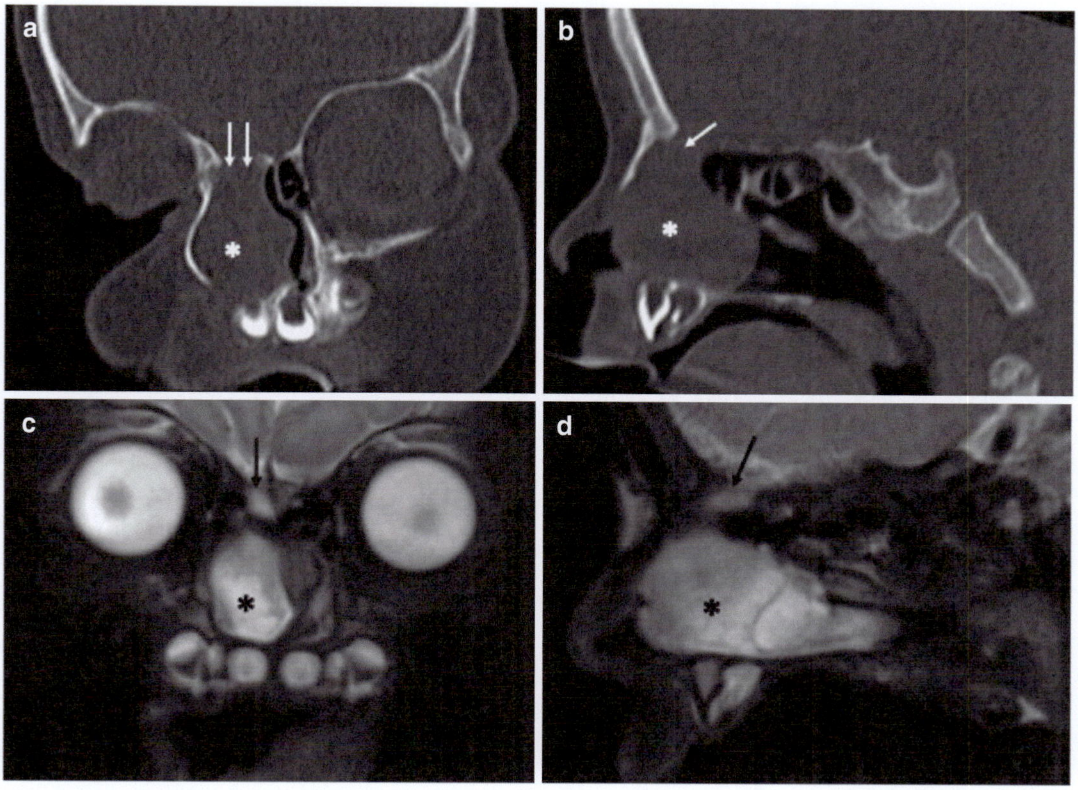

Fig. 31.2 An 8-month-old infant presented with nasal obstruction and cyanotic spells upon feeding. HRCT, bone window, coronal cuts (**a**) and sagittal cuts (**b**), and MRI T2 window, coronal cuts (**c**), and sagittal cuts (**d**) show a large right nasal meningoencephalocele (asterisk) herniating through a defect in the anterior skull base (arrows)

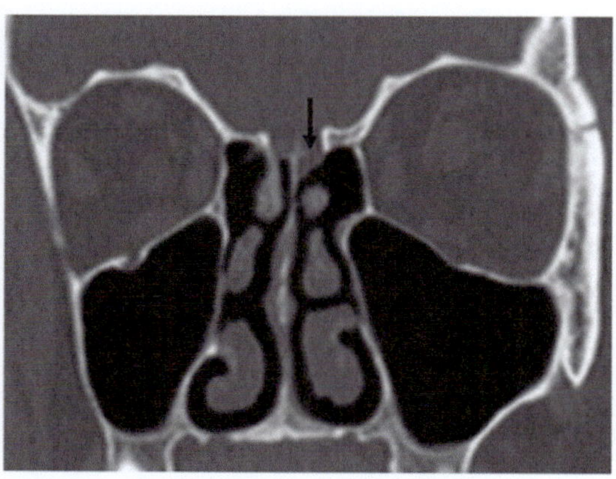

Fig. 31.3 A 16-year-old patient with active CSF rhinorrhea after ESS for CRS. A CT scan of the sinuses with bone window, coronal cuts shows an iatrogenic defect in the lateral lamella of the cribriform plate (arrow)

31.3 Diagnostic Work-Up and Localization of CSF Leaks

Beta-2 transferrin is a noninvasive, highly sensitive, and specific test to confirm CSF rhinorrhea [12]. Beta-2 transferrin is a glycoprotein that is present in CSF but not in nasal drainage and surrounding mucosa. The sensitivity ranges from 87% to 100%, and the specificity ranges from 71% to 100% [12–14]. This lab test is highly recommended to be first-line for CSF confirmation in nasal drainage before more invasive and high-cost studies are done to localize the site of skull base defects and CSF leaks. It is used in both children and adults.

Once CSF leak is confirmed, localization studies are then considered. High-resolution computed tomography scan (HRCT), MR cisternography, CT cisternography, and intrathecal fluorescein are available. HRCT is a common initial study for visualization of the bony skull base, and hence, localization of even small defects. HRCT has an accuracy of 87–93% [12, 15]. It is also important for surgical planning of the sinus anatomy surrounding the skull base. Use of HRCT poses the risk of radiation exposure, which is especially important in children. The risks of using this modality, however, should be weighed against the benefits it provides.

MR cisternography (MRC) is another common noninvasive study that helps with the localization of CSF leak. This scan relies on the bright signal of CSF on T2-weighted images. It is specifically helpful in showing any soft tissue herniation (e.g., meningoceles and meningoencephaloceles) through the defects [12]. The overall accuracy of MRC is reported to be between 78% and 96% [12, 16]. Intrathecal injection of contrast-enhancement (CE) gadolinium can also be added to the MRC protocol to improve the accuracy. The sensitivity and specificity of CE-MRC has been reported to range from 61% to 100% and 66% to 80%, respectively [12, 17]. Compared to MRC, CE-MRC has been found to be more effective in complicated cases [12]. Intrathecal injection of gadolinium is reported to be safe in adults, although theoretically it can cause behavioral and neurological changes, seizures, and allergic reactions [12].

CT cisternography (CTC) involves the use of intrathecal injection of a contrast followed by CT scan to identify the site of active extracranial leak of the contrast material. All the studies comparing CTC to HRCT and MRC showed inferior accuracy which ranged from 33% to 67% for CTC [18, 19]. Because CTC involves the invasive use of intrathecal contrast combined with the relatively lower accuracy it provides, it is not recommended to use in children when trying to localize skull base defects and CSF leaks.

Intrathecal fluorescein injection (IFI) is an excellent test to actively localize the defect and leak during surgical repair. The concentration of fluorescein used for this test in adults is 0.1 ml mixed with 5 ml of CSF and injected back into the subarachnoid space. However, IFI has been reported to cause neurological complications such as seizures, lower extremity weakness, and tactile numbness when used in large doses [20]. In addition, the optimal dose in children has not been studied, and it is rarely used in young children.

As an author recommendation, a combination use of HRCT and MRC is the best imaging strategy for post-CSF leak localization and is the most commonly used imaging modality in children. HRCT provides excellent detail of the skull base and sinus anatomy and allows for surgical planning. MRC is of paramount importance as it shows any soft tissue details and allows for the assessment of any meningoceles/meningoencephaloceles.

Of note, nasal endoscopy is also very essential when evaluating the patient in the office. A 2.7 mm flexible laryngoscope or rigid sinus endoscope is used in children (Fig. 31.4). It has also been suggested that nasal endoscopy can be done simultaneously when children are put under

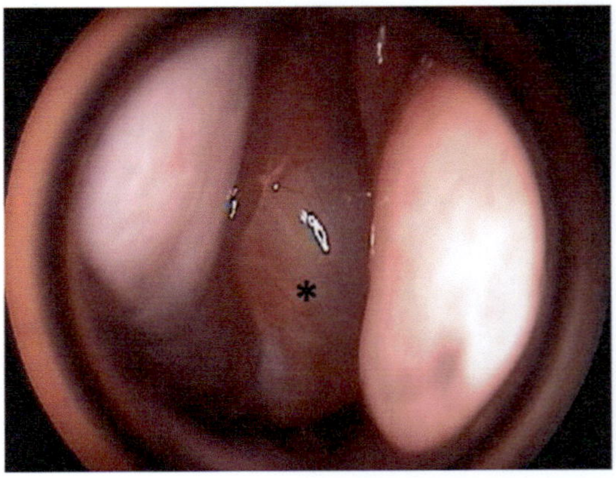

Fig. 31.4 Nasal endoscopy of an 8-month-old infant showing meningoencephalocele (asterisk) filling the right nasal cavity. Pulsation and expansion of the mass can be seen with crying or straining (Furstenberg sign)

sedation for the MRC to prevent additional physical or emotional stress on the patient [21].

31.4 Management of CSF Leaks in Children

Historically, management of CSF rhinorrhea was mostly a surgical endeavor, with attention toward prevention of further complications including meningitis and pneumocephalus [22]. It was not until 1973 when Leech and Paterson published their study on conservative CSF management did alternative methods for treatment develop [23]. While CSF rhinorrhea in children is rare relative to its etiology, treatment algorithms developed from the adult literature have been used in pediatric patients with varying degrees of success. The difficulty with CSF rhinorrhea in children is its diagnosis, as most children who present with rhinorrhea rarely have CSF rhinorrhea unless there has been an obvious traumatic event or other presenting symptomatology concerning for skull base etiology.

31.4.1 Conservative Management

The goal of conservative management is to reduce CSF leak flow with decompression of intracranial pressure in order to allow the cranial defect to heal itself. Patients are recommended to remain on bed rest for 1–2 weeks, with the head of the bed elevated to about 15–30 degrees [2]. Patients are advised against nose blowing, intranasal cannulation/positive pressure, coughing, heavy lifting, and straining with bowel movements. For some patients, medications, including antitussives, antiemetics, and laxatives, maybe necessary. If rhinorrhea persists after 5–7 days of conservative management, continuous subarachnoid drainage via indwelling lumbar catheter or intermittent spinal taps maybe needed to reduce intracranial pressure [2]. CSF drainage via lumbar drain is not without its complications and should be used cautiously in both adult and pediatric patients [24].

A 2010 study by Yadav et al. looked at twelve pediatric patients over a 10-year period (aged 3–14 years) who had resolution of CSF rhinorrhea with conservative management [22]. The majority (58%) of these CSF rhinorrhea patients were admitted following trauma, with the remaining four undergoing endonasal surgery for either infectious or congenital lesion concerns. In their CSF rhinorrhea protocol, all patients were placed on strict bed rest with medications to help with cough and straining. In two patients, a lumbar drain was placed to help reduce the amount of CSF flow. All twelve patients were initially discharged following conservative therapy, but seven patients required readmission for persistent rhinorrhea or meningitis. Definitive surgical repair of persistent rhinorrhea occurred at 6–121 months from date of original injury depending on the date and severity of recurrence [22].

The greatest risk with conservative management in children with a patent skull base defect is the susceptibility to meningitis [25]. A 2005 study looking at adult patients with active CSF rhinorrhea with previous history of ascending bacterial meningitis found that surgical repair of this defect provided excellent long-term results with neither recurrence of ascending meningitis nor incidence of meningitis in the other patients, unless a CSF leak re-appeared [25]. Similarly, a study by Daudia et al. in 2007 found that the overall risk of meningitis in patients with persistent CSF rhinorrhea was 19%, with an annual incidence of 0.3 episodes per year [26].

Results from these studies were consistent with the conclusions by Yadav et al. 2010, who stated the recurrence of CSF rhinorrhea in 58% of their patients firmly established the need for surgical intervention in this patient population despite the initially optimistic hospital discharge rate [22].

31.4.2 Surgical Treatment

Until the advent of endoscopes, intracranial approach with neurosurgical intervention was the standard of therapy for CSF rhinorrhea. The initial rate for successful repair of CSF rhinorrhea was 60–80% per Dr. Walter Dandy in 1926 [27]. An endonasal approach was first described by Dr.

Oskar Hirsch in 1952, which focused on the closure of defects within the sphenoid sinus [28]. In 1981, Dr. Malte Wigand described the first endoscopic repair of CSF rhinorrhea, which has led to success rates of greater than 90% closure with less morbidity than previous studies [9, 29]. All of these studies, however, were focused on adult patients with CSF rhinorrhea.

31.4.3 Surgical Challenges in Pediatric CSF Leakage

Unlike adults, children have constantly evolving head and brain development. Any surgical manipulation of their head can affect their brain development and their facial growth [30]. Young children, especially in their first few years of life, have small nasal cavities, and constantly changing nasal and sinus anatomy. That makes any endoscopic endonasal manipulation quite challenging for the otolaryngologist. That is especially significant in neonates with meningoceles and meningoencephaloceles. These patients often have other comorbidities and can present with failure to thrive.

31.4.4 Surgical Approaches: Intracranial Vs Endoscopic Endonasal

As of writing, the vast majority of modern studies in the otolaryngology and neurosurgical literature focusing on pediatric CSF rhinorrhea are case reports and case series. Endoscopic repair is the standard of care for adult patients. Although there are no specific criteria currently on its use in pediatric patients, it has become the standard approach in children presenting with CSF leak due to its success rate and low morbidity [9]. However, external approaches are still available and occasionally used.

In pediatric patients undergoing external intracranial repair, there are typically two approaches to the anterior cranial fossa: epidural and subdural [31]. The former is suitable for reconstruction of the skull base, while the latter is preferred for intracerebral disease. The standard coronal approach with frontal craniotomy and pericranial flap is the most common external approach used. This approach is associated with many significant morbidities including prolonged hospitalization and significant risks, such as scarring, anosmia, cerebral edema, intracranial hemorrhage, and complications resulting from retraction of the frontal lobe [6, 32]. Current indications for an intracranial approach are secondary to the size of the CSF leak, size and location of bony defect, or recurrence of CSF leak after attempted endoscopic repair [31]. There is no consensus on the size of the defect that would require an external approach, but a 2010 study suggested its use when the defect cannot be entirely sealed and covered by a middle turbinate graft or auricular conchal cartilage graft [8]. Location of the defect also plays a major role in how to approach it. Anterior defects that are less than 1 cm posterior to the posterior wall of the frontal sinus can be approached through a combined craniotomy and endoscopic endonasal approach [8]. Experience of the surgeon and availability of the specialized instruments are important factors when deciding on the best surgical approach for repair.

Age of the child is not an indication for one approach versus the other. The youngest infant reported to have had successful endoscopic endonasal repair of an encephalocele was 1.5-month old [8]. Nevertheless, depending on both the age of the patient and etiology of the CSF rhinorrhea, endoscopic surgical management may not be adequate due to variability and complexity of anatomy which may be better repaired intracranially [9].

The endoscopic endonasal approach is the most commonly used approach for CSF leak repair in adults and children, mostly due to symptoms revolving around CRS. Studies have shown that ESS does not affect facial growth on children over a 10-year follow-up [33, 34]. As stated before, challenges with using this approach include the narrow nasal cavity in children, the constantly evolving skull base anatomy as children grow, the need for special instrumentation to fit the challenging nasal cavity, and the experience of the surgeon.

31.4.5 The Endoscopic Endonasal Approach

The size of the sinus endoscope (2.7 mm vs 4 mm) used during repair depends on the size of the nasal cavity. The older the child is, the larger the nasal cavity. Both 0-degree and 30-degree telescopes are useful for full visualization of the skull base. Smaller, special instrumentations may be needed depending on the age of the child. Neonatal or pediatric sinus instrumentations can be used. In some case reports, otologic micro-instruments (like a circular knife and granulation cupped forceps) had to be used [3, 9].

Exposure is of paramount importance for successful endoscopic repair. In cases of meningoceles or meningoencephaloceles, the intranasal mass must be excised first as the stalk is followed toward skull base. Partial resection of the middle turbinate maybe necessary to improve exposure, especially in nasal cavities [9]. Endoscopic ethmoidectomy is performed as necessary to access the defect in the ethmoid roof or cribriform plate. In older children where the defect is located in the posterior table of the frontal sinus, a Draf III approach, which involves bilateral frontal sinusotomies with superior septectomy, may be performed for access [35]. Defects in the sphenoid sinus are approached through a classic transnasal or transethmoid approach for central or perisellar defects [3]. Defects in the lateral pneumatized sphenoid sinus recesses may need an extended endonasal transpterygoid approach, or even an external pterygoid approach for access [3, 36]. Like in adults, meningoceles and meningoencephaloceles in children are resected along with their stalk using bipolar cautery. The mucosal edges around the defect is freshened also using bipolar cautery.

31.4.6 Materials Used for Repair

Endoscopic repair of skull base defects and resulting CSF leaks can be through an underlay vs overlay approaches (Fig. 31.5). Underlay patching is to place the grafts between the dura and skull base bone. Overlay patching is to place the grafts on the nasal side of the skull base. A combination of both the approaches can also be done. These techniques apply to both adults and children and have been used even in young infants. The best approach is dependent on the size of the defect, materials available, and surgeon's experience and preference.

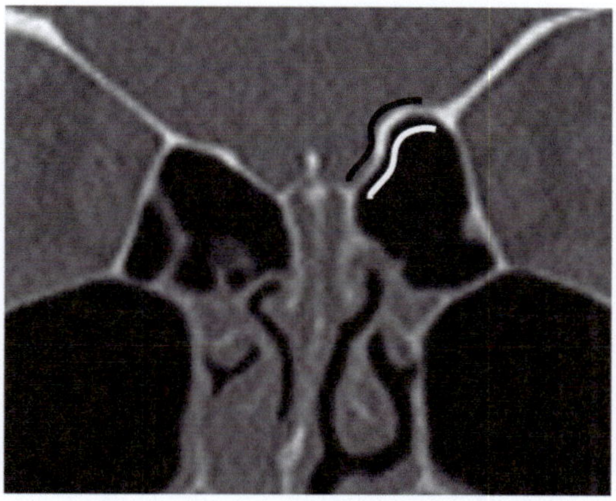

Fig. 31.5 A CT scan of the sinuses with bone window, coronal cuts showing the normal anterior skull base. Underlay patching is placing the graft between the dura and skull base bone (black line), whereas overlay technique is placing the graft on the nasal side of the skull base bone (white line)

There are multiple types of materials that can be used during repair, including fat grafts, bone and cartilage grafts, free tissue grafts (fascia, mucosa), vascularized flaps (middle turbinate flap, nasoseptal flap), and allografts. Theses grafts are usually reinforced with glues and sealants. Nasal packing is applied at the end for various duration to ensure complete healing. Absorbable packing includes Surgicel, Gelfoam, and Merogel (Medtronic). Nonabsorbable packing includes iodoform gauze, Merogel (Medtronic), and finger-cot nasal packing. Multilayered repair increases the likelihood of success especially in larger defects. Stavrakas et al. used two-layered repair for defects <0.5 cm using fat plug intracranially, and mucosal graft or middle turbinate flap on the nasal side [21]. For defects measuring 0.5 cm and larger, three-layered repair was performed with fat plug intracranially, fascia lata intracranially between the dura and skull base, and another layer of fascia lata, free mucosal graft or middle turbinate flap on the nasal side [21].

In pediatric patients, it is preferred to obtain free grafts from the nasal cavity to avoid another incision. Mucosal grafts can be obtained from the septum, inferior turbinate or middle turbinate. Similarly, bone and cartilage can be obtained from the same sites. However, it is not always suitable to obtain adequate grafts from the nasal cavities especially in younger infants. Therefore, donor sites can be used to obtain fascial grafts, including fascia lata or temporalis fascia. Fascia is an excellent choice for grafting because of the rapid healing process [37]. Autologous cartilage can also be harvested from the auricle. Auricular cartilage is adequate to serve as a backbone of an underlay repair in large defects [37].

Pedicled flaps, such as a nasoseptal flap or middle turbinate flap, have also been used in children to close defects within the skull base [38]. However, due to the anatomical difficulty of the procedure in children under 10 years in addition to the risk of postoperative shrinkage, only patients over 14 years with nasal cavities similar to adult patients can reliably have a pedicled flap repair for skull base defects [31, 38].

Endoscopic repair of CSF leaks in children have been highly successful. Most studies have shown success rate close to 100%. Table 31.1 summarizes the outcomes in seven case series with highest number of patients. Follow-up period was not consistent among these studies, with the shortest follow-up being 6 months and longest follow-up being 123 months. In one study by Peng et al., eight children had successful closure on second attempt with endoscopic repair, and three patients required three endoscopic surgeries for successful closure [31].

Table 31.1 Summary of outcomes after endoscopic repair of CSF leak in children

Study/case series	N (patients)	Success rate	Average follow-up (months)
Castelnuovo et al. 2010	11 All congenital	100%	46.7
Di Rocco et al. 2010	28 18 congenital 10 traumatic	96% (1 congenital failure)	26.7
Peng et al. 2011	43 5 congenital 38 traumatic	95% (2 failure)	12–24
Chappity et al. 2015	5 1 congenital 4 traumatic	100%	6
Ma et al. 2015	23 16 congenital 7 traumatic	100%	61
Keshri et al. 2016	6 2 congenital 4 traumatic	100%	6
Stavrakas et al. 2018	5 4 congenital 1 traumatic	100%	59

31.4.7 Timing of Repair of Congenital Meningoencephaloceles

Best of timing of surgical repair of congenital skull base defects in children is of critical importance. As previously mentioned, the youngest infant reported to undergo successful endoscopic repair is 1.5 months [8]. Repair at younger ages raises the theoretical concern of facial growth impairment, but as mentioned before, this controversy has been refuted by studies on ESS for pediatric CRS [33, 34]. Delaying the repair to allow enough growth of the nasal cavity increase the risk of ascending meningitis and encephalitis, which can potentially lead to death. The trend in current practice is to proceed with surgical repair as early as possible to prevent such complications.

31.4.8 Postoperative Management

Endoscopic CSF leak repair has the advantage to shorten hospital stay in both adults and children. Those who underwent purely endoscopic approach for surgical repair did not need pediatric intensive care unit (PICU) stay [3, 7–9, 21, 39]. These children were discharged home within 7–10 days. All studies reviewed suggested postoperative prophylactic antibiotics, preferably third generation cephalosporins [21]. Duration of antibiotics use ranged from 3 to 5 days given through the intravenous route. Postoperative packing is essential to hold the repair material in place and allow healing. When non-absorbable packing is used, it is usually removed in 2–5 days at bed site. When absorbable packing is placed, it is left to dissolve with the help of nasal saline rinses. No debridement under anesthesia is necessary as shown by all studies reviewed. This has also been true for ESS in pediatric CRS, where second look procedures for debridement is not necessary [40].

The specific role and indications for use of lumbar drain postoperatively remain to be determined. However, like in adults, it seems to be rarely used in children. Only two case series mentioned using it in total of two patients (one in each series) [7, 8]. Both the children had high-flow CSF leaks preoperatively. Another suggestion to using the lumbar drain is to use the drain postoperatively in case of leak recurrence, before committing to another repair attempt.

31.5 Summary

There are many details to be aware of when determining the source of CSF rhinorrhea in childhood. The diagnosis, management, and treatment for children are quite similar to the work-up and therapy for CSF leaks adults, but mostly due to lack of published literature and consensus for treating this rare pediatric pathology. While the work-up for children is mostly harmless, a careful balance between benefit and harm for endonasal surgery in children is still be determined at this time. Future research is necessary before endoscopic repair of sinonasal skull base defects becomes the standard of care in pediatric patients as it is for their adult counterparts.

References

1. Omoruyi EA. Practice guideline: approach to the child with rhinorrhea. J Pediatr Health Care. 2018;32(3):319–22.
2. Citardi M, Fakhri S. Cerebrospinal fluid rhinorrhea. In: Flint PW, Haughey BH, Robbins KT, et al., editors. Cummings otolaryngology - head and neck surgery e-book. Elsevier Health Sciences; 2014.
3. Ma J, Huang Q, Li X, Huang D, Xian J, Cui S, Li Y, Zhou B. Endoscopic transnasal repair of cerebrospinal fluid leaks with and without an encephalocele in pediatric patients: from infants to children. Childs Nerv Syst. 2015;31(9):1493–8.
4. Blumenfeld R, Skolnik EM. Intranasal encephaloceles. Arch Otolaryngol. 1965;82:527–31.
5. Suwanwela C, Suwanwela N. A morphological classification of sincipital encephalomeningoceles. J Neurosurg. 1972;36:201–11.
6. Kanowitz SJ, Bernstein JM. Pediatric meningoencephaloceles and nasal obstruction: a case for endoscopic repair. Int J Pediatr Otorhinolaryngol. 2006;70(12):2087–92.
7. Castelnuovo P, Bignami M, Pistochini A, Battaglia P, Loca- telli D, Dallan I. Endoscopic endonasal management of encephaloceles in children: an eight-year experience. Int J Pediatr Otorhinolaryngol. 2009;73(8):1132–6.
8. Di Rocco F, Couloigner V, Dastoli P, Sainte-Rose C, Zerah M, Roger G. Treatment of anterior skull base defects by a transnasal endoscopic approach in children. J Neurosurg Pediatr. 2010;6(5):459–63.
9. Chappity P, Alok T, Rohit V. Endonasal endoscopic approach in management of paediatric CSF rhinorrhoea cases. Indian J Otolaryngol Head Neck Surg. 2015;67(1):88–92.
10. Makary CA, Ramadan HH. The role of sinus surgery in children. Laryngoscope. 2013;123(6):1348–52.
11. Nation J, Schupper AJ, Deconde A, Levy M. CSF leak after endoscopic skull base surgery in children: a single institution experience. Int J Pediatr Otorhinolaryngol. 2019;119:22–6.
12. Oakley GM, Alt JA, Schlosser RJ, Harvey RJ, Orlandi RR. Diagnosis of cerebrospinal fluid rhinorrhea: an evidence-based review with recommendations. Int Forum Allergy Rhinol. 2016;6(1):8–16.
13. Warnecke A, Averbeck T, Wurster U, Harmening M, Lenarz T, Stover T. Diagnostic relevance of beta2-transferrin for the detection of cerebrospinal fluid fistulas. Arch Otolaryngol Head Neck Surg. 2004;130:1178–84.
14. McCudden CR, Senior BA, Hainsworth S, et al. Evaluation of high resolution gel beta(2)-transferrin for detection of cerebrospinal fluid leak. Clin Chem Lab Med. 2013;51:311–5.
15. Zapalac JS, Marple BF, Schwade ND. Skull base cerebrospinal fluid fistulas: a comprehensive diagnostic algorithm. Otolaryngol Head Neck Surg. 2002;126:669–76.
16. Shetty PG, Shroff MM, Sahani DV, Kirtane MV. Evaluation of high-resolution CT and MR cisternography in the diagnosis of cerebrospinal fluid fistula. AJNR Am J Neuroradiol. 1998;19:633–9.
17. Ecin G, Oner AY, Tokgoz N, Ucar M, Aykol S, Tali T. T2-weighted vs. intrathecal contrast-enhanced MR cisternography in the evaluation of CSF rhinorrhea. Acta Radiol. 2013;54:698–701.
18. Goel G, Ravishankar S, Jayakumar PN, et al. Intrathecal gadolinium-enhanced magnetic resonance cisternography in cerebrospinal fluid rhinorrhea: road ahead? J Neurotrauma. 2007;24:1570–5.
19. Eberhardt KE, Hollenbach HP, Deimling M, Tomandl BF, Huk WJ. MR cisternography: a new method

for the diagnosis of CSF fistulae. Eur Radiol. 1997;7:1485–91.
20. Moseley JI, Carton CA, Stern WE. Spectrum of complications in the use of intrathecal fluorescein. J Neurosurg. 1978;48:765–7.
21. Stavrakas M, Karkos PD, Triaridis S, Constantinidis J. Endoscopic management of paediatric meningoencephaloceles: a case series. Eur Arch Otorhinolaryngol. 2018;275(11):2727–31.
22. Yadav JS, Mohindra S, Francis AA. CSF rhinorrhea-feasibility of conservative management in children. Int J Pediatr Otorhinolaryngol. 2011;75(2):186–9.
23. Leech PJ, Paterson A. Conservative and operative management for cerebrospinal-fluid leakage after closed head injury. Lancet. 1973;1(7811):1013–6.
24. Roland PS, Marple BF, Meyerhoff WL, Mickey B. Complications of lumbar spinal fluid drainage. Otolaryngol Head Neck Surg. 1992;107(4):564–9.
25. Bernal-Sprekelsen M, Alobid I, Mullol J, Trobat F, Tomás-barberán M. Closure of cerebrospinal fluid leaks prevents ascending bacterial meningitis. Rhinology. 2005;43(4):277–81.
26. Daudia A, Biswas D, Jones NS. Risk of meningitis with cerebrospinal fluid rhinorrhea. Ann Otol Rhinol Laryngol. 2007;116(12):902–5.
27. Dandy WE. Pneumocephalous (intracranial pneumatocele or aerocele). Arch Surg. 1926;12:949–82.
28. Hirsch O. Successful closure of CSF rhinorrhoea by endonasal surgery. Arch Otolaryngol. 1952;56:1–13.
29. Wigand ME. Transnasal ethmoidectomy under endoscopic control. Rhinology. 1981;19:7–15.
30. Mair EA, Bolger WE, Breisch EA. Sinus and facial growth after pediatric endoscopic sinus surgery. Arch Otolaryngol Head Neck Surg. 1995;121:547–52.
31. Peng A, Li Y, Xiao Z, Wu W. Exploration of endonasal endoscopic repair of pediatric cerebrospinal fluid rhinorrhea. Int J Pediatr Otorhinolaryngol. 2011;75(3):308–15.
32. McCormack B, Cooper PR, Persky M, Rothstein S. Extracranial repair of cerebrospinal fluid fistulas: technique and results in 37 patients. Neurosurgery. 1990;27(3):412–7.
33. Senior B, Wirtschafter A, Mai C, Becker C, Belenky W. Quantitative impact of pediatric sinus surgery on facial growth. Laryngoscope. 2000;110:1866–70.
34. Bothwell MR, Piccirillo JF, Lusk RP, Ridenour BD. Long-term outcome of facial growth after functional endoscopic sinus surgery. Otolaryngol Head Neck Surg. 2002;126:628–34.
35. Wormald PJ, Ananda A, Nair S. The modified endoscopic Lothrop procedure in the treatment of complicated chronic frontal sinusitis. Clin Otolaryngol Allied Sci. 2003;28(3):215–20.
36. Tabaee A, Anand VK, Cappabianca P, et al. Endoscopic management of spontaneous meningoencephalocele of the lateral sphenoid sinus. J Neurosurg. 2010;112(5):1070–7.
37. Martínez-Lage JF, Pérez-Espejo MA, Palaózn JH, López Hernández F, Puerta P. Autologous tissues for dural grafting in children: a report of 56 cases. Childs Nerv Syst. 2006;22:139–44.
38. Shah RN, Surowitz JB, Patel MR, et al. Endoscopic pedicled nasoseptal flap reconstruction for pediatric skull base defects. Laryngoscope. 2009;119(6):1067–75.
39. Keshri AK, Shah SR, Patadia SD, Sahu RN, Behari S. Transnasal endoscopic repair of pediatric meningoencephalocele. J Pediatr Neurosci. 2016;11(1):42–5.
40. Mitchell RB, Pereira KD, Younis RT, Lazar RH. Tric functional endoscopic sinus surgery: is a second look necessary? Laryngoscope. 1997;107(9):1267–9.

Outcomes of Skull Base Reconstruction

32

Stephen C. Hernandez, Peter Papagiannopoulos, Brent A. Senior, and David W. Kennedy

32.1 Introduction

Anterior skull base cerebrospinal fluid (CSF) leaks may be congenital, iatrogenic, traumatic, or idiopathic. Repair of these lesions is of clinical significance for the prevention of complications including pneumocephalus, meningitis, or intracranial abscess [1]. Historically, these defects were repaired by neurosurgeons through a transcranial approach for adequate visualization which frequently required a large degree of brain retraction for access to the skull base [1, 2]. However, in the last 20 years, there has been a rapid advancement in the endoscopic endonasal approach (EEA) to the skull base. While the endoscopic approach was initially used for endoscopic sinus surgery (ESS) for inflammatory disease, indications quickly expanded to include endoscopic repair of encephaloceles and CSF leaks, as well as resection of sinonasal tumors, pituitary lesions, and, more recently, completely intracranial lesions such as meningiomas and craniopharyngiomas [3–7]. Technical and technological advancements have even allowed for the application of EEA techniques to anterior skull base surgery and CSF leak repair in pediatric patients as young as 23 months [3].

These endoscopic advancements are largely due to increased anatomical understanding, newly developed sinonasal instrumentation, and improved image guidance systems. Additionally, advancements in successful skull base reconstruction include the development of different synthetic grafting materials and vascularized pedicled flaps [8]. In this chapter, we will review the success rates of CSF leak repair in general, analyze factors that may affect successful skull base reconstruction, and then review the data available assessing long-term outcomes.

32.2 General Success Rates: Endoscopic Vs. Open Approaches

It is now well demonstrated that endoscopic approaches have become very effective when addressing CSF leaks in most cases. Overall, success rates are excellent regardless of approach, but complication rates and other variables seem to be improved in the setting of endoscopic repair. A systematic review from 2013 compared open and endoscopic surgical series for repair of anterior skull base CSF leaks related to all causes. Seventy-one studies and 1178 patients were included and for all etiologies, by either entirely open or endoscopic approach, the rate of successful repair

S. C. Hernandez · B. A. Senior (✉)
Department of Otolaryngology – Head and Neck Surgery, University of North Carolina at Chapel Hill, Chapel Hill, NC, USA
e-mail: brent_senior@med.unc.edu

P. Papagiannopoulos · D. W. Kennedy
Department of Otorhinolaryngology – Head and Neck Surgery, University of Pennsylvania, Philadelphia, PA, USA

A. A. AlQahtani et al. (eds.), *CSF Rhinorrhea*, https://doi.org/10.1007/978-3-030-94781-1_32

is approximately 90–95% [1]. That same literature review identified no difference in the rate of successful repair between endoscopic and open cohorts but that complications were significantly lower in the endoscopic group, including meningitis (3.9% vs. 1.1%), abscess or wound infection (6.8% vs. 0.7%), and sepsis (3.8% vs. 0%) [1]. Another study comparing endoscopic versus craniotomy outcomes also found no difference in the rate of successful repair between the two techniques but did find that the endoscopic group had a significantly shorter duration of hospitalization, a lower rate of complications, lower cost, and higher patient satisfaction [9].

32.3 Repair Techniques

For larger defects, it is generally well established in the literature that successful skull base reconstruction requires a multilayered approach [3–5, 7, 10–13] with the goal of filling intracranial dead-space when present, utilizing dural underlays, overlays, as well as reconstructing the mucosal surface. For smaller defects, simple free mucosal onlay grafting has been very effective. There are numerous grafts and synthetic materials that can be used for these layers including autologous fat, fascia, free mucosal grafts, pedicled and vascularized flaps, collagen matrix implants, and fibrin glue material (Fig. 32.1). All can be used successfully to repair the anterior skull base; however, the optimal material and/or graft can depend on the flow rate of the CSF leak, the location of the skull base defect, and the size of the defect [14]. We will assess each of these considerations systematically.

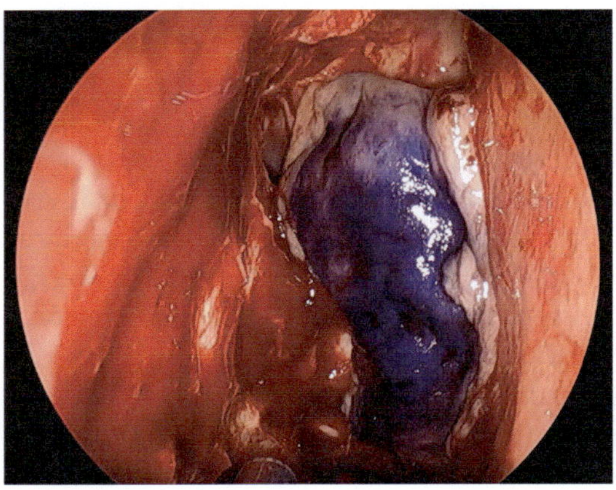

Fig. 32.1 Example of a free mucosal onlay graft. The mucosal surface has been marked to ensure proper orientation

32.3.1 CSF Leak Flow Rate

Studies have established a grading system from 1 to 3 based on the rate of flow in CSF leaks noted endoscopically: grade 1 is defined as a small, "weeping" CSF leak confirmed by Valsalva maneuver; grade 2 is a moderate leak with a visible dural defect; and grade 3 is a large dural defect created as part of an extended suprasellar, transplanum, transtuberculum, transcribriform, or transclival approach or visualization of the ventricular system [4, 5, 15].

For lower flow leaks (grade 1 and 2), no consensus has been reached regarding reconstruction materials chosen [16]. For these leaks, regardless of material chosen and techniques employed, postoperative CSF leaks are reported at 5–10% [4, 14, 17].

We begin to see differences in overall outcomes with larger defects and grade 3 CSF leaks. In this situation, it is clear that the vascularized nasoseptal flap (NSF) is superior to an avascular free mucosal graft (Fig. 32.2). In a recent meta-analysis assessing endoscopic skull base reconstruction of large dural defects,

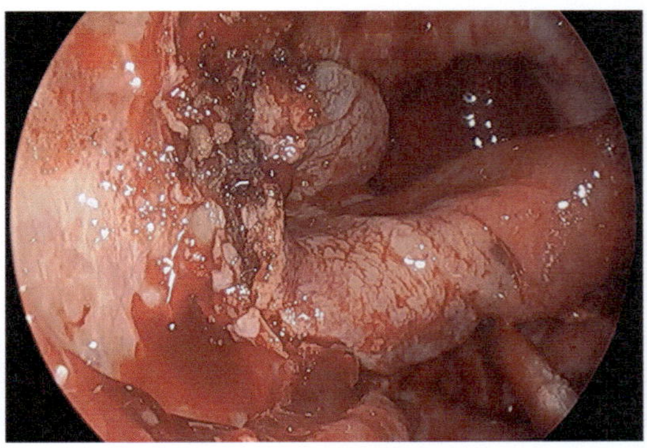

Fig. 32.2 A left-sided nasoseptal flap used for reconstruction of a recurrent right sphenoid lateral recess encephalocele with associated CSF leak

Harvey et al. identified 609 patients who underwent EEA closure. Of those 609 patients, those closed with a free mucosal graft as the most superficial layer had a 15.6% postoperative CSF leak rate (51 leaks out of 326 patients) while NSF-based reconstructions had a 6.7% postoperative CSF leak rate (19 leaks out of 283 patients) ($p = 0.001$) [14, 16]. Further, in case series reported by high-volume skull base centers, an NSF-based reconstructive technique in high-flow CSF leaks has yielded postoperative leak rates of 5–6% [3, 4].

32.3.2 Leak Location

In a review of 22 studies by Soudry et al., an overall postoperative CSF leak rate after skull base repair of 8.5% was found, revealing an overall success rate of 91.5%. To further this evaluation, the authors focused additional inquiry on the role of the location of the skull base defect and degree of intraoperative leak. Utilizing these criteria, no difference between vascularized and non-vascularized reconstruction was identified for any location subsite except the clivus, which demonstrated better reconstructive results with vascularized repair [17, 18]. While CSF leaks and encephaloceles involving the lateral recess of the sphenoid sinus may be more difficult to address, given its challenging access and complex three-dimensional relationships with surrounding neurovascular structures, many series demonstrate that there is no statistically significant difference in success of repair at this location [19].

32.3.3 Dural Defect Size

In a case series of 121 patients who underwent skull base reconstruction, it was found that dural defect size greater than 2 cm^2 is associated with reconstruction failure. Postoperative leak rates in the cohort was 3.8% for defects less than 2.0 cm^2 but 16.7% for defects larger than 2.0 cm^2 [20]. In a case series by Zanation et al., large dural openings trended toward higher reconstructive failure rate but the difference was not found to be significant [4].

32.4 Inpatient Vs. Outpatient Repair of CSF Leaks

With the advent of endoscopic skull base surgery, there has been rapid progression toward expanded approaches and repair of large defects. As these expanded approaches continue to grow with a broader range of indications, we are seeing gradual improvement in outcome measures. With regard to endoscopic CSF leak repair, systematic reviews have demonstrated success rates as high as 91% for primary repair (97% with secondary repair) and complication rates of less than 0.03% [21]. While these success rates continue to improve and morbidity remains exceedingly rare, this has translated into shorter hospitalization stays, lower overall costs, and greater patient satisfaction [9, 21].

As demonstrated, with complication rates remaining less than 1%, we are beginning to see some institutions move toward outpatient repair of CSF leaks in certain situations. Adams et al. have retrospectively reviewed their CSF leak repairs over a 10-year period [22]. This included 39 patients who underwent CSF leak repair in the outpatient setting and 47 patients who underwent repair in the inpatient setting. There were a total of three CSF leak recurrences (7.69%) requiring subsequent management in the ambulatory cohort. Only one complication occurred in this group, requiring readmission. Overall, repair techniques were fairly similar between the two cohorts, but it should be noted that 38 of the 39 repairs in the outpatient setting were for CSF leaks with a skull base defect measuring less than 1 cm^2. For comparison, the inpatient cohort had 12 patients with defects that were greater than 1 cm^2. While complication rates remained low in these patients managed in the outpatient setting, no great statistically significant conclusions can be drawn with regard to overall outcomes.

Although it has been shown that significant complications remain uncommon in the setting of CSF leak repair, it is difficult to recommend repair routinely in the outpatient setting. Certainly, some criteria should be met prior to planning and consideration. In general, large skull base defects should probably be managed in the inpatient setting, given greater risk for recurrence and complication rates. For those select patients with minimal skull base defects, such as those with minimally displaced fractures in the setting of traumatic CSF leak, there can be some discussion for repair in the outpatient setting. However, there remain some factors that one may be unable to account for at the time of surgery. The size of the defect, flow rate of CSF, grafting material available, possible requirement for vascularized pedicled flaps, and patient comorbidities are all things that should be carefully evaluated in the perioperative period. Those with elevated intracranial pressure, obesity, and high-grade leaks all have greater risk for recurrence and complications, as will be discussed. Therefore, those patients under consideration for CSF leak repair in the ambulatory setting should have very minimal to no comorbidities, demonstrate reliability, have adequate support and care at home, and ensure close proximity for follow-up should problems ensue.

32.5 Prognostic Factors for Successful Repair

As has previously been discussed, there are a variety of etiologies leading to the development of CSF leak. These can include iatrogenic, traumatic, congenital, and idiopathic causes. Excluding endonasal resections of anterior cranial base pathology, success rates generally exceed 90% in the primary setting regardless of the underlying etiology [21, 23]. This then begs the question: are there certain risk factors for the remaining 10% that may require a secondary repair?

Looking at case series with reported data on endoscopic repair of CSF leaks, we tend to see a common trend that those patients at higher risk for failure or recurrence seem to have very similar risk factors. Following the advent of endoscopic repair of CSF leaks, early data seemed to suggest that patients with spontaneous CSF leaks recurred more frequently than those CSF leaks related to other etiologies. Kennedy and colleagues have previously reviewed their endoscopic repair of CSF leaks looking as far back as 1987 [24]. Those with spontaneous CSF leaks have a higher BMI in comparison to those patients with traumatic or congenital CSF leaks. In addition, the majority of those patients were middle aged females (77%). Similar studies have since demonstrated comparable risk factors when reviewing spontaneous CSF leaks, linking the underlying etiology to idiopathic intracranial hypertension (IIH) [19, 24, 25]. Lobo et al. have conducted a systematic review of the literature, again defining a clear association with middle-aged obese females, elevated intracranial pressure, and obstructive sleep apnea (Fig. 32.3) [26].

Despite all of the descriptions of these associated factors with spontaneous CSF leaks, there has not been much data reported regarding treatment of the underlying pathophysiology and its potential impact on success rates. As we develop further understanding regarding IIH and spontaneous CSF leaks, there is now some data to suggest appropriately managing these comorbidities may have an impact on outcomes [27]. A recent systematic review has looked at data comparing

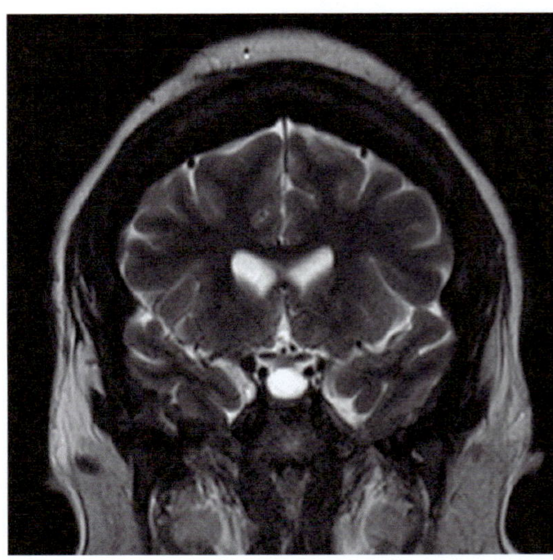

Fig. 32.3 Those with idiopathic intracranial hypertension may also demonstrate imaging findings of CSF expansion in Meckel's cave as well as empty sella, as demonstrated here

success rates between those with no further management of their underlying elevated intracranial pressure (ICP) and those who were under active management for elevated ICP (acetazolamide therapy or CSF diversion procedures) [28]. Primary repair success rates reached 92.82% in those who were actively managed versus just 81.87% of those who received no further management of their underlying elevated ICP. Mean follow-up for these two cohorts was greater than 2 years.

Other risk factors to take into consideration may come into play when discussing CSF leaks that may be created with resection of sinonasal malignancy or other cranial base pathology (Fig. 32.4). This should technically be considered in a different category altogether, as these defects are usually anticipated going into surgical resection and involve much larger dural defects. Needless to say, there remain some risk factors inherent to skull base reconstruction in these scenarios. Namely, the size of the defect, location of the defect, and grade of CSF leak are all inherent factors that may affect overall success. For larger defects and those involving the posterior fossa, there has been reported data that suggests these sites are at greater risk for recurrent CSF leaks and other complications [5, 29]. Furthermore, larger defects are better suited with vascularized pedicled flaps, as has been well demonstrated earlier in this chapter [14].

Regardless of reconstruction techniques utilized or grades of CSF leak present at the time of reconstruction, use of lumbar spinal drains has not demonstrated any statistically significant improvement in successful repairs [5, 19]. A recent meta-analysis reviewing 12 articles and a total of 508 cases corroborated previous findings, with no evidence to suggest that perioperative lumbar spinal drainage reduces recurrence rates following endoscopic repair [30]. There may be some exception to this generalization when discussing endoscopic skull base surgery creating large dural defects. Zwagerman et al. recently published their prospective randomized controlled trial evaluating lumbar drainage in those patients with high flow leaks and a dural defect of greater than 1 cm^2 [31]. A total of 170 patients were randomized during the 4 year period. Results demonstrated that postoperative lumbar spinal drainage was associated with an 8.2% leak rate, as compared to a 21.2% leak rate in those without postoperative lumbar drainage. This trended with increasing defect size and location at the anterior or posterior fossa. These results suggest that creation of large dural defects with communication to CSF cisterns may benefit from postoperative lumbar drainage.

As with any other surgery, there are intrinsic patient factors that may impact overall success. In certain scenarios, it may be difficult to control all of these underlying comorbidities. Regardless, having the knowledge of these risk factors can help in preoperative counseling and perioperative management. In the event that secondary CSF leak repair is required, success rates still remain excellent.

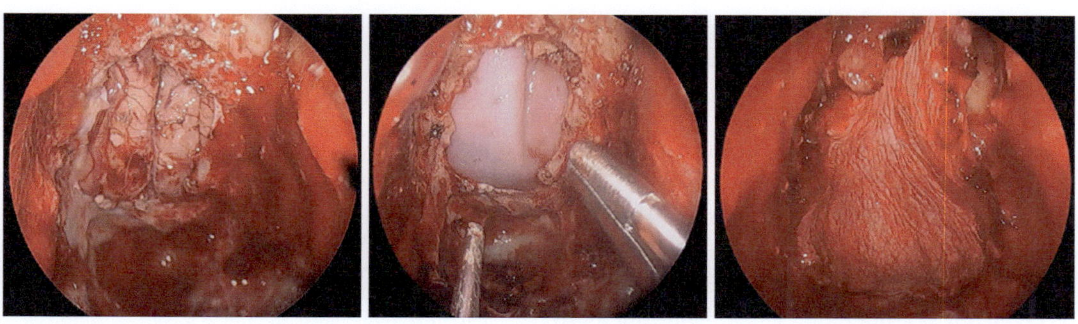

Fig. 32.4 A large anterior skull base defect following resection of sinonasal malignancy. Multilayer reconstruction demonstrated with an acellular inlay graft and an onlay vascularized pericranial flap

32.6 Long-Term Outcomes

Most of what has been discussed thus far in the chapter relates to outcomes in the immediate term, evaluating for those patients and risk factors leading to recurrent leak within the first few months to years. Generally speaking, these success rates remain very high as time goes on. As previously discussed, those patients who are at greatest risk for recurrence in the long term are those that demonstrate idiopathic intracranial hypertension given its known associated comorbidities.

Regardless of a successful primary repair in this patient population, they continue to demonstrate risk for recurrence either at the previous leak site or even at a separate, distant site. Campbell et al. have perhaps published the longest follow-up data regarding those patients with IIH. At a mean follow-up of 10.2 years, 18% of patients required revision surgery either at the initial repair site or at a distant site [32]. One of those patients had evidence of recurrent CSF rhinorrhea 9 years following the initial repair, demonstrating the need for long-term surveillance in this patient population.

Furthermore, adjuvant therapy in those with IIH has proven beneficial in their overall health [33]. This involves conservative measures such as diet, exercise, and weight loss, but also includes pharmacotherapy (acetazolamide) and surgical options for CSF diversion (ventriculoperitoneal shunting or lumboperitoneal shunting). While there is no direct data to suggest that these interventions may reduce incidence of CSF rhinorrhea, there is evidence to suggest that overall weight loss and pharmacotherapy have a direct correlation with reduction in intracranial pressure [34]. One can then infer by maintaining lower baseline intracranial pressures, risk of recurrent CSF rhinorrhea subsequently decreases. However, there are still medication side effects to consider and major complications that can be associated with CSF diversion procedures. These factors should be taken into consideration when reviewing these alternative options with patients.

32.7 Summary

Overall, success rates for primary repair of CSF leaks are excellent regardless of the underlying etiology (>90%). There are certain factors that should be taken into consideration during the perioperative period and reconstructive planning. Generally speaking, free grafts and multilayered reconstruction work very well for small cranial base defects and low-flow CSF leaks. However, high-flow leaks or those defects that are quite large may be better served with upfront vascularized pedicled flap reconstruction. Use of lumbar spinal drains has not shown any statistically significant improvement in success rates (excluding large dural defects created from tumor surgery), and in fact may be associated with more complications and prolonged hospitalizations. Idiopathic intracranial hypertension should be considered in all patients with spontaneous CSF leaks. Their underlying pathophysiology may increase their likelihood of recurrence, and therefore, these patients necessitate long-term follow-up with consideration for pharmacotherapy or CSF diversion in refractory cases.

References

1. Komotar RJ, et al. Endoscopic endonasal versus open repair of anterior skull base CSF leak, meningocele, and encephalocele: a systematic review of outcomes. J Neurol Surg A Cent Eur Neurosurg. 2013;74(4):239–50.
2. Lindstrom DR, et al. Management of cerebrospinal fluid rhinorrhea: the Medical College of Wisconsin experience. Laryngoscope. 2004;114(6):969–74.
3. Khalili S, Palmer JN, Adappa ND. The expanded endonasal approach for the treatment of intracranial skull base disease in the pediatric population. Curr Opin Otolaryngol Head Neck Surg. 2015;23(1):65–70.
4. Zanation AM, et al. Nasoseptal flap reconstruction of high flow intraoperative cerebral spinal fluid leaks during endoscopic skull base surgery. Am J Rhinol Allergy. 2009;23(5):518–21.
5. Conger A, et al. Evolution of the graded repair of CSF leaks and skull base defects in endonasal endoscopic tumor surgery: trends in repair failure and meningitis rates in 509 patients. J Neurosurg. 2018;130(3):861–75.

6. Karnezis TT, et al. Factors impacting cerebrospinal fluid leak rates in endoscopic sellar surgery. Int Forum Allergy Rhinol. 2016;6(11):1117–25.
7. Rawal RB, et al. Endoscopic resection of sinonasal malignancy: a systematic review and meta-analysis. Otolaryngol Head Neck Surg. 2016;155(3):376–86.
8. Lam K, et al. Use of autologous fat grafts for the endoscopic reconstruction of skull base defects: indications, outcomes, and complications. Am J Rhinol Allergy. 2018;32(4):310–7.
9. Christoforidou A, et al. Endonasal endoscopic repair of cerebrospinal fluid leaks versus craniotomy: comparison of the outcomes. Hippokratia. 2016;20(4):299–302.
10. Patel MR, et al. Beyond the nasoseptal flap: outcomes and pearls with secondary flaps in endoscopic endonasal skull base reconstruction. Laryngoscope. 2014;124(4):846–52.
11. Shah RN, et al. Endoscopic pedicled nasoseptal flap reconstruction for pediatric skull base defects. Laryngoscope. 2009;119(6):1067–75.
12. Kuan EC, et al. Lack of sphenoid pneumatization does not affect endoscopic endonasal pediatric skull base surgery outcomes. Laryngoscope. 2019;129(4): 832–6.
13. Ghosh A, et al. Pediatric nasoseptal flap reconstruction for suprasellar approaches. Laryngoscope. 2015;125(11):2451–6.
14. Harvey RJ, et al. Endoscopic skull base reconstruction of large dural defects: a systematic review of published evidence. Laryngoscope. 2012;122(2):452–9.
15. Adappa ND, et al. Radiographic enhancement of the nasoseptal flap does not predict postoperative cerebrospinal fluid leaks in endoscopic skull base reconstruction. Laryngoscope. 2012;122(6):1226–34.
16. Li Z, et al. A stratified algorithm for skull base reconstruction with endoscopic endonasal approach. J Craniofac Surg. 2018;29(1):193–8.
17. Thorp BD, et al. Endoscopic skull base reconstruction: a review and clinical case series of 152 vascularized flaps used for surgical skull base defects in the setting of intraoperative cerebrospinal fluid leak. Neurosurg Focus. 2014;37(4):E4.
18. Soudry E, et al. Endoscopic reconstruction of surgically created skull base defects: a systematic review. Otolaryngol Head Neck Surg. 2014;150(5):730–8.
19. Adams AS, Russell PT, Duncavage JA, et al. Outcomes of endoscopic repair of cerebrospinal fluid rhinorrhea without lumbar drains. Am J Rhinol Allergy. 2016;30:424–9.
20. Gruss CL, et al. Risk factors for cerebrospinal leak after endoscopic skull base reconstruction with nasoseptal flap. Otolaryngol Head Neck Surg. 2014;151(3):516–21.
21. Psaltis AJ, Schlosser RJ, Banks CA, et al. A systematic review of the endoscopic repair of cerebrospinal fluid leaks. Otolaryngol Head Neck Surg. 2012;147: 196–203.
22. Adams AS, Francis DO, Russell PT. Outcomes of outpatient endoscopic repair of cerebrospinal fluid rhinorrhea. Int Forum Allergy Rhinol. 2016;6:1126–30.
23. Hegazy HM, Carrau RL, Snyderman CH, et al. Transnasal endoscopic repair of cerebrospinal fluid rhinorrhea: a meta-analysis. Laryngoscope. 2000;110:1166–72.
24. Banks CA, Palmer JN, Chiu AG, et al. Endoscopic closure of CSF rhinorrhea: 193 cases over 21 years. Otolaryngol Head Neck Surg. 2009;140:826–33.
25. Nyquist GG, Anand VK, Mehra S, et al. Endoscopic endonasal repair of anterior skull base non-traumatic cerebrospinal fluid leaks, meningoceles, and encephaloceles. J Neurosurg. 2010;113:961–6.
26. Lobo BC, Baumanis MM, Nelson RF. Surgical repair of spontaneous cerebrospinal (CSF) leaks: a systematic review. Laryngoscope Investig Otolaryngol. 2017;2:215–24.
27. Konuthula N, Khan MN, Del Signore A, et al. A systematic review of secondary cerebrospinal fluid leaks. Am J Rhinol Allergy. 2017;31:48–56.
28. Teachey W, Grayson J, Cho DY, et al. Intervention for elevated intracranial pressure improves success rate after repair of spontaneous cerebrospinal fluid leaks. Laryngoscope. 2017;127:2011–6.
29. Fraser S, Garder PA, Koutourousiou M, et al. Risk factors associated with postoperative cerebrospinal fluid leak after endoscopic endonasal skull base surgery. J Neurosurg. 2018;128:1066–71.
30. Ahmed OH, Marcus S, Tauber JR, et al. Efficacy of periperative lumbar drainage following endonasal endoscopic cerebrospinal fluid leak repair. Otolaryngol Head Neck Surg. 2017;156:52–60.
31. Zwagerman NT, Wang EW, Shin SS, et al. Does lumbar drainage reduce postoperative cerebrospinal fluid leak after endoscopic endonasal skull base surgery? A prospective, randomized controlled trial. J Neurosurg. 2018;1:1–7.
32. Campbell RG, Farquhar D, Zhao N, et al. Cerebrospinal fluid rhinorrhea secondary to idiopathic intracranial hypertension: long-term outcomes of endoscopic repairs. Am J Rhinol Allergy. 2016;30:294–300.
33. Schuman TA, Senior BA. Long-term management and outcomes after repair of cerebrospinal fluid rhinorrhea related to idiopathic intracranial hypertension. Curr Opin Otolaryngol Head Neck Surg. 2018;26:46–51.
34. Berdahl JP, Fleischman D, Zaydlavora J, et al. Body mass index has a linear relationship with cerebrospinal fluid pressure. Invest Ophthalmol Vis Sci. 2012;53:1422–7.

Abnormal Presentation of CSF Leak

33

Shawkat Abdulrahman and Donata Šukytė-Raubė

The term "abnormal" is a combination of the Latin prefix *ab* that means "away from" and the English word normal. It means "not normal" or "unusual" and is used to describe abnormal or unusual presentation; for example, the transnasal cerebrospinal fluid (CSF) that was first described in 1899 [1], and the temporal bone in 1897 [2], which involves a breakdown of all barriers that separate the subarachnoid space from the upper aerodigestive tract [3–5].

33.1 Unusual Presentation

1. Unusual locations:
   (a) Clival region
   (b) Optic nerve
   (c) Eustachian tube leakage of the middle skull base
   (d) Distant pseudomeningoceles of the ventral skull base
      - Orbit
      - Infratemporal fossa
2. Unusual etiology:
   (a) Systemic disease
   (b) Nonsurgical iatrogenic-induced CSF leak

A skull base cerebrospinal fluid (CSF) leak or fistula, which presents clinically as a clear rhinorrhea or otorrhea, is an abnormal communication between the sterile subarachnoid space and the sinonasal or tympanomastoid cavities as a result of both osseous and dural defects. This chapter introduces rare cases of uncommon clinical presentations of a CSF rhinorrhea. Depending on the perspective, the localization of rhinorrhea, presenting signs and symptoms, or the etiology of rhinorrhea—a rare condition or atypical manifestation (i.e., pseudomeningocele)—can be atypical. The chapter does not include the most common types of rhinorrhea—traumatic or iatrogenic—which should be excluded first when differentiating the cause of rhinoliquorrhea.

Spontaneous liquorrhea is rare, comprising only 3–4% of all cases of liquorrhea [6]. O'Connell developed a classification of spontaneous liquorrhea: primary and secondary CSF leak, depending on whether the cause is known or could not be identified [7]. Ommaya et al., on the contrary, thought that all cases of CSF rhinorrhea have a cause. He subcategorized them as "high

S. Abdulrahman (✉)
Tallaght University Hospital, Dublin, Ireland

D. Šukytė-Raubė
Clinic of Ear, Nose, Throat and Eye Diseases, Vilnius University Hospital Santaros Klinikos, Vilnius, Lithuania

A. A. AlQahtani et al. (eds.), *CSF Rhinorrhea*, https://doi.org/10.1007/978-3-030-94781-1_33

pressure," usually due to tumors and hydrocephalus, and "low pressure," caused by congenital abnormalities, osteomyelitis, and focal atrophy in the cribriform plate and sella [8].

33.2 Clival Lesion

The cribriform plate of the ethmoidal bone—the thinnest place in the skull base—is one of the most common sites of liquorrhea, followed by the sphenoid and frontal sinuses [9–11]. It is important to mention that spontaneous liquorrhea in the sphenoid sinus usually occurs in the lateral pneumatized sphenoid recess that has higher failure repair rate [12]. Those CSF leaks arise lateral to the foramen rotundum and Vidian canal (pterygoid canal) in patients with an extensive pneumatization of the sphenoid are sometimes associated with Sternberg's canal, which is a lateral craniopharyngeal canal resulting from incomplete fusion of different sphenoid bone components [13]. This happens most frequently in middle-aged overweight women, who possibly have increased intracranial pressure (ICP) [13, 14]. A nontraumatic osseous defect in the clivus is an extremely rare site of spontaneous rhinoliquorrhea. The bone in this area of the skull base is usually thick and strong; therefore, only a few cases of transclival CSF leaks have been reported in the scientific literature. Such defects are sometimes associated with intracranial hypertension [15–17]. Information about the condition is limited. Based on these few case reports, it can be summarized that rhinoliquorrhea due to a clival defect can be permanent or episodic, usually one-sided or leaking posterior to the nasopharynx, presenting as recurrent meningitis or headaches.

The etiology usually remains unclear, and individual authors present different theories. Van Zele et al. claim that innate skull base malformations and an over pneumatized sphenoid sinus play an important role together with additional functional factors such as pulsating effect of arteries or increased ICP. It is recommended to accurately assess the ICP in all patients with a spontaneous CSF leak as increased ICP is associated with an increased risk of relapse of liquorrhea after the surgical repair [12, 18, 19]. To date, spontaneous CSF leak is possibly the most common and challenging skull base disorder associated with idiopathic intracranial hypertension [20].

One of the rare causes of clival defect is *Ecchordosis physaliphora*—a benign tumor, arising from the remnants of fetal notochord, and found in the intradural space along the clivus or, rarely, sacrum. Ecchordosis physaliphora has similarities with the chordoma based on both histological and ultrastructural features; however, the latter is characterized by bone invasion, aggressive growth, and intradural localization. Ecchordosis physaliphora is found incidentally in up to 2% of all autopsies and presents with headache and diplopia [21]; however, only 14 cases of ecchordosis physaliphora-related CSF leak have been reported so far [22]. Mcdonald et al. were the first to report a large ecchordosis physaliphora caused rhinorrhea [23]. Allis et al. presented an ecchordosis physaliphora-related CSF liquorrhea case, and sphenoid sinus was approached via a midfacial degloving to repair the defect with a septal mucosal graft and biological glue. However, a relapse occurred 2 months after the surgery; therefore, a transsphenoidal repair of the clival defect was performed using the fascia lata overlay graft, glue, and fat tissue [24]. Transsphenoidal-transclival endoscopic approach has become the gold standard for successful repair and closure [22, 25]. Bolzoni-Villaret et al. also present two cases that are treated by an expanded endoscopic surgical technique, and both patients underwent a transsphenoidal-transclival endoscopic approach (Figs. 33.1, 33.2 and 33.3).

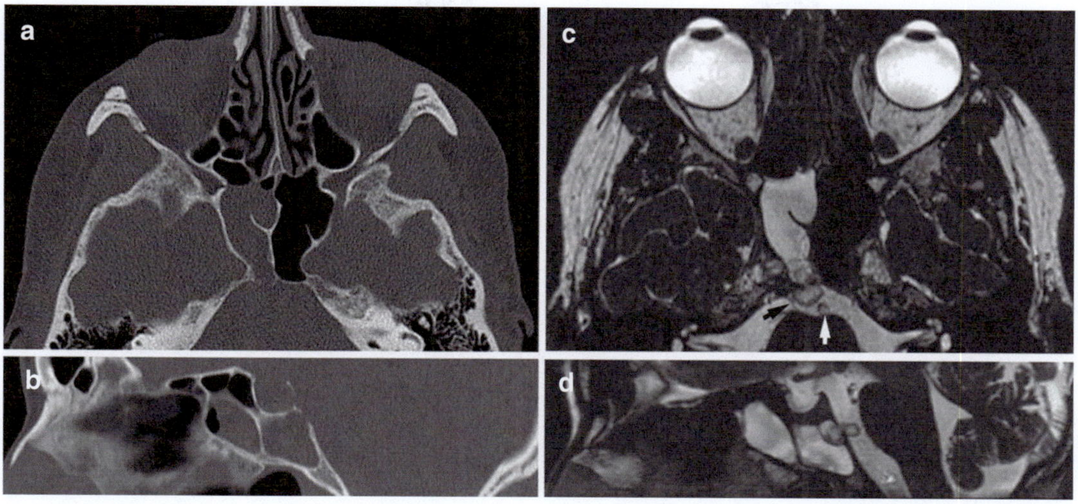

Fig. 33.1 Preoperative axial (**a**) and sagittal (**b**) CT scan images showing bone remodeling of the posterior wall of the right sphenoid sinus and upper clivus. Preoperative axial (**c**) and sagittal (**d**) T2-weighted MRI: The multilobulated lesion appears to be in contact with the basilar artery (white arrow) and the right abducens nerve (black arrow)

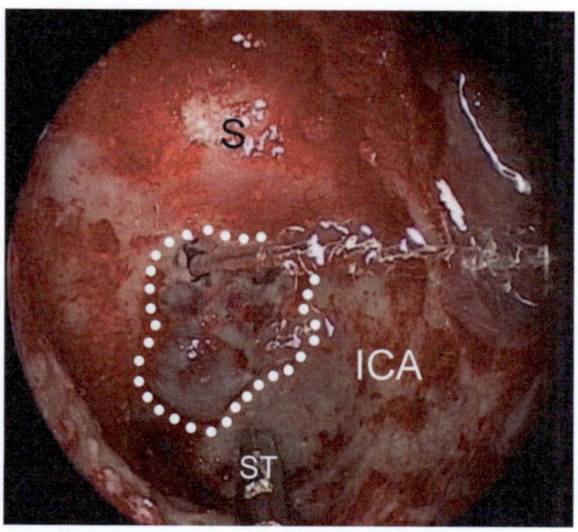

Fig. 33.2 Endoscopic view by 0° endoscope of case 2. Once the lesion (white dots) is opened, high-pressure CSF leakage from the prepontine cistern is clearly evident. ICA, left internal carotid artery in its vertical cavernous portion; S, sella; ST, suction tip

33.3 Optic Nerve

A spontaneous CSF leak originating from the optic canal is a rare site, which has not been previously reported in the literature (Figs. 33.4 and 33.5). It is known that the meninges extend anteriorly through the optic canal and fuse with the sclera of the eyeball such that the intracranial subarachnoid space is contiguous with the intra-orbital subarachnoid space. Thus, the subarachnoid space extends anteriorly along the optic nerve sheath where it terminates as the dura and arachnoid fuse with the periosteum of the orbital cavity.

CSF rhinorrhea originating in the optic canal presents challenges in terms of both delicate preparation of surrounding bone and limited intracranial space that can be involved in repair. For example, grafts used for optic canal defects must be overlaid on the defect to avoid optic nerve compression instead of placed partially within the defect as with the more common dumbbell or

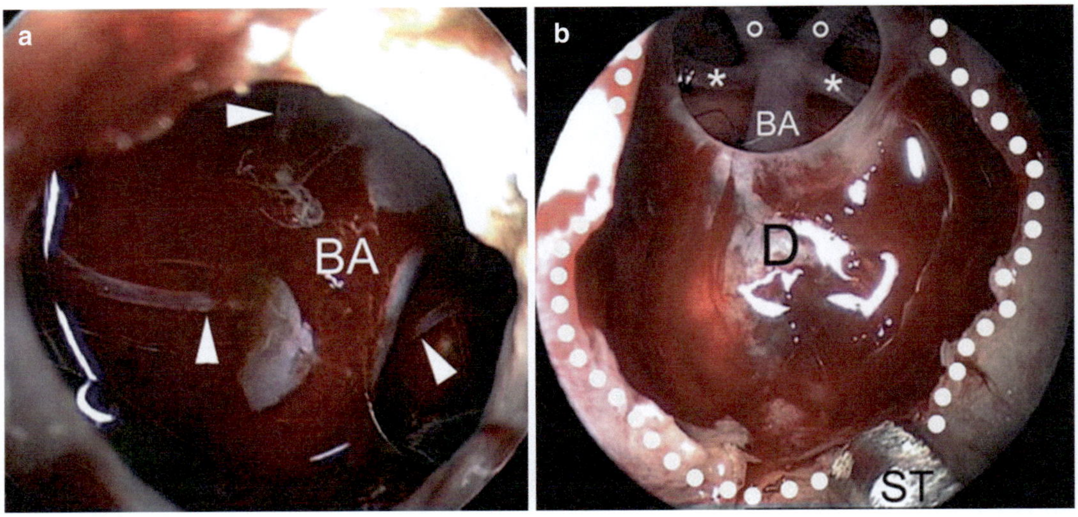

Fig. 33.3 Endoscopic view by 0° endoscope of case 1 (**a**) and case 2 (**b**). A round-shaped medial dural defect is present with exposure of the basilar artery (BA) in both the cases. The white dotted line highlights the bony clival defect. White arrowheads, basilar artery perforators; white circles, posterior cerebral arteries; white asterisks, superior cerebellar arteries. D, dura; ST, suction tip

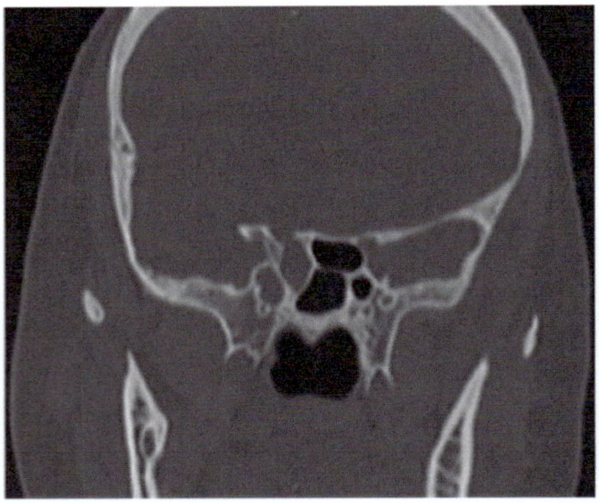

Fig. 33.4 Noncontrast coronal CT of bony defect in the optic canal and opacification in the right sphenoid sinus

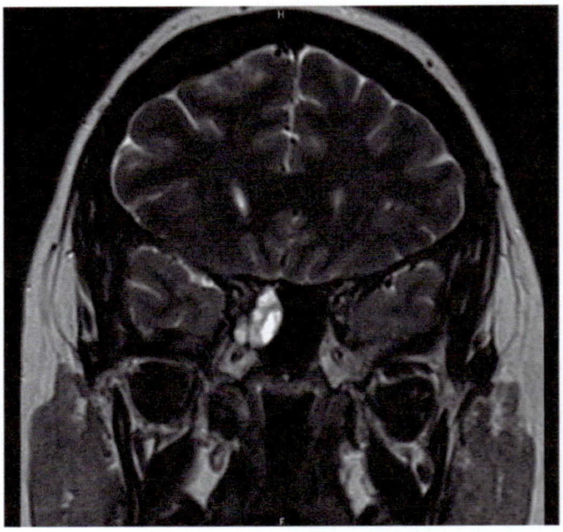

Fig. 33.5 Preoperative coronal T2-weighted MRI showing CSF leak without meningoencephalocele from the right optic nerve canal in the right sphenoid sinus

underlay graft repair, as is commonly employed for ethmoid skull base and lateral sphenoid skull base defects [26].

33.4 Eustachian Tube Leakage of the Middle Skull Base

Cerebrospinal fluid (CSF) otorhinorrhea results from an abnormal communication between subarachnoid spaces and pneumatized parts of the temporal bone through the osteodural defects at the base of the skull [27]. A defect in the middle of the skull base serves as a route for the CSF to reach the tympanic cavity, and then via the auditory tube, the nasopharynx and the nose. CSF otorhinorrhea may be acquired or spontaneous. Acquired temporal bony defects include traumatic injuries (the most common), iatrogenic causes, chronic otitis media with or without cholesteatoma, irradiation, and tumors' invasion of the skull base. A spontaneous otogenic CSF leak, on the other hand, is very rare. Some authors suggest that small bony defects of the middle fossa tegmen originating from imperfect embryologic development may progressively expand with a constant CSF pressure [28]. Another theory suggests the presence of aberrant arachnoid granulations of the dura in the middle and posterior fossa of the skull. Persistent pressure at these arachnoid granulations could erode the underlying bone [29]. Patients with a CSF leak from the temporal bone may complain of aural fullness, hearing loss, tinnitus, vertigo, and headache. Middle ear effusion, otorrhea, rhinorrhea, and pulsatile movement of the tympanic membrane are typical signs of the condition. Medical history might include an episode of meningitis as well [30]. Computed tomography and magnetic resonance imaging provide essential imaging of the encephalocele and suspected CSF otorrhea. b2-Transferrin is a specific marker of the CSF and should be applied as an assay in cases where CSF leakage is suspected [31].

Inner ear dysplasia is another rare cause of CSF otorhinorrhea [32–34]. Congenital inner ear abnormality is also a major cause of sensorineural hearing loss in children [35, 36].

The condition is diagnosed using high-resolution CT images of the temporal bone [37]. Bing Wang et al. reported 18 patients with an otogenic CSF leak secondary to inner ear dysplasia. Two of six patients who complained of rhinorrhea were misdiagnosed with a CSF rhinorrhea and underwent transnasal endoscopy initially. In all 18 cases, a CSF leak was identified during the surgery. The most common defect sites were the stapes footplate (55.6%) and the areas around the oval window (38.9%) [38]. The diagnosis of an otogenic CSF rhinorrhea, in general, is challenging and can be easily misdiagnosed. CT is the diagnostic standard; however, even detailed history and examination can be suggestive of the diagnosis. Authors claim that "for children without symptoms of meningitis, the main presentation is usually a small discharge of clear fluid from the nose that fails to attract the attention of parents and doctors. Even when parents and doctors note the symptoms, if a comprehensive medical examination is not conducted, children with CSF rhinorrhea tend to be misdiagnosed with allergic rhinitis" [38]. Intrathecal gadolinium-enhanced MR cisternography (IGE-MRC) is highly sensitive and can be used for the evaluation of otorhinorrhea as well as to precisely determine the fistula site [39].

Congenital cholesteatoma is a rare entity, but this pathology-related otorhinorrhea is even rarer. Only one case of a 60-year-old patient with a CSF rhinorrhea caused by the congenital cholesteatoma in the petrous apex is reported in the medical literature [40].

CSF otorhinorrhea associated with facial nerve palsy may be indicative of an arachnoid cyst of the fallopian canal. These fistulas are extremely rare. Surgical management includes closure of the fistula with a precise packing of the dilated facial canal to occlude the leak without injuring the facial nerve. Only a few cases have been reported [41–43].

It is important to note that higher body mass index and increased ICP influence the development of spontaneous meningoceles and CSF leak not only in the cribriform plate and lateral recess of the sphenoid sinus but in the temporal bone as well [44, 45]. Kutz et al. suggested that spontaneous CSF fistulas should be suspected in obese female patients with a chronic middle ear effusion, persistent otorrhea after tympanostomy tube placement, or in patients with a history of meningitis [46].

33.5 Distant Pseudomeningoceles of the Ventral Skull Base

A pseudomeningocele is an abnormal collection of cerebrospinal fluid in the soft tissue that is not surrounded by arachnoid membrane. It arises after a fistula from the subarachnoid space causes CSF to leak within an enclosed space such as submucosally or subcutaneously. Most of the available literature on pseudomeningoceles has focused on its occurrence following posterior fossa and spinal surgery; a distant spontaneous pseudomeningocele has been reported by Casiano et al. as two cases of nasopharyngeal and soft palate pseudomeningoceles tracking submucosally from the sphenoid sinus (Fig. 33.6) [47]. Four cases of pseudomeningoceles that masqueraded as sphenoid sinus pathology have also been reported [48]. One patient presented with nasal obstruction secondary to a mucosal covered "polyp" filling the posterior nasal cavity and radiographic expansion of the lateral recess of the sphenoid sinus and posterior maxilla. The CT scan did not show any visible bone defect of the skull base preoperatively; the mass was diagnosed as a mucocele. The patient underwent an endoscopic endonasal transpterygoid approach to the lateral recess of the sphenoid. Intraoperatively, there was elevation of the mucosa from the lateral recess of the sphenoid with a contained collection of fluid. Following removal of the mucosa, drainage of CSF from a 2 mm defect in the lateral recess of the sphenoid sinus was noted with no herniation of meninges. This was repaired successfully.

The second case presented in a middle-aged female with left side clear rhinorrhea positive for beta-2-transferrin. The patient complained of worsening headaches over the past month and intermittent blurred vision. Blunt head trauma occurred 20 years ago. Nasal endoscopy revealed a pulsatile mass of the left sphenoid sinus without evidence of a CSF leak. Computed tomography (CT) showed a total opacification of the left sphenoid sinus without bony erosion. Magnetic resonance imaging (MRI) revealed that the sphenoid sinus opacification was a fluid collection hyperintense on T2-weighted images and hypointense on T1-weighted images (Fig. 33.7).

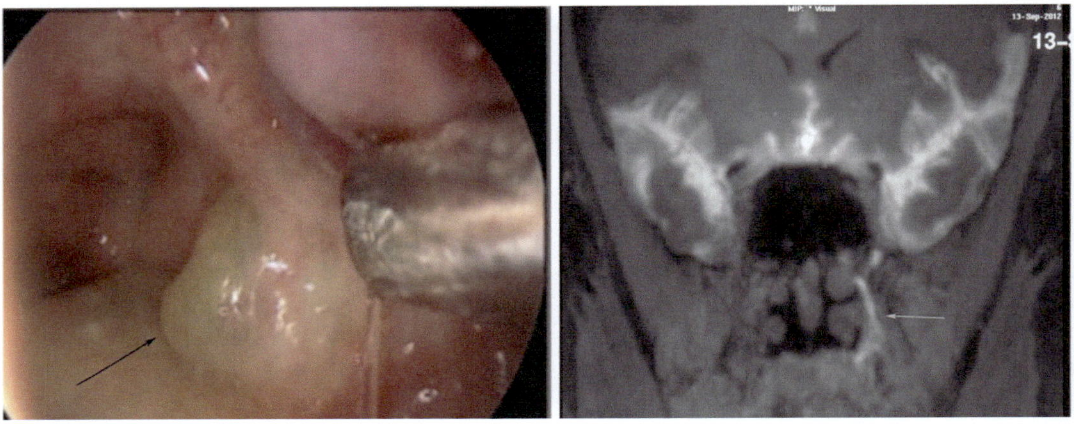

Fig. 33.6 An MRI with intrathecal contrast showed contrast transgressing from the left parasellar area into the nasopharynx (white arrow). MRI, magnetic resonance imaging. Endoscopic picture, pseudomeningocele near the left Eustachian tube (black arrow)

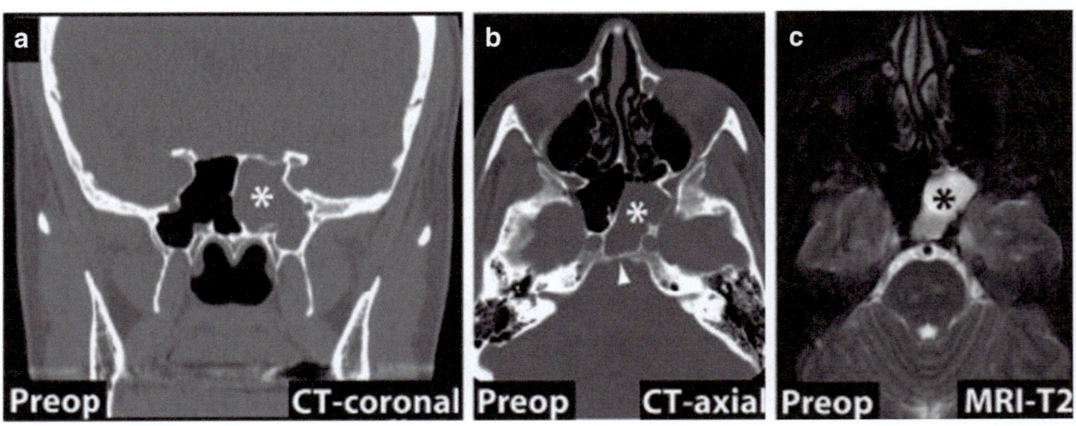

Fig. 33.7 Preoperative CT (**a**, **b**) and MRI (**c**). Computed tomography (CT) showed a total opacification (white asterisk) of the left sphenoid sinus without bony erosion (white arrow). Magnetic resonance imaging (MRI) revealed that the sphenoid sinus opacification was a fluid collection hyperintense on T2-weighted images (black asterisk)

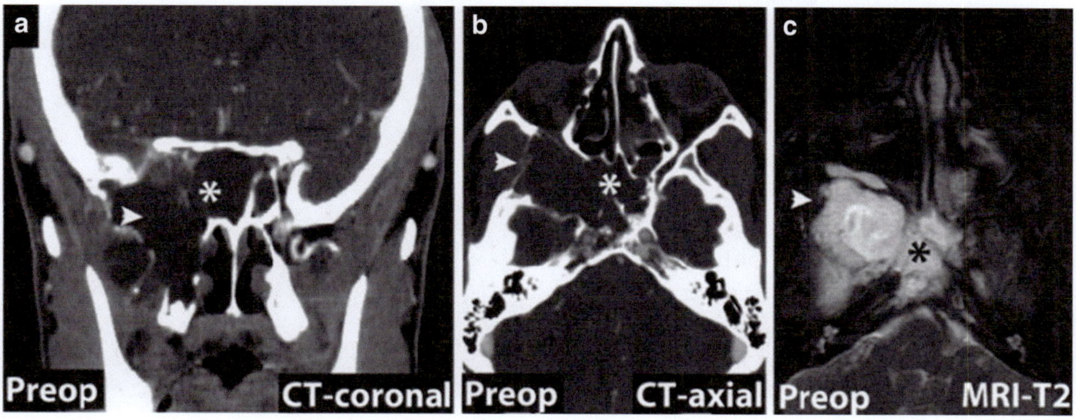

Fig. 33.8 Pre- and postoperative radiographic imaging of case 3. Preoperative CT (**a**, **b**) and MRI (**c**) were obtained immediately prior to surgery. The sphenoid sinuses are opacified (asterisk), and a fluid collection fills part of the right infratemporal fossa (arrowhead). Note the extensive erosion of the sphenoid bone. The opacification is fluid-filled and hyperintense on T2-weighted MRI imaging (MRI-T2)

An expanded endoscopic endonasal approach was performed. A very small opening at the middle part of the clivus was found which caused CSF collection under the sinus mucosa. The skull defect was repaired successfully.

The third case of pseudomeningocele reported by Alec Vaezi et al. was associated with significant bony erosion of the sphenoid bone. It was noted that the CSF leak possibly eroded the bone and caused pseudomeningocele formation. Endoscopic endonasal surgery and closure were performed (Fig. 33.8).

In case 4, the CSF leak originated from a small bony defect in the infero-lateral aspect of the sphenoid sinus and caused distant pseudomeningocele in a 55-year-old woman. Excision of the presumed nasal polyp resulted in clear fluid drainage that was later shown to be beta-2 transferrin positive.

These four reported cases show us that due to the complexity of this pathology, diagnosis is not always easy.

33.6 Systemic Disease

Specific congenital, genetic conditions, predetermining structural changes (anomalies) of a *connective tissue*, may be associated with spontaneous spinal liquorrheas as well as an underlying connective tissue disorder have been hypothesized to cause dural weakness and a predisposition to a CSF leak [49]. Moreover, spontaneous liquorrhea may be the first symptom of these disorders. Reinstein et al. carried out a study including 50 patients with spontaneous spinal liquorrhea and found nine patients with heritable connective tissue disorders, including Marfan syndrome, Ehlers-Danlos syndrome, and other unclassified forms. In seven patients, a spontaneous spinal CSF leak was the first noted manifestation of the genetic disorder [50]. Even though the study included only patients with spinal CSF leaks, there are cases of heritable connective tissue disorders-related skull base CSF leaks. Ramos et al. described the first case of a transclival CSF rhinorrhea in a 36-year-old patient with Marfan syndrome, which is an autosomal dominant genetic disorder caused by a mutation in the fibrillin-1 gene resulting in a reduced structural integrity of connective tissue [51]. The patient presented with 1 month history of rhinorrhea from the left nostril with no history of trauma or iatrogenic injury, but a deficiency in bone development associated with Marfan syndrome gave rise to a clival fenestration and transclival CSF fistula. The defect was closed using the transsphenoidal approach: the defect in the clivus was covered with a graft of abdominal fat and fibrin glue [52].

Arteriovenous malformations are associated with an increased ICP, which therefore can result in the development of meningo/meningoencephalocele and spontaneous liquorrhea [53]. Several cases are reported about this pathology. Dural arteriovenous malformations, possibly caused by an increased ICP, resulted in a CSF rhinorrhea in a 43-year-old female patient [54].

A case of a rare cerebrofacial arteriovenous metameric syndrome (CAMS)-related CSF leak has also been reported in the literature presenting a 45-year-old female patient with a history of rhinorrhea lasting for several months. CAMS is characterized by the presence of retinal, facial, and cerebral arteriovenous malformations with metameric distribution. Radiological examination showed a right-sided facial and orbital arteriovenous malformations extending posteriorly along the optic tract into the suprasellar cistern, and a right-sided meningoencephalocele protruding into the olfactory recess and ethmoid sinus. Endoscopic endonasal surgery was performed to remove the meningoencephalocele and to repair the CSF leak. The authors concluded that "the combination of a congenital osseous defect and the elevated intracranial pressure secondary to the arteriovenous malformations are responsible for the unusual clinical presentation of this patient" [55].

Another rare *systemic disease*, which can be the cause of a CSF leak, is *amyloidosis*—a condition characterized by deposits of altered proteins in the tissues [56]. Two distinct forms exist: localized amyloidosis that can be managed conservatively or surgically with a good prognosis, and systemic, associated with significant morbidity and mortality. Localized amyloidosis of the head and neck is a slowly progressing disease that does not respond to medical therapy. Nevertheless, the treatment of choice is conservative management unless symptomatic. Then, local excision is recommended when necessary. Isolated sinonasal amyloidosis is extremely rare [57]. Ali et al. reported a patient with a localized amyloidosis of the sphenoid sinus, presenting with a cerebrospinal fluid rhinorrhea. An endonasal endoscopic approach was used to remove the lesion and perform multilayered obliteration of the sphenoid sinus. Twelve months follow-up showed no evidence of recurrence [58].

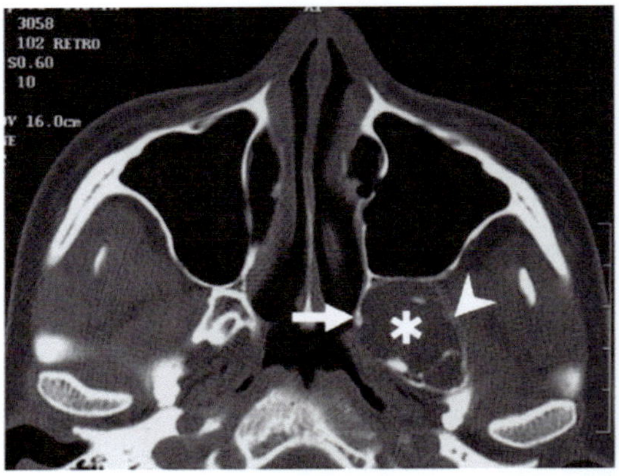

Fig. 33.9 Axial CT at the level of the inferior turbinate. A dense, oval soft tissue mass (asterisk) is present in the left pterygoid fossa. Arrow, medial pterygoid plate; arrowhead, lateral pterygoid plate

Nasal tuberculosis, a localized presentation of a systemic condition, has also been shown to be the cause of a CSF liquorrhea, which should be suspected in the differential in endemic areas [59].

Calvarial encephaloceles occur most frequently in the occipital region and are usually noted at birth. In contrast, basal meningoencephaloceles are extremely rare congenital malformations and are frequently occult. A rare case of basal meningoencephalocele that protruded into the left pterygoid fossa from the middle cranial fossa has been reported (Fig. 33.9) [60].

33.7 Nonsurgical Iatrogenic-Induced CSF Leak

A CSF leak can develop following a nonsurgical treatment of skull base tumors. The literature presents cases when cerebrospinal fluid (CSF) rhinorrhea appears after a medical treatment of a pituitary adenoma, especially with a dopamine agonist therapy of invasive prolactinomas. It has been estimated that rates of rhinorrhea after initiating dopamine agonist therapy are 6–7% [36, 61]. The mean time from the initialization of a medical treatment to the onset of rhinorrhea is about 3 months [62–66]. Priddy et al. presented the case of a CSF rhinorrhea caused by a systemic erlotinib chemotherapy for anterior skull base metastases in a 66-year-old woman presented with stage IV adenocarcinoma of the lung [67]. Chemotherapy of the tumor is rarely complicated by a CSF leak; therefore, the exact rate of the condition is not known. It is thought that a CSF leak is associated with the invasion of a tumor to the bone and dura mater: when tumor cells disappear or shrink in size as a result of treatment, a defect remains in the skull for a CSF leak [67]. It has also been reported that a CSF leak is a rare complication following flutamide therapy, especially if large areas of the anterior skull base are involved [68].

Stereotactic radiosurgery and radiotherapy are becoming increasingly common in the management of skull base tumors and other disorders. The literature presents cases of CSF rhinorrhea as a complication of such treatment methods: CSF rhinorrhea occurred 4 months after a stereotactic radiosurgery treatment of a metastatic renal cell carcinoma in the petroclival region [69]. A case report of a patient with a GH-secreting adenoma, treated with gamma knife surgery, described a CSF rhinorrhea, which occurred 11 years after the treatment. However, the authors tended to relate the complication to the empty sella observed in the MR images, and just then to "the other potential causes, may be the original invasiveness of the tumor or delayed radiation damage to the mucous membranes of the skull" [70]. It was noticed that radiosurgery is more frequently complicated with the CSF rhinorrhea in patients who already underwent a transsphenoidal surgical tumor excision. Perry et al. reported two cases of a delayed CSF leak after gamma knife radiosurgery for pituitary adenoma. Notably, both the patients had a transsphenoidal tumor resection in the history. The authors concluded that CSF leaks of this origin "have the potential to be refractory," and thus, it is recommended to perform an "aggressive reconstruction preferably with a vascularized flap, and potentially supplemented by placement of a lumbar drain and acetazolamide. Current evidence is scant and provides little insight regarding an underlying mechanism, which may include bony destruction by the tumor, delayed radiation necrosis, or a secondary empty sella syndrome."

It can be summarized that a clear rhinorrhea for a patient treated with medication or radiotherapy for a cerebral or skull base tumor should be investigated for a potential CSF leak. If rhinoliquorrhea is confirmed, an urgent surgical management is needed to prevent such severe complications as meningitis.

References

1. Thomson SC. The cerebrospinal fluid: its spontaneous escape from the nose. London: Cassell; 1899.
2. Escat E. Ecoulement spontane de liquide cephalorachidien par le conduit auditif externe, fistule congénitale probable. Arch Int Laryngol. 1897;10:653–9.
3. Dandy WD. Pneumocephalus. Arch Surg. 1926;12:949–82.
4. Dohlman G. Spontaneous cerebrospinal rhinorrhea. Acta Otolaryngol Suppl. 1948;67:20–3.
5. El-Banhawy OA, Halaka AN, El-Hafiz Shehab El-Dien A, Ayad H. Subcranial transnasal repair of cerebrospinal fluid rhinorrhea with free autologous grafts by the combined overlay and underlay techniques. Minim Invasive Neurosurg. 2004;47:197–202.
6. Loew F, Pertuiset B, Chaumier EE, Jaksche H. Traumatic, spontaneous and postoperative CSF rhinorrhea. Adv Tech Stand Neurosurg. 1984;11:169–207.
7. O'Connell JE. Primary spontaneous cerebrospinal fluid rhinorrhoea. J Neurol Neurosurg Psychiatry. 1964;27:241–6.
8. Ommaya AK. Non-traumatic cerebrospinal fluid rhinorrhoea. J Neurol Neurosurg Psychiatry. 1968;31: 214–25.
9. Joo JD. Isolated abducens nerve palsy due to cerebrospinal fluid leakage following lumbar discectomy: a rare clinical entity. Eur Spine J. 2013;22(Suppl 3):S421–3. https://doi.org/10.1007/s00586-012-2545-z; Epub 2012 Oct 16
10. Psaltis AJ, Schlosser RJ, Banks CA, Yawn J, Zachary M. Soler a systematic review of the endoscopic Repair of cerebrospinal fluid leaks. Otolaryngol Head Neck Surg. 2012;147:196. https://doi.org/10.1177/0194599812451090; originally published online 15 June 2012
11. Schlosser RJ, Bolger WE. Nasal cerebrospinal fluid leaks: critical review and surgical considerations. Laryngoscope. 2004;114:255–65.
12. Konuthula N, et al. A systematic review of secondary cerebrospinal fluid leaks. Am J Rhinol Allergy. 2017;31:e48–56. https://doi.org/10.2500/ajra.2017.31.4487.
13. Castelnuovo P, et al. Endonasal endoscopic repair of Sternberg's canal cerebrospinal fluid leaks.

Laryngoscope. 2007;117(2):345–9. https://doi.org/10.1097/01.mlg.0000251452.90657.3a.
14. Prashant G, et al. A retrospective analysis of spontaneous sphenoid sinus fistula: MR and CT Findings. AJNR Am J Neuroradiol. 2000;21:337–42.
15. Schuknecht B, et al. Nontraumatic skull base defects with spontaneous CSF rhinorrhea and arachnoid herniation: imaging findings and correlation with endoscopic sinus surgery in 27 patients. AJNR Am J Neuroradiol. 2008;29:542–9.
16. Van Zele T, et al. Primary spontaneous cerebrospinal fluid leaks located at the clivus. Allergy Rhinol. 2013;4:e100–4. https://doi.org/10.2500/ar.2013.4.0053.
17. Pagella F, et al. Endoscopic management of spontaneous clival cerebrospinal fluid leaks: case series and literature review. World Neurosurg. 2016;86:470–7.
18. Goddard JC, Meyer T, Nguyen S, Lambert PR. New considerations in the cause of spontaneous cerebrospinal fluid otorrhea. Otol Neurotol. 2010;31:940–5.
19. Carrau RL, Snyderman CH, Kassam AB. The management of cerebrospinal fluid leaks in patients at risk for high-pressure hydrocephalus. Laryngoscope. 2005;115:205–21.
20. Stevens SM, et al. Idiopathic intracranial hypertension: contemporary review and implications for the otolaryngologist. Laryngoscope. 2018;128:248–56.
21. Yamamoto T, Yano S, Hide T, et al. A case of ecchordosis physaliphora presenting with an abducens nerve palsy: a rare symptomatic case managed with endoscopic endonasal transsphenoidal surgery. Surg Neurol Int. 2013;4:13.
22. Bolzoni-Villaret A, et al. Transnasal endoscopic resection of symptomatic ecchordosis physaliphora. Laryngoscope. 2013;124(6):1325–8.
23. Macdonald RL, et al. Cerebrospinal fluid fistula secondary to ecchordosis physaliphora. Neurosurgery. 1990;26(3):515–8.
24. Alli A, et al. Cerebrospinal fluid rhinorrhea secondary to ecchordosis physaliphora. Skull Base. 2008;18(6):395–9. https://doi.org/10.1055/s-0028-1087221).
25. Galloway L, Hayhurst C. Spontaneous cerebrospinal fluid rhinorrhoea with meningitis secondary to ecchordosis physaliphora. Br J Neurosurg. 2019 Feb;33(1):99–100.
26. Hannabass K, Justice JM. Spontaneous cerebrospinal fluid leak from the optic canal. SAGE Open Med Case Rep. 2017;5:1–3.
27. Yi HJ, Zhao L-D, Guo W, Wu N, Li JN, Ren LL, Liu PN, Yang SM. The diagnosis and surgical treatment of occult otogenic CSF leakage. Acta Otolaryngol. 2013;133:130–5.
28. Brown NE, et al. Diagnosis and management of spontaneous cerebrospinal fluid-middle ear effusion and otorrhea. Laryngoscope. 2004;114(May (5)):800–5.
29. Gacek RR, Gacek MR. Arachnoid granulations of the temporal bone. Am J Otol. 1999;20(May (3)):405–6.
30. Patel RB, Kwartler JA, Hodosh RM, Baredes S. Spontaneous cerebrospinal fluid leakage and middle ear encephalocele in seven patients. Ear Nose Throat J. 2000;79(5):372–3, 376–8
31. Chan D, et al. How useful is glucose detection in diagnosing cerebrospinal fluid leak? The rational use of CT and Beta-2 transferrin assay in detection of cerebrospinal fluid fistula. Asian J Surg. 2004;27(1):39–42.
32. Tyagi I, et al. Cerebrospinal fluid otorhinorrhoea due to inner-ear malformations: clinical presentation and new perspectives in management. J Laryngol Otol. 2005 Sep;119(9):714–8.
33. Mehdi E, et al. CSF otorhinorrhea in a child with inner ear dysplasia: diagnosis with T2-weighted and intrathecal contrast-enhanced MR cisternography. Jpn J Radiol. 2014;32(7):437–40.
34. Joseph ST, Bhalodiya NH, Ghosh R. Simultaneous cerebrospinal fluid otorrhea and rhinorrhea as a cause of recurrent meningitis in a patient with cochlear dysplasia. Eur J Pediatr. 2012;171(8):1277–9.
35. Robson CD. Congenital hearing impairment. Paediatr Radiol. 2006;36:309–24.
36. Suliman SG, et al. Nonsurgical cerebrospinal fluid rhinorrhea in invasive macroprolactinoma: incidence, radiological, and clinicopathological features. J Clin Endocrinol Metab. 2007;92(10):3829–35.
37. Yiin RS, Tang PH, Tan TY. Review of congenital inner ear abnormalities on CT temporal bone. Br J Radiol. 2011;84(1005):859–63.
38. Wang B, et al. Cerebrospinal fluid otorrhea secondary to congenital inner ear dysplasia: diagnosis and management of 18 cases. J Zhejiang Univ Sci B. 2019;20(2):156–63.
39. Nacar Dogan S, et al. Intrathecal gadolinium-enhanced MR cisternography in patients with otorhinorrhea: 10-year experience of a tertiary referral center. Neuroradiology. 2018;60(5):471–7.
40. Dzaman K, et al. Non-classical presentation of congenital cholesteatoma as cerebrospinal fluid rhinorrhea - case report and systematic review of the literature. Neurol Neurochir Pol. 2015;49(3):183–8.
41. Isaacson JE, Linder TE, Fisch U. Arachnoid cyst of the fallopian canal: a surgical challenge. Otol Neurotol. 2002;23(4):589–93.
42. Teufert KB, Slattery WH. Cerebrospinal fluid leak of the fallopian canal. Ear Nose Throat J. 2013;92(3):E20–3.
43. Dey JK, Van Gompel JJ, Lane JI, Carlson ML. Fallopian canal meningocele with spontaneous cerebrospinal fluid otorrhea: case report and systematic review of the literature. World Neurosurg. 2019;122:e285–90.
44. Stucken EZ, Selesnick SH, Brown KD. The role of obesity in spontaneous temporal bone encephaloceles and CSF leak. Otol Neurotol. 2012;33(8):1412–7.
45. Burduk PK, Mierzwiński J, Burduk D, Winkler P, Bilewicz R. Spontaneous temporal bone meningoencephalocele. Otolaryngol Pol. 2008;62(2):199–203.
46. Kutz JW Jr, Johnson AK, Wick CC. Surgical management of spontaneous cerebrospinal fistulas and

encephaloceles of the temporal bone. Laryngoscope. 2018;128(9):2170–7.
47. Lieberman SM, Ojo RB, Casiano RR. Distant pseudomeningoceles of the ventral skull base: a report of 2 cases. Int Forum Allergy Rhinol. 2013;3(12): 1021–4.
48. Vaezi A, Snyderman CH, Saleh HA, Carrau RL, Zanation A, Gardner P. Pseudomeningoceles of the sphenoid sinus masquerading as sinus pathology. Laryngoscope. 2011;121:2507–13.
49. Liu FC, et al. Connective tissue disorders in patients with spontaneous intracranial hypotension. Cephalalgia. 2011;31(6):691–5.
50. Reinstein E. Connective tissue spectrum abnormalities associated with spontaneous cerebrospinal fluid leaks: a prospective study. Eur J Hum Genet. 2013;21(4):386–90.
51. Judge DP, Dietz HZ. Marfan's syndrome. Lancet. 2005;366(9501):1965–76.
52. Ramos A, et al. Transclival cerebrospinal fluid fistula in a patient with Marfan's syndrome. Acta Neurochir. 2007;149:723–5.
53. Vorstman EBA, et al. Benign intracranial hypertension associated with arteriovenous malformation. Dev Med Child Neurol. 2002;44(2):133–5.
54. Willems PWA, et al. Aggressive intracranial dural arteriovenous fistula presenting with cerebrospinal fluid rhinorrhea: case report. Neurosurgery. 2009;65(6):E1208–9.
55. Fernandez-Gajardo R, et al. Ethmoid meningoencephalocele in a patient with cerebrofacial arteriovenous metameric syndrome. World Neurosurg. 2018;114:1–3.
56. Benson MD. Amyloid nomenclature 2018: recommendations by the International Society of Amyloidosis (ISA) nomenclature committee. Amyloid. 2018;25(4):215–9.
57. Rauba D, Sukytė D, et al. Isolated nasal amyloidosis: a case report. Medicina (Kaunas). 2013;49(11): 497–503.
58. Ali EA, et al. Cerebrospinal fluid rhinorrhea secondary to amyloidosis of the sphenoid sinus. Med J Malaysia. 2008;63(4):341–2.
59. Baig WW, et al. Spontaneous cerebrospinal fluid rhinorrhea with pneumocephalus: an unusual manifestation of nasal tuberculosis. Korean J Intern Med. 2012;27(3):350–2; Epub 2012 Sep 1
60. Nishikawa T, Ishida H, Nibu K-i. A rare spontaneous temporal meningoencephalocele with dehiscence into the pterygoid fossa. Auris Nasus Larynx. 2004;31:429–31.
61. Leong KS, et al. CSF rhinorrhoea following treatment with dopamine agonists for massive invasive prolactinomas. Clin Endocrinol. 2000;52(1):43–9.
62. Lam G, Mehta V, Zada G. Spontaneous and medically induced cerebrospinal fluid leakage in the setting of pituitary adenomas: review of the literature. Neurosurg Focus. 2012;32:E2.
63. Singh P, Singh M, Cugati G, Singh AK. Bromocriptine or cabergoline-induced cerebrospinal fluid rhinorrhea: a life-threatening complication during management of prolactinoma. J Hum Reprod Sci. 2011;4:104–5.
64. de Lacy P, Benjamin S, Dixon R, Stephens JW, Redfern R, Price DE. Is surgical intervention frequently required for medically managed macroprolactinomas? A study of spontaneous cerebrospinal fluid rhinorrhea. Surg Neurol. 2009;72:461–3.
65. Thakur B, Jesurasa AR, Ross R, Carroll TA, Mirza S, Sinha S. Transnasal trans-sphenoidal endoscopic repair of CSF leak secondary to invasive pituitary tumours using a nasoseptal flap. Pituitary. 2011;14:163.
66. Prague JK, Ward CL, Mustafa OG, Whitelaw BC, King A, Thomas NW, et al. Delayed presentation of late-onset cerebrospinal fluid rhinorrhoea following dopamine agonist therapy for giant prolactinoma. Endocrinol Diabetes Metab Case Rep. 2014;2014:140020.
67. Priddy B, Hardesty DA, Beer-Furlan A, Otto B, Prevedello DM. Cerebrospinal fluid leak rhinorrhea after systemic Erlotinib chemotherapy for metastatic lung cancer: a familiar problem from an unfamiliar culprit. World Neurosurg. 2017;108:992.e11–4.
68. Panda S, Phalak M, Thakar A, Dharanipathy S. CSF leak in juvenile nasopharyngeal angiofibroma – rare sequelae of flutamide induced tumour shrinkage. World Neurosurg. 2018;120:78–81. https://doi.org/10.1016/j.wneu.2018.07.288.
69. Kim CH, Chung SK, Dhong HJ, Lee JI. Cerebrospinal fluid leakage after gamma knife radiosurgery for skull base metastasis from renal cell carcinoma: a case report. Laryngoscope. 2008;118: 1925–7.
70. Hongmei Y, Zhe W, Jing W, Daokui W, Peicheng C, Yongjie L. Delayed cerebrospinal fluid rhinorrhea after gamma knife surgery in a patient with a growth hormone-secreting adenoma. J Clin Neurosci. 2012;19:900–2.

Management of Idiopathic Intracranial Hypertension

34

Ehtesham Ghani, Mahmoud AlYamany, and Fahad Alfawwaz

34.1 Definition

Idiopathic intracranial hypertension (IIH) is characterized by symptoms and signs of raised intracranial pressure (ICP) with normal cerebrospinal fluid (CSF) composition and no other cause of intracranial hypertension evident on neuroimaging [1].

34.2 Terminology

The first report of idiopathic intracranial hypertension came from Heinrich Quincke in 1893 with the diagnosis of serous meningitis [2]. The term pseudotumor cerebri was introduced by Max Nonne in 1904 [3]. Its name was changed to benign intracranial hypertension in 1955 [4]. The terms "pseudotumor cerebri" and "benign" were used at that time as mostly intracranial hypertension was linked with brain tumors. "Benign" means not fatal, nonthreatening or not harmful. In contrast, it can threaten the vision and affect the activity of daily living. The term benign intracranial hypertension is now obsolete as it is associated with significant morbidity of visual impairment [5]. Therefore, it was revised to idiopathic intracranial hypertension (IIH) in 1989 [6].

34.3 Epidemiology

The incidence of IIH is approximately 1/100,000/year to 13/100,000/year in women between 20 to 40-year who are 10% above the ideal body weight and 19/100,000/year in those 20% above the ideal body weight [5]. In simple words, it mainly affects obese women of child bearing age [7]. However, it is also seen in males [5]. Children as young as 4-months can be affected [8]. The prevalence is higher reflecting the chronic nature of the condition.

34.4 Associations

Diseases like hypothyroidism, hyperthyroidism, anemia, chronic hypocalcemia due to vitamin D deficiency and hypoparathyroidism are linked with IIH. Drugs related IIH have been reported which include tetracycline, isotretinoin, thyroxine, nitrofurantoin, oral contraceptives and steroid withdrawal. Medical conditions including obstructive sleep apnea, systemic lupus erythematosis, and Behcet's disease also have some association with IIH [5, 8].

E. Ghani (✉) · M. AlYamany
Department of Neurosurgery, National Neuroscience Institute, King Fahad Medical City, Riyadh, Saudi Arabia
e-mail: ighani@kfmc.med.sa

F. Alfawwaz
Otolaryngology Head and Neck Surgery Department, King Fahad Medical City, Riyadh, Saudi Arabia

A. A. AlQahtani et al. (eds.), *CSF Rhinorrhea*, https://doi.org/10.1007/978-3-030-94781-1_34

34.5 Pathogenesis

There are different theories that are related to the pathogenesis of IIH. These are related to impaired CSF dynamics which include decreased CSF absorption, increase CSF secretion, increased blood volume, increased dural venous sinus pressure and brain edema [8, 9].

34.6 Diagnosis

Diagnosis of IIH is not simple as it can occur in the absence of classical signs including papilledema. CSF pressure at the time of lumbar puncture may be normal. Therefore, IIH has wide clinical spectrum. Diagnosis depends on clinical presentation, ophthalmological assessment, radiological findings and the results of lumbar puncture.

Dandy [10] described the original criteria of IIH including:

- Signs and symptoms of increased ICP–CSF pressure more than 25 cmH_2O.
- No localizing signs with the exception of abducens nerve palsy.
- Normal CSF production.
- Normal to small ventricles on imaging with no intracranial mass.

In 1985 Smith revised the criteria of IIH by including computer tomography (CT) scan instead of ventriculography [11].

Friedman and Jacobson [1] introduced the Modified Dandy criteria in 2002 that include:

- High-pressure headache and papilledema.
- CSF opening pressure of more than 25 cmH_2O.
- Awake and alert patient.
- No localizing signs other than lateral rectus paresis.
- Normal CSF constituents.
- Normal brain imaging with no evidence of venous obstruction.
- Benign clinical course apart from visual deterioration.
- No other cause of raised intracranial pressure.

Moreover, they stated that lumbar puncture should be performed in lateral lying position as lumbar puncture in sitting position can lead to falsely high CSF pressure.

Mollan et al. [12] divided IIH into the following three types;

1. Fulminant IIH: the patient has imminent risk to vision.
2. Typical IIH: the patient is a woman of reproductive age with body mass index (BMI) of more than 30 kg/m^2.
3. Atypical IIH: the patient is not female, or if the patient is female, she is not of reproductive age and her BMI is less than 30 kg/m^2.

34.7 Symptoms

Symptoms of IIH are nonspecific. These are related to raised ICP. Headache and visual disturbances are the main presenting symptoms. Headache is predominantly frontal in location. It worsens while lying down. It may wake the patient at night. It is also more in the early morning. Visual disturbances include blurring of vision, transient visual loss and diplopia. Patient may present with seizures or neck pain [8].

CSF rhinorrhea is a rare presentation of IIH. The long-standing pulsatile effect of CSF under high pressure leads to expansion and eventual rupture of arachnoid sleeve surrounding the olfactory rootlets which pass through cribriform plate, results in CSF rhinorrhea. It may also lead to the rupture of arachnoid in the empty sella due to downward herniation of diaphragma sella. CSF pressure measurements after sealing the defect confirms the diagnosis of IIH if there is no papilledema. The persistent elevated ICP causes remodeling of skull base, that may result in meningo-encephaloceles which also in turn leads to CSF rhinorrhea. CSF rhinorrhea with IIH must be considered as high-pressure CSF leaks and should be treated accordingly [13–15].

34.8 Signs

As per definition and diagnostic criteria, neurological examination is normal except for papilledema and or sixth cranial nerve palsy. Occulomotor and trochlear nerves palsies can also be seen occasionally. Other rare findings include facial paresis, hyper-reflexia, bruit, hypoglossal nerve palsy, nystagmus and choreiform movements. However, features other than papilledema and or sixth cranial nerve palsy are rare. The level of consciousness and intellectual functions remain normal in IIH [8]. Diagnosis of intracranial lesion (tumor, infection, inflammatory process) must be ruled out if such rare features are present.

Papilledema is the hallmark feature of IIH. It is usually bilateral but it may be unilateral or asymmetrical despite the global nature of disease. Fluorescein angiography differentiates between papilledema and pseudo-papilledema (optic nerve drusen). Persistent papilledema will lead to secondary optic atrophy [16].

The enlargement of blind spot is the most common visual field change. It is followed by central scotomas, inferior nasal field defect and peripheral visual field constriction. The visual field assessment is the most sensitive indicator of impending visual impairment [8, 12].

Visual loss is the main serious and threatening complication of IIH. A number of retinal changes may also contribute to visual impairment that includes choroidal compression folds across macula, choroidal neovascularization and serous retinal elevation around optic nerve head in severely acute cases. Flattening of the globe may lead to refractive changes as well [5].

34.9 Imaging

CT scan is the initial screening test. Magnetic resonance imaging (MRI) assists in the diagnosis of IIH. Intracranial lesion must be ruled out before making the diagnosis of IIH. Radiological features of IIH include undilated, small or slit ventricles, hydrops of optic nerve sheath, tortuous course of optic nerve, flattening of posterior aspect of globe and empty or partial empty sella as shown in Fig. 34.1 [12]. Magnetic resonance venography should be done to diagnose venous sinus thrombosis. It must be considered if the patient does not improve after lumbar puncture. Orbital ultrasound is also a useful tool as it helps in assessing the diameter of optic nerve [8].

34.10 Diagnostic Lumbar Puncture

Lumbar puncture is done after excluding intracranial lesion on MRI. CSF pressure varies normally as it does in IIH [8]. It may be normal with papilledema. In such cases, repeated lumbar punctures or lumbar CSF pressure monitoring can be useful. It can work as diagnostic and therapeutic modality. If the pressure is more than 30 cm H_2O, CSF can be drained gradually to reduce the pressure below 15 cm H_2O.

34.11 Management

IIH causes significant short term and long-term morbidity with no proven effective treatment available. A prospective study is needed to establish the indications and the efficacy of the treatment. The main goal of treatment is to save the vision. The other aim is to alleviate the symptoms. CSF pressure may remain high despite of resolved papilledema. Asymptomatic papilledema with progressive visual loss has been reported in the literature [8]. Most cases respond to medical treatment at least temporarily. Gradual improvement or stabilization of the symptoms occurs with the treatment. Many of the patients with IIH have persistent papilledema, visual field defects and raised ICP.

34.12 Acetazolamide

Acetazolamide is a carbonic anhydrase inhibitor. It is the first choice in the medical management of IIH. Its usual dose is 1-g/day. It may be raised to 4-g/day in refractory cases. It is a diuretic agent that acts on proximal renal tubules. It lowers intracranial and intra-orbital pressures. Side effects are dose related which include gastrointestinal upset, peri-oral and digital tingling, loss of appetite, electrolyte imbalance, metabolic

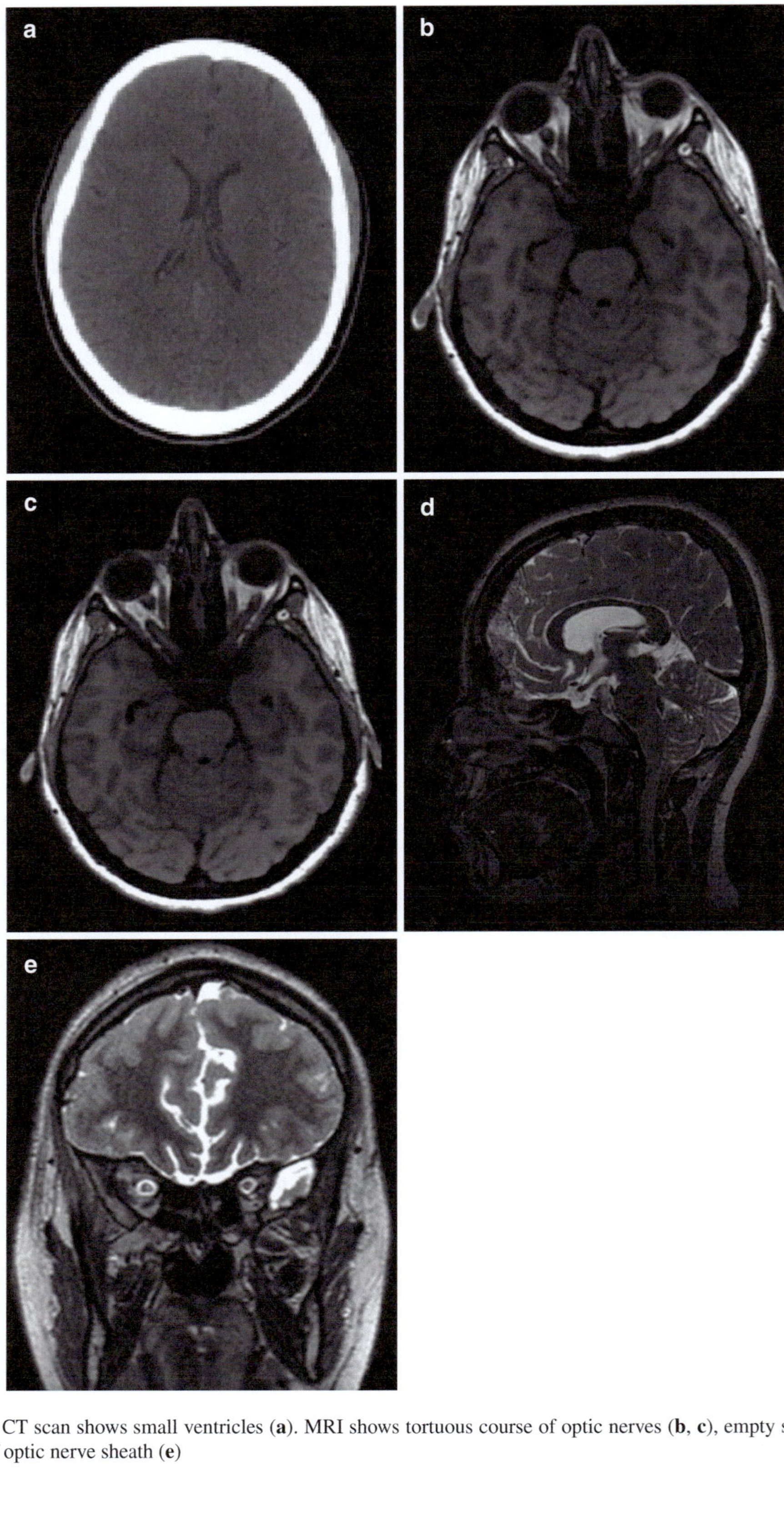

Fig. 34.1 CT scan shows small ventricles (**a**). MRI shows tortuous course of optic nerves (**b**, **c**), empty sella (**d**) and hydrops of optic nerve sheath (**e**)

acidosis and renal stones [8]. It is contraindicated in patients who have sulfa allergy. It belongs to FDA class C. Therefore, it should only be used if potential benefits are more than risks during pregnancy. It is associated with teratogenic effects during the first trimester in animal studies.

34.13 Topiramate

It is a striking option for the treatment of IIH. It has similar efficacy to acetazolamide with regard to improvement in visual field and symptom relief. It reduces the CSF production by acting on carbonic anhydrase. It also helps in reducing the weight which is one of the treatment modalities of the condition [17].

34.14 Steroids

Resolution of IIH symptoms and papilledema usually takes two weeks with acetazolamide. If this does not occur, steroids may be added as these help in reducing the brain edema and swelling. On the other hand, steroids cause weight gain which may worsen IIH. Steroid withdrawal may result in severe rebound IIH [8]. There are other systemic side effects as well. Therefore, steroids should be avoided in the treatment of IIH.

34.15 Other Medications

Furosemide and indomethacin have also shown some effect in the treatment of IIH [18, 19].

34.16 Therapeutic Lumbar Puncture

Repeated lumbar punctures are used for diagnosis as well as for symptomatic relief. Effect of repeated spinal taps is usually short lived. It may be a painful and distressing procedure for the patient. It can result in chronic back pain and carries a theoretical risk of developing intraspinal epidermoid tumors [8]. Moreover, it will be difficult to do in obese patients. In such circumstances, interventional radiologist will be of great help. However, it may be valuable in patients who are pregnant and who wishes to delay the surgical treatment. Theoretically repeated lumbar puncture using large bore spinal needle may create a path for the CSF to the spinal epidural space where it can be absorbed by the paraspinal muscles.

34.17 Surgery

Surgery is considered for the patients with deteriorating vision and who have severe incapacitating headaches that are not responding to medical treatment. Surgical options include subtemporal decompression, CSF diversion surgery and bariatric surgery.

Potential indications for surgery include: [6].

- Poor vision due to papilledema.
- Worsening visual field defect despite medical therapy.
- Intractable headache.
- Anticipated hypotension (as with antihypertensive medications and renal dialysis).
- Difficult follow-up.

34.18 Cranial Decompression

Historically, subtemporal decompression was tried for the treatment of IIH but it was ineffective in reducing the CSF pressure [20].

34.19 Optic Nerve Sheath Fenestration

Optic nerve sheath fenestration (ONSF) was first performed for the relief of papilledema via transconjunctival approach in 1871. CSF was drained into the orbit after making incision in optic nerve sheath [21].

ONSF provides successful resolution of papilledema and rapidly reverses the visual impairment. The fundamental steps to success with ONSF are early intervention and appropriate expertise [8]. Patient may be treated with second ONSF after initial failure. Eyes that need more than one ONSF rarely improve after surgery due to the vascular insult to optic nerves [16]. The most common complications are transient diplopia, pupillary dysfunction and visual loss. Blindness is reported in 1–2% of the cases [5, 22]. Therefore, the procedure is recommended for those who have threat to vision or in those who did not get benefit from the CSF diversion.

34.20 Shunt Surgery

Headache, diplopia, visual impairment and papilledema improve after CSF diversion surgery. Headache resolves almost immediately after the CSF diversion procedure. Lumbo-peritoneal shunts were used in the past. Now the trend is toward ventriculo-peritoneal (VP) shunt surgery.

34.21 Lumbo-Peritoneal Shunts

It is a satisfactory treatment method for the majority of the patients with IIH. However, some of them require multiple shunt revisions. It effectively lowers raised ICP, relieves headaches and improves vision and papilledema. Shunt obstruction and low pressure headaches are the main complications. It also carries the risks of cerebellar tonsillar herniation, syringomyelia, subdural hematoma, lumbar radiculopathy and infection [5, 8, 16].

34.22 Ventriculo-Peritoneal Shunts

VP shunt surgery is another option in the surgical treatment of IIH. Frameless stereotactic image guidance techniques for the insertion of VP shunt in the presence of small ventricles are published in the literature. Problems that are related to overdrainage from lumbo-peritoneal shunts are avoided through VP shunt [5]. Moreover, by using this technique, chances of optimal placement of ventricular catheter are improved. When this technique is used, ventricular cannulation rate reaches up to 100% [23]. Various intraoperative modalities have been employed in addressing the challenges of accurate insertion of ventricular catheter. These modalities include the use of navigation, stereotaxic guidance, ultrasound, endoscope and intraoperative CT (iCT) scan. Frameless stereotaxy has some limitations including head fixation, intraoperative cost of the equipment and added operating time. With the help of iCT, adjustment of the ventricular catheter can be easily made. Although, increased intraoperative time is an important factor for shunt infection. These additional intraoperative modalities do not effect the rate of shunt infection [24]. VP shunt may be less prone to shunt obstruction than lumbo-peritoneal shunts [25]. In recently published article, authors stated that stereotactic placement of bilateral VP shunt catheters improves shunt survival rates and the presenting symptoms in patients with IIH [26]. It may be more effective and functionally sustained method for the treatment of IIH.

34.23 Endoscopic Repair

The chances of spontaneous resolution of CSF rhinorrhea with IIH are less. Endonasal endoscopic repair is the standard of care. The rate of recurrence is higher due to IIH. Early recurrence was noted at same site. However, late recurrence was noted at distant site [27]. Therefore, IIH should be treated at the same time either with medications or with surgical intervention [14, 28].

34.24 Venous Sinus Stenting

In IIH with venous sinus stenosis, venous sinus stenting is an alternative approach. There may be some technical problems related to stent delivery in the area of stenosis. It can be overcome by appropriate selection of the stent and operator dependent technique [29]. It also helps in relieving headache and improving vision [30].

Although it improves the symptomatology, it can result in stenosis proximal to the stent, stent-migration, in-stent thrombosis and intracranial bleeding [31].

34.25 Weight Loss

Vision, visual field and papilledema improve rapidly in patients who have weight loss after diagnosis. In obese patients, resolution of symptoms can be achieved with bariatric surgery in 95% of the cases [32]. Weight gain may be a contributing risk factor for the recurrence.

34.26 Conclusion

IIH can affect the normal life and cause significant visual catastrophe. Early recognition, prompt diagnosis, quick and timely intervention either medical or surgical may preserve vision. There are no randomized controlled trials to guide the decision as to which procedure or the treatment is best.

References

1. Friedman DI, Jacobson DM. Diagnostic criteria for idiopathic intracranial hypertension. Neurology. 2002;59:1492.
2. Quincke HI. Meningitis serosa. Sammlung Linisher Vortrage. 1893;67:655.
3. None M. Ueber falle vom symptomkomplex "tumor cerebri" mit ausgang in heilung (pseudotumor cerebri). Deutsche Zeitschrift fur Nervenheilkunde (in Germany). 1904;27:169–216.
4. Foley J. Benign forms of intracranial hypertension; toxic and otitic hydrocephalus. Brain. 1955;78:1–41.
5. Acheson JF. Idiopathic intracranial hypertension and visual function. Br Med Bull. 2006;79-80:233–44.
6. Corbett J, Thompson HS. The rational management of idiopathic intracranial hypertension. Arch Neurol. 1989;46:1049–51.
7. Biousse V, Bruce BB, Newman NJ. Update on the pathophysiology and management of idiopathic intracranial hypertension. J Neurol Neurosurg Psychiatry. 2012;83:488.
8. Soler D, Cox T, Bullock P, et al. Diagnosis and management of benign intracranial hypertension. Arch Dis Child. 1998;78:89–94.
9. Go G. Pseudotumor cerebri: incidence, management and prevention. CNS Drugs. 2000;14:33–49.
10. Dandy WE. Intracranial pressure without brain tumor – diagnosis and treatment. Ann Surg. 1937;106:492–513.
11. Smith JL. Whence pseudotumor cerebri? J Clin Neuroophthalmol. 1985;5:55–6.
12. Mollan SP, Davies B, Silver NC, Shaw S, Mallucci CL, Wakerley BR, et al. Idiopathic intracranial hypertension: consensus guidelines on management. J Neurol Neurosurg Psychiatry. 2018;89:1088–100.
13. Saifudheen K, Gafoor A, Arun G, Abdurahiman P, Jose J. Idiopathic intracranial hypertension presenting as CSF rhinorrhea. Ann Indian Acad Neurol. 2010;13:72–3.
14. Perez MA, Bialer OY, Bruce BB, Newman NJ, Biousse V. Primary spontaneous cerebrospinal fluid leaks and idiopathic intracranial hypertension. J Neuroophthalmol. 2013;33:330–7.
15. Clark D, Bullock P, Hui T, Firth J. Benign intracranial hypertension: a cause of CSF rhinorrhea. J Neurol Neurosurg Psychiatry. 1994;57:847–9.
16. Eggenberger ER, Miller NR, Vitale S. Lumboperitoneal shunt for the treatment of pseudotumor cerebri. Neurology. 1996;46:1524–30.
17. Celebisoy N, Gokcay F, Sirin H, Akyurekli O. Treatment of idiopathic intracranial hypertension: topiramate vs acetazolamide, an open-label study. Acta Neurol Scand. 2007;116:322.
18. Lee AG, Anderson R, Kardon RH, Wall M. Presumed "sulfa allergy" in patients with intracranial hypertension treated with acetazolamide or furosemide: cross-reactivity, myth or reality? Am J Ophthalmol. 2004;138:114.
19. Rasmussen M. Treatment of elevated intracranial pressure with indomethacin: friend or foe? Acta Anaesthesiol Scand. 2005;49:341.
20. Johnston I, Paterson A, Besser M. The treatment of benign intracranial hypertension: a review of 134 cases. Surg Neurol. 1981;16:218–24.
21. De Wecker L. On the incision of the optic nerve in cases of neuroretinitis. Int Ophthalmol Cong Reps. 1872;4:11–4.
22. Banta JT, Farris BK. Pseudotumor cerebri and optic nerve sheath decompression. Ophthalmology. 2000;107:1907–12.
23. Heyman J, Ved R, Amato-Watkins A, Bhatti I, Te Water NJ, Gibbon F, et al. Outcomes of ventriculoperitoneal shunt insertion on the management of idiopathic intracranial hypertension in children. Childs Nerv Syst. 2017;33:1309–15.
24. Yim B, Gooch R, Dalfino JC, Adamo MA, Kenning TJ. Optimizing ventriculoperitoneal shunt placement in the treatment of idiopathic intracranial hypertension: an analysis of neuroendoscopy, frameless stereotaxy and intraoperative CT. Neurosurg Focus. 2016;40:1–8.
25. McGirt MJ, Woodworth G, Thomas G, et al. Cerebrospinal fluid shunt placement for pseudotumor cerebri associated intractable headache: predictors of

treatment response and an analysis of long-term outcomes. J Neurosurg. 2004;101:627.
26. Karsy M, Abou-al-Shaar H, Bowers CA, Schmidt RH. Treatment of idiopathic intracranial hypertension via stereotactic placement of bi-ventriculoperitoneal shunts. J Neurosurg. 2018;130:136–44.
27. Campbell RG, Farquhar D, Zhao N, Chiu AG, Adappa ND, Palmer JN. Cerebrospinal fluid rhinorrhea secondary to idiopathic intracranial hypertension: long term outcomes of endoscopic repairs. Am J Rhinol Allergy. 2016;30:294–300.
28. Teachey W, Grayson J, Cho DY, Riley KO, Woodworth BA. Intervention for elevated intracranial pressure improves success rate after repair of spontaneous cerebrospinal fluid leaks. Laryngoscope. 2017;127:2011–6.
29. Dandapat S, Siddiqui F, Qureshi M, Elias A, Kale S, Qureshi A. Venous sinus stenting for pseudotumor cerebri: a multicenter experience with various stents and deployment techniques. Neurology. 2015;84(14 supplement):120.
30. Puffer RC, Mustafa W, Lanzino G. Venous sinus stenting for idiopathic intracranial hypertension: a review of the literature. J Neurointerv Surg. 2013;5:483.
31. Kanagalingam S, Subramanian PS. Cerebral venous sinus stenting for pseudotumor: a review. Saudi J Ophthalmol. 2015;29:3–8.
32. Binder DK, Lawton MT, McDermott MW. Idiopathic intracranial hypertension. Neurosurgery. 2004;54: 538–51.

35 Olfaction and CSF Leak

Carl Philpott, Naif Alotaibi, and Philippe Rombaux

35.1 Introduction

The olfactory system is considered the most sensitive system for detection and identification of odours. It influences the quality of life and plays an innate role of safety by warning about the dangers of environmental and occupational hazards. It also has a major role in food intake and perception of odours [1–3].

Around 6–10 million bipolar olfactory receptor cells are located at the superior recess of nasal cavity (olfactory cleft) including the middle and the superior turbinate, at the upper nasal septum, and below the cribriform plate [3–5] (Fig. 35.1). The olfactory cells within the pseudostratified columnar epithelium contribute in recovery of the sense of smell after infections or trauma due to their ability of regeneration from the basal and the globose cells [3].

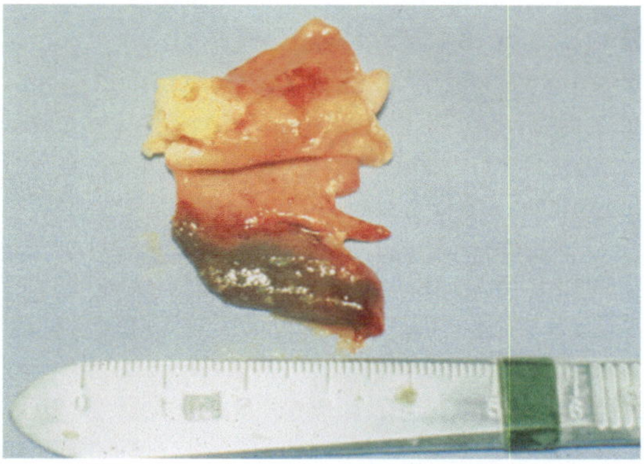

Fig. 35.1 The superior recess of nasal cavity (olfactory cleft) including the middle and the superior turbinate, at the upper nasal septum, and below the cribriform plate, the majority of olfactory epithelium is located in this anatomical area. (Reproduced with permission from: Aaron I. Brescia and Allen M. Seiden (2009) The Anatomy and Physiology of Olfaction and Gustation In Rhinology and Facial Plastic Surgery. F.J. Stucker, C. de Souza, G. S. Kenyon, T. S. Lian, W. Draf, B. Schick (Eds.). Springer)

Normal olfactory function requires a normal nasal physiological environment along with normal anatomical nasal and olfactory groove patency [3]. These factors are affected by common disorders including chronic rhinosinusitis, upper respiratory infections, toxic exposure, head injury, aging, genetic factors, smoking, and drugs [4–6]. These disorders might cause an altered

C. Philpott (✉)
Rhinology & ENT Research Group, University of East Anglia, Norwich, UK

James Paget University Hospital, Great Yarmouth, UK
e-mail: C.Philpott@uea.ac.uk

N. Alotaibi
King Faisal Specialist Hospital & Research Center, Alfaisal University, Riyadh, Kingdom of Saudi Arabia

P. Rombaux
Department of Otorhinolaryngology, Cliniques Universitaires Saint-Luc, Brussels, Belgium

Institute of Neuroscience, Université Catholique de Louvain, Brussels, Belgium

A. A. AlQahtani et al. (eds.), *CSF Rhinorrhea*, https://doi.org/10.1007/978-3-030-94781-1_35

sense of smell, which might be temporary or permanent [6].

Olfaction is considered an important diagnostic and prognostic factor in rhinology and general otolaryngology practice. Disorders related to olfactory system might negatively affect certain professionals such as chefs, firefighters, electricians, military personnel, and nutritionists and might affect their personal safety [7]. A growing amount of evidence suggests that the olfactory disorders manifest as early symptoms (mainly associated with identification and discrimination of odours) and signs of neurodegenerative diseases including the Alzheimer's disease and the Parkinson's disease [4].

Olfactory dysfunction can be classified into quantitative (hyperosmia, hyposmia, and anosmia) or qualitative (parosmia, phantosmia) disorders [8].

Clinicians should evaluate the olfactory abilities with different diagnostic tools available, not limited to the Sniffin' Sticks test (Burghardt®, Wedel, Germany) and The University of Pennsylvania Smell Identification Test [9, 10]. Objective evaluation provides the patients and the clinicians with the ability of baseline assessment to measure the disease progression or the treatment outcomes (medical or surgical or both). It also helps in better documentation for medicolegal purposes and in better standardization of tools for research.

35.1.1 Cerebrospinal Fluid Rhinorrhoea and Olfaction

Cerebrospinal fluid (CSF) rhinorrhea commonly results following head injuries. It may also be iatrogenic, idiopathic, or related to anterior skull base tumours. CSF leak may occur more frequently due to a defect in the meningeal layers or due to destruction at the anterior skull base. The dura at this site is more adherent than at the other parts of the skull base. Due to this anatomical feature, the CSF leak is more frequently associated with this site compared to injuries at other sites such as temporal bone fractures [11].

35.1.2 Head Trauma, CSF, and Olfaction

Olfactory nerve palsy is commonly observed following anterior cranial fossa fractures [12]. The olfactory cleft is located at the roof of the nasal fossa and is attached to anterior cranial fossa (cribriform plate). Altered olfactory function is associated with CSF rhinorrhoea following trauma to the anterior skull base that mainly originated from the ethmoidal areas and the cribriform plate [13]. It can be predicted during the physical examination with signs such as periorbital ecchymosis and telecanthus [13]. CSF leaks following head trauma are encountered in 1–3% of all closed traumatic brain injuries in adult population as a result of different types of trauma that are not limited to falls, assaults, and motor vehicle accidents. On the other hand, 80–90% of all the instances of CSF leaks in adult patients are due to head injuries. The altered olfactory sense might be observed within 48 h after the surgery and manifests in 95% of the patients within the following 3 months [3, 11, 12, 14]. Fractures at the cribriform plate and at the junction of the ethmoidal bones bilaterally, are believed to be the most frequent sites of CSF leak following head trauma. Trauma at these sites along with other factors including arachnoid tearing and dural disruption contribute to CSF leak [11]. Trauma and brain injuries are considered some of the commonest causes of olfactory disorders after upper respiratory tract infections, with an estimated frequency of 5–17%. The variability in frequency among different studies might be influenced by the variety of tools used for diagnosis and evaluation of the olfactory function [13, 15]. Injury to the olfactory nerve is often complicated by CSF leak. Jin et al. [16] reported that 74.2% of the olfactory nerve injuries were associated with the CSF leak. It is important to highlight that while repairing the CSF leak at the olfactory cleft, surgeons have to consider the olfactory function without jeopardizing the treatment outcomes [16]. Patients and /or health care practitioners might miss the signs and symptoms of the olfactory disorders for months after head trauma or brain injuries in contrast to CSF leak which appears earlier, starting at or investigated at 48 h following trauma [7, 12, 13].

Olfactory disorders following head trauma or brain injuries are believed to be elicited by stretching, distortion, or direct injury to the olfactory or the central nervous system [7, 17, 18]. Direct shift of the brain position relative to the skull base (coup-contrecoup injuries) or bony disruption of the cribriform plate and the ethmoidal bones unilaterally or bilaterally [13], might also be among the mechanisms responsible for the olfactory disorders [19]. These pathomechanisms are more frequently associated with motor vehicle accidents. The foramina (filia in cribriform plate) that the olfactory nerves traverse to reach the olfactory bulb are vulnerable to injury in head trauma. Given the fact that this site has adhered meninges, CSF leak might be present in such scenarios of nerve shearing or coup-contrecoup injuries [13].

Skull base defects following trauma are believed to be one of the major factors contributing to the formation of encephaloceles or meningoencephaloceles. Encephaloceles or meningoencephaloceles located in the olfactory clefts might result in the olfactory disorders as well. Shearing of the olfactory nerves or fractures of the cribriform plate with CSF leak may cause bilateral smell disorder. It is less likely in cases of unilateral skull base tumours. The sense of smell on the normal side is less likely to be affected in cases of limited (small size) unilateral tumours and even in case of postsurgical resection according to some reports [20, 21].

It is important to note that the altered sense of smell might be associated with multiple factors prior to or after the incidence of traumas including previous sinonasal or brain pathologies and surgeries, skull base defects, viral infections, chemotherapy, radiation treatment to the head and neck, Alzheimer's disease, and Parkinson's disease [5, 13]. Therefore, detailed history and review of the medical reports are imperative. During acute trauma conditions, the focus of the treatment is on emergencies such as hematoma and severe brain injuries with CSF leak. Understandably, olfactory sensory loss might not be adequately evaluated even after months following the primary acute event. Therefore any objective or subjective olfactory assessment will be useful to determine the baseline olfactory function [13, 20].

35.1.3 Iatrogenic

CSF leak following functional endoscopic sinus surgery (FESS), skull base surgeries, and craniofacial surgeries is a known risk that should be anticipated and discussed with patients. The most common site to be injured during FESS is the lateral cribriform lamella. Although the experience of the surgeons, surgical tools and equipment, and severity of the pathology (Chronic sinusitis, tumour size, and tumour extensions) influence the surgical outcomes, the anatomy of the anterior skull base also plays a major role during FESS. The surgeon dissecting the ethmoidal sinuses is operating above the lower level of the anterior skull base, making it a relatively challenging step during FESS [22].

CSF leak post FESS usually presents as unilateral CSF rhinorrhoea immediately following the surgery, or may be delayed. Various authors have reported that patients had objective anosmia following FESS or septoplasty (anosmia caused by surgery, and not disease-related anosmia). Although the published literature involved case reports, altered sense of olfaction or complete loss of olfaction should not be neglected due to medical and legal aspects [23–25].

35.1.4 Idiopathic Intracranial Hypertension (IIH)

Idiopathic intracranial hypertension (IIH) is a medical condition associated with elevation in CSF pressure with normal brain parenchyma, or obstructive hydrocephalus, and has no known cause. Chronic severe headache and visual impairment (papilloedema) are the main presenting symptoms of IIH [21, 26]. Majority of the patients with IIH are obese (90%) and female (80%) [27–29]. Increasing amount of literature has reported impaired olfactory sense as one of the manifestations of IIH [21]. Dilatation of the arachnoid sheath of the first and second cranial nerve was found to be associated with increased CSF pressure and CSF leak in cases with IIH [30].

Osteo-dural defects at the cribriform plate are believed to be the most common cause of spontaneous CSF rhinorrhoea [31, 32]. These defects create a communication between the subarachnoid space and the sinonasal spaces (the nasal and the paranasal cavities) [31–33].

35.1.5 Tumours

Benign or malignant tumours located at the anterior skull base commonly affect the olfactory sense. Meningiomas affecting the olfactory bulb commonly result in such a comorbidity because of the nature and the evolution of the disease, or as a sequela of surgical treatment or radiotherapy. Esthesioneuroblastoma is a rare neoplasm originating from the olfactory neuroepithelium primarily in the superior nasal cavity. It involves the anterior skull base and grows along the cranial nerves into and out of the skull base [6, 34]. Risk of CSF leak and anosmia (unavoidable) might be significant comorbidities due to the necessity of total tumour resection, which includes the cribriform plate and the olfactory bulb. In certain conditions, unlike the extensive involvement of the anterior cranial fossa, unilaterally located malignant tumours including esthesioneuroblastomas with negative resection margins sparing the contralateral side, might preserve the sense of smell [20, 35].

Olfactory groove meningiomas (OGMs) account for 4–13% of all the intracranial meningiomas. Surgical resection is the primary mode of treatment (endoscopic or transcranial approach). When the surgical resection is not an option, other treatment modalities such as radiotherapy and stereotactic radiosurgery [36–38] are available. Jang et al. [39] found that olfaction was preserved in 55% of the studied patients who underwent resection of OGM; the patients had meningioma less than 4 cm in size and did not complain of olfactory disorder previously. However, the small sample size might decrease the statistical power of this study. High rates of CSF leaks following endoscopic resection of OGM in suboptimal reconstruction are a major concern [40]. CSF leak and anosmia were important sequelae of the surgery. Therefore, controversies regarding surgical approaches for OGM, preservation of olfaction, and CSF leak were reported by different authors. Shetty et al. [38] believed that the endoscopic endonasal approaches usually result in anosmia, and the transcranial approach might have a better chance of preserving the olfactory sense. Smaller benign tumours are less likely to invade the cribriform plate and consequently, less likely to be removed in cases with OGM [41]. Incidence of CSF leak while resecting the benign tumours of the anterior skull base is believed to be higher when compared with the other skull base locations. This outcome may be related to multiple factors including tumours at the posterior wall of the frontal sinus and crista galli that are difficult to repair, the experience of the surgeon, techniques and material for the anterior skull base defect closure, and the learning curves [38].

35.2 Preventative Management

In order to attempt to avoid poor olfactory function after treatment for CSF leaks or skull base surgery, planning of the surgical approach and opportunities to avoid unnecessary injury to the olfactory apparatus are needed. The approach utilized will depend on the experience of the surgical team involved, but increasingly skull base lesions in the anterior cranial fossa will be managed endoscopically. Patients undergoing endoscopic skull base surgery (ESBS) typically have less problems with preexisting inflammatory sinonasal disease and as such with preexisting olfactory loss, although this will of course depend on the site of the lesion. A CSF leak occurring in the olfactory niche has a higher chance of any repair being associated with olfactory dysfunction postoperatively than other locations such as the ethmoid roof (orbital process of the frontal bone). Endoscopic approaches nonetheless typically create far less potential trauma to the olfactory apparatus than open approaches where traction on the frontal lobes can lead to damage of olfactory fila passing through the cribriform plate. Inevitably any surgery involving the olfactory apparatus directly or necessitating resection of the cribriform plate will be associated with a much higher potential for postoperative olfactory dysfunction.

35.2.1 Olfactory Assessment

Ideally, where there is a potential for the surgical intervention to have a deleterious effect on olfaction, patients should undergo preoperative psychophysical testing such as with the Sniffin' Sticks or the UPSIT to provide a baseline performance. This will also help identify patients with preexisting olfactory loss and guide counselling of postoperative outcomes and expectations.

35.2.2 Imaging

Patients undergoing ESBS typically receive both CT and MRI imaging prior to surgery, which will have been utilized to discuss the treatment options for the individual patient and to plan the surgery. Skull base units may also have access to image guidance systems, allowing use of the preoperative imaging during the ESBS. Appropriate use of imaging for careful planning in conjunction with sound anatomical knowledge and surgical finesse can help to anticipate and avoid unnecessary injury to the olfactory apparatus [42, 43]. Of course, this will be dependent on the planned procedure and any potential need to sacrifice parts of the olfactory apparatus in the name of a sound oncological resection. In cases where the pathology is confined unilaterally, preservation of olfactory function may prove more attainable [44], especially with modern endoscopic techniques [45, 46].

35.2.3 Technique and Sequelae

35.2.3.1 Direct Trauma and Reconstruction

Clearly direct injury to the olfactory apparatus will inevitably lead to deleterious outcomes, but the extent of the injury may be crucial. Traditional craniotomy approaches with retraction of the frontal lobes, typically results in tearing of olfactory fibres and anosmia. Endoscopic approaches lend themselves to a more conservative approach and the potential to avoid injury. The use of vascularized flaps have become commonplace in ESBS but the technique in relation to these may be critical for postoperative olfactory function. Griffiths et al. compared the techniques of bilateral nasoseptal rescue flaps with pedicled nasoseptal or middle turbinate flaps [47]. Neither approach favoured better olfactory outcomes with the former being associated with a lower risk of epistaxis. Furthermore, they recommended that superior olfactory strip preservation during elevation of the flaps maintained adequate surgical exposure as well as helping to preserve olfactory function. In contrast, another study demonstrated that there was a significant ***decrease*** in olfactory function of the side of the nasoseptal flap donor in comparison with the opposite side [48] and similarly another study showing decreased olfactory function on the UPSIT test in both comparator groups, showed that the patients who had the nasoseptal flap utilized fared worse [49]. Greig et al. were quite clear to recommend avoidance of nasoseptal flaps for reconstruction due to evidence from their systematic review for adverse olfactory outcomes [50].

In a study looking specifically at pituitary adenomas, this revealed ***worse*** olfactory performance in the group receiving cautery compared to those where cold steel was used [51]. A large case series of 513 patients undergoing ESBS for a variety of reasons including CSF leak repair found that failures were not significantly related to the reconstruction technique ($p = 0.28$) but unfortunately did not consider olfaction within this remit [52]. A series of 113 cases of endoscopic transsphenoid pituitary adenoma resection using a nasoseptal "rescue" flap for reconstruction, reported a 15% incidence of postoperative olfactory dysfunction although no formal assessment of olfaction was undertaken [53]. Matano et al. proposed the fibrin-gelatin fixation method to attempt to avoid the olfactory bulbs peeling away from the cribriform plate during an open anterior interhemispheric approach with 2 of 45 cases (4.4%) reporting permament postoperative anosmia [54].

35.2.3.2 Inflammation and Obstruction

Management of concurrent sinonasal disease and good postoperative care will be crucial to ensuring good olfactory outcomes after surgery. Preexisting sinonasal disease will be evident from the imaging and in cases of skull base tumours, may often represent secondary infection/stagnation of sinuses due to the mass effect of the tumour obstructing drainage pathways. Whilst postoperative debridement has not been shown to achieve more than prevent postoperative adhesions [55], there is a need for higher quality studies to underpin this and in the context of olfactory function, synechiae that obstruct the olfactory clefts may lead to deleterious olfactory function in the postoperative period. Saline irrigations should be recommended in all patients once initial precautions over the repair site have waned and in the presence of inflammatory sinus disease [56, 57]. Where needed for persistent inflammation, intranasal corticosteroids may also be required.

35.2.3.3 Evidence for Prognosis of Postoperative Olfactory Function

Due to limitations in the literature for olfaction and CSF leak repair per se, the evidence considered here includes that for ESBS in general. A recent meta-analysis looked specifically at olfactory outcomes following ESBS and found 29 studies reporting outcomes using one of either UPSIT, CCSIT, Smell Diskettes or Sniffin' Sticks [58]. Overall, the analysis did not demonstrate any evidence that olfactory outcomes are adversely affected in the long-term, however there was high heterogeneity within this demonstrating significant variation amongst the studies analysed. Looking into the details of the individual studies assessed, a large series of 535 patients with a variety of sella/parasellar lesions including pituitary adenomas, showed that after ESBS there was significant impairment of olfaction on two psychophysical tests as well as on visual analogue scores [59]. Whilst the Forest plots of the meta-analysis sit in favour of good overall long-term olfactory outcomes, there are clearly considerations regarding the techniques utilized for the ESBS that should prompt skull base units to ensure auditing of olfactory outcomes, especially in relation to the use of nasoseptal flaps, and allow surgeons to counsel their patients accordingly [60, 61]. One of the limitations of the meta-analysis was also the small sample size of most of the included studies and is a limitation with the wider literature available. In a series of 27 patients with planum sphenoidale meningiomas, 2 reported anosmia at presentation and remained unchanged after surgery [62]. A recent study looking at a cohort of 28 patients with anterior midline skull base meningiomas found that although 26 of the cohort underwent a craniotomy, olfaction was preserved in 87.5%, however there was only a 50% return rate on the postoperative UPSIT scores [63]. Again, a small sample size limits the interpretation of these results. In another recent case series of meningiomas, the risk of postoperative ipsilateral anosmia was significantly increased in olfactory groove meningiomas (odds ratio of 11.1) with a recommendation of ipsilateral olfactory testing to help guide surgical planning [64]. Surgical complications predisposed patients to loss of olfaction on the opposite or both sides. Older patients and those where the meningioma produces a midline shift preoperatively were more likely to have preexisting olfactory dysfunction prior to any surgical intervention.

References

1. Doty RL. Olfactory dysfunction and its measurement in the clinic and workplace. Int Arch Occup Environ Health. 2006;79(4):268–82. Epub Jan 21
2. Papon JF, Coste A. Physiology of the nose. In: Arnold W, Ganzer U, editors. European Manual of Medicine. Otolaryngology &Head and Neck Surgery. New York: Springer- Verlag Berlin Heidelberg; 2010.
3. Coelho DH, Costanzo RM. Posttraumatic olfactory dysfunction. Auris Nasus Larynx. 2016;43:137–43.
4. Doty RL. Olfactory dysfunction in neurodegenerative diseases: is there a common pathological substrate? Lancet Neurol. 2017;16:478–88.
5. O'Brien EK, Leopold DA. Olfaction and gustation: implications of viral, toxic exposure, Head injury, aging, and drugs. In: Stucker FJ, de Souza C, Kenyon GS, Lian TS, Draf W, Schick B, editors. Rhinology and facial plastic surgery. Berlin: Springer; 2009.
6. Abolmaali N, Gudziol V, Hummel T. Pathology of the olfactory nerve. Neuroimaging Clin N Am. 2008;18:233–42.
7. Frasnelli J, Lague-Beauvais M, LeBlanc J, Alturki AY, Champoux MC, Couturier C, et al. Olfactory function in acute traumatic brain injury. Clin Neurol Neurosurg. 2016;140:68–72.
8. Hummel T, Whitcroft KL, Andrews P, et al. Position paper on olfactory dysfunction. Rhinol Suppl. 2017;54:1–30.
9. Doty RL, Shaman P, Dann M. Development of the University of Pennsylvania Smell Identification Test: a standardized microencapsulated test of olfactory function. Physiol Behav. 1984;32(3):489–502.
10. Hummel T, Sekinger B, Wolf SR, Pauli E, Kobal G. 'Sniffin' sticks': olfactory performance assessed by the combined testing of odor identification, odor discrimination and olfactory threshold. Chem Senses. 1997;22(1):39–52.
11. Oh JW, Kim SH, Whang K. Traumatic cerebrospinal fluid leak: diagnosis and management. Korean J Neurotrauma. 2017;13:63–7.
12. Lin DT, Lin AC. Surgical treatment of traumatic injuries of the cranial base. Otolaryngol Clin N Am. 2013;46:749–57.
13. Howell J, Costanzo RM, Reiter ER. Head trauma and olfactory function. World J Otorhinolaryngol Head Neck Surg. 2018;4(1):39–45. . Published 2018 Mar 14. https://doi.org/10.1016/j.wjorl.2018.02.001.
14. Costanzo RM, Becker DP. Smell and taste disorders in head injury and neurosurgery patients. In: Meiselman HL, Rivlin RS, editors. Clinical measurements of taste and smell. New York, NY: MacMillan Publishing Company; 1986. p. 565–78.
15. Schriever VA, Studt F, Smitka M, Grosser K, Hummel T. Olfactory function after mild head injury in children. Chem Senses. 2014;39:343–7.
16. Jin H, Wang S, Hou L, Pan C, Li B, Wang H, et al. Clinical treatment of traumatic brain injury complicated by cranial nerve injury. Injury. 2010;41:918–23.
17. Reiter ER, DiNardo LJ, Costanzo RM. Effects of head injury on olfaction and taste. Otolaryngol Clin N Am. 2004;37:1167–84.
18. Wu AP, Davidson T. Posttraumatic anosmia secondary to central nervous system injury. Am J Rhinol. 2008;22:606–7.
19. Delank KW, Fechner G. Pathophysiology of post-traumatic anosmia. Laryngorhinootologie. 1996;75(3): 154–9.
20. Tajudeen B, Adappa N, Kuan E, et al. Smell preservation following endoscopic unilateral resection of esthesioneuroblastoma: a multi-institutional experience. Int Forum Allergy Rhinol. 2016;6: 1047–50.
21. Julayanont P, Karukote A, Ruthirago D, Panikkath D, Panikkath R. Idiopathic intracranial hypertension: ongoing clinical challenges and future prospects. J Pain Res. 2016;9:87–99.
22. Mantravadi AV, Welch KC. Repair of cerebrospinal fluid leak and encephalocele of the cribriform plate. In: Chiu AG, Palmer JN, editors. Atlas of endoscopic sinus and skull base surgery. Philadelphia: Elsevier Saunders; 2013. p. 241–50.
23. Kimmelman CP. The risk to olfaction from nasal surgery. Laryngoscope. 1994;104:981–8.
24. Stevens CN, Stevens MH. Quantitative effects of nasal surgery on olfaction. Am J Otolaryngol. 1985;6: 264–7.
25. Fiser A. Changes of olfaction due to aesthetic and functional nose surgery. Acta Otorhinolaryngol Belg. 1990;44:457–60.
26. Schmidt C, Wiener E, Hoffmann J, et al. Structural olfactory nerve changes in patients suffering from idiopathic intracranial hypertension. PLoS One. 2012;7(4):e35221.
27. Wall M. Idiopathic intracranial hypertension (pseudotumor cerebri). Curr Neurol Neurosci Rep. 2008;8:87–93.
28. Jindal M, Hiam L, Raman A, Rejali D. Idiopathic intracranial hypertension in otolaryngology. Eur Arch Otorhinolaryngol. 2009;266:803–6.
29. Stevens S, Rizk H, Golnik K, Andaluz N, Samy R, Meyer T, et al. Idiopathic intracranial hypertension: contemporary review and implications for the otolaryngologist. Laryngoscope. 2017;128:248–56.
30. Hansen HC, Helmke K. Validation of the optic nerve sheath response to changing cerebrospinal fluid pressure: ultrasound findings during intrathecal infusion tests. J Neurosurg. 1997;87(1):34–40.
31. Shetty PG, Shroff MM, Sahani DV, Kirtane MV. Evaluation of high-resolution CT and MR cisternography in the diagnosis of cerebrospinal fluid fistula. AJNR Am J Neuroradiol. 1998;19(4):633–639 5.
32. Schuknecht B, Simmen D, Briner HR, Holzmann D. Nontraumatic skull base defects with spontaneous CSF rhinorrhea and arachnoid herniation: imaging findings and correlation with endoscopic sinus surgery in 27 patients. AJNR Am J Neuroradiol. 2008;29(3):542–9.

33. Gharzouli I, Verillaud B, Tran H, Blancal JP, Sauvaget E, Kania R, Guichard JP, Herman P. Value of systematic analysis of the olfactory cleft in case of cerebrospinal rhinorrhea: incidence of olfactory arachnoid dilatation. Eur Arch Otorhinolaryngol. 2015:18.
34. Dulguerov P, Allal AS, Calcaterra TC. Esthesioneuroblastoma: a meta-analysis and review. Lancet Oncol. 2001;2(11):683–90.
35. Gardner P, Snyderman C. In: Mayers EN, editor. Endonasal Transcribriform approach to the anterior cranial fossa. In master techniques in otolaryngology - Head and neck surgery: Skull Base surgery. Philadelphia. USA: Wolters Kluwer; 2014. p. 130–24.
36. Adappa ND, Lee JYK, Chiu AG, Palmer JN. Olfactory groove meningioma. Otolaryngol Clin N Am. 2011;44(4):965–980 ix 2.
37. Aguiar PHP, Tahara A, Almeida AN, Simm R, Silva MMVC, Panagopoulos AT, Zicarelli CA, Silva PG. Olfactory groove meningiomas: approaches and complications. J Clin Neurosci. 2009;16(9):1168–73.
38. Shetty SR, Ruiz-Treviño AS, Omay SB, Almeida JP, Liang B, Chen YN, et al. Limitations of the endonasal endoscopic approach in treating olfactory groove meningiomas. A systematic review. Acta Neurochir. 2017;159(10):1875–85.
39. Jang W-Y, Jung S, Jung T-Y, Moon K-S, Kim I-Y. Preservation of olfaction in surgery of olfactory groove meningiomas. Clin Neurol Neurosurg. 2013;115(8):1288–92.
40. Banu MA, Mehta A, Ottenhausen M, Fraser JF, Patel KS, Szentirmai O, Anand VK, Tsiouris AJ, Schwartz TH. Endoscope-assisted endonasal versus supraorbital keyhole resection of olfactory groove meningiomas: comparison and combination of 2 minimally invasive approaches. J Neurosurg. 2016;124(3):605–20.
41. Koutourousiou M, Fernandez-Miranda JC, Wang EW, Snyderman CH, Gardner PA. Endoscopic endonasal surgery for olfactory groove meningiomas: outcomes and limitations in 50 patients. Neurosurg Focus. 2014;37:E8.
42. Thompson CF, Kern RC, Conley DB. Olfaction in endoscopic sinus and Skull Base surgery. Otolaryngol Clin N Am. 2015;48(5):795–804. https://doi.org/10.1016/j.otc.2015.05.007.
43. Knopp U, Sepehrnia A. Preservation of olfaction in bifrontal craniotomies for lesions of the anterior and middle cranial fossa. Laryngorhinootologie. 2005;84(5):319–22. https://doi.org/10.1055/s-2004-826074.
44. Browne JD, Mims JW. Preservation of olfaction in anterior skull base surgery. Laryngoscope. 2000;110(8):1317–22. https://doi.org/10.1097/00005537-200008000-00017.
45. Youssef AS, Sampath R, Freeman JL, et al. Unilateral endonasal transcribriform approach with septal transposition for olfactory groove meningioma: can olfaction be preserved? Acta Neurochir. 2016;158(10):1965–72. https://doi.org/10.1007/s00701-016-2922-1.
46. Hayhurst C, Sughrue ME, Gore PA, et al. Results with expanded Endonasal resection of Skull Base Meningiomas technical nuances and approach selection based on an early experience. Turk Neurosurg. 2016;26(5):662–70. https://doi.org/10.5137/1019-5149.JTN.16105-15.3.
47. Griffiths CF, Barkhoudarian G, Cutler A, et al. Analysis of olfaction after bilateral Nasoseptal rescue flap Transsphenoidal approach with olfactory mucosal preservation. Otolaryngol Head Neck Surg. 2019;161(5):881–9. https://doi.org/10.1177/0194599819861340.
48. Soyka MB, Serra C, Regli L, et al. Long-term olfactory outcome after nasoseptal flap reconstructions in midline skull base surgery. Am J Rhinol Allergy. 2017;31(5):334–7. https://doi.org/10.2500/ajra.2017.31.4463.
49. Tam S, Duggal N, Rotenberg BW. Olfactory outcomes following endoscopic pituitary surgery with or without septal flap reconstruction: a randomized controlled trial. Int Forum Allergy Rhinol. 2013;3(1):62–5. https://doi.org/10.1002/alr.21069.
50. Greig SR, Cooper TJ, Sommer DD, et al. Objective sinonasal functional outcomes in endoscopic anterior skull-base surgery: an evidence-based review with recommendations. Int Forum Allergy Rhinol. 2016;6(10):1040–6. https://doi.org/10.1002/alr.21760.
51. Hong SD, Nam DH, Park J, et al. Olfactory outcomes after endoscopic pituitary surgery with nasoseptal "rescue" flaps: electrocautery versus cold knife. Am J Rhinol Allergy. 2014;28(6):517–9. https://doi.org/10.2500/ajra.2014.28.4109.
52. Turri-Zanoni M, Zocchi J, Lambertoni A, et al. Endoscopic Endonasal reconstruction of anterior Skull Base defects: what factors really affect the outcomes? World Neurosurg. 2018;116:e436–e43. https://doi.org/10.1016/j.wneu.2018.04.225.
53. Zhang C, Yang N, Mu L, et al. The application of nasoseptal "rescue" flap technique in endoscopic transsphenoidal pituitary adenoma resection. Neurosurg Rev. 2018; https://doi.org/10.1007/s10143-018-1048-8.
54. Matano F, Murai Y, Mizunari T, et al. Olfactory preservation during anterior interhemispheric approach for anterior skull base lesions: technical note. Neurosurg Rev. 2016;39(1):63–8.; ; discussion 69. https://doi.org/10.1007/s10143-015-0647-x.
55. Tzelnick S, Alkan U, Leshno M, et al. Sinonasal debridement versus no debridement for the postoperative care of patients undergoing endoscopic sinus surgery. Cochrane Database Syst Rev. 2018;11:CD011988. https://doi.org/10.1002/14651858.CD011988.pub2.
56. Chen XZ, Feng SY, Chang LH, et al. The effects of nasal irrigation with various solutions after endoscopic sinus surgery: systematic review and meta-analysis. J Laryngol Otol. 2018;132(8):673–9. https://doi.org/10.1017/S0022215118000919.
57. Chong LY, Head K, Hopkins C, et al. Saline irrigation for chronic rhinosinusitis (Review). Cochrane Database Syst Rev. 2016;4:CD011995. https://doi.org/10.1002/14651858.CD011995.pub2.
58. Yin LX, Low CM, Puccinelli CL, et al. Olfactory outcomes after endoscopic skull base surgery: a sys-

tematic review and meta-analysis. Laryngoscope. 2019;129(9):1998–2007. https://doi.org/10.1002/lary.28003.
59. Kim DH, Hong YK, Jeun SS, et al. Endoscopic Endonasal Transsphenoidal approach from the surgeon point of view. J Craniofac Surg. 2017;28(4):959–62. https://doi.org/10.1097/SCS.0000000000003423.
60. Patel ZM, DelGaudio JM. Olfaction following endoscopic skull base surgery. Curr Opin Otolaryngol Head Neck Surg. 2016;24(1):70–4. https://doi.org/10.1097/MOO.0000000000000216.
61. Alobid I, Ensenat J, Marino-Sanchez F, et al. Impairment of olfaction and mucociliary clearance after expanded endonasal approach using vascularized septal flap reconstruction for skull base tumors. Neurosurgery. 2013;72(4):540–6. https://doi.org/10.1227/NEU.0b013e318282a535.
62. Mortazavi MM, Brito da Silva H, Ferreira M Jr, et al. Planum sphenoidale and tuberculum Sellae Meningiomas: operative nuances of a modern surgical technique with outcome and proposal of a new classification system. World Neurosurg. 2016;86:270–86. https://doi.org/10.1016/j.wneu.2015.09.043.
63. Ung TH, Yang A, Aref M, et al. Preservation of olfaction in anterior midline skull base meningiomas: a comprehensive approach. Acta Neurochir. 2019;161(4):729–35. https://doi.org/10.1007/s00701-019-03821-8.
64. Hendrix P, Fischer G, Linnebach AC, et al. Perioperative olfactory dysfunction in patients with meningiomas of the anteromedial skull base. Clin Anat. 2019;32(4):524–33. https://doi.org/10.1002/ca.23346.

Part VI

CSF Rhinorrhea and Infection

36

Oweida F. Aldosary, M. Rizwan Sohail,
and Imad M. Tleyjeh

36.1 Introduction

Cerebrospinal fluid (CSF) rhinorrhea is a symptom caused by the leakage of CSF into the nasal sinus, resulting from a defect in the skull base [1].

Since its first description by Galen in 200 BC [2] and Bidloo the elder in the seventeenth century [3], CSF rhinorrhea has been a well-known entity, occurring spontaneously [4–6] or resulting from congenital malformations, postinfectious hydrocephalus, and skull base erosion from intracranial tumors [7–10].

O. F. Aldosary
Department of Medicine, Infectious Diseases Section, King Fahad Medical City, PO, Riyadh, Saudi Arabia

M. R. Sohail
Division of Infectious Diseases, Mayo Clinic College of Medicine and Science, Rochester, MN, USA

Department of Cardiovascular Diseases, Mayo Clinic College of Medicine and Science, Rochester, MN, USA

I. M. Tleyjeh (✉)
Department of Medicine, Infectious Diseases Section, King Fahad Medical City, PO, Riyadh, Saudi Arabia

Division of Infectious Diseases, Mayo Clinic College of Medicine and Science, Rochester, MN, USA

Department of Epidemiology, Mayo Clinic, Rochester, MN, USA

College of Medicine, AlFaisal University, Riyadh, Saudi Arabia
e-mail: itleyjeh@kfmc.med.sa

CSF rhinorrhea is a major complication following traumatic head injuries associated with basilar skull fractures and skull base surgeries with an estimated incidence of 10–30% and 2–64% from nonpenetrating head trauma [11, 12] and after endonasal skull base surgery [13–20], respectively, despite recent advances in skull base surgery and the introduction of functional endoscopic sinus surgery (FESS) [1].

CSF leakage has been associated with serious, and potentially fatal, infectious sequelae such as meningitis, ventriculitis, and intracranial abscess formation. These complications may increase the duration of hospital stay, readmission rate, and mortality risk [21]. The risk of intracranial infection developing in the setting of CSF leakage, regardless of the etiology, is very concerning and has drawn the attention of surgeons for many years [22].

Majority of post-traumatic CSF leaks resolve spontaneously within 24–48 h after their onset without complications [23, 24]. However, some persist and may lead to an increased risk of life-threatening intracranial infections particularly meningitis (7–30%) [12, 25–27].

Surprisingly, the presentation and risk of meningitis after posttraumatic CSF leakage could be delayed for years and develop after a minor trauma while the leak might not be apparent or may be occurring intermittently [28–34].

A. A. AlQahtani et al. (eds.), *CSF Rhinorrhea*, https://doi.org/10.1007/978-3-030-94781-1_36

36.2 Pathophysiology

CSF is a physiologic fluid that is a major component of the central nervous system (CNS) and serves as a shock absorber to protect the brain, cerebellum, and meninx. It also helps to maintain the intracranial pressure (ICP). Approximately, 70% CSF is produced at the choroid plexus located at the lateral, third, and fourth ventricles. Another 18% is produced by capillary ultrafiltrate, whereas 12% is produced by the metabolism of water. An average volume of 140 mL (range 90–150 mL) actively circulates and turns over daily [35–37].

The blood–brain barrier separates the CNS, including the CSF, from the circulation and is an important defense mechanism against bacteria invading the CNS. It also maintains a stable environment inside the nervous system and potentiates molecular transport between blood and brain.

Disruption of this barrier can occur following trauma, surgery, congenital defects, or ear and sinus infections [23, 25]. Clinically such disruption manifests as CSF rhinorrhea which occurs as a result of an abnormal communication between the subarachnoid space and a pneumatized area in the skull base that includes the sinonasal tract. This communication or fistula must involve a breach of the arachnoid and dura matter, the bone of skull base, and the underlying mucosa [38]. CSF fluid fistulas occurring from various causes can render the individual vulnerable to invasion of the intradural space by microorganisms inhabiting the nasopharyngeal spaces especially when they persist [23].

36.3 Risk Factors

Studies evaluating risk factors implicated in the development of infectious complications in various etiologic causes of CSF leaks particularly in traumatic and nontraumatic head injuries are limited. Nonetheless, there are few studies in the literature which assessed some risk factors after certain kinds of otorhinologic procedures and trauma.

36.3.1 CSF Leakage

The mere presence of CSF leakage is known to carry a high risk of developing CNS infections [24, 39–42]. It is also a potential risk factor for once or recurrent bacterial meningitis in both community-acquired and nosocomial settings [43–46]. Despite lower estimated incidence of meningitis (1.8%) in a large study by Kono et al. [47], there was a significant association between the development of meningitis in patients who experienced postoperative CSF leak (9.3%).

36.3.2 Duration of the CSF Leakage

Risk of meningitis increases with the duration of CSF leakage [23]. Recent data suggest that risk is greatest during the first week (9.1%) after the head trauma and may continue to increase at around 8% per month for the first 6 months and about 8–9.8% per year thereafter [48, 49]. However, this is contrary to an old study showing an increased risk of about 11% within the first week and 88% risk when CSF rhinorrhea persisted longer than 7 days [33]. Besides the high chance of recurrence, there can be several years of delay between trauma and development of bacterial meningitis [39, 50, 51].

36.3.3 Gender, Type of Surgery, Complex Tumors, Presence of an External Ventricular Drain or Shunt

In the study by Kono et al. [47], male sex, history of surgery (craniotomy or endonasal surgery), long duration of surgery (×4 h), procedures with a higher level of complexity (level IV or V), lumbar drain placement immediately after surgery, the presence of an external ventricular device (EVD) or ventriculoperitoneal (VP) shunt at the time of surgery, and their placement after surgery were risk factors for infection in the univariable analysis and in the multivariable analysis [47]. On the contrary, in one analysis, the routine insertion of an external lumbar drain (ELD) in patients in whom intraoperative CSF leakage was observed led to significantly reduced incidence of postoperative meningitis [52].

36.3.4 Lumbar Drain Duration

A recent study by Ivan et al. [16] found a statistically significant difference in the duration of lumbar drain present in patients who developed meningitis associated with a postoperative CSF leak compared to those who did not develop infection (8.0 days versus 5.7 days, $p = 0.04$). However, the authors concluded that the increased risk of infection can be either associated with the lumbar drain itself or perhaps the increased exposure of CSF leakage postoperatively [16].

36.3.5 Reoperation

In a large 5-year retrospective review of the 916 patients undergoing transsphenoidal surgery, an increased incidence of CSF leak and meningitis was observed in patients who had repeat surgery. The authors postulated that this increased risk likely reflects increasing difficulty in obtaining a successful resection while preserving the diaphragm sellae, which separates CSF from the resection cavity throughout the immediate postoperative period [53].

36.3.6 Increased BMI

Obesity has been implicated as a major contributor of morbidity and mortality in various medical and surgical conditions. Spontaneous and iatrogenic CSF leaks are no exceptions. Although many studies have clearly shown that increasing BMI ($\geq$30) is associated with an increased risk of CSF leakage [16, 54, 55], a multivariate analysis in one study found an increased BMI to be independently associated with both CSF leak and postoperative meningitis [16].

36.3.7 Pneumocephalus and Diaphragmatic Defects

Pneumocephalus after endoscopic endonasal transsphenoidal surgery is not uncommon finding, and its presence indicates there are clear links between the cranial cavity and the external environment, as do the postoperative CSF leaks. Pneumocephalus (maximum bubble diameter of $\geq$1 cm) and diaphragmatic defects (an intraoperative CSF leak, Kelly grade $\geq$1) are risk factors for a postoperative intracranial infection [41].

36.4 Epidemiology and Incidence of Infection in CSF Rhinorrhea

Since Cairns, a British neurosurgeon, first proposed it in 1937, many classifications of CSF rhinorrhea have been published and are based on the timing and the etiologic causes [56–58]. However, the current classification of CSF rhinorrhea has the same scheme [59] without assessing the risk for infection due to the different causes of CSF rhinorrhea. Identifying the types of skull fractures that would suggest an increased risk for persistent CSF leaks and/or meningitis and those refractory to conservative management is crucial in determining appropriate management [59].

36.4.1 Incidence of Infection in Spontaneous CSF Rhinorrhea

Several studies have evaluated the incidence and risk for developing bacterial meningitis following spontaneous CSF leaks. Daudia et al. found an overall risk of 10%. Regardless of spontaneous resolution of CSF rhinorrhea, the risk of meningitis remains, and most commonly occurs within the first year of the CSF leak [60]. Eljamel et al. [61] found that the risk of meningitis in nontraumatic CSF leakage was 26% prior to attempted repair. Other studies suggested that regardless of the location, spontaneous CSF fistulas increase the risk for meningitis, though encephalitis and parenchymal abscess were reported with much lesser frequency [62–64].

36.4.2 Incidence and Type of Infection in Posttraumatic CSF Rhinorrhea

36.4.2.1 Accidental Trauma

Meningitis

Previous studies have reported a high overall risk of meningitis in patients with CSF rhinorrhea occurring after accidental trauma and in patients whose CSF leak does not close spontaneously. In 1966 Mincy et al. [33] published a series of 54 patients with posttraumatic CSF rhinorrhea and found an 11% risk of meningitis among patients in whom CSF leak stopped spontaneously in 7 days, compared with 88% among patients in whom drainage lasted longer than 7 days [65]. Similarly, Eljamel and Foy [48] in their study reported an overall 30.6% risk of meningitis before surgical repair and a risk of 1.3% per day in the first 2 weeks after injury, 7.4% per week in the first month after injury, and a cumulative risk of 85% at the 10-year follow-up. More recently, Daudia et al. reported an overall risk of meningitis of 32% in the same category of patients, regardless of spontaneous resolution of CSF rhinorrhea and observed that the risk of meningitis remains and most commonly occurs within the first year of the CSF leak [60]. Furthermore, Horst showed in her study an increased incidence of community-acquired meningitis of 37% that was due to a previously identified CSF leak [66].

Recurrent Meningitis

Recurrent meningitis is defined as two separate episodes of meningitis that are separated by a period of convalescence and full recovery [23]. This definition seems to be widely accepted. The persistence of CSF fistulae in patients with head trauma is the commonest cause of recurrent meningitis in adults [67]. The risk of recurrent meningitis after posttraumatic CSF leakage has been reported to range from 12.5% to 50%, with a 29.4% neurological complication rate [68, 69]. In a recent retrospective study, the rate of recurrent meningitis was found to be high (8.5%) in patients with previous head trauma, although there was no clear documentation of CSF rhinorrhea [70]. Horst showed in her study an incidence of recurrent community-acquired meningitis of (53%) and observed that recurrence occurred despite previous surgery aimed at closing the leak [66].

Finally, a nationwide observational cohort study in the Netherlands estimated incidence of meningitis of 53% and 32% among patients with community acquired pneumonia who have remote head injury and CSF leakage, respectively.

Penetrating Injury

CSF leakage is a common complication of penetrating head injuries. Aarabi [71] and Meirowsky et al. [72] reported that at the time of penetrating injury, CSF leakage occurred at a frequency of 8.7% and 8.9%, respectively, and infectious complication happened at an increased rate of 36% and 49.5%, respectively.

Iatrogenic Trauma

There have been several advances in image-guided technology, surgical instrumentation, and skull base reconstructive techniques over the past decade, and endoscopic endonasal skull base surgery has emerged as an alternative approach for the treatment of many skull base lesions [15]. However, iatrogenic CSF rhinorrhea remains a potential complication with significant morbidity and mortality regardless of the type of the surgery [73].

The rate of postoperative intracranial infection is variable and reported incidence of CSF rhinorrhea and intracranial infection rates range from 0% to 36.5% [16, 47, 52, 60, 74–80] (see Table 36.1). Development of intracranial infection in this setting can be fatal [81].

Table 36.1 Summary of studies reporting percentages of CNS infections in patients with CSF leakage

Study	Risk of CNS infection in patient with leakage (%)
Ivan [16] 2015	10
Kono [47] 2014	9.3
Kryzanski [80] 2008	2
Daudia [60] 2007	22
Dumont [74] 2005	1.5
Bernal-Sprekelsen [79] 2005	36.5
van Aken [75] 1997	3.1
Black [76] 1987	0.4
Kennedy [78] 1984	1.75
Ciric [77] 1983	0.8

36.4.2.2 Types of Surgery

Endonasal Transsphenoidal Surgery

According to one estimate, the incidence of meningitis was 36.5% in patients with CSF leak or skull base defect of various origins [79]. In another retrospective analysis of 149 patients who underwent endoscopic CSF rhinorrhea repair, three patients developed frontal brain abscesses giving an incidence of 2.0%. Most abscesses formed within 10 days after surgery [82].

Endonasal Transsphenoidal Surgery vs Sublabial Transsphenoidal Surgery

Meningitis occurs in 3% or less of patients undergoing transsphenoidal surgery [83, 84]. In a meta-analysis of studies comparing endoscopic versus sublabial pituitary surgery, the authors found that the incidences of meningitis in both approaches remained the same (1% vs 1%), despite that the proportion of patients who had a CSF leak was significantly lower in those who had endoscopic surgery (5% vs 7%) [13].

Endoscopic Endonasal (EE) Versus Microscopic Transsphenoidal (MT) Versus Open Transcranial (OT) Resection of Craniopharyngiomas

In a systemic review, CSF leak and meningitis were among the postoperative complications in all the three approaches for resection of craniopharyngiomas with incidences of 2.6% and 2.3% in the OT cohort, 9.0% and 1.8% in the TM cohort, and 18.4% and 5.1% in the EE cohort, respectively [85].

36.5 Microbiology

Bacterial meningitis in patients with CSF leakage can be classified as community-acquired, in case of anatomic defects or contiguous spread of infection, or nosocomial or healthcare-associated meningitis, after surgery or trauma [16, 86–89].

36.5.1 Community-Acquired Pathogens

Organisms associated with single or recurrent community-acquired meningitis secondary to CSF leaks are those commonly found in the upper respiratory tract. Most cases are caused by *S. pneumoniae* followed by *H. influenzae*, *Neisseria meningitidis*, and *S. aureus* [44, 48, 66, 90, 91]. It is reported that *Streptococcus pneumoniae* accounts for 80% of CNS infections associated with bony anatomical defects in the skull [67]. Previous studies have also suggested to consider a disruption of the blood–brain barrier when *S. pneumoniae* is cultured from CSF [25, 44].

36.5.2 Nosocomial-Acquired Pathogens

Specific bacterial pathogens causing meningitis in nosocomial setting may vary according to the timing and pathogenesis of the infection and the mechanism of head injury [39, 92–97]. The majority of bacterial meningitis cases that occur after skull base fracture or early after otorhinologic surgery are caused by organisms that colonize the nasopharynx (especially S. pneumoniae) while Staphylococcal species and facultative and/or aerobic gram-negative bacilli are

Table 36.2 Cerebrospinal fluid culture results according to underlying conditions in adults with nosocomial bacterial meningitis

Cerebrospinal fluid culture results	All episodes ($N = 50$)	History of neurosurgery ($N = 32$)	Distant focus of infection ($N = 9$)	Immunocompromised state[a] ($N = 14$)
Streptococcus pneumoniae	13 (26)	4 (13)	6 (67)	4 (29)
Staphylococcus aureus	12 (24)	10 (31)	2 (22)	2 (14)
Haemophilus influenzae	4 (8)	3 (9)	1 (11)	1 (7)
Staphylococcus epidermidis	3 (6)	2 (6)	0	0
Escherichia coli	3 (6)	2 (6)	0	0
Klebsiella pneumoniae	2 (4)	2 (6)	0	1 (7)
Pseudomonas aeruginosa	2 (4)	2 (6)	0	2 (14)
Other bacterial pathogens[b]	11 (22)	7 (22)	0	4 (29)

Data are number (%). Numbers do not add up to a total of 50 episodes due to the presence of multiple comorbid conditions in several patients

Reproduced with permission from: Weisfelt M, van de Beek D, Spanjaard L, de Gans J. Nosocomial bacterial meningitis in adults: a prospective series of 50 cases. J Hosp Infect. 2007 May;66(1):71–8

[a] Defined as the use of immunosuppressive drugs, a history of splenectomy, the presence of diabetes mellitus, alcoholism, or infection with the human immunodeficiency virus

[b] α-Hemolytic streptococci in four; group B streptococcus, *Neisseria meningitidis, "streptococcus," Listeria monocytogenes, Bacillus* species, *Enterococcus faecalis,* and "not viable" each in one

among the common bacterial pathogens causing nosocomial meningitis in patients who undergo neurosurgical procedures or have prolonged hospital stay following penetrating head trauma or fractures involving the skull base [87].

M. Weisfelt et al., in their prospective series of 50 patients with nosocomial meningitis following neurosurgery, CSF leakage, or recent head trauma, reported the following distribution of causative organisms: *S. aureus* in 11 of 40 episodes (28%), *S. pneumoniae* in nine episodes (23%), *H. influenzae* in four episodes (10%), *S. epidermidis* in three episodes (8%), and other bacterial pathogens in 13 episodes (33%) [96] (see Table 36.2).

36.6 Diagnosis of CNS Infections in Patient with CSF Leakage

CNS infections following CSF leakage, including meningitis, encephalitis, and brain abscess, are rare but time-sensitive diagnoses. These infections can develop in both community-acquired and nosocomial settings [43, 44].

The diagnosis of CNS infections requires vigilance and a high index of suspicion based on the history and physical examination which must be confirmed with appropriate imaging and laboratory evaluation [98].

The acuteness, type, and severity of the iatrogenic or noniatrogenic trauma-associated CSF rhinorrhea is an essential element to assess when patient is presenting with an intracranial infectious complication.

36.6.1 Clinical Presentation

Before the infection ensues and depending on the acuteness and etiology of the event leading to the CSF leakage and the mental status of the patients, the symptoms may vary. In majority of patients, the only presenting symptom may be salty or even sweet taste in the retropharyngeal space [65, 99]. However, CSF rhinorrhea might be unnoticeable in some patients. Patients may present with other symptoms suggestive of acute craniofacial trauma including epistaxis, nasal discharge, anosmia, peri-orbital ecchymosis, chemosis, oculomotor impairment, open-head injury or surgery, loss of vision, cranial nerve or motor deficits. However, in the chronic phase, patients may present with intermittent nasal discharge, headaches, salty or sweet taste in the retropharyngeal space [59].

When CNS infection occurs, it can manifest with a host of nonspecific signs and symptoms, including headache, fever, altered mental status, and behavioral changes [98]. The classic triad of fever, neck stiffness, and altered mental status may occur in only a third (32%) of the patients, and the duration of symptoms may be shorter than 24 h in patient with CSF leakage complicated by community-acquired meningitis [66].

While patients are being hospitalized for recent trauma or in the setting of neurosurgical procedures, the development of new headache, fever, evidence of meningeal irritation, seizures, and/or worsening mental status may suggest nosocomial meningitis [100].

Immunologically competent individuals presenting with recurrent meningitis should prompt further assessment to rule out the presence of CSF fistula [51] owing to their close association [69].

Development of a single episode or recurrent episodes of meningitis associated with CSF leakage in patients with remote history of accidental head trauma, basilar skull fractures, and or surgery has been reported in the literatures occurring few months to several years after injury [69, 101–104].

36.6.2 Physical Examination

CSF rhinorrhea is usually detected by nasal endoscopy and/or endonasal examination [1]. β2-Transferrin provides an accurate, noninvasive method to establish the diagnosis of an active CSF leak with great sensitivity and specificity but does not provide information on the location of the leak [105].

Classically, Battle's sign (ecchymosis over the mastoid process) and periorbital ecchymosis have been associated with skull base fractures. Battle's sign and unilateral blepharohematoma have positive predictive values (PPVs) for skull base fractures of 100% and 90%, respectively [106].

Classic physical examination maneuvers in patient with meningitis, such as Kernig's and Brudzinski's signs, are relatively insensitive although specific for predicting CNS infection.

Patients with parenchymal involvement, as occurs with encephalitis and brain abscess, may also have focal neurologic deficits or seizures [98].

36.6.3 Laboratory

36.6.3.1 Routine Laboratory

Initial laboratory workup should include complete blood counts, coagulation profile, and renal function tests to exclude contraindication to lumbar puncture and to help with antimicrobial dosing. Blood culture should also be obtained prior to antibiotic administration.

36.6.3.2 Lumbar Puncture and CSF Analysis

If no contradictions, lumbar puncture should be performed in all cases of suspected intracranial infections [86]. CSF should be submitted for battery of tests including CSF leukocyte count with differential, glucose and protein concentration, bacterial cultures, and other special tests. Occasionally, CSF analysis can appear benign early in the course of meningitis and encephalitis, and the clinicians should not be falsely reassured if clinical suspicion is strong [98]. Repeat testing 24–48 h later may be necessary in these cases if symptoms persist or worsen.

36.6.3.3 Specific CSF Diagnostic Tests

CSF Color

The CSF fluid may appear cloudy; however, this color change depends largely on the degree and the concentrations of white blood cells (WBCs), red blood cells (RBCs), bacteria, and/or protein levels in the CSF sample [88].

WBC Count

Elevated CSF WBC count in untreated bacterial meningitis is usually seen in the range of 1000–5000 cells/mm^3. However, WBC counts of <100 or >110,000 cells/mm^3 can also be seen. CSF neutrophils are typically observed between 80% and 95% in most of the bacterial meningitis cases; however, in 10% of patients presenting with acute bacterial meningitis, a lymphocyte rather than neutrophile predominance (defined as >50% of lymphocytes or monocytes) might occur [88].

CSF Glucose Concentration

Hypoglycorrhachia defined as CSF glucose concentration below 40 mg/dL is seen in the setting of untreated bacterial meningitis in approximately half to two-third of patients [88].

CSF Protein Concentration

Most patients with bacterial meningitis have some degree of elevated CSF protein levels [88].

CSF Cultures

While 70-85% of CSF cultures in patients who have not yet received any empirical antibiotics can turn positive, however, results may take up to 48 h for microorganism identification and subsequent susceptibility testing. Therefore, utilization of other nonculture rapid diagnostic tests is encouraged to help with the identification of the culprit bacterial pathogen (see below) [88].

36.6.3.4 Gram Stain

Routine Gram staining of CSF sample is inexpensive, and rapid test that shows an accuracy of 60–90% and specificity of more than 97% in identifying the causative bacterial pathogen in patients with suspected bacterial meningitis; therefore, it is strongly recommended in all patients with suspected bacterial meningitis [107]. While, the use of cytospin techniques can increase the probability of microscopic detection of bacteria on a Gram stain up to 100-fold [108]; however, prior antimicrobial therapy may lower the yield of CSF Gram stain by around 20%. Factors contributing to false-positive CSF Gram stain results include observer misinterpretation, reagent contamination, or contamination of the needle during lumbar puncture by the skin flora [109, 110].

Latex Agglutination

Latex agglutination test is simple and rapid with short turnaround time (results are usually available in less than 15 min). It has shown good sensitivity in detecting antigens of common bacterial pathogens causing meningitis [111]. However, it is important to know that a negative latex agglutination test does not necessarily rule out bacterial meningitis. The test may be most useful for the patient who receive antimicrobial therapy prior to lumbar puncture and whose Gram stain and CSF culture results are negative.

PCR

Although, several broad-range PCR kits have a great sensitivity (100%) and specificity (98.2%) with a positive predictive value reaching up to 98.2% and an excellent negative predictive value of 100% [112]; however, these tests are not readily available in all hospitals. This technique may be useful to rule out the diagnosis of bacterial meningitis, subsequently aiding to stop the empiric antimicrobial therapy.

36.6.4 Imaging Studies

Modern cranial imaging techniques such as CT scan and MRI 3D-CISS can effectively be used to localize the anatomical location of the CSF leakage [113, 114]. Advances in CT and MR imaging techniques have improved sensitivity, which amounted to 88.25% [115] and 93% [116] for high-resolution CT and for MR cisternography to 89% [116, 117], 93.6% [118], and 100% [119, 120] even in patients with inactive leaks.

Neuroimaging is also useful in revealing expanding masses (i.e., brain abscess, subdural empyema, or hydrocephalus) and midline shift, which should be identified before lumbar puncture [87]. CNS imaging is also recommended in specific group of patients owing to their high risk of brain herniation after lumbar puncture (see Table 36.3) [88].

Table 36.3 Recommended criteria for doing CT scan brain before lumbar puncture for adults with suspected bacterial meningitis

Criterion	Comment
• Immunocompromised state	• HIV infection or AIDS, receiving immunosuppressive therapy, or after transplantation
• History of CNS disease	• Mass lesion, stroke, or focal infection
• New onset seizure	• Within 1 week of presentation; some authorities would not perform a lumbar puncture on patients with prolonged seizures or would delay lumbar puncture for 30 min in patients with short, convulsive seizures
• Papilledema	• Presence of venous pulsations suggests absence of increased intracranial pressure
• Focal neurologic deficit	• Including dilated nonreactive pupil, abnormalities of ocular motility, abnormal visual fields, gaze palsy, arm or leg drift
• Abnormal level of consciousness	• Unable to assess focal neurological deficits on physical examination in patients with altered level of consciousness

Reproduced with permission from: Tunkel AR, Hartman BJ, Kaplan SL, Kaufman BA, Roos KL, Scheld WM, Whitley RJ. Practice guidelines for the management of bacterial meningitis. Clin Infect Dis. 2004 Nov 1;39(9):1267–84, page 1271

36.7 Medical Management of CNS Infections

Early detection of CSF leaks is of utmost importance as it determines the outcome of the patient. The decision of whether to observe or to surgically intervene is mainly based on the cause, site of leak, and timing of the leak.

The traditional treatment of postoperative or posttraumatic CNS infections associated with CSF leakage involves immediate administration of intravenous antibiotic therapy as well as primary closure or repair of dural defect if the definite injury is suspected.

36.7.1 Community-Acquired Meningitis

Treatment of patients with suspected bacterial CNS infection (e.g., meningitis) with antimicrobial therapy generally requires careful assessment of the patient age, immune status, clinical setting, the most common bacteria causing the disease and on patterns of antimicrobial susceptibility [88, 121].

Empiric therapy using agents with adequate CSF concentrations is recommended when microbiological data are still insufficient based on the patient risk factors (see Table 36.4). With the worldwide increase in the prevalence of penicillin-resistant pneumococci, combination therapy with intravenous vancomycin plus a third-generation cephalosporin (either ceftriaxone or cefotaxime) has become the standard approach to empirical antimicrobial therapy [122, 123].

Table 36.4 Empirical therapy in adults with community-acquired bacterial meningitis

Predisposing factor	Common bacterial pathogen	Antimicrobial regimen
Age 16–50 years	*Neisseria meningitidis, Streptococcus pneumoniae*	Vancomycin plus either cefotaxime or ceftriaxone
Age >50 years	*S. pneumoniae, N. meningitidis, Listeria monocytogenes, aerobic gram-negative bacilli*	Vancomycin plus either cefotaxime or ceftriaxone plus ampicillin
Presence of a risk factor[a]	*S, pneumoniae. L. monocytogenes. Haemophilus influenzae*	

Reproduced with permission from: Diederik van de Beek, Jan de Gans, Allan R. Tunkel, et al. N Engl J Med 2006;354:44–53

[a] Risk factors include alcoholism and altered immune status

Table 36.5 Preemptive antimicrobial therapy in adults with presumptive pathogen identification by positive Gram stain

Microorganism	Recommended therapy	Alternative therapies
Streptococcus pneumoniae	Vancomycin plus ceftriaxone or cefotaxime[a]	Meropenem, gatifloxacin, or moxifloxacin.
Neisseria meningitidis	Ceftriaxone or cefotaxime	Penicillin G, ampicillin, chloramphenicol, gatifloxacin, or moxifloxacin, aztreonam
Listeria monocytogenes	Ampicillin[b] or penicillin G[b]	Trimethoprim-sulfamethoxazole, meropenem
Streptococcus agalactiae	Ampicillin[b] or penicillin G[b]	Ceftriaxone or cefotaxime
Haemophilus influenza	Ceftriaxone or cefotaxime	Chloramphenicol, cefepime, meropenem, gatifloxacin, or moxifloxacin
Escherichia coli	Ceftriaxone or cefotaxime	Cefepime, meropenem, aztreonam, gatifloxacin or moxifloxacin, trimethoprim-sulfamethoxazole

Reproduced with permission from: Tunkel AR, Hartman BJ, Kaplan SL, Kaufman BA, Roos KL, Scheld WM, Whitley RJ. Practice guidelines for the management of bacterial meningitis. Clin Infect Dis. 2004 Nov 1;39(9):1267–84, page 1274

[a] Some experts would add rifampin if dexamethasone is also given

[b] Addition of an aminoglycoside should be considered

Recommended preemptive and definitive therapies according to the partial or complete availability of the culture result are summarized in (Tables 36.5 and 36.6, respectively).

36.7.1.1 Duration of Therapy

In patients with bacterial meningitis, the duration of antibiotic therapy should be individualized and guided by the clinical response. Surprisingly, evidence-based data on the exact duration of therapy has been lacking, and most of the recommendations have often been based more on tradition [124, 125]. Recommended duration of therapy is shown in Table 36.7.

36.7.1.2 Adjunctive Dexamethasone Therapy

Experimental studies in animal models of infection have shown that the subarachnoid space inflammation during bacterial meningitis has a major impact on morbidity and mortality [107]. Controlling this inflammation with steroids may be of benefit in decreasing many of the pathophysiologic sequelae of the meningeal bacterial infection, such as cerebral edema, elevated intracranial pressure, disrupted cerebral blood flow, cerebral vasculitis, and neuronal injury, as mediated by proinflammatory cytokine release and expression [126–128].

Adjunctive treatment with dexamethasone before or with the first dose of antimicrobial in adult patients with suspected bacterial meningitis especially in the presence of cloudy CSF, positive CSF Gram stain, or a CSF WBC count of more than 1000 cells per cubic millimeter has been reported in several studies to have a significant reduction in mortality and neurologic sequelae [129–132].

The benefit was greatest in patients with intermediate disease severity, as defined by a score on the Glasgow Coma Scale (GCS) of 8–11 on admission, and in those with pneumococcal meningitis, in whom unfavorable outcomes and mortality declined from 52% to 26% and from 34% to 14%, respectively. This beneficial effect was a result of reduced mortality from systemic causes. Moreover, the benefits of dexamethasone use were not offset by any concerning side effects of dexamethasone therapy.

Table 36.6 Definitive antimicrobial therapy for adults with bacterial meningitis based on isolated pathogen and susceptibility testing

Microorganism	Standard therapy	Alternative therapies
Streptococcus pneumoniae		
• Penicillin MIC <0.1 μg/mL	• Penicillin G or ampicillin	• Ceftriaxone or cefotaxime, chloramphenicol
• Penicillin MIC 0.1–1.0 μg/mL	• Ceftriaxone or cefotaxime	• Cefepime, meropenem
• Penicillin MIC ≥2.0 μg/mL	• Vancomycin plus ceftriaxone or cefotaxime[a]	• Gatifloxacin or moxifloxacin
• Cefotaxime or ceftriaxone MIC ≥1.0 μg/mL	• Vancomycin plus ceftriaxone or cefotaxime	• Gatifloxacin or moxifloxacin
Neisseria meningitidis		
• Penicillin MIC <0.1 μg/mL	• Penicillin G or ampicillin	• Ceftriaxone or cefotaxime, chloramphenicol
• Penicillin MIC 0.1–1.0 μg/mL	• Ceftriaxone or cefotaxime	• Chloramphenicol, fluoroquinolone, meropenem
Listeria monocytogenes	• Ampicillin or penicillin G[b]	• Trimethoprim-sulfamethoxazole, meropenem
Streptococcus agalactiae	• Ampicillin or penicillin G[b]	• Ceftriaxone or cefotaxime
Escherichia coli and other Enterobacteriaceae[c]	• Ceftriaxone or cefotaxime	• Aztreonam, gatifloxacin or moxifloxacin, meropenem, trimethoprim-sulfamethoxazole, ampicillin
Pseudomonas aeruginosa[c]	• Cefepime[b] or ceftazidime[b]	• Aztreonam,[b] ciprofloxacin,[b] meropenem[b]
Haemophilus influenzae		
• β-Lactamase negative	• Ampicillin	• Ceftriaxone or cefotaxime, cefepime, chloramphenicol, gatifloxacin, or moxifloxacin
• β-Lactamase positive	• Ceftriaxone or cefotaxime	• Cefepime, chloramphenicol, gatifloxacin, or moxifloxacin
Staphylococcus aureus		
• Methicillin susceptible	• Nafcillin or oxacillin	• Vancomycin, meropenem
• Methicillin resistant	• Vancomycin[d]	• Trimethoprim-sulfamethoxazole, linezolid
Staphylococcus epidermidis	• Vancomycin[d]	• Linezolid
Enterococcus species		
• Ampicillin susceptible	• Ampicillin plus gentamicin	• …
• Ampicillin resistant	• Vancomycin plus gentamicin	• …
• Ampicillin and vancomycin resistant	• Linezolid	• …

Reproduced with permission from: Tunkel AR, Hartman BJ, Kaplan SL, Kaufman BA, Roos KL, Scheld WM, Whitley RJ. Practice guidelines for the management of bacterial meningitis. Clin Infect Dis. 2004 Nov 1;39(9):1267–84, page 1276

[a] Consider addition of rifampin if the MIC of ceftriaxone is >2 μg/mL

[b] Addition of an aminoglycoside should be considered

[c] Choice of a specific antimicrobial agent must be guided by in vitro susceptibility test results

[d] Consider addition of rifampin

Table 36.7 Duration of antimicrobial therapy for bacterial meningitis based on isolated pathogen

Microorganism	Duration of therapy in days
Neisseria meningitidis	7
Haemophilus influenzae	7
Streptococcus pneumoniae	10–14
Streptococcus agalactiae	14–21
Aerobic gram-negative bacilli[a]	21
Listeria monocytogenes	≥21

Reproduced with permission from: Tunkel AR, Hartman BJ, Kaplan SL, Kaufman BA, Roos KL, Scheld WM, Whitley RJ. Practice guidelines for the management of bacterial meningitis. Clin Infect Dis. 2004 Nov 1;39(9):1267–84, page 1281

[a] Duration in the neonate is 2 weeks beyond the first sterile CSF culture or ≥3 weeks, whichever is longer

In the subgroup of patients with meningococcal meningitis, mortality (relative risk, 0.9; 95% confidence interval, 0.3–2.1) and neurologic sequelae (relative risk, 0.5; 95% confidence interval, 0.1–1.7) were both reduced; however, the result did not reach statistical significance.

36.7.1.3 Outpatient Antimicrobial Therapy in Patients with Bacterial Meningitis

Intravenous antimicrobial therapy is often given to patients with bacterial meningitis during their hospitalization for the duration of treatment. Outpatient antimicrobial therapy can be given and may be appropriate in selected patients. This strategy may contribute to reduce the costs of hospitalization, minimize the occurrence of nosocomial infections, and improve the quality of life [133, 134]. The potential risk of serious complications in patients with bacterial meningitis usually happen within the first 2–3 days and are exceedingly rare after 3 or 4 days of appropriate antimicrobial therapy. Therefore, it is essential to carefully select and closely follow-up patients eligible for outpatient antimicrobial therapy.

Recommended criteria for patients with bacterial meningitis who are eligible and can receive outpatient antimicrobial therapy are shown in Table 36.8.

Table 36.8 Selection criteria for outpatient antimicrobial therapy in patients diagnosed with bacterial meningitis

• Inpatient antimicrobial therapy for ≥6 days
• Absence of fever for at least 24–48 h prior to initiation of outpatient therapy
• No significant neurologic dysfunction, focal findings, or seizure activity
• Clinical stability or improving condition
• Ability to take fluids by mouth
• Access to home health nursing for antimicrobial administration
• Reliable intravenous line and infusion device (if needed)
• Availability of a physician, as needed
• Established plan for physician visits, nurse visits, laboratory monitoring, and emergencies
• Patient and/or family compliance with the program
• Safe environment with access to a telephone, utilities, food, and refrigerator

Reproduced with permission from: Tunkel AR, Hartman BJ, Kaplan SL, Kaufman BA, Roos KL, Scheld WM, Whitley RJ. Practice guidelines for the management of bacterial meningitis. Clin Infect Dis. 2004 Nov 1;39(9):1267–84, page 1281

36.7.2 Nosocomial Meningitis

The choice of empirical antibiotic therapy in the setting of nosocomial bacterial meningitis is guided by suspected pathogen and the pathogenesis of the infection. For example, bacterial meningitis following basilar skull fracture or early after otorhinologic procedure should be treated empirically with a regimen containing vancomycin and a third-generation cephalosporin (either cefotaxime or ceftriaxone) [39, 44, 94]. Antibiotic therapy can be modified according to the isolation of the specific bacterial pathogen [87].

However, for nosocomial meningitis developing in the setting of neurosurgery or after prolonged hospitalization especially after penetrating head trauma or basilar skull fracture, empiric therapy should consist of vancomycin plus an antipseudomonal beta lactam antibiotic such as cefepime, ceftazidime, or meropenem (see Table 36.9) [88].

Adding the second agent should be based on the local antibiogram profiles of the Gram-negative

Table 36.9 Recommended empirical antimicrobial therapy for nosocomial bacterial meningitis, according to the pathogenesis of the infection

Pathogenesis	Common bacterial pathogens	Antimicrobial therapy
Postneurosurgical infection	Facultative and aerobic Gram-negative bacilli (including *Pseudomonas aeruginosa*), *Staphylococcus aureus*, and coagulase-negative *staphylococci* (especially *S. epidermidis*)	Vancomycin plus cefepime, ceftazidime, or meropenem[a]
Ventricular or lumbar catheter	Coagulase-negative *staphylococci* (especially *S. epidermidis*), *S. aureus*, facultative and aerobic Gram-negative bacilli (including *P. aeruginosa*), *Propionibacterium acnes*	
Penetrating trauma	*S. aureus*, coagulase-negative staphylococci (especially *S. epidermidis*), facultative and aerobic Gram-negative bacilli (including *P. aeruginosa*)	
Basilar skull fractures	*Streptococcus pneumoniae*, *Haemophilus influenzae*, group A β-hemolytic *streptococci*	Vancomycin plus a third-generation cephalosporin (i.e., ceftriaxone or cefotaxime)

Reproduced with permission from: van De Beek D et al. N Engl J Med 2010;362:146–54

[a] The choice of the specific agent should be based on local antimicrobial susceptibility of aerobic Gram-negative bacilli

bacilli. Among the carbapenems, meropenem is the agent of choice, given the lower risk of seizure compared to imipenem and its usefulness in the treatment of nosocomial bacterial meningitis which has been shown in several clinical studies [88].

36.7.2.1 Duration of Therapy

Duration of antibiotic therapy is guided by the findings on initial or repeat sampling, CSF glucose, and clinical symptoms and systemic features.

Infections caused by a coagulase-negative *staphylococcus* or *P. acnes* with no or minimal CSF pleocytosis, normal CSF glucose, and few clinical symptoms or systemic features should be treated for 10 days. Duration should be longer (10–14 days) if there is significant CSF pleocytosis, CSF hypoglycorrhachia, or clinical symptoms or systemic features.

Infections caused by *S. aureus* or Gram-negative bacilli with or without significant CSF pleocytosis, CSF hypoglycorrhachia, or clinical symptoms or systemic features should be treated for 10–14 days; some experts suggest treatment of infection caused by Gram-negative bacilli for 21 days.

In patients with repeatedly positive CSF cultures on appropriate antimicrobial therapy, treatment should be continued for 10–14 after the last positive culture.

36.7.3 Repeated Lumbar Puncture

The analysis of the cerebrospinal fluid should be repeated only in patients whose condition has not responded clinically after 48 h of appropriate antimicrobial therapy [86]. Due to the anti-inflammatory effect of dexamethasone therapy, vancomycin penetration into subarachnoid spaces might be compromised [135, 136] leading to treatment failures [137]; therefore, it is prudent to repeated lumbar puncture especially in patients with pneumococcal meningitis caused by penicillin-resistant or cephalosporin-resistant strains and who receive adjunctive dexamethasone therapy and vancomycin [88, 135].

Suggested algorithm for the diagnosis and management of suspected meningitis in patient with confirmed or suspected CSF leakage.

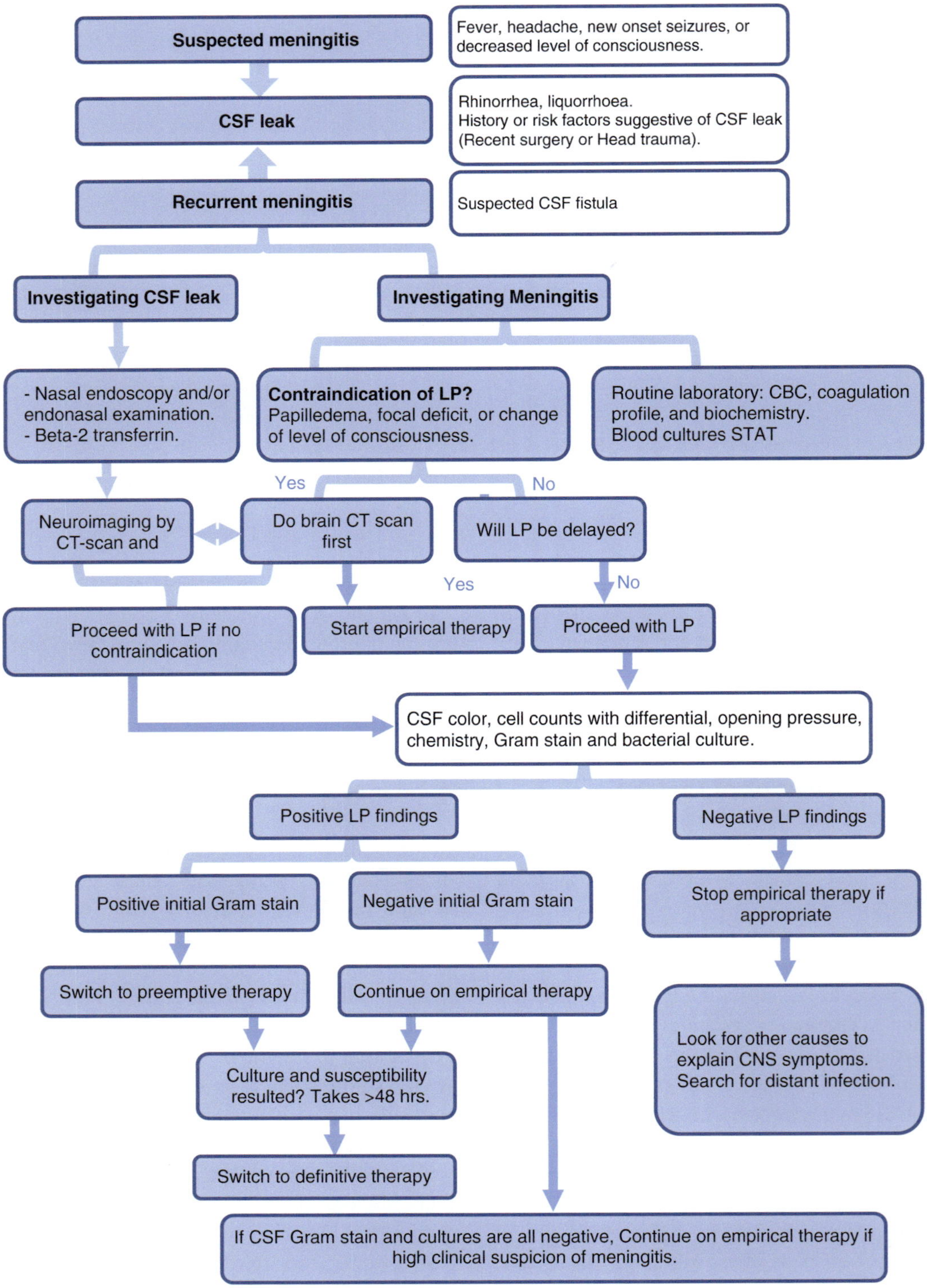
Suspected meningitis
Fever, headache, new onset seizures, or decreased level of consciousness.
CSF leak
Rhinorrhea, liquorrhoea.
History or risk factors suggestive of CSF leak (Recent surgery or Head trauma).
Recurrent meningitis
Suspected CSF fistula
Investigating CSF leak
Investigating Meningitis
- Nasal endoscopy and/or endonasal examination.
- Beta-2 transferrin.
Contraindication of LP?
Papilledema, focal deficit, or change of level of consciousness.
Routine laboratory: CBC, coagulation profile, and biochemistry.
Blood cultures STAT
Yes
No
Neuroimaging by CT-scan and
Do brain CT scan first
Will LP be delayed?
Yes
No
Proceed with LP if no contraindication
Start empirical therapy
Proceed with LP
CSF color, cell counts with differential, opening pressure, chemistry, Gram stain and bacterial culture.
Positive LP findings
Negative LP findings
Positive initial Gram stain
Negative initial Gram stain
Stop empirical therapy if appropriate
Switch to preemptive therapy
Continue on empirical therapy
Look for other causes to explain CNS symptoms.
Search for distant infection.
Culture and susceptibility resulted? Takes >48 hrs.
Switch to definitive therapy
If CSF Gram stain and cultures are all negative, Continue on empirical therapy if high clinical suspicion of meningitis.

36.8 Antibiotic Prophylaxis

36.8.1 In Patient with Preoperative CSF Leakage

Antibiotic prophylaxis has not been rigorously studied in this setting and remains controversial in CSF leakage without infection. The routine use of prophylactic antibiotics in patients with skull base fractures even appears to be associated with a higher risk of meningitis [39]. While one study showed no statistical difference among patients treated with antibiotics versus those not treated with antibiotics for CSF leakage [40], several other studies highlighted an increased incidence of infection [27, 138, 139] in patients receiving prophylactic antibiotics compared to those not treated and greater incidence of resistant organisms with use of prophylactic antibiotics [51]. Furthermore, most experts recommend against using antibiotics to prevent the emergence of resistant organisms [140, 141].

36.8.2 In Patient with Intra and Post-operative CSF Leakage

The paucity of quality data for the type of perioperative antibiotic prophylaxis and duration has left this issue to the discretion of the surgical team. However, studies have shown no added benefit of extending antibiotics beyond 48 h postoperatively in the setting of open cranial base surgery as well as head and neck surgeries [142–144]. Prophylactic antibiotics are routinely administered before skin incision and continue its use until the nasal packing is removed. The most commonly used prophylactic agents are nafcillin or cefazolin. Infection rates have been acceptable (rate of meningitis less than 1%) [74]. Clindamycin or vancomycin is typically used for patients with penicillin allergy.

36.9 Role of Vaccination in CSF Rhinorrhea

Vaccination is minimally invasive intervention with a low risk for adverse reaction. Multiple studies reported on the effect of vaccination in the reduction of all-age-specific incidence of pneumococcal meningitis, *H. influenzae* type b meningitis, and meningococcal meningitis [145, 146]. The expert opinion is that vaccination is indicated in this small subgroup of adults with community-acquired bacterial meningitis with high risk of recurrence.

36.9.1 Pneumococcal Vaccination

The two widely used types of pneumococcal vaccine are the 23-valent polysaccharide vaccine (PPSV-23) and the 13-valent conjugate vaccines (PCV-13). Patients with a persistent communication between the CSF and oropharynx or nasopharynx should receive both PCV-13 and PPSV-23, preferably ≥8 weeks after the receipt of PCV-13. A second dose of PPSV-23 can be considered in those patients 5 years after the initial dose, although this is not recommended by the ACIP or AAP [147].

Although not supported by evidence, it is recommended to use Hib, Men-ACYW, and Men-B vaccines in patients presenting with community-acquired bacterial meningitis and CSF leak (see Table 36.10).

Table 36.10 Recommended adult immunization for meningitis in individuals with or without CSF leak

Vaccination	Medical indication	How to administer?
Pneumococcal vaccinations	Recommended for patients with CSF leak	• 1 dose PCV-13 followed by 1 dose PPSV-23 at least 8 weeks later
Meningococcal vaccination	Recommended for general population	*Meningococcal A, C, W, Y* (MenACWY) • 1 or 2 doses depending on indication, then booster every 5 years if risk remains *Meningococcal B (MenB)* • 2 or 3 doses depending on vaccine and indication
Influenza vaccination	Recommended for patients with CSF leak	Influenza inactivated (IIV) or influenza recombinant (RIV) • 1 dose annually Or Influenza live attenuated • 1 dose annually
Haemophilus *influenzae*	Recommended for general population	Haemophilus influenza type b (Hib) • 1 dose

References

1. Tohge R, Takahashi M. Cerebrospinal fluid rhinorrhea and subsequent bacterial meningitis due to an atypical clival fracture. Intern Med. 2017;56(14):1911–4.
2. Wax MK, Ramadan HH, Ortiz O, Wetmore SJ. Contemporary management of cerebrospinal fluid rhinorrhea. Otolaryngol Head Neck Surg. 1997;116(4):442–9.
3. Lewin W. Cerebrospinal fluid rhinorrhea in nonmissile head injuries. Neurosurgery. 1966;12(CN_suppl_1):237–52. http://academic.oup.com/neurosurgery/article/12/CN_suppl_1/237/4099203.
4. Wang EW, Vandergrift WA, Schlosser RJ. Spontaneous CSF leaks. Otolaryngol Clin North Am. 2011;44(4):845–56. https://doi.org/10.1016/j.otc.2011.06.018.
5. Thomson SC. The cerebrospinal fluid. Its spontaneous escape from the nose. With observations on its position and function in the human subject. J Nerv Ment Dis. 1900;27(2):125.
6. Aarabi B, Leibrock LG. Neurosurgical approaches to cerebrospinal fluid rhinorrhea. Ear Nose Throat J. 1992;71(7):300–5. http://journals.sagepub.com/doi/10.1177/014556139207100704.
7. Singh R, Bandyopadhyay M. Median defect in the skull. Singapore Med J. 2008;49(2):92–4.
8. Boseley ME, Tami TA. Endoscopic management of anterior skull base encephaloceles. Ann Otol Rhinol Laryngol. 2004;113(1):30–3. http://journals.sagepub.com/doi/10.1177/000348940411300106.
9. Miller C. Case of hydrocephalus chronicus, with some unusual symptoms and appearances on dissection. Trans Med Chir Soc Edinb. 1826;2:243–8. https://www.ncbi.nlm.nih.gov/pmc/articles/PMC5406566/.
10. Hegazy HM, Carrau RL, Snyderman CH, Kassam A, Zweig J. Transnasal endoscopic repair of cerebrospinal fluid rhinorrhea: a meta-analysis. Laryngoscope. 2000;110(7):1166–72. http://doi.wiley.com/10.1097/00005537-200007000-00019.
11. Ratilal BO, Costa J, Sampaio C, Pappamikail L. Antibiotic prophylaxis for preventing meningitis in patients with basilar skull fractures. Cochrane Database Syst Rev. 2011;(8).
12. Yilmazlar S, Arslan E, Kocaeli H, Dogan S, Aksoy K, Korfali E, et al. Cerebrospinal fluid leakage complicating skull base fractures: analysis of 81 cases. Neurosurg Rev. 2006;29(1):64–71.
13. Deklotz TR, Chia SH, Lu W, Makambi KH, Aulisi E, Deeb Z. Meta-analysis of endoscopic versus sublabial pituitary surgery. Laryngoscope. 2012;122(3):511–8.
14. Tabaee A, Anand VK, Barrón Y, Hiltzik DDH, Brown SM, Kacker A, et al. Endoscopic pituitary surgery: a systematic review and meta-analysis: clinical article. J Neurosurg. 2009;111:545–54.
15. Naunheim MR, Sedaghat AR, Lin DT, Bleier BS, Holbrook EH, Curry WT, et al. Immediate and delayed complications following endoscopic skull base surgery. J Neurol Surg Part B Skull Base. 2015;76(5):390–6.
16. Ivan ME, Bryan Iorgulescu J, El-Sayed I, McDermott MW, Parsa AT, Pletcher SD, et al. Risk factors for postoperative cerebrospinal fluid leak and meningitis after expanded endoscopic endonasal surgery. J Clin Neurosci. 2015;22(1):48–54. https://doi.org/10.1016/j.jocn.2014.08.009.
17. Chowdhury T, Prabhakar H, Bithal PK, Schaller B, Dash HH. Immediate postoperative complications in transsphenoidal pituitary surgery: a prospective study. Saudi J Anaesth. 2014;8(3):335–41.
18. Kumar S, Darr A, Hobbs CG, Carlin WV. Endoscopic, endonasal, trans-sphenoidal hypophysectomy: ret-

rospective analysis of 171 procedures. J Laryngol Otol. 2012;126(10):1033–40.
19. Karnezis TT, Baker AB, Soler ZM, Wise SK, Rereddy SK, Patel ZM, et al. Factors impacting cerebrospinal fluid leak rates in endoscopic sellar surgery. Int Forum Allergy Rhinol. 2016;6(11):1117–25.
20. Jakimovski D, Bonci G, Attia M, Shao H, Hofstetter C, Tsiouris AJ, et al. Incidence and significance of intraoperative cerebrospinal fluid leak in endoscopic pituitary surgery using intrathecal fluorescein. World Neurosurg. 2014;82:E513–23. https://doi.org/10.1016/j.wneu.2013.06.005.
21. Narayan V, Nanda A. 15—Skull base surgery complications: an overview. In: Complications in neurosurgery. Elsevier Inc. p. 77–8. https://doi.org/10.1016/B978-0-323-50961-9.00015-3.
22. Lewin W. Cerebrospinal fluid rhinorrhœa in closed head injuries. Br J Surg. 1954;42(171):1–18. http://doi.wiley.com/10.1002/bjs.18004217102.
23. Tebruegge M, Curtis N. Epidemiology, etiology, pathogenesis, and diagnosis of recurrent bacterial meningitis. Clin Microbiol Rev. 2008;21(3):519–37. http://cmr.asm.org/cgi/doi/10.1128/CMR.00009-08.
24. Friedman JA, Ebersold MJ, Quast LM. Persistent posttraumatic cerebrospinal fluid leakage. Neurosurg Focus. 2008;9(1):1–5.
25. Adriani KS, Brouwer MC, van de Beek D. Risk factors for community-acquired bacterial meningitis in adults. Neth J Med. 2015;73(2):53–60. http://www.embase.com/search/results?subaction=viewrecord&from=export&id=L602940133%0Ahttp://limo.libis.be/resolver?&sid=EMBASE&issn=03002977&id=doi:&atitle=Risk+factors+for+community-acquired+bacterial+meningitis+in+adults&stitle=Neth.+J.+Med.&title=Neth.
26. Koso-Thomas AK, Harley EH. Traumatic cerebrospinal fluid fistula presenting as recurrent meningitis. Otolaryngol Head Neck Surg. 1995;112(3):469–72.
27. Friedman JA, Ebersold MJ, Quast LM. Posttraumatic cerebrospinal fluid leakage. World J Surg. 2001;25(8):1062–6.
28. Davis CEDD. Discussion on Injuries of the Frontal and Ethmoidal Sinuses. Proc R Soc Med. 1942;35(12):805–10. https://www.ncbi.nlm.nih.gov/pmc/articles/PMC1998470/.
29. Adson AW. Repair of defects in ethmoid and frontal sinuses resulting in cerebrospinal rhinorrhea. Arch Surg. 1949;58(5):623. http://archsurg.jamanetwork.com/article.aspx?doi=10.1001/archsurg.1949.01240030633006.
30. Dandy WE. Pneumocephalus (intracranial penumatocele or aerocele). Arch Surg. 1926;12(5):949. http://archsurg.jamanetwork.com/article.aspx?doi=10.1001/archsurg.1926.01130050003001.
31. Dandy WE. Treatment of rhinorrhea and otorrhea. Arch Surg. 1944;49(2):75. http://archsurg.jamanetwork.com/article.aspx?doi=10.1001/archsurg.1944.01230020080001.
32. Jamieson KG, Yelland JDN. Surgical repair of the anterior fossa because of rhinorrhea, aerocele, or meningitis. J Neurosurg. 1973;39(3):328–31. https://thejns.org/view/journals/j-neurosurg/39/3/article-p328.xml.
33. Mincy JE. Posttraumatic cerebrospinal fluid fistula of the frontal fossa. J Trauma Inj Infect Crit Care. 1966;6(5):618–22. https://insights.ovid.com/crossref?an=00005373-196609000-00007.
34. Russell T, Cummins BH. Cerebrospinal fluid rhinorrhea 34 years after trauma: a case report and review of the literature. Neurosurgery. 1984;15(5):705–6. https://academic.oup.com/neurosurgery/article-lookup/doi/10.1227/00006123-198411000-00013.
35. Oh J-W, Kim S-H, Whang K. Traumatic cerebrospinal fluid leak: diagnosis and management. Korean J Neurotrauma. 2017;13(2):63.
36. Schlosser RJ, Bolger WE. Nasal cerebrospinal fluid leaks: critical review and surgical considerations. Laryngoscope. 2004;114(2):255–65. http://ovidsp.ovid.com/ovidweb.cgi?T=JS&PAGE=reference&D=emed6&NEWS=N&AN=2004068325.
37. Hasheminia D, Kalantar Motamedi MR, Hashemzehi H, Nazeri R, Movahedian B. A 7-year study of 1,278 patients with maxillofacial trauma and cerebrospinal fluid leak. J Maxillofac Oral Surg. 2015;14(2):258–62. https://doi.org/10.1007/s12663-014-0630-z.
38. Zapalac JS, Marple BF, Schwade ND. Skull base cerebrospinal fluid fistulas: a comprehensive diagnostic algorithm. Otolaryngol Head Neck Surg. 2002;126(6):669–76.
39. Choi D, Spann R. Traumatic cerebrospinal fluid leakage: risk factors and the use of prophylactic antibiotics. Br J Neurosurg. 1996;10(6):571–6. http://www.tandfonline.com/doi/full/10.1080/02688699646880.
40. Clemenza JW, Kaltman SI, Diamond DL. Craniofacial trauma and cerebrospinal fluid leakage. A retrospective clinical study. J Oral Maxillofac Surg. 1995;53(9):1004–7.
41. Guo K, Heng L, Zhang H, Ma L, Zhang H, Jia D. Risk factors for postoperative intracranial infections in patients with pituitary adenoma after endoscopic endonasal transsphenoidal surgery: pneumocephalus deserves further study. Neurosurg Focus. 2019;47(2):E5.
42. Vaz-Guimaraes F, Koutourousiou M, de Almeida JR, Tyler-Kabara EC, Fernandez-Miranda JC, Wang EW, et al. Endoscopic endonasal surgery for epidermoid and dermoid cysts: a 10-year experience. J Neurosurg. 2019;130(2):368–78.
43. Durand ML, Calderwood SB, Weber DJ, Miller SI, Southwick FS, Caviness VS, et al. Acute bacterial meningitis in adults—a review of 493 episodes. N Engl J Med. 2002;328(1):21–8. http://www.nejm.org/doi/abs/10.1056/NEJM199301073280104.
44. Adriani KS, van de Beek D, Brouwer MC, Spanjaard L, de Gans J. Community-acquired recurrent bacterial meningitis in adults. Clin Infect Dis. 2007;45(5):e46–51.
45. Bijlsma MW, Brouwer MC, Kasanmoentalib ES, Kloek AT, Lucas MJ, Tanck MW, et al. Community-

acquired bacterial meningitis in adults in the Netherlands, 2006-14: a prospective cohort study. Lancet Infect Dis. 2016;16(3):339–47. https://doi.org/10.1016/S1473-3099(15)00430-2.

46. Dzupova O, Rozsypal H, Prochazka B, Benes J. Acute bacterial meningitis in adults: predictors of outcome. Scand J Infect Dis. 2009;41(5):348–54.
47. Kono Y, Prevedello DM, Snyderman CH, Gardner PA, Kassam AB, Carrau RL, et al. One thousand endoscopic skull base surgical procedures demystifying the infection potential: incidence and description of postoperative meningitis and brain abscesses. Infect Control Hosp Epidemiol. 2014;32(1):77–83.
48. Eljamel MS, Foy PM. Acute traumatic CSF fistulae: the risk of intracranial infection. Br J Neurosurg. 1990;4(5):381–5. http://ovidsp.ovid.com/ovidweb.cgi?T=JS&PAGE=reference&D=emed2&NEWS=N&AN=1990381027.
49. Nandapalan V, Watson ID, Swift AC. Beta-2-transferrin and cerebrospinal fluid rhinorrhoea. Clin Otolaryngol. 1996;21(3):259–64. http://doi.wiley.com/10.1111/j.1365-2273.1996.tb01737.x.
50. Giunta G, Piazza I. Recurrent bacterial meningitis occurring five years after closed head injury and caused by an intranasal post-traumatic meningo-encephalocele. Postgrad Med J. 1991;67(786):377–9. http://pmj.bmj.com/cgi/doi/10.1136/pgmj.67.786.377.
51. Pappas DG, Hammerschlag PE, Hammerschlag M. Cerebrospinal fluid rhinorrhea and recurrent meningitis. Clin Infect Dis. 1993;17(3):364–8. https://academic.oup.com/cid/article-lookup/doi/10.1093/clinids/17.3.364.
52. Van Aken MO, Feelders RA, De Marie S, Delwel EJ, Romijn JA, Van Der Lely AJ, et al. Surgery: postoperative external lumbar drainage reduces the risk for meningitis. Pituitary. 2004;7(2):89–93.
53. Jahangiri A, Wagner J, Han SW, Zygourakis CC, Han SJ, Tran MT, et al. Morbidity of repeat transsphenoidal surgery assessed in more than 1000 operations. J Neurosurg. 2014;121(1):67–74. https://thejns.org/view/journals/j-neurosurg/121/1/article-p67.xml.
54. Lindstrom DR, Toohill RJ, Loehrl TA, Smith TL. Management of cerebrospinal fluid rhinorrhea: the Medical College of Wisconsin experience. Laryngoscope. 2004;114(6):969–74. http://mail.google.com/mail/?ui=2&view=bsp&ver=1qygpcgurkovy%5Cnpapers2://publication/uuid/24E7E450-3BF3-40B0-A139-C7F0BB1006CF.
55. Dunn CJ, Alaani A, Johnson AP. Study on spontaneous cerebrospinal fluid rhinorrhoea: its aetiology and management. J Laryngol Otol. 2005;119(1):12–5.
56. Cairns H. Injuries of the frontal and ethmoidal sinuses with special reference to cerebrospinal rhinorrhœa and aeroceles. J Laryngol Otol. 1937;52(9):589–623. https://www.cambridge.org/core/product/identifier/S0022215100043991/type/journal_article.
57. Ommaya AK. Cerebrospinal fluid rhinorrhea. Neurology. 1964;14(2):106. http://www.neurology.org/cgi/doi/10.1212/WNL.14.2.106.
58. Vrabec DP, Hallberg OE. Cerebrospinal fluid rhinorrhea: intranasal approach, review of the literature, and report of a case. Arch Otolaryngol Head Neck Surg. 1964;80(2):218–29. http://archotol.ama-assn.org/cgi/doi/10.1001/archotol.1964.00750040224022.
59. Ziu M, Savage JG, Jimenez DF. Diagnosis and treatment of cerebrospinal fluid rhinorrhea following accidental traumatic anterior skull base fractures. Neurosurg Focus. 2012;32(6):E3.
60. Daudia A, Biswas D, Jones NS. Risk of meningitis with cerebrospinal fluid rhinorrhea. Ann Otol Rhinol Laryngol. 2007;116(12):902–5. http://ovidsp.ovid.com/ovidweb.cgi?T=JS&PAGE=reference&D=emed8&NEWS=N&AN=2007625131.
61. Eljamel MSM, Foy PM. Non-traumatic CSF fistulae: clinical history and management. Br J Neurosurg. 1991;5(3):275–9.
62. Lloyd KM, DelGaudio JM, Hudgins PA. Imaging of skull base cerebrospinal fluid leaks in adults. Radiology. 2008;248:725–36.
63. Meco C, Oberascher G. Comprehensive algorithm for skull base dural lesion and cerebriospinal fluid fistula diagnosis. Laryngoscope. 2004;114(6):991–9. http://doi.wiley.com/10.1097/00005537-200406000-00007.
64. Wind JJ, Caputy AJ, Roberti F. Spontaneous encephaloceles of the temporal lobe. Neurosurg Focus. 2008;25(6):1–6.
65. Kerr JT, Chu FWK, Bayles SW. Cerebrospinal fluid rhinorrhea: Diagnosis and management. Otolaryngol Clin North Am. 2005;38:597–611.
66. ter Horst L, Brouwer MC, van der Ende A, van de Beek D. Community-acquired bacterial meningitis in adults with cerebrospinal fluid leakage. Clin Infect Dis. 2019;70(11):2256–61. https://academic.oup.com/cid/advance-article/doi/10.1093/cid/ciz649/5531894.
67. Ansari S, Carron DB, Smith MJ. Recurrent late onset post-traumatic meningitis. J Pak Med Assoc. 1994;44(8):193–4.
68. Eljamel MSM, Foy PM. Post-traumatic CSF fistulae, the case for surgical repair. Br J Neurosurg. 1990;4(6):479–83. http://www.tandfonline.com/doi/full/10.3109/02688699008993796.
69. Levin S, Nelson KE, Spies HW, Lepper MH. Pneumococcal meningitis: the problem of the unseen cerebrospinal fluid leak. Am J Med Sci. 1972;264(4):319–27. http://content.wkhealth.com/linkback/openurl?sid=WKPTLP:landingpage&an=00000441-197210000-00010.
70. Deveci Ö, Uysal C, Varol S, Tekin R, Bozkurt F, Bekçibaşı M, et al. Erişkin posttravmatik tekrarlayan menenjitlerin değerlendirilmesi. Ulus Travma ve Acil Cerrahi Derg. 2015;21(4):261–5.
71. Aarabi B. Causes of infections in penetrating head wounds in the Iran-Iraq war. Neurosurgery. 1989;25(6):923–6. http://content.wkhealth.com/

linkback/openurl?sid=WKPTLP:landingpage&an=00006123-198912000-00011.
72. Meirowsky AM, Caveness WF, Dillon JD, Rish BL, Mohr JP, Kistler JP, et al. Cerebrospinal fluid fistulas complicating missile wounds of the brain. J Neurosurg. 1981;54(1):44–8. https://thejns.org/view/journals/j-neurosurg/54/1/article-p44.xml.
73. Abuabara A. Cerebrospinal fluid rhinorrhoea management. Injury. 2004;14(6):561.
74. Dumont AS, Nemergut EC, Jane JA, Laws ER. Postoperative care following pituitary surgery. J Intens Care Med. 2005;20:127–40.
75. van Aken MO, de Marie S, van der Lely A, Singh R, van den Berge JH, Poublon RML, et al. Risk factors for meningitis after transsphenoidal surgery. Clin Infect Dis. 1997;25(4):852–6. https://academic.oup.com/cid/article-lookup/doi/10.1086/515533.
76. Black PM, Zervas NT, Candia GL. Incidence and management of complications of transsphenoidal operation for pituitary adenomas. Neurosurgery. 1987;20(6):920–4. https://academic.oup.com/neurosurgery/article-lookup/doi/10.1227/00006123-198706000-00017.
77. Ciric I, Mikhael M, Stafford T, Lawson L, Garces R. Transsphenoidal microsurgery of pituitary macroadenomas with long-term follow-up results. J Neurosurg. 1983;59(3):395–401.
78. Kennedy DW, Cohn ES, Papel ID, Holliday MJ. Transsphenoidal approach to the sella. Laryngoscope. 1984;94(8):1066–74. http://doi.wiley.com/10.1288/00005537-198408000-00015.
79. Bernal-Sprekelsen M, Alobid I, Mullol J, Trobat F, Tomás-Barberán M. Closure of cerebrospinal fluid leaks prevents ascending bacterial meningitis. Rhinology. 2005;43(4):277–81. http://doi.wiley.com/10.1097/00005537-199912000-00012.
80. Kryzanski JT, Annino DJ, Gopal H, Heilman CB. Low complication rates of cranial and craniofacial approaches to midline anterior skull base lesions. Skull Base. 2008;18(4):229–42.
81. Laws ER, Trautmann JC, Hollenhorst RW. Transsphenoidal decompression of the optic nerve and chiasm. Visual results in 62 patients. J Neurosurg. 1977;46(6):717–22.
82. Li HY, Yu HX, Liu G. [Clinical analysis of brain abscess after endoscopic repairment of cerebrospinal fluid rhinorrhea]. Zhonghua Er Bi Yan Hou Tou Jing Wai Ke Za Zhi. 2018;53(9):650–4. http://www.ncbi.nlm.nih.gov/pubmed/30293255.
83. Jane JA, Laws ER. The surgical management of pituitary adenomas in a series of 3,093 patients. J Am Coll Surg. 2001;193(6):650–9. http://ac.els-cdn.com.ezproxy.auckland.ac.nz/S1072751501011012/1-s2.0-S1072751501011012-main.pdf?_tid=3f26a8ec-61f6-11e7-af39-00000aab0f01&acdnat=1499309771_77ddce1e3545adc3132bf20323c94776.
84. Blennow K, Fredman P. Detection of cerebrospinal fluid leakage by isoelectric focusing on polyacrylamide gels with silver staining using the PhastSystem™. Acta Neurochir (Wien). 1995;136(3–4):135–9.
85. Komotar RJ, Starke RM, Raper DMS, Anand VK, Schwartz TH. Endoscopic endonasal compared with microscopic transsphenoidal and open transcranial resection of craniopharyngiomas. World Neurosurg. 2012;77(2):329–41. https://doi.org/10.1016/j.wneu.2011.07.011.
86. van de Beek D, de Gans J, Tunkel AR, Wijdicks EFM. Community-acquired bacterial meningitis in adults. N Engl J Med. 2006;354(1):44–53. https://academic.oup.com/cid/article-lookup/doi/10.1086/425368.
87. van de Beek D, Drake JM, Tunkel AR. Nosocomial bacterial meningitis. N Engl J Med. 2010;362(2):146–54. http://www.nejm.org/doi/abs/10.1056/NEJMra0804573.
88. Tunkel AR, Hartman BJ, Kaplan SL, Kaufman BA, Roos KL, Scheld WM, et al. Practice guidelines for the management of bacterial meningitis. Clin Infect Dis. 2004;39(9):1267–84. https://academic.oup.com/cid/article-lookup/doi/10.1086/425368.
89. Asad S, Peters-Willke J, Brennan W, Asad S. Clival defect with primary CSF rhinorrhea: a very rare presentation with challenging management. World Neurosurg. 2017;106:1052.e1–4. https://doi.org/10.1016/j.wneu.2017.07.011.
90. Maitra S, Ghosh SK. Recurrent pyogenic meningitis—a retrospective study. QJM. 1989;73(1):919–29.
91. Kaufman BA, Tunkel AR, Pryor JC, Dacey RG. Meningitis in the neurosurgical patient. Infect Dis Clin North Am. 1990;4(4):677–701.
92. Korinek AM, Baugnon T, Golmard JL, Van Effenterre R, Coriat P, Puybasset L. Risk factors for adult nosocomial meningitis after craniotomy: role of antibiotic prophylaxis. Neurosurgery. 2006;59(1):126–32.
93. McClelland S, Hall WA. Postoperative central nervous system infection: incidence and associated factors in 2111 neurosurgical procedures. Clin Infect Dis. 2007;45(1):55–9.
94. Baltas I, Tsoulfa S, Sakellariou P, Vogas V, Fylaktakis M, Kondodimou A. Posttraumatic meningitis: bacteriology, hydrocephalus, and outcome. Neurosurgery. 1994;35(3):422–7. https://academic.oup.com/neurosurgery/article/35/3/422/2757632.
95. Baer ET. Post-dural puncture bacterial meningitis. Anesthesiology. 2006;105:381–93. http://insights.ovid.com/crossref?an=00000542-200608000-00022.
96. Weisfelt M, van de Beek D, Spanjaard L, de Gans J. Nosocomial bacterial meningitis in adults: a prospective series of 50 cases. J Hosp Infect. 2007;66(1):71–8.
97. Mayhall CG, Archer NH, Lamb VA, Spadora AC, Baggett JW, Ward JD, et al. Ventriculostomy-related infections. N Engl J Med. 1984;310(9):553–9. http://www.nejm.org/doi/abs/10.1056/NEJM198403013100903.
98. Dorsett M, Liang SY. Diagnosis and treatment of central nervous system infections in the emer-

gency department. Emerg Med Clin North Am. 2016;34(4):917–42. https://linkinghub.elsevier.com/retrieve/pii/S0733862716300542.
99. Scholsem M, Scholtes F, Collignon F, Robe P, Dubuisson A, Kaschten B, et al. Surgical management of anterior cranial base fractures with cerebrospinal fluid fistulae. Neurosurgery. 2008;62(2):463–71. https://academic.oup.com/neurosurgery/article/62/2/463/2558524.
100. Tunkel AR, Hasbun R, Bhimraj A, Byers K, Kaplan SL, Scheld WM, et al. 2017 Infectious Diseases Society of America's clinical practice guidelines for healthcare-associated ventriculitis and meningitis*. Clin Infect Dis. 2017;64(6):701–6.
101. Romanowski B, Tyrrell DL, Weir BK, Goldsand G. Meningitis complicating transsphenoidal hypophysectomy. Can Med Assoc J. 1981;124(9):1172–5. http://www.ncbi.nlm.nih.gov/pubmed/7237338.
102. Blomstedt GC. Infections in neurosurgery: a retrospective study of 1143 patients and 1517 operations. Acta Neurochir (Wien). 1985;78(3–4):81–90.
103. Buckwold FJ, Hand R, Hansebout RR. Hospital acquired bacterial meningitis in neurosurgical patients. J Neurosurg. 1977;46(4):494–500.
104. Flad TM, McKenna TJ. Meningitis as a late complication of surgically and medically treated pituitary adenoma. Clin Endocrinol (Oxf). 1991;35(5):419–22.
105. Skedros DG, Cass SP, Hirsch BE, Kelly RH. Sources of error in use of beta-2 transferrin analysis for diagnosing perilymphatic and cerebral spinal fluid leaks. Otolaryngol Neck Surg. 1993;109(5):861–4.
106. Pretto Flores L, De Almeida CS, Casulari LA, Andrioli G, De Divitiis E, Foroglou G. Positive predictive values of selected clinical signs associated with skull base fractures. J Neurosurg Sci. 2000;44(2):77–82.
107. Tunkel AR, Scheld WM. Bacterial meningitis. Philadelphia: Lippincott Williams & Wilkins; 2001.
108. Chapin-Robertson K, Dahlberg SE, Edberg SC. Clinical and laboratory analyses of cytospin-prepared gram stains for recovery and diagnosis of bacteria from sterile body fluids. J Clin Microbiol. 1992;30(2):377–80.
109. Swartz MN. Infections of the central nervous system Edited by W. Michael Scheld, Richard J. Whitley, and David T. Durack. 2nd ed. Philadelphia: Lippincott-Raven Publishers, 1997. 1,039 pp., illustrated. $205. Clin Infect Dis. 1997;24(6):1288.
110. Feigin RD, McCracken GH, Klein JO. Diagnosis and management of meningitis. Pediatr Infect Dis J. 1992;11(9):785. https://insights.ovid.com/crossref?an=00006454-199209000-00039.
111. Gray LD, Fedorko DP. Laboratory diagnosis of bacterial meningitis. Clin Microbiol Rev. 1992;5(2):130–45.
112. Saravolatz LD, Manzor O, VanderVelde N, Pawlak J, Belian B. Broad-range bacterial polymerase chain reaction for early detection of bacterial meningitis. Clin Infect Dis. 2003;36(1):40–5.
113. Oakley GM, Alt JA, Schlosser RJ, Harvey RJ, Orlandi RR. Diagnosis of cerebrospinal fluid rhinorrhea: an evidence-based review with recommendations. Int Forum Allergy Rhinol. 2016; 6(1):8–16.
114. Algin O, Hakyemez B, Gokalp G, Ozcan T, Korfali E, Parlak M. The contribution of 3D-CISS and contrast-enhanced MR cisternography in detecting cerebrospinal fluid leak in patients with rhinorrhoea. Br J Radiol. 2010;83(987):225–32.
115. Mostafa BE, Khafagi A. Combined HRCT and MRI in the detection of CSF rhinorrhea. Skull Base. 2004;14(3):157–62.
116. Shetty PG, Shroff MM, Sahani DV, Kirtane MV. Evaluation of high-resolution CT and MR cisternography in the diagnosis of cerebrospinal fluid fistula. Am J Neuroradiol. 1998;19(4):633–9.
117. Tuntiyatorn L, Laothammatas J. Evaluation of MR cisternography in diagnosis of cerebrospinal fluid fistula. J Med Assoc Thail. 2004;87(12):1471–6.
118. Eberhardt KEW, Hollenbach HP, Deimling M, Tomandl BF, Huk WJ. MR cisternography: a new method for the diagnosis of CSF fistulae. Eur Radiol. 1997;7(9):1485–91.
119. Eljamel MS, Pidgeon CN, Toland J, Phillips JB, O'Dwyer AA. MRI cisternography, and the localization of CSF fistulae. Br J Neurosurg. 1994;8(4):433–7. https://www.tandfonline.com/doi/abs/10.3109/02688699408995111.
120. Stafford Johnson DB, Brennan P, Toland J, O'Dwyer AJ. Magnetic resonance imaging in the evaluation of cerebrospinal fluid fistulae. Clin Radiol. 2005;51(12):837–41.
121. van de Beek D, de Gans J, Spanjaard L, Vermeulen M, Dankert J. Antibiotic guidelines and antibiotic use in adult bacterial meningitis in The Netherlands. J Antimicrob Chemother. 2002;49(4):661–6.
122. Whitney CG, Farley MM, Hadler J, Harrison LH, Lexau C, Reingold A, et al. Increasing prevalence of multidrug-resistant Streptococcus pneumoniae in the United States. N Engl J Med. 2000;343(26):1917–24. http://www.nejm.org/doi/abs/10.1056/NEJM200012283432603.
123. Fraser A, Gafter-Gvili A, Paul M, Leibovici L. Antibiotics for preventing meningococcal infections. In: Fraser A, editor. Cochrane database of systematic reviews. Wiley: Chichester; 2006. http://doi.wiley.com/10.1002/14651858.CD004785.pub3.
124. Radetsky M. Duration of treatment in bacterial meningitis. Pediatr Infect Dis J. 1990;9(1):2–9. https://insights.ovid.com/crossref?an=00006454-199001000-00002.
125. O'Neill P, Heath C, Shann F, Henry D, Hilton-Jones D, Squier MV, et al. Meningitis. Lancet. 1993;341(8844):530. https://linkinghub.elsevier.com/retrieve/pii/014067369390287Q
126. Scheld WM, Koedel U, Nathan B, Pfister H. Pathophysiology of bacterial meningitis: mechanism(s) of neuronal injury. J Infect Dis. 2002;186(s2):S225–33.

127. Van der Flier M, Geelen SPM, Kimpen JLL, Hoepelman IM, Tuomanen EI. Reprogramming the host response in bacterial meningitis: how best to improve outcome? Clin Microbiol Rev. 2003;16(3):415–29.
128. Tunkel AR, Scheld WM. Pathogenesis and pathophysiology of bacterial meningitis. Clin Microbiol Rev. 1993;6(2):118–36.
129. Van De Beek D, De Gans J. Dexamethasone and pneumococcal meningitis. Ann Intern Med. 2004;141:327. http://annals.org/article.aspx?doi=10.7326/0003-4819-141-4-200408170-00028.
130. Brouwer MC, Mcintyre P, Prasad K, van de Beek D. Corticosteroids for acute bacterial meningitis. Cochrane Database Syst Rev. 2015;2016(3).
131. de Gans J, van de Beek D. Dexamethasone in adults with bacterial meningitis. N Engl J Med. 2002;347(20):1549–56. http://www.nejm.org/doi/abs/10.1056/NEJMoa021334.
132. Assiri AM, AlAsmari FA, Zimmerman VA, Baddour LM, Erwin PJ, Tleyjeh IM. Corticosteroid administration and outcome of adolescents and adults with acute bacterial meningitis: a meta-analysis. Mayo Clin Proc. 2009;84(5):403–9.
133. Tice AD, Strait K, Ramey R, Hoaglund PA. Outpatient parenteral antimicrobial therapy for central nervous system infections. Clin Infect Dis. 1999;29(6):1394–9.
134. Waler JA, Rathore MH. Outpatient management of pediatric bacterial meningitis. Pediatr Infect Dis J. 1995;14(2):89.
135. Van De Beek D, De Gans J, McIntyre P, Prasad K. Steroids in adults with acute bacterial meningitis: a systematic review. Lancet Infect Dis. 2004;4(3):139–43.
136. Klugman KP, Friedland IR, Bradley JS. Bactericidal activity against cephalosporin-resistant Streptococcus pneumoniae in cerebrospinal fluid of children with acute bacterial meningitis. Antimicrob Agents Chemother. 1995;39(9):1988–92.
137. Viladrich PF, Gudiol F, Linares J, Pallares R, Sabate I, Rufi G, et al. Evaluation of vancomycin for therapy of adult pneumococcal meningitis. Antimicrob Agents Chemother. 1991;35(12):2467–72.
138. Tos M. Course of and sequelae to 248 petrosal fractures. Acta Otolaryngol. 1973;75(2–6):353–4.
139. Price DJE, Sleigh JD. Control of infection due to Klebsiella aerogenes in a neurosurgical unit by withdrawal of all antibiotics. Lancet. 1970;296(7685):1213–5.
140. Rathore MH. Do prophylactic antibiotics prevent meningitis after basilar skull fracture? Pediatr Infect Dis J. 1991;10(2):87–8. https://insights.ovid.com/crossref?an=00006454-199102000-00001.
141. Stankiewicz JA. Cerebrospinal fluid fistula and endoscopic sinus surgery. Laryngoscope. 1991;101:250–6.
142. Carrau RL, Snyderman C, Janecka IP, Sekhar L, Sen C, D'Amico F. Antibiotic prophylaxis in cranial base surgery. Head Neck. 1991;13(4):311–7.
143. Carroll WR, Rosenstiel D, Fix JR, De la Torre J, Solomon JS, Brodish B, et al. Three-dose vs extended-course clindamycin prophylaxis for free-flap reconstruction of the head and neck. Arch Otolaryngol Head Neck Surg. 2003;129(7):771–4.
144. Coskun H, Erisen L, Basut O. Factors affecting wound infection rates in head and neck surgery. Otolaryngol Head Neck Surg. 2000;123(3):328–33.
145. McIntyre PB, O'Brien KL, Greenwood B, Van De Beek D. Effect of vaccines on bacterial meningitis worldwide. Lancet. 2012;380:1703–11.
146. Brouwer MC, Tunkel AR, Van De Beek D. Epidemiology, diagnosis, and antimicrobial treatment of acute bacterial meningitis. Clin Microbiol Rev. 2010;23:467–92.
147. Rubin LG, Levin MJ, Ljungman P, Davies EG, Avery R, Tomblyn M, et al. 2013 IDSA clinical practice guideline for vaccination of the Immunocompromised Host. Clin Infect Dis. 2014;58(3):e44–100. https://academic.oup.com/cid/article/58/3/e44/336537.

Evidence-Based Medicine in Cerebrospinal Fluid Leak and Skull Base Reconstruction

37

Seth M. Lieberman and Michael G. Stewart

37.1 Evidence-Based Diagnosis of Cerebrospinal Fluid Rhinorrhea

There are clearly different techniques for the diagnosis of cerebrospinal fluid (CSF) rhinorrhea—and these techniques have evolved over time. There is some good evidence supporting the effectiveness of certain methods, however experience also plays a role since the evidence is not high-level or definitive. That statement is not a critique of the authors that have published on the topic; rather, it is a reflection of the rarity of the condition, and the difficulty in performing true randomized or controlled trials in this diagnosis. We have divided this section of the chapter into discussion on the diagnosis of CSF rhinorrhea—whether or not it is present—and the localization of the leak—after the diagnosis has been established—and a section on intrathecal fluorescein, which is used for both diagnosis and localization.

S. M. Lieberman (✉)
Department of Otolaryngology-Head and Neck Surgery, NYU Langone Health, New York, NY, USA
e-mail: Seth.Lieberman@nyulangone.org

M. G. Stewart
Department of Otolaryngology-Head and Neck Surgery, Vice Dean of the Medical College, Weill Cornell Medical College, Otolaryngologist-in-Chief, NewYork-Presbyterian Hospital/Weill Cornell Medical Center, New York, NY, USA

37.1.1 Diagnosis

It is important to first identify that CSF is present in the rhinorrhea, since non-CSF rhinorrhea is a common symptom and finding. The possible techniques are the ring sign, glucose testing, beta-2 transferrin testing, beta trace protein testing, fluorescein testing, and radionucleotide testing.

Oakley et al. performed an evidence-based review with recommendations in 2016, based on studies from 1990 to 2014 [1]. They used standard search methodology and identified 68 possible studies and evaluated them for study methodology and quality, and then created evidence tables summarizing the level of evidence and the findings. As is typical in such reports, multiple authors worked independently and if there was disagreement it was resolved using a standardized methodology. The highest collective grade of evidence they identified was Grade C, so there is not high-level evidence available for any of these tests. Nevertheless, the findings tended to be consistent across studies and also supported by clinical experience, so the pooled evidence is still quite helpful.

37.1.1.1 Ring Sign

There is no good published evidence to support this diagnostic technique, which is not surprising as it is a subjective tool that was used before more specific and sensitive studies were available [1]. The authors "Recommended Against"

A. A. AlQahtani et al. (eds.), *CSF Rhinorrhea*, https://doi.org/10.1007/978-3-030-94781-1_37

the use of ring testing in the diagnosis of CSF rhinorrhea.

37.1.1.2 Glucose Test

It was originally believed that there was no glucose in nasal rhinorrhea, so the presence of glucose in the fluid would indicate the presence of CSF, however this was disproved many years ago by studies identifying the presence of glucose in nasal secretions in certain medical conditions. In addition, some authors used glucose test strips (designed for use in urinalysis) and said a positive result was abnormal. Others sent the fluid for glucose level testing, but the cutoff for an elevated test was never established. The specificity and sensitivity of glucose strip testing were determined to be specificity from 20% to 45%, and sensitivity from 80% to 100% [1]. High sensitivity is not surprising because most patients do not have a CSF leak, so there are many true negative tests and very few false negatives. The low specificity is very concerning however, as the test generates many false positive results. The evidence-based recommendation was "Recommend Against."

37.1.1.3 Beta-2 Transferrin

This is a protein which is present in CSF but not in nasal secretions, so the detection of beta-2 transferrin should have a high specificity for CSF rhinorrhea. There were nine different studies on the accuracy of beta-2 transferrin testing, and the pooled data found very high sensitivity and specificity of >90%, when the testing results were all verified using surgical findings. In addition to the high specificity and sensitivity, the cost of testing was very low compared to some other methodologies, and the risk was also very low since the test is noninvasive. Based on this evidence, the authors "Recommended For" the use of beta-2 transferrin testing in the diagnosis of CSF rhinorrhea [1]. Interestingly, the authors identified one study which evaluated whether the specimen must be kept refrigerated (which many believe), and that study found no difference in positive testing rates whether the specimens were stored and delivered at room temperature or were kept refrigerated, so in fact there is evidence that the fluid can be sent for testing even if not refrigerated [2].

37.1.1.4 Beta Trace Protein

Beta trace protein is also present in the CSF in high concentrations; it is also present in blood but at much lower concentrations. In some medical conditions the protein levels are altered, for example renal failure increases blood levels, and bacterial meningitis decreases CSF levels. Nevertheless, there are several studies which show that sensitivity (91–100%) and specificity (86–100%) of beta trace protein are about as high as beta-2 transferrin, and the test is also inexpensive and has a rapid turnaround time of 15 min. Based on the evidence, the authors "Recommended For" the use of beta trace protein. The authors also quoted prices of about $38 for beta-2 transferrin, and about $20 for beta trace protein testing in the 2016 article [1].

In the opinion of the chapter authors, there do not seem to be significant advantages of beta trace protein compared to beta-2 transferrin, and no reason to recommend one test over the other. In practice, beta trace protein seems to be used more frequently in Europe, and beta-2 transferrin more frequently in the United States, likely due to test availability.

37.1.1.5 Radionuclide Cisternography

The authors also reviewed the evidence supporting this test as a diagnostic tool, however it is expensive, invasive, and has only moderate accuracy, so the authors "Recommended against" its use as a diagnostic test [1].

37.1.1.6 Other Radiologic Testing

Typically, the diagnosis of CSF rhinorrhea is performed with markers within the fluid itself, however sometimes the fluid cannot be collected and tested, so the diagnosis of CSF rhinorrhea remains unproven. In those cases, radiologic testing can be considered for the diagnosis of CSF rhinorrhea. The evaluation of the evidence on radiologic testing for diagnosis and localization is very difficult to parse, because the tests are done for both reasons, often within the same series. So, using radiologic evaluation can prove the presence of a leak, and can also identify or confirm the location of that leak. If the diagnosis is confirmed by examination of the fluid, then the radiologic testing is performed for localization only.

The next section covers the evidence on radiologic evaluation, which includes both localization and diagnosis.

37.1.2 Localization

Marker testing will often not localize the exact leak site, although it can narrow down the potential sites. Once the diagnosis has been established, radiologic testing is frequently used for the anatomic localization of the leak.

A systematic review was reported in 2019 on the radiologic evaluation for CSF leak [3]. It was a more comprehensive assessment than just CSF rhinorrhea, and included traumatic injuries and CSF otorrhea. Nevertheless, the findings are useful for any case where radiologic localization is needed. The authors screened 2125 papers and identified 38 studies for review, which included 1000 total patients.

37.1.2.1 Radionuclide Cisternography

The authors pooled the data from different modalities and reported sensitivity ranges. Radionuclide cisternography had only 2 studies, and only one reported sensitivity, which was 76%. These were older studies, and the more contemporary reports did not use this technology.

37.1.2.2 Computed Tomography Scanning

CT imaging will show bony detail and help localize a leak's location, but will not demonstrate actual CSF. It is typically performed without IV contrast. CT cisternography requires a lumbar puncture and injection of radiopaque contrast material with subsequent CT imaging.

CT imaging for localization and/or diagnosis was reported in 24 studies, and included both high-resolution CT and CT cisternography with intrathecal contrast [3]. Sensitivities ranged from 58.8% to 100% for high-resolution CT, and from 37.5% to 72.3% for cisternography.

The Oakley et al. evidence-based review with recommendation from 2016 found some conflicting data on the sensitivity and specificity of high-resolution CT scanning in identifying the location of a CSF leak, primarily because natural bony dehiscences can occur with no leak [1]. Overall sensitivity and specificity ranged from 44% to 100% (sensitivity) and 45% to 100% (specificity), but some studies found high-resolution CT to be 100% accurate. The cost was moderate and the harm was minimal (radiation exposure), and based on their review, they made a "Recommendation for" high-resolution CT scanning as an initial test for localization. CT cisternography with intrathecal contrast requires a lumbar puncture, and actually has lower sensitivity than MR cisternography, which is a noninvasive, high-resolution T2-weighted MR, so the authors made a "Recommendation against" CT cisternography with intrathecal contrast.

37.1.2.3 Magnetic Resonance Imaging

Eljazzar et al. identified 29 studies which evaluated Magnetic Resonance Imaging, but there were variations on the theme: 3-D techniques, T1 and T2 weighted images, and MR cisternography with intrathecal contrast were all studied [3]. "MR cisternography" can be performed without contrast using the CSF enhancing characteristics of T2 imaging sequences, or MR cisternography can include intrathecal injection of gadolinium. Sensitivity ranges of MRI were broad: 3D techniques from 74.7% to 100%, T1 and T2 techniques from 11.8% to 100%, and cisternography with injected contrast from 56% to 100%.

The Oakley review concluded that MR imaging with T2-weighted images was more expensive and had similar sensitivity and specificity as high-resolution CT. The addition of intrathecal contrast to MR scanning added more cost and invasiveness (lumbar puncture is of course required). However, when the diagnosis is in doubt, you do get the potential added benefit of demonstrating CSF outside the cranial cavity. The authors concluded with a "Recommendation for" noninvasive MR cisternography, ".....where cheaper or less invasive studies have failed to diagnose or localize the site of a leak," and they did not make a recommendation on MR with intrathecal contrast [1].

37.1.2.4 Combination Studies

Eljazzar et al. also reviewed 6 studies which combined CT and MRI studies, and found sensitivities from 89.7% to 95% [3]. They commented that MRI and CT are of course complementary because of the differences in soft tissue and bony detail offered by each modality.

The authors' overall conclusion was that MRI studies had higher overall sensitivity to detect a leak, but lacked the bony detail to fully localize the leak, and they recommended consideration of a strategy of MRI first, followed by CT if needed [3]. There are also fusion technologies which overlay the MR and CT images. The authors commented that the studies often did not distinguish between active and inactive leaks, and there was no stratification based on etiology. Based on the heterogeneity of the studies and the techniques, the authors were also unable to make evidence-based recommendations on which specific CT or MRI technique (contrast vs. cisternography, etc.) was preferred for individual cases [3].

37.1.3 Intrathecal Fluorescein

Finally, fluorescein injected intrathecally can be used for both diagnosis and localization of CSF rhinorrhea. This is an off-label application of fluorescein, which is not approved for intrathecal use. However, there is a lot of published evidence supporting the use and safety of <u>dilute</u> fluorescein intrathecally. Adverse neurologic events from intrathecal fluorescein have been reported after doses from 100 mg to 700 mg, and the Otolaryngology and Neurosurgery communities generally use no more than 50 mg total and often as little as 10–20 mg [4]. When used outside the operating room, fluorescein can be diluted with sterile saline for injection, and when used in the operating room setting, it is usually diluted with CSF which was extracted from the lumbar drain, and the mixture is then reinjected into the CSF [4]. In the United States, fluorescein is available as a 10% solution, intended for intravenous injection, and it states on the bottle "Not for intrathecal use." So the patient must be counseled about the indications, risks, and the off-label use. Nevertheless, dilute fluorescein is used intrathecally by large numbers of Otolaryngologists, and survey studies have indicated similar popularity in the Neurosurgery community.

If you dilute 0.2 ml of 10% fluorescein into 9.8 ml of withdrawn CSF, then you have created a 2 mg/ml fluorescein solution. Injection of all 10 ml of this solution would be a total dose of 20 mg—a dose that the literature supports to be safe with minimal risk of major complication.

The evidence on the effectiveness of fluorescein as an intraoperative localization tool is very limited because comparative studies have not been performed. Anecdotally many surgeons report it to be very useful—attesting to their perception of benefit which is worth the risk—and they use it routinely even when they are confident about the location, often to confirm that the leak has been closed intraoperatively. However there is no pooled or comparative evidence on which to make an evidence-based recommendation.

Fluorescein could be used as a preoperative diagnostic or localization test, but it would require lumbar puncture and evaluation in a non-operative setting, and there are no data on this application. There are three studies which reported the use of topical fluorescein: it is placed into the nasal cavity, and then a CSF leak can be identified by a color change of the fluorescein at that site. Obviously this is subjective, and cannot be used if the potential leak site is not visible with intranasal endoscopy, and although the studies reported "100% accuracy" there are no comparative or saline-controlled trials, and the results are likely not consistently reproducible.

The overall evidence-based recommendation on the use of intrathecal fluorescein for localization and/or diagnosis was "Option." [1].

37.2 Evidence-Based Management of CSF Rhinorrhea and Skull Base Reconstruction

Management of ventral skull base cerebrospinal fluid leaks has evolved considerably over the past few decades as the technology and techniques of endoscopic skull base surgery have been developed. Based on the published literature, the trend has been toward less invasive surgery, decreased rates of recurrent CSF leaks, and decreased morbidity. Our patients have truly benefitted from these advancements. There are many decisions that must be made when managing these patients that go beyond whether to use an endoscopic or open approach. Here we will address the recent and pertinent literature related to such topics, including some of the gaps in the literature.

37.2.1 Spontaneous CSF Rhinorrhea

Spontaneous CSF rhinorrhea in patients with Idiopathic intracranial hypertension (IIH) has been increasing in the proportion of all CSF rhinorrhea patients, most likely due to the worsening obesity epidemic [5]. The postoperative management of these patients pertains primarily to the outcome of recurrent CSF leak. Given the pathophysiology behind spontaneous CSF rhinorrhea, controlling intracranial pressures is plausibly an important intervention to minimize recurrence of CSF leaks whether through behavioral (i.e., diet and exercise), pharmacologic (e.g., acetazolamide), or surgical interventions (e.g., bariatric surgery, shunting procedure).

37.2.1.1 Weight Loss

Data on the effect of weight loss in the IIH patient population mainly come from patients who do not have concomitant CSF rhinorrhea. Weight loss has been shown to improve the symptoms and signs of idiopathic intracranial pressure in both retrospective and prospective studies. Sinclair et al. performed a prospective study of 25 women with IIH treated with a low-energy diet [6]. These women served as their own controls after 3 months of a low-energy diet with an average weight loss of 16 kg (15% of body weight). Papilledema grade also improved, as did headaches, tinnitus, and diplopia. Though the group's intracranial pressure decreased on average, only 4 of 20 (5 refused follow-up lumbar puncture) patients developed normal intracranial pressure. Therefore the majority of patients experienced improvement in symptoms despite persistently elevated intracranial pressure. Manfield et al., performed a systematic review and comparison of meta-analyses evaluating bariatric surgery or nonsurgical weight loss for idiopathic intracranial hypertension, and both weight loss interventions resulted in a decrease in CSF pressure [7]. While we can only infer the effect of weight loss on outcomes after CSF leak repair from the available literature, the beneficial effects on CSF pressure and other IIH symptoms, not to mention the more globally positive health effects, suggests that this issue should be addressed in overweight and obese patients treated for spontaneous CSF rhinorrhea.

37.2.1.2 Acetazolamide and Shunt

The use of acetazolamide in the postoperative management of IIH patients with spontaneous CSF rhinorrhea is also a controversial topic. The most recent and scientifically rigorous evaluation of this population was the Idiopathic Intracranial Hypertension Treatment Trial (IIHTT) which evaluated 165 participants at 38 sites in North America with IIH who were randomized to 2 treatment arms: *acetazolamide + weight loss* versus *placebo + weight loss*. Of the 165 patients, 85 agreed to undergo repeat LP at 6 months. The acetazolamide group had a significantly greater decrease in CSF pressure (treatment effect (-)59.9 mm H_2O; 95% CI (-)96.4 to (-)23.4 mm H_2O, $p = 0.002$) [8].

The dosing used was 1 tablet (250 mg) of acetazolamide twice daily with subsequent dosage increases of 1 tablet every week up to a maximum of 8 tablets twice daily (4 g/d of acetazolamide). Dosage escalation was stopped if the subject reported related symptoms. Thirty-eight of 86 (44.1%) tolerated the maximum dosage [9]. Therefore, while acetazolamide does appear to have the effect of lowering elevated intracranial pressure in patients with IIH, it is unclear from the literature the efficacy of lowering recurrence of CSF leaks in patients with spontaneous CSF rhinorrhea. Dosing regimens vary widely and, in addition to its utility in managing patients with spontaneous CSF leaks, would be considered another gap in our knowledge regarding this intervention.

Teachey et al. put forth a large prospective case series and systematic review of the literature with a total of 679 patients undergoing treatment for CSF rhinorrhea to evaluate whether postoperative control of intracranial pressure in this patient population affected outcomes. The interventions included lumbar puncture, lumbar drain, ventriculostomy, acetazolamide, or permanent CSF diversion with shunt. Lumbar drain alone was not considered an intervention unless used as an assessment for long-term intervention. They found the success rate for the active intervention cohort was 92.8% versus 81.9% in the no active ICP management group ($P < 0.001$) [10].

While controlling intracranial pressure is plausibly an effective and widely accepted intervention for reducing recurrence rates of CSF rhinorrhea in the IIH population, this specific outcome has not been evaluated in a prospective randomized fashion, likely in part due to the rarity of this disease process. Future research endeavors can evaluate the most clinically- and cost-effective means for realizing this outcome. A few examples of lingering questions that can potentially be addressed with prospective randomized trials include the following: How effective is weight loss at preventing recurrent leaks and is this intervention equivalent to weight loss plus pharmacologic intervention? Is bariatric surgery more effective than behavioral modification at preventing recurrent leak? Does acetazolamide decrease the rates of leak recurrence and what is the optimal dosing? How do shunting procedures compare with these procedures in terms of leak prevention and quality of life outcomes?

37.2.2 Lumbar Drainage in the Management of CSF Rhinorrhea

Lumbar drainage carries a risk of persistent drainage after removal, overdrainage and subsequent pneumocephalus or subdural hemorrhage, and retained catheter [11]. On the topic of its utility in postoperative management of CSF leak repair, the literature predominantly consists of retrospective case series. Ahmed et al. performed a meta-analysis dedicated to evaluating the efficacy of perioperative lumbar drainage following CSF leak repair for anterior cranial fossa defects, with all etiologies included. They found that there was insufficient evidence that lumbar drainage decreases CSF leak recurrence after endoscopic repair of anterior skull base defects [12].

37.2.2.1 High-Flow Leaks

Zwagerman et al. performed a randomized controlled trial (RCT) of lumbar drain placement after endoscopic skull base surgery [13]. The drains were placed after the surgical closure was completed, and surgeons were blinded to which patients would receive the drain until after the repair. Inclusion criteria included patients with high-flow leaks, dural defects greater than 1 cm^2 and either extended arachnoid dissection, and/or dissection into a ventricle or cistern. One hundred seventy patients were randomized into the study. Skull base repair consisted of multilayer reconstruction including a vascularized flap. Lumbar drainage was performed at 10 cm^3/h for 72 h. Primary outcome was the presence of a CSF leak during the 30 day follow-up period. There was a significant difference in CSF leak rate between the 2 groups, with the LD group at 8.2% and the no-LD at 21.2% prompting early cessation of the study.

37.2.2.2 Low-Flow Leaks

Albu et al. performed a prospective randomized study evaluating use of lumbar drainage in 150 patients with CSF rhinorrhea from trauma, iatrogenic etiology, or spontaneous CSF rhinorrhea [14]. In contrast to the Zwagerman et al. study, patients were excluded if they had high-flow leaks with exposed cisterns or ventricles. One hundred fifty patients were randomized over a 12 years period to either postoperative lumbar drain for 72 h versus no lumbar drain. The method of repair did not include a vascularized flap, but mainly an underlay with bone or cartilage for large defects followed by a mucosal graft. Seventy-five patients were randomized to each group. In patients with LDs, success rate was 95%, compared to 92% in the control group, and the difference was not statistically significant ($p = 0.2$). The only factors found to be significantly associated with recurrent leak was the presence of elevated intracranial pressure (77% vs. 96%).

Taking the results of both studies, these data suggest that lumbar drainage may provide benefit in large defects with high-flow leaks, but not with low-flow leaks. Future studies to address the gaps in our knowledge would include continued stratification of clinical factors such as defect size and flow rates, as well as patient specific factors, such as BMI and sleep apnea.

37.2.3 Vascularized Flap Versus Free Graft

The improvement in the success rate of skull base reconstruction has allowed endoscopic skull base surgery to grow as a field. Perhaps the biggest contribution was the development of the nasoseptal flap, first described in 2006 [15]. The innovation of an intranasal vascularized pedicled flap has led to the development of a variety of other local and regional vascularized flaps that are options when the nasoseptal flap is unavailable or inadequate. While there have been no RCTs evaluating vascularized versus avascular grafts in skull base reconstruction, their utility is supported by the literature in the form of case series and meta-analyses.

37.2.3.1 Large Versus Small Skull Base Defects

Harvey et al. performed a systematic review evaluating reconstruction of large skull base defects defined as 3 cm or greater [16]. Of 609 patients with large dural defect, the overall rate of CSF leak was 11.5%, with 15.6% for free grafts and 6.7% for vascularized reconstruction ($x^2 = 11.88$, $P = 0.001$). Soudry et al. performed a systematic review of the literature evaluating reconstruction of surgically-created anterior skull base defects [17]. Of 673 patients, the overall success rate was 91.5%. When comparing outcomes by subsite of defect, there were no clear differences between vascularized and nonvascularized reconstruction techniques for any individual subsite apart from the clivus, for which a vascularized pedicled flap was associated with a higher success rate. For any given subsite, higher flow leaks were repaired with greater success rates when vascularized tissue was used (94% vs. 82%), but were equivalent in low-flow leaks.

When considering the appropriate technique for skull base reconstruction, the surgeon must take into account patient factors (e.g., body habitus, presence of IIH, sleep apnea, age), defect factors (e.g., location, size, flow rate, entry of tumor into cistern or ventricle), and disease factors (e.g., need for radiation, mucosal involvement of tumor, risk of recurrent disease). The current literature supports that utilizing vascularized tissue will improve the success rate of skull base reconstruction for large skull base defects, but this may not hold true for smaller defects. There are many reconstructive algorithms available [18, 19], and future studies with stratification of defect and patient specific factors will further delineate the most appropriate and least morbid reconstructive approach for smaller defects.

37.2.4 Non-iatrogenic Traumatic CSF Rhinorrhea

37.2.4.1 Antibiotics

There have been several RCTs and meta-analyses evaluating the use of antibiotics in patients with traumatic CSF rhinorrhea. The majority has not found a significant difference between the antibiotic and no antibiotic groups in terms of infectious complications [20–23]. The most recent meta-analysis on this topic was a Cochrane review, evaluating 5 RCTs, comprising a total of 208 participants with basilar skull fracture comparing groups with and without preventative antibiotic therapy [24]. The study found no significant difference for incidence of infection (OR 0.69; 95% confidence interval = 0.29 to 1.61). When evaluating subgoups of patients with and without CSF leakage, again no difference was found. The authors also performed a meta-analysis of controlled nonrandomized studies. This meta-analysis consisted of 2168 participants with the frequency of meningitis 6.92% in the treatment group and 6.52% in the control group, with an OR 1.13; (95% CI = 0.67 to 1.88). In a subgroup analysis of the nonrandomized studies, the authors analyzed subgroups of patients with and without CSF leakage. For participants with CSF leakage, the OR was 0.61 (95% CI 0.37 to 0.99) and for patients without CSF leakage it was 0.86 (95% CI 0.27 to 2.78). Based on this analysis, the authors state that there is insufficient evidence to support or refute the use of antibiotics to prevent meningitis in patients with basilar skull fractures. Better stratification in future studies would be necessary to elucidate whether antibiotic prophylaxis prevents meningitis in patients with active CSF rhinorrhea or presence of pneumocephalus.

37.2.4.2 Lumbar Drain

Most leaks will resolve within 7–10 days with conservative treatment [25]. Management options include conservative management with bed rest, lumbar drain, or primary repair. Most of the current data regarding this topic are based on cohort studies. Albu et al., however, performed a RCT to evaluate the utility of lumbar drainage versus conservative therapy on outcomes in patients with traumatic CSF leaks [26]. The patients included in the study were highly selected and had to meet the following criteria: persistent rhinorrhea beyond 48 h, absence of pneumocephalus on presentation, blunt cranial trauma, and admitted within 24 h following the start of rhinorrhea. Patients were excluded if they presented with CSF otorrhea, or had evidence of pneumocephalus, meningitis, intracranial hemorrhage, cerebral edema or cerebral contusion. Thirty patients were randomly allocated to each treatment arm—lumbar drainage or bed rest—and drained at 10 ml/h. The lumbar drain was removed once the CSF rhinorrhea stopped, or after a maximal time period of 10 days. Antibiotics were not used in either group. Mean time interval of CSF leak in patients managed with LDs was 4.83 ± 1.88 days while in the conservatively managed patients leakage persisted for 7.03 ± 2.02 days (95% CI 3.05–1.35, $p < 0.0001$). In addition, 2 patients in the conservative arm ultimately needed endoscopic repair while none in the treatment arm underwent operative repair. Rates of recurrent CSF rhinorrhea and meningitis were not different between groups.

Therefore, while a small sample, this study does provide level 1b evidence showing some benefit to LD in terms of leak duration and need for operative repair in a select group of patients with traumatic CSF rhinorrhea. While there were not significant adverse effects of LD amongst the 30 patients receiving this intervention, we know that these risks do exist, and so risks and benefits of this intervention must be considered.

37.2.5 Antibiotics in Surgical Defects

While there was initial concern that endoscopic skull base surgery would increase the risk of postoperative intracranial infections due to the communication between the sinonasal and intracranial cavities, the actual rates of infection have been shown to be quite low at around 2% or less [27–30]. While prevention of postoperative infection largely relies on prevention of postoperative CSF leak, there is no consensus on appropriate perioperative antibiotics management [31]. Based on a survey sent out by Johans et al., there is considerable variation in perioperative antibiotic regimens among different institutions and surgeons [30]. The data are largely based on retrospective or prospective nonrandomized studies with a heterogeneous mixture of skull base pathologies.

Therefore, the optimal perioperative antibiotic regimen remains elusive in endoscopic skull base surgery. It is not clear whether there is benefit to continuing antibiotics into the postoperative period, and if so, for which patients. We also do not know if there are patient, pathologic, or intraoperative factors that can help us to determine this. For example, the postoperative infection risk for a patient undergoing a 5-h resection of a large tuberculum sellae meningioma is likely higher than for a patient undergoing a routine pituitary adenoma resection with a small tear of the diaphragma sella or a patient with a spontaneous CSF leak through a 1 mm defect of the cribriform plate. It is also unclear if reconstruction technique affects risk of infection; for example, do we need antibiotics in patients with nonabsorbable packing? These are just a few gaps in our knowledge which cannot be answered using the existing observational studies.

References

1. Oakley GM, Alt JA, Schlosser RH, Harvey RJ, Orlandi RR. Diagnosis of cerebrospinal fluid rhinorrhea: an evidence-based review with recommendations. Int Forum Allergy Rhinol. 2016;6:8–16.
2. Bleier BS, Debnath I, et al. Preliminary study on the stability of beta-2 transferrin in extracorporeal cerebrospinal fluid. Otolaryngol Head Neck Surg. 2011;144:101–3.
3. Eljazzar R, Loewenstern J, Dai JB, Shrivastava RK, Iloreta AM. Detection of cerebrospinal fluid leaks: is there a radiologic standard of care? A systematic review. World Neurosurg. 2019;127:307–15.
4. Keerl R, Weber RK, Draf W, Wienke A, Schaefer SD. Use of sodium fluorescein solution for detection of cerebrospinal fluid fistulas: an analysis of 420 administrations and reported complications in Europe and the United States. Laryngoscope. 2004;114:266–72.
5. Nelson RF, Gantz BJ, Hansen MR. The rising incidence of spontaneous cerebrospinal fluid leaks in the United States and the association with obesity and obstructive sleep apnea. Otol Neurotol. 2015;36:476–80.
6. Sinclair AJ, Burdon MA, Nightingale PG, Ball AK, Good P, Matthews TD, Jacks A, Lawden M, Clarke CE, Stewart PM, Walker EA, Tomlinson JW, Rauz S. Low energy diet and intracranial pressure in women with idiopathic intracranial hypertension: prospective cohort study. BMJ. 2010;341:c2701. https://doi.org/10.1136/bmj.c2701.
7. Manfield JH, Yu KK, Efthimiou E, Darzi A, Athanasiou T, Ashrafian. Bariatric surgery or non-surgical weight loss for idiopathic intracranial hypertension? A systematic review and comparison of meta-analyses. Obes Surg. 2017;27(2):513–21.
8. Kattah JC, Pula JH, Mejico LJ, McDermott MP, Kupersmith MJ, Wall M. CSF pressure, papilledema grade, and response to acetazolamide in the idiopathic intracranial hypertension treatment trial. J Neurol. 2015;262(10):2271–4.
9. ten Hove MW, Friedman DI, Patel AD, Irrcher I, Wall M, McDermott MP, et al. Safety and tolerability of acetazolamide in the idiopathic intracranial hypertension treatment trial. J Neuroophthalmol. 2016;36(1):13–9.
10. Teachey W, Grayson J, Cho DY, Riley KO, Woodworth BA. Intervention for elevated intracranial pressure improves success rate after repair of spontaneous cerebrospinal fluid leaks. Laryngoscope. 2017;127(9):2011–6.
11. Ransom ER, Palmer JN, Kennedy DW, Chiu AG. Assessing risk/benefit of lumbar drain use for endoscopic skull-base surgery. Int Forum Allergy Rhinol. 2011;1:173–7.
12. Ahmed OH, Marcus S, Tauber JR, Wang B, Fang Y, Lebowitz RA. Efficacy of perioperative lumbar drainage following Endonasal endoscopic cerebrospinal fluid leak repair. Otolaryngol Head Neck Surg. 2017;156(1):52–60.
13. Zwagerman NT, Wang EW, Shin SS, Chang YF, Fernandez-Miranda JC, Snyderman CH, et al. Does lumbar drainage reduce postoperative cerebrospinal fluid leak after endoscopic endonasal skull base surgery? A prospective, randomized controlled trial. J Neurosurg. 2018:1–7.
14. Albu S, Emanuelli E, Trombitas V, Florian IS. Effectiveness of lumbar drains on recurrence rates in endoscopic surgery of cerebrospinal fluid leaks. Am J Rhinol Allergy. 2013;27(6):e190–4.
15. Hadad G, Bassagasteguy L, Carrau RL, Mataza JC, Kassam A, Snyderman CH, Mintz AH. A novel reconstructive technique after endoscopic expanded endonasal approaches: vascular pedicle nasoseptal flap. Laryngoscope. 2006;116:1882–6.
16. Harvey RJ, Parmar P, Sacks R, Zanation AM. Endoscopic skull base reconstruction of large dural defects: a systematic review of published evidence. Laryngoscope. 2012;122(2):452–9.
17. Soudry E, Turner JH, Nayak JV, Hwang PH. Endoscopic reconstruction of surgically created skull base defects: a systematic review. Otolaryngol Head Neck Surg. 2014;150(5):730–8.
18. Turri-Zanoni M, Zocchi J, Lambertoni A, Giovannardi M, Karligkiotis A, Battaglia P, et al. Endoscopic Endonasal reconstruction of anterior Skull Base defects: what factors really affect the outcomes? World Neurosurg. 2018;116:e436–e43.

19. Patel MR, Stadler ME, Snyderman CH, Carrau RL, Kassam AB, Germanwala AV, et al. How to choose? Endoscopic skull base reconstructive options and limitations. Skull Base. 2010;20(6):397–404.
20. Brodie HA. Prophylactic antibiotics for posttraumatic cerebrospinal fluid fistulae. A meta-analysis. Arch Otolaryngol Head Neck Surg. 1997;123(7):749–52.
21. Eftekhar B, Ghodsi M, Nejat F, Ketabchi E, Esmaeeli B. Prophylactic administration of ceftriaxone for the prevention of meningitis after traumatic pneumocephalus: results of a clinical trial. J Neurosurg. 2004;101(5):757–61.
22. Villalobos T, Arango C, Kubilis P, Rathore M. Antibiotic prophylaxis after basilar skull fractures: a meta-analysis. Clin Infect Dis. 1998;27(2):364–9.
23. Rathore MJ. Do prophylactic antibiotics prevent meningitis after basilar skull fracture? Pediatr Infect Dis J. 1991;10:87–8.
24. Ratilal BO, Costa J, Pappamikail L, Sampaio C. Antibiotic prophylaxis for preventing meningitis in patients with basilar skull fractures. Cochrane Database Sys Rev. 2015; https://doi.org/10.1002/14651858.CD004884.pub4.
25. Bell RB, Dierks EJ, Homer L, Potter BE. Management of cerebrospinal fluid leak associated with craniomaxillofacial trauma. J Oral Maxillofac Surg. 2004;62:676–84.
26. Albu S, Florian IS, Bolboaca SD. The benefit of early lumbar drain insertion in reducing the length of CSF leak in traumatic rhinorrhea. Clin Neurol Neurosurg. 2016;142:43–7.
27. Dehdashti AR, Ganna A, Karabatsou K, Gentili F. Pure endoscopic endonasal approach for pituitary adenomas: early surgical results in 200 patients and comparison with previous microsurgical series. Neurosurgery. 2008;62:1006–115.
28. Brown SM, Anand VK, Tabaee A, Schwartz TH. Role of perioperative antibiotics in endoscopic skull base surgery. Laryngoscope. 2007;117:1528–32.
29. Kassam AB, Prevedello DM, Carrau RL, Snyderman CH, Thomas A, Gardner P, et al. Endoscopic endonasal skull base surgery: analysis of complications in the authors' initial 800 patients. J Neurosurg. 2011;114:1544–68.
30. Johans SJ, Burkett DJ, Swong KN, Patel CR, Germanwala AV. Antibiotic prophylaxis and infection prevention for endoscopic endonasal skull base surgery: our protocol, results, and review of the literature. J Clin Neurosci. 2018;47:249–53.
31. Horowitz G, Fliss DM, Margalit N, Wasserzug O, Gil Z. Association between cerebrospinal fluid leak and meningitis after skull base surgery. Otolaryngol Head Neck Surg. 2011;145:689–93.

Quality of Life in CSF Leak

38

G. F. J. P. M. Adriaensen, S. Reitsma, and W. J. Fokkens

38.1 Introduction

Quality of life (QOL) is a multidimensional construct that describes an individual's overall perception of well-being [1]. Over the past decades, measuring QOL and using it as an outcome parameter for (surgical) therapies has become more and more common practice in many areas of medicine. When considering cerebrospinal fluid (CSF) rhinorrhea, it seems very likely that this condition impacts a patient's QOL in multiple ways. The burden of CSF rhinorrhea is formed by symptoms of (intermittent) watery discharge from the nose and, in case of a severe leak, symptoms of CSF hypotension. Furthermore, the communication between the intracranial contents and the nasal cavity produces a risk of meningitis (about 10% per year) [2], which gives rise to uncertainty and worrying. Depending on the size and location of the defect, and on the underlying pathology causing the CSF rhinorrhea, less or more extensive surgery is needed. All have their own morbidity and therefore effect on QOL.

G. F. J. P. M. Adriaensen (✉) · S. Reitsma
W. J. Fokkens
Department of Otorhinolaryngology, Amsterdam UMC location University of Amsterdam, Amsterdam, The Netherlands
e-mail: G.F.Adriaensen@amsterdamumc.nl

38.2 Measuring Quality of Life

QOL assessments provide patient-reported estimates of well-being that may be clinically relevant [3]. They eliminate possible observer bias introduced by the clinician via directed questioning and subjective estimation. The surgeon's perception of the patient's QOL has been shown to be inaccurate in the postoperative period after skull base surgery [4]. Therefore, using QOL assessments may play an important role in the balanced evaluation of the efficacy of surgical interventions. This in turn could help the clinician to provide appropriate preoperative counseling and postoperative care, resulting in better anticipation, recovery, and acceptance of the procedure by the patient.

QOL instruments can be divided into generic and disease-specific health-related questionnaires. Generic assessments focus more broadly on the patient's overall perception of their well-being concerning health. They often make use of multiple domains to cover all aspects of human well-being, e.g., physical, social, emotional, or mental. Disease-specific instruments are more focused on a specific subgroup of patients in which they are validated.

A. A. AlQahtani et al. (eds.), *CSF Rhinorrhea*, https://doi.org/10.1007/978-3-030-94781-1_38

38.3 Relevant Available QOL Instruments in CSF Rhinorrhea

38.3.1 Generic Instruments

Generic questionnaires often used in sinonasal or skull base studies are the Short Form 36 Health Survey (SF-36), the EQ-5D, or the Karnofsky performance scale. The SF-36 consists of 36 items in eight domains (vitality, physical functioning, bodily pain, general health perceptions, physical role functioning, emotional role functioning, social role functioning, and mental health) [5]. As such, it is a rather complete questionnaire of generic quality of life. Furthermore, it can be used to study cost-effectiveness of interventions.

The EQ-5D encompasses five domains (mobility, self-care, usual activities, pain/discomfort, and anxiety/depression) and an overall VAS-score to indicate self-perceived health status. Whereas older versions of this questionnaire used three-level scales for every item (EQ-5D-3L), currently five levels are used (EQ-5D-5L) enabling better differentiation between patient states. The EQ-5D can also be used in cost-effectiveness studies [6].

The Karnofsky performance scale is a rough indication of limitations in daily activities, and mostly used in oncological cases. It does not cover multiple domains. It is easy to use, but for CSF rhinorrhea itself hardly applicable, as this condition will generally not have major impact on the ability to perform daily activities.

38.3.2 Disease-Specific Instruments

Ideally, for patients suffering from CSF rhinorrhea a disease-specific QOL instrument is used to assess the impact on patient perceived health and the merits of (endonasal) surgery for closure of the leak. The complaints tested should include the nasal (e.g., patency, crusting, smell), the psychological (e.g., anxiety, depression, worrying), as well as the neurological domain (e.g., CSF hypotension symptoms, headache). However, no such instrument has been developed yet. Therefore, other disease-specific QOL questionnaires could be used, each separately relating to the type of surgery, nasal complaints, anxiety, headache etc.

Two validated instruments concerning skull base surgery have been developed so far.

The anterior skull base quality of life questionnaire (ASBQ) is an instrument validated for patients undergoing open anterior skull base tumor surgery [7]. It has multiple dimensions comprising subscale scores for performance, physical function, vitality, pain, specific symptoms (taste, smell, appearance, epiphora, nasal secretions and visual disturbance), influence on emotion and a total score. It is also used to report on outcomes of patients treated with the endoscopic resection of sinonasal malignancies [8]. The endoscopic endonasal sinus and skull base surgery questionnaire (EESQ) is developed for patients undergoing endoscopic endonasal surgery for sinus or skull base pathology. It assesses nasal morbidity after treatment and covers physical, psychological and social functioning [9].

Another option is the 22 item sinonasal outcome test (SNOT-22) which is a validated disease-specific questionnaire designed to assess QOL related to benign sinonasal disease. It is originally devised for the context of chronic rhinosinusitis and therefore focuses on nasal symptoms as well as some social and emotional consequences [10]. However, specific symptoms of CSF hypotension, like headache relieved when lying flat, nausea, vomiting and double vision, and especially the fear of getting serious complications like meningitis are not included.

Given the lack of a disease-specific instrument for CSF rhinorrhea, other domains such as anxiety, depression, and headache, could be investigated using separate validated questionnaires for each domain.

38.4 Quality of Life in Endoscopic Endonasal Surgery Techniques in CSF Rhinorrhea

The chosen technique for closure can influence QOL. During surgical endoscopic repair, healthy sinonasal structures are resected which induces nasal morbidity. The same is true for anterior skull base pathology warranting endoscopic surgery even without CSF rhinorrhea. In these cases, using the SNOT-22 would make sense, as it deals extensively with the nasal domain. On the other hand, it also encompasses items not relevant to anterior skull base surgery, such as ear-related symptoms. Still, many authors have used this instrument to obtain QOL measurements peri-operatively (for example Ransom 2012, Pant 2010, McCoul 2012, McCoul 2012, Thompson 2014, Patel 2015, Jones 2016, Riley 2019, Ahn 2019) [3, 11–18]. The general tendency is that the QOL in nasal domains decreases postoperatively in the first few weeks or months, after which it will again improve, and in some studies increases to better levels than preoperatively. A good overview of the various QOL outcomes in anterior skull base surgery is given by Kirkman et al. [19].

There is debate in the literature regarding the influence of a nasoseptal flap for skull base repair on the postoperative QOL. Some studies identify the use of such a flap as a negative factor for QOL [16, 20, 21], although others do not confirm this finding [11].

Another important issue is olfactory functioning and its influence on QOL. It has been suggested that using a nasoseptal flap impairs olfaction [22]. From an anatomical point of view, middle turbinate resection could also negatively impact olfactory performance. As such, some authors have modified their endoscopic approach to preserve middle turbinate anatomy and restrict the use of a nasoseptal flap where possible, thus obtaining improved postoperative QOL [13]. Others have chosen to use a unilateral transethmoidal and paraseptal approach where possible, thus retaining olfactory function and good sinonasal QOL [23].

In light of CSF rhinorrhea, currently available studies on QOL after (endoscopic) surgery hardly ever deal will CSF rhinorrhea per se. It seems logical that the influences of specific approaches/techniques on QOL that are found in non-leaking subjects are also true for those with CSF rhinorrhea. Still, no real data exist on this issue.

38.5 Conclusions

The QOL in CSF rhinorrhea can be influenced on several levels (current complaints and risks, type of (surgical) therapy). Not surprisingly, the impact of CSF rhinorrhea alone on QOL is not well known. Given the expanding range of indications for endonasal surgery in skull base pathology, the incidence of CSF rhinorrhea might well increase. Therefore, a newly validated disease-specific questionnaire could be of value. This disease-specific questionnaire ideally contains items in the sinonasal, neurological, and psychological domain. The impact of endonasal surgery on healthy sinonasal structures and related QOL should not be overlooked and be kept in mind while performing the procedure. In the rapidly evolving field of endonasal surgical techniques and indications such a validated instrument specific to the CSF leak population may play an important role in the balanced evaluation of the surgical intervention, and thus patient counseling.

References

1. Van Wijk R. Assessment of quality of life: advantages and pitfalls. Clin Exp All Rev. 2005;5:32–5.
2. Tebruegge M, Curtis N. Epidemiology, etiology, pathogenesis, and diagnosis of recurrent bacterial meningitis. Clin Microbiol Rev. 2008;21(3):519–37.
3. McCoul ED, Anand VK, Bedrosian JC, Schwartz TH. Endoscopic skull base surgery and its impact on sinonasal-related quality of life. Int Forum Allergy Rhinol. 2012;2(2):174–81.
4. Gil Z, Abergel A, Spektor S, Khafif A, Fliss DM. Patient, caregiver, and surgeon perceptions of quality of life following anterior skull base surgery. Arch Otolaryngol Head Neck Surg. 2004;130(11):1276–81.

5. Ware J. SF-36 health survey: Manuel and interpretation guide. Boston, MA: Boston New England Medical Center, Health Institute; 1993.
6. Devlin NJ, Brooks R. EQ-5D and the EuroQol group: past, present and future. Appl Health Econ Health Policy. 2017;15(2):127–37.
7. Gil Z, Abergel A, Spektor S, Shabtai E, Khafif A, Fliss DM. Development of a cancer-specific anterior skull base quality-of-life questionnaire. J Neurosurg. 2004;100(5):813–9.
8. Castelnuovo P, Lepera D, Turri-Zanoni M, Battaglia P, Bolzoni Villaret A, Bignami M, et al. Quality of life following endoscopic endonasal resection of anterior skull base cancers. J Neurosurg. 2013;119(6):1401–9.
9. ten Dam E, Feijen RA, van den Berge MJC, Hoving EW, Kuijlen JM, van der Laan BFAM, et al. Development of the endoscopic Endonasal sinus and Skull Base surgery questionnaire. Int Forum Allergy Rhinol. 2017;7(11):1076–84.
10. Hopkins C, Gillett S, Slack R, Lund VJ, Browne JP. Psychometric validity of the 22-item Sinonasal outcome test. Clin Otolaryngol. 2009;34(5):447–54.
11. McCoul ED, Anand VK, Schwartz TH. Improvements in site-specific quality of life 6 months after endoscopic anterior skull base surgery: a prospective study. J Neurosurg. 2012;117(3):498–506.
12. Ransom ER, Doghramji L, Palmer JN, Chiu AG. Global and disease-specific health-related quality of life after complete endoscopic resection of anterior skull base neoplasms. Am J Rhinol Allergy. 2012;26(1):76–9.
13. Thompson CF, Suh JD, Liu Y, Bergsneider M, Wang MB. Modifications to the endoscopic approach for anterior skull base lesions improve postoperative sinonasal symptoms. J Neurol Surg B Skull Base. 2014;75(1):65–72.
14. Patel KS, Raza SM, McCoul ED, Patrona A, Greenfield JP, Souweidane MM, et al. Long-term quality of life after endonasal endoscopic resection of adult craniopharyngiomas. J Neurosurg. 2015;123(3):571–80.
15. Riley CA, Tabaee A, Conley L, Amine M, Soneru CP, Anand VK, et al. Long-term sinonasal outcomes after endoscopic skull base surgery with nasoseptal flap reconstruction. Laryngoscope. 2019;129(5):1035–40.
16. Pant H, Bhatki AM, Snyderman CH, Vescan AD, Carrau RL, Gardner P, et al. Quality of life following endonasal skull base surgery. Skull Base. 2010;20(1):35–40.
17. Jones SH, Iannone AF, Patel KS, Anchouche K, Raza SM, Anand VK, et al. The impact of age on long-term quality of life after Endonasal endoscopic resection of Skull Base Meningiomas. Neurosurgery. 2016;79(5):736–45.
18. Ahn JC, Cho SW, Kim DK, Han DH, Kim DY, Rhee CS, et al. Recovery period of sinonasal quality of life and its associated factors after endoscopic endonasal approach for anterior skull base tumors. Acta Otolaryngol. 2019;139(5):461–6.
19. Kirkman MA, Borg A, Al-Mousa A, Haliasos N, Choi D. Quality-of-life after anterior Skull Base surgery: a systematic review. J Neurol Surg B Skull Base. 2014;75(2):73–89.
20. Georgalas C, Badloe R, van Furth W, Reinartz S, Fokkens WJ. Quality of life in extended endonasal approaches for skull base tumours. Rhinology. 2012;50(3):255–61.
21. Alobid I, Ensenat J, Marino-Sanchez F, Rioja E, Notaris M, Mullol J, et al. Expanded endonasal approach using vascularized septal flap reconstruction for skull base tumors has a negative impact on sinonasal symptoms and quality of life. Am J Rhinol Allergy. 2013;27(5):426–31.
22. Greig SR, Cooper TJ, Sommer DD, Nair S, Wright ED. Objective sinonasal functional outcomes in endoscopic anterior skull-base surgery: an evidence-based review with recommendations. Int Forum Allergy Rhinol. 2016;6(10):1040–6.
23. Eordogh M, Briner HR, Simmen D, Jones N, Reisch R. Endoscopic unilateral transethmoid-paraseptal approach to the central skull base. Laryngoscope Investig Otolaryngol. 2017;2(5):281–7.

39 Surgical Competencies and Simulation Models in CSF Leak Repair

Abeer Albathi, Saud Alromaih, and Abdulaziz A. AlQahtani

39.1 Introduction

The surgical approaches, techniques, and materials used for endoscopic skull base reconstructions vary widely. In the hands of an expert surgeon, skull base reconstructions can be successful. However, a steady learning curve is necessary to master different techniques [1, 2]. Smith et al. examined one team's first 51 endoscopic CSF leak repair cases and found that there was a significant decrease in the risk of Diabetes Insipidus and CSF leak in the last group of patients ($p = 0.039$) [2]. Snyderman and Gardner reported a retrospective quantitative analysis of CSF leaks in 1000 consecutive cases of endoscopic endonasal surgeries. When they compared the recurrence rate of CSF leak, they found that there is a significant decrease in CSF leaks ($p = 0.002$) between the first half (88/500) and the second half (53/500) of the series. They concluded that continued improvement in second half of the series may reflect a learning curve of the surgeons [1].

Training performed on simulation models that mimic real situations enables trainees to receive hands-on experience at an earlier stage of training, before operating on patients [3–5]. Simulation models allow residents and fellows to perform different procedures under lifelike conditions, in a safe environment, without time restrictions [6, 7]. There are many simulation models available for endoscopic sinus surgery that have demonstrated positive impacts on actual operating room performance [6]. However, limited simulation models exist for skull base surgery, especially for CSFL repair [8–11].

In the following section, authors will describe a novel CSFL repair simulation model that has been designed to train surgeons and facilitate the acquisition of the fundamental skills necessary for skull base reconstruction [10]. The feasibility and validity of the model has been reported [10, 12].

39.2 The CSF Leak Simulation Model

39.2.1 Settings

The surgical model was prepared to simulate a real CSF leak scenario. This model has utilized Fresh-frozen human cadaveric heads, standard sinus and skull base endoscopic instruments, 4-mm 0° and 45° endoscopes, and a high-speed drill.

A. Albathi
Department of Otorhinolaryngology/Head and Neck Surgery, Prince Sultan Military City, Riyadh, Saudi Arabia

S. Alromaih
Department of Otorhinolaryngology/Head and Neck Surgery, Faculty of Medicine, King Saud University, Riyadh, Saudi Arabia

A. A. AlQahtani (✉)
Department of Otorhinolaryngology/Head and Neck Surgery, King Fahad Medical City, Riyadh, Saudi Arabia

A. A. AlQahtani et al. (eds.), *CSF Rhinorrhea*, https://doi.org/10.1007/978-3-030-94781-1_39

39.2.2 Steps

1. *The control holes:* Two 10-mm skin incisions were made in the right and left uppermost areas of the frontal bone, followed by a bur hole approach, using a size 6 cutting bur. The dura was incised, and two tubes with free ends were inserted, to drain the intracranial space when the fluid fills the space (Fig. 39.1). The use of two control holes in the forehead is the benchmark design of this model. These two holes are necessary to flow off intracranial air during the initial fluid loading process and ensure that the fluid fills the intrathecal space. Additionally, rising the fluid through the control holes works as an indicator of watertight closure after the reconstruction. The control holes also decrease the fluid pressure over the skull base/neck foramina, as the control holes provide an outlet for excess fluid.
2. *Fluid infusion:* The spinal canal at the cervical end was explored, and the epidural space was identified and spaced from the spinal cord. A Foley's catheter, French size 14, was inserted into the epidural space at a 10–11 cm depth until it reached the intracranial space. The catheter's balloon was inflated with 8 cm of air to fix the tube in place. We applied a commercial glue to seal the dura over the catheter. Subsequently, the skin of the neck was collected around the spinal canal and sutured together tightly, with 3.0 silk sutures (Fig. 39.2). This additional measure was necessary to prevent any fluid leakage through different neck foramina during the fluid infusion. The other end of the Foley's catheter was connected to an infusion pump containing a normal saline bag, to deliver the fluid in pulsating mode. Fluorescein dye was injected into the fluid to enhance endoscopic visualization and to test the closure of the defect. The intracranial space was filled with fluid until it drained through the control holes at the forehead. The average time necessary to prepare the model was 43 min (33–55 min).

In the initial version of this model, we connected one of the control holes to the infusion pump instead of the cervical route, to deliver

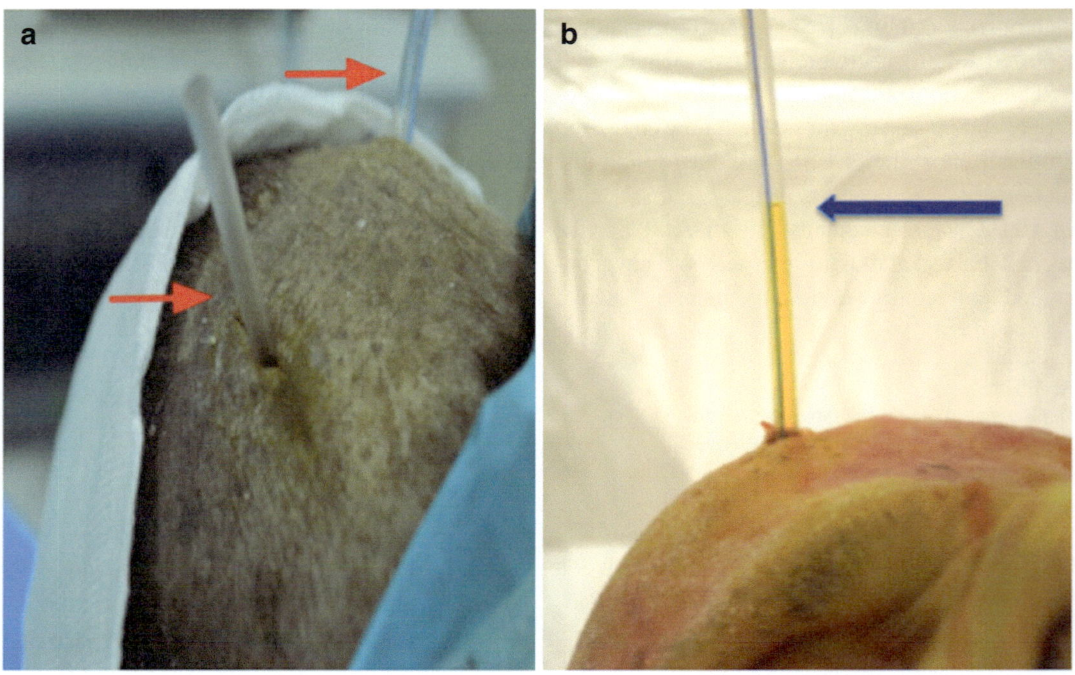

Fig. 39.1 (**a**) Open-ended tubes (red arrows) are inserted in the frontal bur holes. (**b**) Fluorescein-dyed fluid is drained through the forehead tube (blue arrow) when the intracranial space is filled with fluid

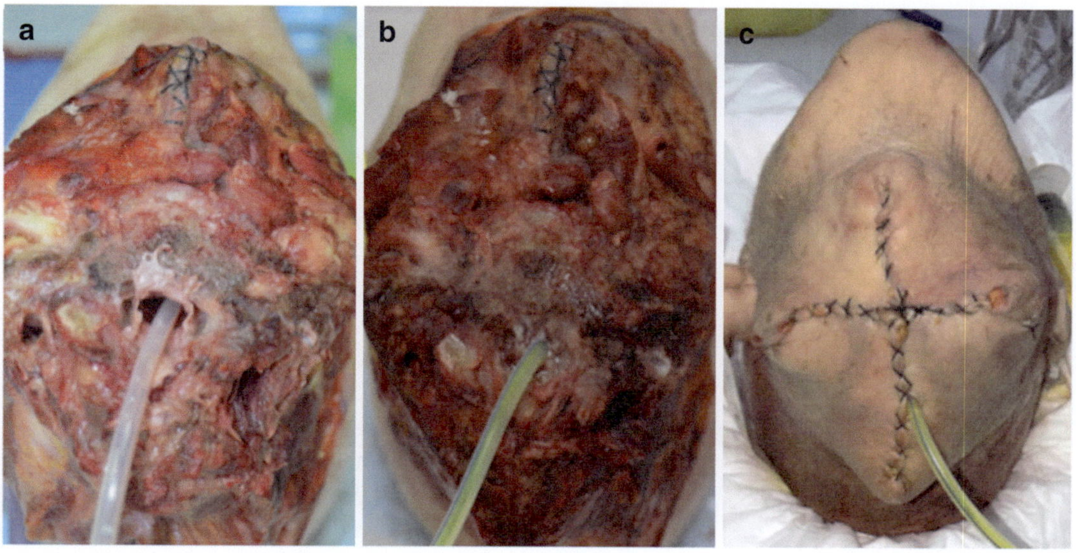

Fig. 39.2 (**a**) Foley catheter is inserted into the spinal canal. (**b**) The spinal canal dura is sutured around the tube. (**c**) The neck skin is sutured around the tube to prevent a fluid leak from the neck

fluid, and sealed the neck with "melted wax." We found that this technique was useful for chemically embalmed specimens, where the brain is smaller and wax adherence to the neck skin is feasible. Fresh frozen specimens offer very similar conditions to live humans. However, the brain is often swollen, and the neck skin is wet and difficult to seal with wax. For these reasons, we have modified the infusion system from the transcranial route to the spinal canal route.

3. *Surgical dissection:* Standard functional endoscopic sinus surgery, transclival, and transsellar approaches were performed in all specimens. Afterward, one skull base defect was created at a time, in the ethmoid roof, cribriform plate, sella, and clivus. A fluorescein-dyed fluid leak was observed (Fig. 39.3).
4. *Reconstruction:* The participant then identified the defect, smoothened the bony edges, skeletonized the mucosa around the defect, undermined the dura, applied the reconstruction material, and then applied glue at the edges. The participant performed skull base reconstruction using local flaps/grafts and human fascia temporalis. The graft used in the reconstruction was the muco-periostium of the middle turbinate or floor of the nose while nasoseptal muco-periostium was used as a pedicled flap. A multilayer technique (inlay and overlay) was used for the ethmoid roof, sella, and clival defects, while the overlay technique was used for cribriform defects (Fig. 39.4).

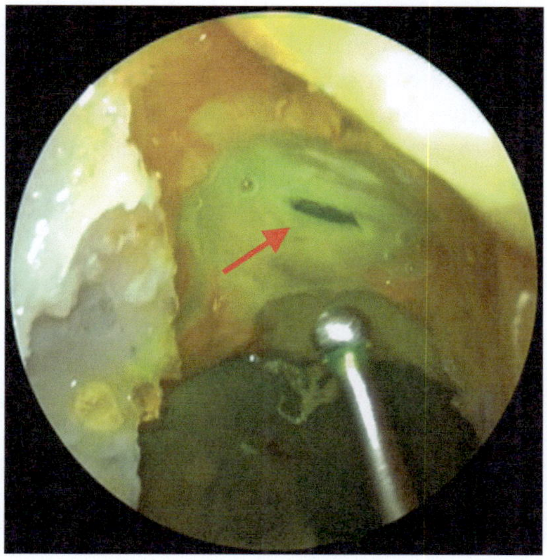

Fig. 39.3 The fluorescein-dyed fluid is leaking through an iatrogenic skull base defect in the left ethmoid roof

5. *Testing the reconstruction:* The fluid infusion pump was then operated to deliver the fluid.

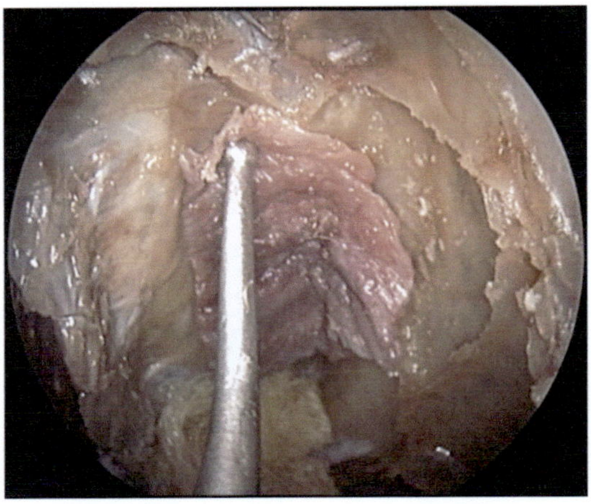

Fig. 39.4 The muco-periosteal graft of middle turbinate is applied over the left ethmoid roof defect. The seeker helps in positioning the graft

The reconstruction was labeled as a watertight closure if the fluid drained from the control holes at the forehead and as a failure if it leaked through the defect. The participant performed each skull base reconstruction separately before introducing an additional iatrogenic defect, to test the sealing of each area independently.

39.2.3 Validation

This simulation model underwent face, content, and construct validity [12].

Eight novices (residents- PGY3) and eight experts have participated in the validation process. The experts completed a post-study 21-item questionnaire to assess the face and content validity. The performances of the participants were recorded and scored by two independent investigators who were blinded to the participant's level. Global Rating Scale of Operative Performance (GRSOP) and a Specific Skull Base Reconstruction Checklist (SBRC) were used to score the performances.

Face and content validation represent subjective processes during which experts in the field review and examine the contents of a simulator, in detail, to determine if the simulator measures what it is designed to measure. Validation includes testing the logical steps and the skills used in the procedure. Whereas face validity tests the realism of the model and the degree of similarity between the model and real conditions, the content validity tests the ability of the model to teach the participants the principle surgical skills necessary for skull base reconstruction [13]. For this simulation model, the face and content validity showed high response rates among the experts. The responses from the expert group for the 21-item questionnaire were high for all items (4.13–4.88 out of 5). The internal consistency reliability of the questionnaire and the intra-class correlation, which was derived by Cronbach's Alpha, were 0.913 and 0.941, respectively. Seven experts (87%) agreed or strongly agreed that the model mimics real CSFL conditions. All of the experts (100%) agreed or strongly agreed that the model helps to develop the skills necessary for skull base reconstructions and believe that the model can increase competency among the residents/fellows. All other questionnaire items received high response rates (minimum 87%), regarding the reality of the model, whether the model helps teach how to harvest different flaps/grafts and different reconstruction methods, the reality of the fluid pulsation, and the development of hand-eye coordination.

Construct validation is an objective test of simulator power, to identify the quality of the model to differentiate between participants according to proficiency levels. The model showed high construct validity, with a statistically significant difference (p-value <0.001) when comparing the performances of participants according to their general and specific surgical skills (GRSOP and SBRS). This validity confirms the assumption that the performance associated with a high-proficiency level under real conditions will be similar during the simulation and vice versa.

39.2.4 Limitations

The model lacks CSF pressure measurements, which could help determine the actual intracranial pressure after the reconstruction. We opted not to add a CSF pressure-measuring tool because doing so would increase the complexity of the model. Additionally, under real conditions, the surgeons do not measure the pressure after the reconstruction. The closure of skull base defect depends mostly on the healing process rather than the intracranial pressure fluctuation. The healing can take days after the surgery, which is not applicable in the simulation model that requires a prompt watertight closure. This model relies on the amount of fluid, rather than the pressure to confirm the watertight closure, which is the rationale for the use of control holes that allow the fluid to drain when the intracranial space is full. Another limitation is lacking the dedicated instruments used for skull base reconstruction that are available for human use but not for cadaver dissection.

39.3 Other Models

The first simulation model for skull base reconstruction was developed by a group of researchers from the University of South Carolina in 2017. They performed a cervical laminectomy and durotomy, followed by the insertion of an arterial catheter into the intradural space for Intrathecal perfusion of fluorescein-infused saline into the ventricular/subarachnoid space [8, 9]. The model has been validated for different neurosurgical procedures, as well as skull base reconstruction. The significant limitation of this model that it was based on full-body human cadavers, which are difficult to obtain for regular educational programs. Our model in 2018 overcomes this limitation by utilizing cadaveric heads only to make it easier for uses in dissection courses [10].

In 2020, Mattavelli et al. reported a similar preclinical model, in which they injected a fluorescein-dyed fluid in the subarachnoid space through the cervical route. Measuring CSFL pressure points was the merit of the model [11]. It was achieved by connecting the cervical catheter to a vertical graded tube. Graduation of the tube was adapted to have the "0" value at the same height of the predicted skull base defect. Once the skull base reconstruction is done, they inject the fluid and measure the height of the fluid in the vertical tube at the level when it leaks from the defect. This measure is labeled as "CSF leak pressure point." However, the authors concluded that correlation between the expert surgeon's impression and the measured CSF leak pressure point was suboptimal.

Muhamed et al. in 2021 evaluated the use of a three-dimensional (3D) printed, anatomically accurate model to simulate CSF leak closure [14]. The volunteers (Thirteen otolaryngologists and eleven neurosurgeons) performed two sessions of skull base repair. They showed significant improvement in the surgical skills; time to close the defect and an increase in confidence after the second attempt.

In conclusion, the CSFL simulation models allow trainees to perform multiple skull base reconstructions, using different techniques and materials, under conditions similar to live surgeries. These models could be implemented in the training curriculum for rhinology, neurosurgery, and skull base surgery.

References

1. Snyderman CH, Gardner PA. Quality control approach to cerebrospinal fluid leaks. Adv Otorhinolaryngol. 2013;74:130–7. https://doi.org/10.1159/000342289.
2. Smith SJ, Eralil G, Woon K, Sama A, Dow G, Robertson I. Light at the end of the tunnel: the learning curve associated with endoscopic transsphenoidal skull base surgery. Skull Base. 2010;20:69–74. https://doi.org/10.1055/s-0029-1238214.
3. Tolsdorff B, Pommert A, Höhne KH, et al. Virtual reality: a new paranasal sinus surgery simulator. Laryngoscope. 2010;120:420–6. https://doi.org/10.1002/lary.20676.
4. Delgado-Vargas B, Romero-Salazar AL, Reyes Burneo PM, et al. Evaluation of resident's training for endoscopic sinus surgery using a sheep's head. Eur Arch Otorhinolaryngol. 2016;273:2085–9. https://doi.org/10.1007/s00405-015-3877-1.
5. Zuckerman JD, Wise SK, Rogers GA, Senior BA, Schlosser RJ, DelGaudio JM. The utility of cadaver dissection in endoscopic sinus surgery training courses. Am J Rhinol Allergy. 2009;23:218–24. https://doi.org/10.2500/ajra.2009.23.3297.

6. Edmond CV Jr. Impact of the endoscopic sinus surgical simulator on operating room performance. Laryngoscope. 2002;112:1148–58. https://doi.org/10.1097/00005537-200207000-00002.
7. Fried MP, Sadoughi B, Gibber MJ, et al. From virtual reality to the operating room: the endoscopic sinus surgery simulator experiment. Otolaryngol Head Neck Surg. 2010;142:202–7. https://doi.org/10.1016/j.otohns.2009.11.023.
8. Christian EA, Bakhsheshian J, Strickland BA, et al. Perfusion-based human cadaveric specimen as a simulation training model in repairing cerebrospinal fluid leaks during endoscopic endonasal skull base surgery. J Neurosurg. 2017;3:1–5. https://doi.org/10.3171/2017.5.JNS162982.
9. Zada G, Bakhsheshian J, Pham M, et al. Development of a perfusion-based cadaveric simulation model integrated into neurosurgical training: feasibility based on reconstitution of vascular and cerebrospinal fluid systems. Oper Neurosurg. 2017;14:72–80. https://doi.org/10.1093/ons/opx074.
10. AlQahtani AA, Albathi AA, Alhammad OM, Alrabie AS. Innovative real CSF leak simulation model for rhinology training: human cadaveric design. Eur Arch Otorhinolaryngol. 2018;275:937–41. https://doi.org/10.1007/s00405-018-4902-y.
11. Mattavelli D, Ferrari M, Rampinelli V, et al. Development and validation of a preclinical model for training and assessment of cerebrospinal fluid leak repair in endoscopic skull base surgery. Int Forum Allergy Rhinol. 2020;10:89–96. https://doi.org/10.1002/alr.22451.
12. AlQahtani A, Albathi A, Castelnuovo P, Alfawwaz F. Cerebrospinal fluid leak repair simulation model: face, content, and construct validation. Am J Rhinol Allergy. 2021;35(2):264–71. https://doi.org/10.1177/1945892420952262. Epub 2020 Aug 20
13. Evgeniou E, Walker H, Gujral S. The role of simulation in microsurgical training. J Surg Educ. 2018;75:171–81. https://doi.org/10.1016/j.jsurg.2017.06.032.
14. Masalha MA, VanKoevering KK, Latif OS, Powell AR, Zhang A, Hod KH, Prevedello DM, Carrau RL. Simulation of cerebrospinal fluid leak repair using a 3-dimensional printed model. Am J Rhinol Allergy. 2021;20:19458924211003537. https://doi.org/10.1177/19458924211003537. Epub ahead of print

Patient Advocacy and Medicolegal Issues In CSF Rhinorrhea

40

Jonathan R. Mallen, Eric H. Holbrook, and Seth M. Brown

40.1 Informed Consent

The importance of informed consent is derived from the ethical principle of patient autonomy. Given the significant difference of medical knowledge and power differential inherent to the patient–doctor relationship, there is ample opportunity for physicians to guide their patients' decision making. For surgeons, this includes understanding both the underlying medical knowledge as well as patients' values to help them decide when to undergo surgery and perhaps just as importantly, when not to. To do this, the surgeon must concurrently play the role of advisor, advocate, and confidant. Patients are entitled to make informed decisions, and it is their physician's responsibility to provide them with the requisite information needed to make such choices. It is helpful to view informed consent as a process instead of a contract to be signed. To be valid, a truly *informed* consent must contain three key elements: adequate information, a process free of coercion, and patient capacity of understanding. While the term "adequate" is subject to interpretation, and can differ culturally and geographically, it typically involves a standard involving what either a "prudent doctor" would discuss with a patient or what a "reasonable layperson" would want to know to make a decision. Secondly, the process must be free of coercion—namely, the patient should not feel pressured one way or the other (though this does not necessarily preclude physician paternalism in the form of medical expertise and recommendation). Finally, the person must have capacity, which is loosely defined as the ability to both recognize that a decision must be made, and reflect on the risks and benefits and alternatives as they relate to their personal values [1].

Documentation is increasingly essential. Insofar as there is validity to the expression "if it isn't in the chart, it didn't happen," it is likely particularly relevant with regards to the surgical informed consent. While the discussion is arguably more important than the documentation, it is insufficient to simply note, "risks, benefits, and alternatives discussed." These conversations should be explicitly documented in the same way that they are discussed. While time consuming, in the event that a patient develops a postoperative cerebral spinal fluid (CSF) leak, or has a complication throughout the course of treatment, the documentation of the consent can significantly affect liability. Demonstrating that appropriate medical therapy was trialed first can also stave off questions regarding the necessity of the procedure. Part of explain-

J. R. Mallen
Department of Otorhinolaryngology, University of Pennsylvania, Philadelphia, PA, USA

E. H. Holbrook
Department of Otolaryngology, Massachusetts Eye and Ear Infirmary, Boson, MA, USA

S. M. Brown (✉)
Department of Surgery, Division of Otolaryngology, University of Connecticut, Farmington, CT, USA
e-mail: sbrown1@prohealthmd.com

A. A. AlQahtani et al. (eds.), *CSF Rhinorrhea*, https://doi.org/10.1007/978-3-030-94781-1_40

ing the proposed benefits of surgery and managing expectations is noting that it is imprudent, if not impossible, to guarantee a cure or specific outcome. Additionally, we recommend explicit inclusion of the phrase "risks include but are not limited to 'need for additional surgery', CSF leak, and meningitis" in the consent for sinonasal procedures. These complications have specifically been cited in malpractice cases alleging that failure to discuss them constituted consent inadequacy. In regards to the use of repair grafts, it is good practice to inform the patient of possible graft material such as acellular dermis from human cadavers or membranes synthesized from animal tissue (porcine or bovine) since religious, cultural, or ideologic beliefs should be respected and adhered to.

Some physicians worry that listing rare, but potentially very serious complications may cause patients undue anxiety, but this does not appear to be the case [2]. This is particularly true when the patient is counseled on what to expect in the event of a given complication and how that would subsequently alter the treatment plan and long-term outcomes [1]. There are notable geographic differences based on country of practice. Historically, a formal consent form was not signed in France, Sweden, or the Netherlands, though they tended to document a discussion took place. Conversely, in Germany, documentation is required even for notably atypical severe complications, such as MI following local anesthetic injection [3]. In any case, even with patients who request to "leave the decision" in the surgeon's hands and are quick to sign the form, it is the physicians responsibility to ensure the patient has understood all aspects of the discussion.

Patient comprehension and recall of the consent process tends to be poor. Despite a 97% satisfaction rate with his consent process, Godwin found that on average patients could only recall 25% of discussed potential complications with a maximum of 50% observed [4]. It is a matter of preference which member of the surgical team obtains the consent and the American College of Surgeons goes so far as to explicitly state that the surgeon "responsible for obtaining informed consent from the patient need not personally obtain the patient's signature on the consent form." [5] Irrespective of the specific team member obtaining consent, in order to maximize comprehension, it is recommend that 15–30 min is needed for the average patient, though this clearly differs based on a host of patient and procedure-specific factors [6]. Supplemental information sheets can be helpful to standardize consent among patients, increase patient recall, and serve as further documentation of the consent process [7]. Along these lines, a printed or digital copy of post-op instructions on signs/symptoms of potential complications such as CSF leak can decrease the delay in postoperative patient recognition of relevant issues.

Since first described in 1985, Functional Endoscopic Sinus Surgery (FESS) has come a long way. Not only have complication rates for standard procedures decreased in the last 30 years, but our understanding of the risks of surgery are also better appreciated, even as the rate of injury has decreased. Current rates of CSF leak for FESS have been estimated to be as low as 0.17% at a high volume center, though rates of occult leak with spontaneous closure have been estimated at closer to 3% [8, 9]. In 1994, 76% of otolaryngologists regularly discussed the risk of CSF leak with patients [10]. By 2002, this number appropriately increased to greater than 99% [11].

With the advent of endoscopic techniques, patients are able to avoid the added morbidity of a craniotomy for many skull-base procedures. While the potential for improved outcomes and lack of incisions are no doubt a positive for patients, they can lull a patient into underestimating the risks of a skull-base procedure in a way which would be difficult to do with an open approach. It is thus perhaps even more vital for surgeons performing such minimally invasive approaches to stress that the risks include, but are certainly not limited to, CSF leak, meningitis, brain abcess and hemorrhage. Additionally, in regards to endoscopic skull-base approaches, the patient must also understand the degree of surgery "hidden" by the nose. It should be clear that although there may be no external incisions or bruising, the extent of surgery is significant requiring similar lengths of post-op recovery as with craniotomy.

It is important to resist any urge to alter documentation after the fact, a practice known legally as record spoliation. From a legal perspective, this is considered a premeditated act exposing the physician to punitive damages in addition to malpractice. Not only is this fraudulent and unethical, it is also easily uncovered by time stamps in electronic health records or analysis by handwriting experts. Such punitive damages have exceeded $1 million previously, and may not be covered by malpractice insurance. Further, it can lead to disciplinary action from professional boards and medical licensing authorities, including license revocation [12, 29].

40.2 Intraoperative Tools

The use of intraoperative navigation has expanded rapidly in recent years as technological advances have made CT and MRI-guided surgery more accurate, user-friendly, and cost effective. There are clear potential benefits including identification of critical structures, particularly in patients with altered anatomy such as those who have undergone prior surgery. The American Academy of Otolaryngology Head and Neck Surgery (AAO-HNS) endorses the use of image guidance for complex cases including in the treatment of patients with CSF rhinorrhea, skull-base pathology, extensive polyposis, and a history of prior surgery, as well as in patients with posterior ethmoid, frontal, and/or sphenoid pathology. Importantly, the official position statement stresses that this is not intended as a mandate, a standard of care, or medical/legal advice [13]. The decision to forgo the use of navigation does not appear to be a risk factor for litigation in cases which result in iatrogenic CSF leak [14]. While many surgeons prefer to use navigation during surgical repair, it is not strictly necessary in every situation from a patient care nor medicolegal perspective. Conversely, having on-demand access to the images as needed, such as on a computer in the operating room, has been implicated in legal proceedings before and is more difficult to justify forgoing [15].

Fluorescein can safely and effectively be used intrathecally to localize CSF leaks and/or ensure water-tight closure [16]. At higher doses or concentrations, however, it can be neurotoxic owing to chemical irritation of the meninges [17]. It is for this reason that the drug package insert includes an advisory warning against intrathecal use despite its demonstrated safety and efficacy profile [16, 17]. Of note, the US Food and Drug Administration (FDA) neither approves nor condemns its usage. FDA approval of a medication for a specific indication is notably not required for doctors to use it to treat patients, however the potential harms of its use should be noted and communicated to the patient. Many physicians thus include the off-label use of intrathecal flourescein in the informed consent process.

40.3 Communication After Iatrogenic Leak

Disclosure of an error can be frightening and humbling for a physician. Patel et al. propose an outline for a straightforward approach [18]. The first step typically comes at the conclusion of a procedure once an error is identified. Disclosure should occur as soon as is reasonably possible, even if not all information is yet available. The communication process following a medical error such as an iatrogenic CSF leak is a continual one and patients and their families should be told as much. Failure to do so, or delegation of such a task to another team member, can lead to feelings of resentment by the patient, in addition to raising concerns about the motives and transparency on the part of the surgeon. The initial conversation in particular should focus on facts available, and avoid the temptation to speculate as to prognosis or fault [1]. Next, one should explain in simple terms how and why an injury occurred. An explanation of the plan of action should follow with the understanding that the plan may involve additional team members and may change over time. There should be a low threshold for involving neurosurgical consultation for the patient either during surgery or in the immediate post-op period. Not only is this good medical-legal practice, but it can assure proper and timely care for the patient at a time when the surgeon may unconsciously minimize the extent of the complication.

It is important during this process to continually provide emotional support. Patients' negative feelings should be openly acknowledged and legitimized. It is never easy for patients and their families to hear about complications, but this is likely even more challenging for patients undergoing FESS given its elective and outpatient nature, and the historically high satisfaction rates. Finally, apologize without assigning blame. Patients and family members expect and appreciate an apology following an adverse outcome [19]. While there are conflicting viewpoints on whether this suggests an admission of guilt [20, 21], it is entirely feasible to structure an apology in a way which acknowledges the patient's feelings without admitting culpability. Body language can be exceedingly important, particularly the decision to sit down next to a patient. This simple act leads patients to rate interactions as being longer and more meaningful, and to consider their physicians to be more compassionate and accessible [22, 23].

The importance of patient relationships and communication to preventing lawsuits cannot be overstated [24]. With regard to medical quality, in some ways, patient perception is more relevant than reality—objective measures of medical care quality correlate poorly with patient satisfaction [1]. Strong rapport between doctors and patients on the other hand, is independently associated with patient perception of physician competence. Further, a good relationship is associated with decreased patient perception of physician responsibility for an adverse outcome as well as decreased likelihood of litigation [24]. That is not to suggest that actual quality is unimportant, but rather that the importance of a strong relationship with patients should not be underestimated.

The level of communication with the patient and their family should be dependent on an understanding of the patient's desires and fears. Particularly with CSF leak, the fear of the unknown with regard to potential neurological sequelae are often more distressing than the actual physical manifestations. It is important to avoid isolating oneself from the patient. In addition to the moral obligation to be available to our patients, particularly those with iatrogenic injury, it is notable that patients and family who feel abandoned are more likely to sue [18]. Conversely, it can come across as disingenuous interest when a physician suddenly is smotheringly attentive. Follow-up office visits and phone calls should be appropriate for proper medical care of the patient without appearing over-attentive.

With regard to the disclosure of asymptomatic complications such as in the case of a CSF leak identified and repaired intraoperatively, some physicians may be inclined to be less forthcoming, believing that doing so may invite unnecessary scrutiny. Such obfuscation is difficult to justify ethically and is potentially a violation of the American Medical Association's Principles of Medical Ethics [25]. Additionally, this strategy is often ultimately self-damaging, as patients are more understanding of errors which are disclosed honestly, directly, and in a timely manner. In fact, this was a protective factor against eventual litigation and from a risk management perspective when compared to patients who learned of complications through other means [26–28].

Finally, we should consider the needs of the surgeon who would be best served avoiding self-isolation during a vulnerable time. Research shows that the doctor is often the second victim after a medical error [29]. Shame, and fear of retribution, litigation, or damage to reputation can lead doctors to withdraw from the patient and their colleagues. Such isolation can lead to counterproductive decisions such as attempting to hide errors, which often serves only to compound mistakes. It is important to understand which kinds of professional communication can be helpful versus those which may be damaging. Formal discussion of errors with colleagues, as occurs in a Morbidity and Mortality conference, is importantly immune from legal discovery and should be considered a safe space to solicit objective advice on managing a complication. This legal exemption does NOT, however, have blanket applicability to most other formal and informal communications with colleagues when discussing specific case-related details of a case.

40.4 Legal Considerations

40.4.1 Logistics

In the United States, for doctors practicing in high-risk specialties, which encompasses surgeons operating near the skull-base, litigation is all but a guarantee. Such doctors have an 88% likelihood of being sued before the age of 45, and a 99% chance of being sued for malpractice at some point in their careers [30]. When considering just neurosurgeons, this rate is even more dramatic, as this group traditionally has an annual risk of lawsuit of 19% [30]. It is worth noting that even among patients who have suffered injury from negligent care, the litigation rate is a meager 1.53% (CI 0–3.24%) [31]. A similar study found such litigation rates to be 2.5% (CI 0.1–4.9%) with a modest increase to 3.8% when considering patients with significant or major disability [32].

Legal precedent and norms are notably regional in their application and impact. We will herein focus on the United States (US), with the understanding that there are considerable differences seen in other countries (which often have out-of-court, no-fault systems) and even between jurisdictions within the US. Malpractice law is based on the historical English Common Law [33]. Put simply, court rulings are based on historical precedent, applying similar reasoning and decisions from past comparable cases when possible. These rules have been influenced over time by legislative actions as well. Malpractice law is under the authority of individual states (Veterans Affairs care notwithstanding), leading to notable geographic differences, though most states have significant overlap in their underlying principles.

Medical malpractice suits require proof that care was provided negligently and that this care resulted in harm. To prove negligence, four elements must be demonstrated. (1) A professional duty was owed to the patient, (2) this duty was breached through a violation of the standard of care, (3) injury was caused by that breach of duty, and (4) damages resulted from said breach of duty [33, 34]. Element one is implicit with any physician–patient relationship. The standard of care is regionally determined and is based on what a reasonable, similarly-situated physician would do in the same scenario. This is traditionally determined by expert testimony. There is also a variable time constraint on when a suit can be filed with relation to the alleged malpractice, known as the statute of limitations.

Plaintiffs' lawyers are typically hired on contingency and are only paid if they secure an award. Because of this payment structure, there is a disincentive to file suits in which they feel they are unlikely to prevail. These decisions are made by individual legal firms and are based on how similar cases have historically been decided, with outcomes often recorded in public legal databases. Defense lawyers alternatively are typically assigned and paid for by the insurance company. Nearly all malpractice trials are decided by a jury, as opposed to by a judge. The standard of proof is "more likely than not" or "preponderance of the evidence" which is easier to prove than the standard for criminal trials which require "proof beyond a reasonable doubt." [33] Post-trial appeals are rarely successful [33]

The process of case selection often starts with evidence of a disability and works backwards through the use of medical record discovery to determine whether there was antecedent negligence leading to harm or if the case is frivolous. If the plaintiffs feel there is a case to be made, the case will proceed and will eventually reach deposition, which is sworn testimony, recorded outside of court in a mutually agreed upon setting, commonly the defendant doctor's office. The goal of this arrangement is to have both parties come to an understanding of the facts and merits of the case early in the process. This is by design to encourage out of court settlement, potentially saving all involved parties substantial time, money, and stress, and to reduce the risk associated with an uncertain outcome. This is not fool-proof however, as a study of cases from five different liability insurers found that 37% of malpractice cases brought were frivolous, in that they did not involve any medical errors. Such claims, while less likely to result in compensation, still accounted for 13–16% of the system's total monetary costs. Notably, 54 cents of every dollar spent on patient compensation goes toward administrative costs [35].

Unfortunately, the only factor correlated with payment in a malpractice suit is extent of disability; specifically, there is no correlation appreciated between payment to the plaintiff and history of any adverse event (injury sustained secondary to medical treatment) [36]. Shockingly, this is true regardless of the presence or absence of negligence. While it may be expected that a portion of lawsuits are initiated in response to a suboptimal outcome with discovery used to determine the merits of a suit, absence of negligence or even of adverse event were not protective [36]. Notably, there is a degree of selection bias as cases settled early in the process or quickly dropped by the plaintiffs are inherently not included in the public record.

40.4.2 Financial Considerations

Like many aspects of the American medical system, the malpractice system and risk pooling are largely handled within the private domain. Malpractice insurance rates and availability have fluctuated significantly over time. As with many other types of insurance, the financial viability lies in the timing discrepancy between when premiums are received and when claims are paid out. Even a company which pays out a similar amount in claims as it collects in premiums is able to invest this money and collect interest in the intervening years. In the 1970s, the West entered an economic recession and interest rates fell. This occurred at a time when malpractice claims were increasing nationally and many insurers abandoned medical malpractice markets. The task of insurance fell largely on professional societies, state run Joint Underwriting Associations, and publicly administered programs which offered umbrella coverage. In the 1980s commercial insurance was more widely available but rates for premiums climbed dramatically [37]. Since that time, malpractice filings have continued to increase. The reasons for this are myriad but include a litigious society, improvements in medicine and subsequent increased patient expectations with regards to outcomes, and a relatively new (over several decades) willingness of physicians to act as expert witnesses and testify on behalf of plaintiffs. Outlier awards, while uncommon, have reached into the hundreds of millions of dollars. This makes it difficult for even large insurance companies to adequately prepare and ultimately increases premiums and makes malpractice coverage for physicians a costlier and riskier financial proposition. Employed physicians often have their insurance premiums covered, though it is worth noting that from an employers' perspective, this is included in the total calculated compensation and benefits package, such that over time if insurance rates rise, other compensation is likely to decrease commensurately.

Importantly, malpractice insurance rates are tied to both geographic location as well as type of practice. Perhaps not surprisingly, neurosurgeons most commonly have the highest premiums, surpassing even high-risk obstetricians. General otolaryngologists can expect significantly lower premiums in line with the median of all medical specialties [38] Malpractice administration in the US has substantial financial cost. In 1991, the World Bank estimated the annual cost at $4.9B [39] By 2003, that cost was estimated to have grown by 29% to $6.3B in addition to an estimated $60-108B in unneeded medical care provided in the practice of defensive medicine [40]. Furthermore, there are substantial indirect costs of even an unsuccessful lawsuit which include time lost, stress, and damage to reputation and mental health.

Malpractice monetary awards typically take into account both economic and noneconomic damages. Economic damages are comparatively straightforward and encompass such factors as income lost from inability to work, and further medical bills accrued. Loss of future income is calculated by projecting a patient's pre- and post-injury income prospects over a lifetime, which can add up quickly for a younger patient with a high income potential. It is perhaps not surprising then that the elderly and the poor have traditionally been less likely to bring suit [32].

Noneconomic damages are often more contentious and involve more nebulous calculations of the monetary cost of "pain and suffering." In the case of CSF leak with subsequent neurologic insult, a given patient could claim pain and suffering compensation for loss of enjoyment from not being able to play tennis or cook, mental anguish from being injured, the cost of potentially life-long neurogenic pain, and loss of social contact with friends. This is in addition to potential claims by family members who are legally entitled to seek compensation as a result of damage to their relationship with their spouse or parent. This is known as loss of consortium. This component of awards is naturally more abstract and subjective with a very wide array of possible outcomes for any given jury. The movement to regulate these noneconomic damages is referred to as tort reform. Evidence suggests such efforts to cap noneconomic damages reduce malpractice premiums with the potential to decrease medical costs associated with defensive medicine and encourage doctors to practice in a given area [41, 42]. The data is not unanimously in support of this notion however [43]. Predictably, it is difficult to isolate the extent to which fear of litigation discourages surgeons from operating on, and caring for patients with complex medical issues such as skull-base tumors or CSF leaks.

40.4.3 Legal Outcomes by Type of Surgery

Rhinology is the most litigated field within otolaryngology with claim numbers continually increasing over time [44]. Rhinologic claims compromise 70% of all otolaryngological indemnity compensation paid out, with most cases involving FESS [45, 46] examining lawsuits stemming from endoscopic sinus surgery over a 15 year period, Lynn-Macrae et al. found that CSF leak was the cause of lawsuit in 10% of all cases reported. In lawsuits brought secondary to iatrogenic injury, CSF leak was the single most common injury implicated, with a prevalence of 24%. Informed consent inadequacy was claimed in 37%, and unnecessary surgery alleged in 27%, which is in line with previously reported rates 47–49. Recent work by Tolisano utilized the legal database LexisNexis Jury Verdicts and Settlements. Their work found that two-thirds of all rhinology malpractice cases had an unfavorable outcome for the defendant. Half of their identified cases were settled, with out-of-court settlement payments averaging $1.3Million, as compared with $2Million for jury verdicts [45].

Kovalerchik utilized another preeminent legal database (the Westlaw legal database, Thomson Reuters, New York, NY) to specifically examine lawsuits brought as a consequence of iatrogenic CSF leaks [47]. Their group identified 18 lawsuits from 1990 to 2010. Notably, these include only cases which made it to trial, though cases which were resolved prior to judgment are included in the database. Of these, 10 were decided in the defendant's favor, two were decided in the plaintiff's favor, and 6 were settled out of court. Mean damages awarded for cases were approximately $1M regardless of whether it was decided in court or settled before trial. 78% of these suits involved patients who had undergone endoscopic sinus surgery. The most frequent alleged factors cited for litigation were need for additional surgery (88.9%), meningitis (50%), and failure to recognize complications in a timely manner (44.4%). Additionally, allegations of the initial procedure being unnecessary and informed consent inadequacy were cited in one-third of cases each [47] Importantly, CSF leaks identified intraoperatively and repaired without neurologic sequelae, rarely result in litigation [50].

When considering litigation for cases involving the anterior skull-base, only 33% are related to surgical intervention with the rest related to missed or delayed diagnosis [51]. Wang et al. found that of the surgical cases, permanent injury (17%) and intraoperative complications (13%) were among the most commonly alleged factors prompting litigation. Thirty percent of cases were settled out of court for an average of $2.5M. Of the remaining 16 cases, 13% were decided in the plaintiff's favor for an average of $11.9M and 57% of cases were decided in the defendants favor. There was no statistically significant difference based on open versus endoscopic approach.

When looking at legal outcomes for all otolaryngology cases, a trend was found between the patient's age and likelihood of negative outcome for the defendant, such that pediatric patients were more likely to successfully obtain compensation (80% vs. 52.2%, respectively). Despite increased likelihood of legal success by the plaintiff's representing pediatric patients, the total amount of compensation was irrespective of age [52].

40.5 Conclusion

Patients with CSF rhinorrhea are often medically complex and require multidisciplinary treatment. To provide comprehensive care, we are tasked with understanding not just the medical and technical details, but also the ethical and medicolegal nuances involved. Much of the information covered in this chapter, particularly regarding consent, relationships with patients, and disclosure of adverse events, is widely applicable. While the legal landscape can seem daunting, the fact that most skull-base surgeons will almost certainly be affected at some point in their careers, should serve as motivation to understand the medicolegal environment of our time. For our patients' sake, we should strive to avoid making medical decisions rooted predominantly in fear of litigation and remember that clear communication with our patients ultimately results in better care and stronger patient–physician relationships.

References

1. Snissarenko EP, Church CA. Informed consent process and patient communication after complications in sinus surgery. Otolaryngol Clin N Am. 2010;43(4):915–27. https://doi.org/10.1016/j.otc.2010.04.015.
2. Kerrigan D, Thevasagayam R, Woods T, et al. Who's afraid of informed consent? BMJ. 1993;306:298–300.
3. Lund VJ, Wright A, Yiotakis J. Complications and medicolegal aspects of endoscopic sinus surgery. J R Soc Med. 1997;90:422–8.
4. Godwin Y. Do they listen? Br J Plast Surg. 2000;53:121–5.
5. Statement on principles underlying perioperative responsibility American college of surgeons. Bull Am Coll Surg. 1996;81(9):39–40.
6. Fink AS, Prochazka AV, Henderson WG, et al. Predictors of comprehension during surgical informed consent. J Am Coll Surg. 2010;210(6):919–26.
7. Stacey D, Bennett CL, Barry MJ, Col NF, Eden KB, HolmesRovner M, et al. Decision aids for people facing health treatment or screening decisions. Cochrane Database Syst Rev. 2011;5:CD001431.
8. Ramakrishnan VR, Kingdom TT, Nayak JV, et al. Nationwide incidence of major complications in endoscopic sinus surgery. Int Forum Allergy Rhinol. 2012;2(1):34–9.
9. Bachmann G, Dienabri U, Jungehulsing M, Peterit H, Michel V. Incidence of occult CSF fistula during paranasal sinus surgery. Arch Otolaryngol Head Neck Surg. 2002;128:1299–302.
10. Kennedy DW, Shaman P, Han W, Selman H, Deems DA, Lanza DC. Complications of ethmoidectomy: a survey of fellows of the American Academy of Otolaryngology-Head and Neck Surgery. Otolaryngol Head Neck Surg. 1994;111(5):589–99.
11. Wolf JS, Malekzadeh S, Berry JA. O'Malley, BW informed consent in functional endoscopic sinus surgery. Laryngoscope. 2002;112:774–8.
12. Weintraub MI. Medicolegal aspects of iatrogenic injuries. Neurol Clin. 1998;16(1):217–27.
13. American Academy of Otolaryngology–Head and Neck Surgery. Intra-operative use of computer aided surgery: updated. http://www.entnet.org/Practice/policyIntraOperativeSurgery.cfm.
14. Eloy JA, Svider PF, D'aguillo CM, Baredes S, Setzen M, Folbe AJ. Image-guidance in endoscopic sinus surgery: is it associated with decreased medicolegal liability? Int Forum Allergy Rhinol. 2013;3(12):980–5.
15. Stankiewicz JA, Hotaling J. Medicolegal issues in endoscopic sinus surgery and complications. Otolaryngol Clin N Am. 2015;48(5):827–37. https://doi.org/10.1016/j.otc.2015.05.014. Epub 2015 Jun 26. Review
16. Felisati G, Bianchi A, Lozza P, Portaleone S. Italian multicentre study on intrathecal fluorescein for craniosinusal fistulae. Acta Otorhinolaryngol Ital. 2008;28(4):159–63.
17. Carrau RL, Snyderman CH, Kassam AB. The management of cerebrospinal fluid leaks in patients at risk for high-pressure hydrocephalus. Laryngoscope. 2005;115(2):205–12.
18. Patel AM, Still TE, Vaughan W. Medicolegal issues in endoscopic sinus surgery. Otolaryngol Clin North Am. 2010;43(4):905–14. https://doi.org/10.1016/j.otc.2010.04.014.
19. Vincent C, Young M, Phillips A. Why do people sue doctors? A study of patients and relatives taking legal action. Lancet. 1994;343:1609–13.
20. Gallagher TH, Waterman AD, Ebers AG. Patients' and physicians' attitudes regarding disclosure of medical errors. JAMA. 2003;289:1001–7.
21. Boothman RC. Apologies and a strong defense at the University of Michigan Health System. Physician Exec. 2006;32(2):7–10.

22. Bruera E, Palmer JL, Pace E, et al. A randomized, controlled trial of physician postures when breaking bad news to cancer patients. Palliat Med. 2007;21(6): 501–5.
23. Swayden KJ, Anderson KK, Connelly LM, Moran JS, Mcmahon JK, Arnold PM. Effect of sitting vs. standing on perception of provider time at bedside: a pilot study. Patient Educ Couns. 2012;86(2):166–71.
24. Moore PJ, Adler NE, Robertson PA. Medical malpractice: the effect of doctorpatient relations on medical patient perceptions and malpractice intentions. West J Med. 2000;173:244–50.
25. Wu AW, Cavanaugh TA, McPhee SJ, Lo B, Micco GP. To tell the truth— ethical and practical issues in disclosing medical mistakes to patients. J Gen Intern Med. 1997;12:770–5.
26. Witman AB, Park DM, Hardin SB. How do patients want physicians to handle mistakes? Arch Intern Med. 1996;156:2565–9.
27. Witman AB, Park DM, Hardin SB. How do patients want physicians to handle mistakes? A survey of internal medicine patients in an academic setting. Arch Intern Med. 1996;156:2565–9.
28. Kraman SS, Hamm G. Risk management: extreme honesty may be the best policy. Ann Intern Med. 1999;131:963–7.
29. Wu AW. Medical error: the second victim. BMJ. 2000;320:726–7.
30. Jena AB, Seabury S, Lakdawalla D, Chandra A. Malpractice risk according to physician specialty. N Engl J Med. 2011;365:629–36.
31. Localio AR, Lawthers AG, Brennan TA, et al. Relationship between malpractice claims and adverse events due to negligence: results of the Harvard medical practice study III. N Engl J Med. 1991;325: 245–51.
32. Studdert DM, Thomas EJ, Burstin HR, et al. Negligent care and malpractice claiming behavior in Utah and Colorado. Med Care. 2000;38:250–60.
33. Bal BS. An introduction to medical malpractice in the United States. Clin Orthop Relat Res. 2009;467(2):339–47.
34. Moffett P, Moore G. The standard of care: legal history and definitions: the bad and good news. West J Emerg Med. 2011;12:109–12.
35. Studdert DM, Mello MM, Gawande AA. Claims, errors, and compensation payments in medical malpractice litigation. N Engl J Med. 2006;354(19): 2024–33.
36. Brennan CM, Burstin HR. Relation between negligent adverse events and the outcomes of medical-malpractice litigation. N Engl J Med. 1996;335: 1963–7.
37. Sage WM. The forgotten third: liability insurance and the medical malpractice crisis. Health Aff (Millwood). 2004;23(4):10–21.
38. MLMIC Insurance Company. Medical Liability Mutual Insurance Company Rating Classifications. www.health.ny.gov/health_care/medicaid/redesign/docs/mlmic_mrt_medical_malpractice_wg_presentation.pdf. Accessed on March 17 4, 2019.
39. Medical Malpractice Systems around the Globe: Examples from the US tort liability system and the Swedish no fault system. Washington, DC: World Bank. 2004. Available at: http://194.84.38.65/files/esw_files/malpractice_systems_eng.pdf. Accessed Feb. 17, 2019.
40. Medical Malpractice. Implications of rising premiums on access to health care. Washington, D.C. U.S. General Accounting Office. August 2003. Available at: http://www.gao.gov/new.items/d03836.pdf. Accessed Feb. 17, 2019.
41. Medical malpractice litigation raises health-care cost, reduces access, and lowers quality of care. J Med Pract Manage. 2004;20:44–51.
42. Guirguis-blake J, Fryer GE, Phillips RL, Szabat R, Green LA. The US medical liability system: evidence for legislative reform. Ann Fam Med. 2006;4(3): 240–6.
43. Hellinger FJ, Encinosa WE. The impact of state laws limiting malpractice damage awards on health care expenditures. Am J Public Health. 2006;96(8): 1375–81.
44. Harris AS, Edwards SJ, Pope L. Litigation in English rhinology. J Laryngol Otol. 2015;129(03):244–9. https://doi.org/10.1017/S0022215115000286.
45. Tolisano AM, Justin GA, Ruhl DS, Cable BB. Rhinology and medical malpractice: an update of the medicolegal landscape of the last ten years. Laryngoscope. 2016;126(1):14–9.
46. Re M, Magliulo G, Romeo R, Gioacchini FM, Pasquini E. Risks and medico-legal aspects of endoscopic sinus surgery: a review. Eur Arch Otorhinolaryngol. 2014;271(8):2103–17.
47. Kovalerchik O, Mady LJ, Svider PF, et al. Physician accountability in iatrogenic cerebrospinal fluid leak litiga-tion. Int Forum Allergy Rhinol. 2013;3:722–5.
48. Lynn-macrae AG, Lynn-macrae RA, Emani J, Kern RC, Conley DB. Medicolegal analysis of injury during endoscopic sinus surgery. Laryngoscope. 2004;114(8):1492–5.
49. Winford TW, Wallin JL, Clinger JD, Graham AM. Malpractice in treatment of Sinonasal disease by otolaryngologists. Otolaryngol Head Neck Surg. 2015;152(3):536–40. https://doi.org/10.1177/0194599814566787.
50. Stankiewicz JA, Lal D, Connor M, Welch K. Complications in endoscopic sinus surgery for chronic rhinosinusitis: a 25-year experience. Laryngoscope. 2011;121:2684–701.
51. Wang AC, Darlin S, Lai W, Svider PF, Jacob JT, Liu JK, Eloy JA, Folbe AJ. Pituitary and skull-base lesions and the litigious patient. Int Forum Allergy Rhinol. 2017;7(10):1022–8.
52. Svider PF, Blake DM, Sahni KP, Folbe AJ, Liu JK, Baredes S, Eloy JA. Meningitis and legal liability: An otolaryngology perspective. Am J Otolaryngol. 2014;35(2):198–203.

MIX
Papier aus verantwortungsvollen Quellen
Paper from responsible sources
FSC® C105338

If you have any concerns about our products,
you can contact us on
ProductSafety@springernature.com

In case Publisher is established outside the EU,
the EU authorized representative is:
Springer Nature Customer Service Center GmbH
Europaplatz 3, 69115 Heidelberg, Germany

Printed by Libri Plureos GmbH
in Hamburg, Germany